VOLUME

1

Depressive Disorders

Second Edition

WPA Series
Evidence and Experience in Psychiatry

Other Titles in the *WPA Series* Evidence and Experience in Psychiatry

VOLUME

1

Depressive Disorders

Second Edition

Edited by

Mario Maj
University of Naples, Italy

Norman Sartorius
University of Geneva, Switzerland

WPA Series
Evidence and Experience in Psychiatry

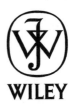

WILEY

Contents

Review Contributors

Dr David Ames   *Academic Unit for Psychiatry of Old Age, St George's Health Service, University of Melbourne, 283 Cotham Road, Kew, Victoria 3101, Australia*

Professor Per Bech   *Psychiatric Research Unit, Frederiksborg General Hospital, Dyrehavevej 48, DK-3400 Hillerød, Denmark*

Dr Edmond Chiu   *Academic Unit for Psychiatry of Old Age, St George's Health Service, University of Melbourne, 283 Cotham Road, Kew, Victoria 3101, Australia*

Dr Brian Draper   *Academic Department of Psychogeriatrics, Prince of Wales Hospital, Randwick, Sydney, NSW 2031, Australia*

Dr Richard Harrington   *Department of Child and Adolescent Psychiatry, Royal Manchester Children's Hospital, Pendlebury, Manchester M27 1HA, UK*

Dr Timothy R. Hylan   *Research Scientist, Lilly Research Laboratories, Lilly Corporate Center, Indianapolis, IN 46285, USA*

Dr Jerrold F. Rosenbaum   *Department of Psychiatry, Massachusetts General Hospital, 15 Parkman Street, WAC 812, Boston, MA 02114-3117, USA*

Professor A. John Rush   *Department of Psychiatry, University of Texas Southwestern Medical Center, 5323 Harry Hines Blvd, Dallas, TX 75235-9086, USA*

Dr John Snowdon   *Central Sydney Area Health Service, Rozelle Hospital, PO Box 1, Rozelle, NSW 2039, Australia*

Professor Costas N. Stefanis   *University Mental Health Research Institute, Eginition Hospital, 74 Vasilissis Sophias Avenue, Athens 11528, Greece*

Dr Nicholas C. Stefanis   *University Mental Health Research Institute and Department of Psychiatry, University of Athens, Eginition Hospital, 74 Vasilissis Sophias Avenue, Athens 11528, Greece*

Dr Michael E. Thase   *Department of Psychiatry, University of Pittsburgh Medical Center and Western Psychiatric Institute and Clinic, 3811 O'Hara Street, Pittsburgh, PA 15213, USA*

Preface

Among the most serious difficulties that beset the field of psychiatry are the stigma marking mental illness and all that is connected with it (from its treatments and institutions to mental health workers and families of people with mental illness), disunity within the profession, and the gaps between findings of research and practice. These three sets of problems are interconnected: the disregard of research findings contributes to the persistence of differences in the orientation of psychiatric schools, and this diminishes the profession's capacity to speak out with one voice and to demonstrate that most mental illnesses can be successfully treated and are not substantially different from other diseases.

The diagnosis and treatment of depressive disorders illustrate the gaps that exist between research evidence, clinical experience, and guidelines for practice and quality assurance. Although clinicians, for example, feel that there are significant difficulties in the application of research criteria to the diagnosis of depression in people who suffer from a severe physical illness, current classifications of mental disorders contain no provisions that would make them easier to apply in such instances. Psychodynamic psychotherapies, the efficacy of which is not supported by empirical evidence, are still widely used in many countries, whereas other forms of psychotherapy, for which research evidence of effectiveness is available, remain unknown or scarcely used. Many clinicians continue to believe that there are significant differences in the effectiveness of antidepressant drugs, although research tends to demonstrate that they are equivalent, and some claim that tricyclic antidepressants are active when given in doses that are below the range that research has proved to be effective.

Differences of opinion between skilled clinicians and discussions about reasons for the gaps between research findings and practice are not reflected in the current psychiatric literature. The experience of skilled clinicians is only rarely published in psychiatric journals, while the best of scientific evidence is only infrequently presented in a manner and in a place that would make it immediately accessible to clinicians. Reports on clinical practice in different countries—possibly enriching knowledge by providing a range of experience and a powerful commentary on the applicability of research findings in everyday work—are not easily found in accessible psychiatric literature. In the current era of promotion of evidence-based medicine, these separations between research evidence, experience, and practice are a dangerous anachronism.

The series *Evidence and Experience in Psychiatry* has been initiated as part of the effort of the World Psychiatric Association to bridge the gaps within psychiatry and between psychiatry and the rest of medicine. The series aims to be the forum in which major issues for psychiatry and mental health care will be discussed openly by psychiatrists from many countries and different schools of thought. Each volume will cover a group of mental disorders, by means of a set of systematic reviews of the research evidence, each followed by a number of commentaries.

No publication can expect to cover everything, or to present all possible views on a matter. The WPA series is not an exception to this rule. It is the editors' hope that the volumes will inform and stimulate further discussion, attract attention to controversial issues, and help to recreate respect for clinical experience and differences of opinion between psychiatrists in different parts of the world, all united in their wish to find a consensus that will make it possible to move psychiatry forward, and make it even more useful in diminishing the burden of mental illnesses and the plight of the many suffering from them.

Mario Maj
Norman Sartorius

1

Diagnosis of Depressive Disorders: A Review

Costas N. Stefanis[1] and Nicholas C. Stefanis[2]

[1]*University Mental Health Research Institute, Athens, Greece;* [2]*University Mental Health Research Institute and Department of Psychiatry, University of Athens, Greece*

INTRODUCTION

Depression is a complex diagnostic construct, applied to individuals with a particular set of symptoms among which the essential ingredients are a depressed mood and a loss of interest [1–10]. The general issues surrounding the diagnosis of depression will be briefly addressed as an introduction to this chapter.

Issues on Nomenclature

Depression as a diagnostic and clinically meaningful term has a short history. No one has claimed fame for coining it and, whoever he was, might not feel justified in introducing it. It is a term widely used, not only in psychopathology but also in economics, in meteorology, in life sciences and in several other areas of human exercise. In psychiatry, it has been used with variable meanings and over the years has gradually lost its initial semantic value. All the varieties of emotional reactions to actual or anticipated loss, all feelings of distress and sorrow arising from the adversities and vicissitudes of life, have been associated with depression. The individual today views depression as a part of life experience, an unavoidable condition that everyone has to go through at least once in his or her lifetime, and considers it subject to self-cure by will power. This attitude, by failing to distinguish between transient dysphoric loss-related emotional states and clinical depression leading to profound disturbance of mental and social functioning, is both misleading and hazardous. In contrast to the normal emotional responses to unwanted and stressful events, clinical depression is a mental disorder which, due to its severity, its tendency to recur and its high

Depressive Disorders, Second Edition. Edited by Mario Maj and Norman Sartorius.
© 2002 John Wiley & Sons Ltd.

cost for the individual and for society, is a medically significant condition that needs to be diagnosed and properly treated.

Names and terms have to convey a distinct meaning applicable only or principally to the things or the items they designate. This is not the case with the term "depression". The proliferation of the term, with its use in multiple contexts, has considerably reduced its diagnostic specificity and its psychological meaning. The term "depressive disorders", denoting the psychopathological nature of depression, may have lessened but has not removed the confusion.

It is to be hoped that, in the near future, more appropriate terms will be adopted that will satisfy taxonomic criteria based on single, psychologically meaningful, parent terms from which the subordinate subtypes will derive. "Thymos" might be considered as an appropriate candidate parent term for mood disorders in general and for depression (catathymia) in particular.

The elimination of the term "unipolar" from both DSM and ICD systems is largely justified, mainly due to the observation that there are latent bipolar cases occupying a significant part of the depressive spectrum. Patients diagnosed as unipolars in one or several past depressive episodes may turn out as bipolars even in late age, particularly if dysthymia preceded the major depressive episodes.

Issues on Diagnosis and Classification

Depression, like many other mental disorders, is characterized by the presence of a number of symptoms which are changeable over time. These symptoms cluster together in several combinations and they present an infinite variability at the individual patient level. Grouping these symptoms and signs together, according to their shared features, is a necessary step to understanding their psychopathological substrate, to uncovering their underlying consistencies and eventually their common mechanisms, as well as to accomplishing our clinical responsibility to predict their course and effectively control them. Up to now no common causes for depressive disorders are known that would allow for an etiologically based (true) classification. Neither are there any biological markers available, which would by themselves reliably and validly secure a biologically based diagnostic classification. We have, therefore, to rely mainly on symptoms and the clinical and familial characteristics of the patient in order to formulate a typological diagnostic categorization. The assessment of symptoms, on the other hand, is judgement-based, since there are no pathognomonic symptoms or categorical cut-off points on depression measurements that would adequately define and diagnose a "case" of depression [1, 4, 7, 8, 11–13].

One of the major conceptual issues that has been haunting psychiatrists since the middle of this century, and is still debated, is whether a categorical or a dimensional approach would better explain the nature of mood disorders. In other words, whether to divide depressive disorders into a number of autonomous, distinct and mutually exclusive categories or to assign them to specified dimensions. The dispute has mainly centered in the past on the question as to whether the distinction between endogenous and reactive or neurotic and psychotic depression, including their variants, is valid or whether all are part of a wide spectrum, in an uninterrupted symptom continuum [11–18]. The dispute — albeit not as vigorous as in the past — has not ceased up to this day. The pros and cons for each of the two approaches have their advocates who, however, in contrast with their forerunners, are not theorists but empirical researchers providing new methods and new data in support of their views [19–28].

The introduction of operationally defined diagnostic criteria had an impact on both camps. The merit of the categorical approach is that it is closer to the way the human mind conceives nature, seeing it divided into distinct objects, identifiable by the specific name attached to them. Physicians in particular are more familiar with categories than with dimensionally defined constructs. If depressive disorders and their subtypes were to be documented in the future as existing in nature as separate entities with impermeable boundaries, it would be a welcome development that would lead to a "true" and etiologically based diagnosis. Since, evidently, such developments are not readily foreseeable, the categorical approach has still to rely on indirect methods of reliability and validity measures, which up to now do not provide for a sharp demarcation of the various types of depressive disorders. There is still considerable overlap and the gray areas between even the major diagnostic categories are large enough to include patients who qualify for multiple allocations and for diagnostic hybridization. There is also a risk that, through application of the operational criteria, a number of patients may not be eligible for any of the categories and thus will remain "operationally" undefined.

The disadvantages of the rigid categorical approach are not sufficiently offset by the dimensional (or spectrum) alternative, which, however, has several merits, cardinal among them being its flexibility in application and its capacity to include all "typical and atypical" cases. Moreover, by broadening the diagnostic boundaries, the latter approach provides an evolutionary perspective in our understanding of depressive disorders from temperament (idiosyncrasis) to depressive personality, and from the subsyndromal and the mild to the psychotic depressive episodes [29, 30].

Recently, two general population epidemiological studies have addressed the issue. The first, based on data from the National Comorbidity Survey, has shown that across the minor, major and severe categories of depression (depending on the number of symptoms) there was a "monotonic" increase for a number of indices (i.e. average number of episodes, impairment, comorbidity and parental psychopathology) [31]. The second study, extending a previous one in a population-based sample of female twins, yielded findings which enabled the authors to conclude that there is little empirical support for the DSM-IV requirement for 2-week duration, five symptoms and clinically significant impairment to validate the syndromal autonomy of major depression with sharply defined boundaries. Most functions appeared continuous across symptom, severity, duration and impairment measures. The authors concluded that DSM-IV major depression may be a diagnostic construct imposed on a continuum of depressive symptoms of varying severity and duration [32].

Issues on Secondary or Comorbid Depression

The concept of primary-secondary depressive disorder was introduced by the Washington University group in 1972, together with the formulation of diagnostic criteria which led to the development of the current operationalized major diagnostic systems [18].

In the Washington group's criteria the primary-secondary depression distinction is entirely based on the temporal relationship of depression to another psychiatric illness, especially schizophrenia and alcoholism. The concept was later expanded to include physical illness and drug-related conditions. It is, however, acknowledged that the concept of secondary depression, if based only on temporal sequence, may not be easily validated. Temporal sequences are complex and the succession of syndromes or illnesses is often not clear, particularly if information relies on retrospective reporting. The situation is further complicated when two individual distinct episodes (depressive and non-depressive) have a concurrent (or difficult to discern) onset of symptoms. The term "complicated depression" may not overcome the definitional and practical diagnostic difficulties.

The introduction of multiaxial classification in current diagnostic systems greatly facilitated the establishment of the comorbidity concept, which progressively substituted the primary-secondary distinction. However, comorbidity itself has its own definitional and practical shortcomings. Its conceptual clarity is poor [33]. The term strictly refers to distinct disease entities within a well-defined time-window and should not be loosely applied — as it often is — to variously defined syndromal and subsyndromal conditions, with an undetermined time relationship with the "comorbid" depression. Furthermore, the issue of nosological hierarchy is not resolved by the comorbidity concept. Adherents of primary-secondary distinction still argue that this is more appropriate than the comorbidity concept and it does serve the clinician better, on the grounds that in the majority of cases depression is preceded by another mental and/or physical illness [34, 35]. Also to be considered is the possibility that what appears to be a comorbid relationship of two discrete conditions may well be the polymorphic presentation of one single nosological entity [33]. Despite theoretical and clinical limitations, the comorbidity concept has been tested and proved particularly useful in psychiatric clinical studies [36] and epidemiological investigations such as the Epidemiologic Catchment Area (ECA) study [37, 38], the US National Comorbidity Survey [39], and the WHO Study on Psychological Disorders in Primary Health Care [40, 41].

CLASSIFICATION OF DEPRESSIVE DISORDERS

Historical Background

From Hippocrates to Kraepelin

Descriptions of depression and depression-related mental disorders date back to antiquity (Summerian and Egyptian documents date back to 2600 BC). However, it was Hippocrates (460–370 BC) and his disciples who first studied these conditions systematically and introduced the term "melancholia" to describe the symptoms and to provide a physiological explanation of their origin. The Hippocratic School attempted to link the balance of the postulated four humors (blood, yellow bile, black bile and phlegm) with the temperament and personality, and the latter two with the propensity to develop one of the four diseases (mania, melancholia, phrenitis and paranoia). It is interesting that Hippocrates considered symptom duration as a diagnostic criterion for melancholia by stating in one of his aphorisms (the 23rd) that "if sorrow persists, then it is melancholia".

Subsequent eminent authors of antiquity (Aretaeus of Capadokia, Galen and others) continued using the term melancholia and elaborated further on its symptomatology, its causation and its delineation from related disorders. The essentials of the traditional views on melancholia were retained during the middle ages and long after. The publication of Robert Burton's *Anatomy of Melancholy* in 1621, in addition to presenting an excellent description of a sufferer's feelings, provided an informative review of the prevailing concepts on the nature of the illness at the time.

The term "melancholia" survived as the only specifier of morbid mood and disposition until Kraepelin, at the end of the nineteenth century, introduced the term "manic-depression" to separate nosologically mood disorders from dementia praecox, known after Bleuler as schizophrenia.

From Kraepelin to DSM-IV and ICD-10

The eighth revision of the WHO *International Classification of Diseases, Injuries and Causes of Death* (ICD-8) signaled the beginning of a systematic effort at an international level to develop a unified system of diagnosis and classification of mental disorders. Despite improvements brought about in the ninth revision (ICD-9), both these WHO systems limited their diagnostic guidelines to narrative descriptions that did not particularly enhance the diagnostic reliability of mental disorders.

This was also true for the first two editions of the American Psychiatric Association's (APA) *Diagnostic and Statistical Manual of Mental Disorders*, which in addition to narrative presentation of symptoms attempted to associate clinical features with psychopathological mechanisms. The advent of DSM-III in 1980 marked the contemporary era in diagnosis and classification of mental disorders. Every diagnostic category was given an operational definition, strictly descriptive and "neutral", and this substantially increased the diagnostic reliability. The subsequent revisions (DSM-IIIR and DSM-IV) were based on the extensive experience derived from the application of DSM-III. An additional feature of the latest edition (DSM-IV) [5] is that it was initially designed to be compatible with the WHO's tenth revision (ICD-10) of the *Classification of Mental and Behavioural Disorders* [2, 3]. The latter is structured in alphanumerical format and is the product of almost 10 year-long deliberations and extensive field trials [42].

Comparison of ICD-10 with DSM-IV

As shown in Table 1.1, ICD-10 and DSM-IV are basically similar in their orientation, and despite their differences, mainly in terminology, may be used interchangeably in clinical practice. They converge on the following major features: (a) the previously dispersed depressive disorders are grouped together under a common name signifying a unified syndromal entity; (b) the term "affective disorders" is replaced by the term "mood disorders", thus narrowing the depression's boundaries by not subsuming anxiety disorders under the same roof; (c) while the clear intraclass distinction between bipolar and depressive disorders is retained, the term "unipolar" is abandoned; (d) the diagnostic criteria are symptom-based, descriptive and not explanatory; (e) symptom severity and recurrence are used as subtyping and specifying criteria; (f) diagnostic threshold is determined by a constellation of core and supplementary symptoms, which have to fulfill the number and duration criteria in order to qualify for a distinct diagnostic entity; (g) dysthymia is classified as a separate entity within the general frame of depressive disorders.

CLINICAL PRESENTATION OF DEPRESSION

Depression signifies an affective experience (mood state), a complaint (reported as a symptom) as well as a syndrome defined by operational

TABLE 1.1 Depressive disorders in ICD-10 and DSM-IV

ICD-10		DSM-IV (ICD-9-CM)	
F32	*Depressive episode (single)*	*296.2x*	*Major depressive disorder, single episode*
F32.0	Mild depressive episode .00 Without somatic syndrome .01 With somatic syndrome		With melancholic features
F32.1	Moderate depressive episode .10 Without somatic syndrome .11 With somatic syndrome		With melancholic features
F32.2	Severe depressive episode without psychotic symptoms		
F32.3	Severe depressive episode with psychotic symptoms		
F32.8	Other depressive episodes		With catatonic/atypical features
F32.9	Depressive episode, unspecified		.20 Unspecified
F33	*Recurrent depressive disorder*	*296.3x*	*Major depressive disorder, recurrent*
F33.0	Recurrent depressive disorder, current episode mild .00 Without somatic syndrome .01 With somatic syndrome		With melancholic features
F33.1	Recurrent depressive disorder, current episode moderate .10 Without somatic syndrome .11 With somatic syndrome		With melancholic features
F33.2	Recurrent depressive disorder, current episode severe without psychotic symptoms		
F33.3	Recurrent depressive disorder, current episode severe with psychotic symptoms		
F33.4	Recurrent depressive disorder, currently in remission		
F33.8	Other recurrent depressive disorders		With catatonic/atypical features
F33.9	Recurrent depressive disorder, unspecified		.30 Unspecified
F34	*Persistent mood (affective) disorders*		
F34.0	Cyclothymia	301.13	Cyclothymic disorder
F34.1	Dysthymia	300.4	Dysthymic disorder
F34.8	Other persistent mood (affective) disorders	300.4	Dysthymic disorder with atypical features
F34.9	Persistent mood (affective) disorder, unspecified		

continues overleaf

TABLE 1.1   (*continued*)

ICD-10		DSM-IV (ICD-9-CM)	
F38	*Other mood (affective) disorders*		
F38.0	Other single mood (affective) disorders		
	.00 Mixed affective episode	296.0x	Bipolar I disorder, single mixed episode
			.01 Mild
			.02 Moderate
			.03 Severe without psychotic symptoms
			.04 Severe with psychotic symptoms
F38.1	Other recurrent mood (affective) disorders		
	.10 Recurrent brief depressive disorder		See Appendix B: Recurrent brief depressive disorder
F38.8	Other specified mood (affective) disorders		
F39	*Unspecified mood (affective) disorder*	*296.90*	*Mood disorders NOS*

criteria. As an affective experience of sadness, it is common to all humans; as a symptom, it is present in several mental and physical illnesses and, as a syndrome, it is associated with specific mental and physical disorders.

The prototype of the syndromal entity of depressive disorders is the depressive episode (DE) in ICD-10 and the corresponding major depressive episode (MD) in DSM-IV. In both systems, it serves as the qualifying yardstick for all the other forms of depression.

Depressive Episode — Major Depression

As shown in Table 1.1, both DE and MD are specified according to their severity (mild, moderate, severe) and course (single or recurrent). Furthermore, both systems share two fundamental features for identifying depressive episodes: (a) a minimum number of typical and associated symptoms; (b) a minimum duration of symptoms of 2 weeks. In DSM-IV, but not in ICD-10, a third feature is added, that is the impairment in important areas of functioning.

The symptom criteria for the DE according to ICD-10 are listed in Table 1.2. The typical symptoms are depressed mood and lack of interest, pleasure and energy. The typical symptoms are combined with the additional ones in many patterns, each one of them determining the clinical picture of a depressive episode at the individual's level. Symptoms may not be stable during the

TABLE 1.2   Depressive episode according to ICD-10

General criteria
- The depressive episode should last for at least 2 weeks
- No hypomanic or manic symptoms sufficient to meet the criteria for hypomanic or manic episode at any time in the individual's life
- Not attributable to psychoactive substance use or to any organic mental disorder

Typical symptoms
- Depressed mood to a degree that is definitely abnormal for the individual, present for most of the day and almost every day, largely unresponsive to circumstances, and sustained for at least 2 weeks
- Loss of interest or pleasure in activities that are normally pleasurable
- Decreased energy or increased fatigability

Additional symptoms
- Loss of confidence or self-esteem
- Unreasonable feelings of self-reproach or excessive and inappropriate guilt
- Recurrent thoughts of death or suicide, or any suicidal behavior
- Complaints or evidence of diminished ability to think or concentrate, such as indecisiveness or vacillation
- Bleak and pessimistic views of the future
- Sleep disturbance of any type
- Change in appetite (decrease or increase) with corresponding weight change

episode, and their change over time adds to the polymorphic presentation of each particular depressed patient.

There is no one single pathognomonic symptom that in itself would identify DE/MD depression and would allow its monothetic classification. However, the symptoms listed in Table 1.2 and described more extensively below, are considered as core symptoms which, if present in sufficient number and duration, provide for a reliable and valid diagnosis of DE/MD as a distinct psychopathological syndrome.

Depressed Mood

Depressed mood is the hallmark of all depressions, regardless of their additional specifying features and of their intensity, duration and variation. "Depressio sine depressione" (a term proposed to signify depression masked by somatic symptoms) does not exist. The depressed mood is always there, it only needs to be elicited. It is therefore in the authors' view inexplicable why in both the DSM and the ICD criteria the depressed mood, instead of being considered as essential, is recorded as an optional symptom.

Depressed mood is a sustained emotional state that is characterized by sadness, low morale, misery, discouragement, hopelessness, emptiness, unhappiness, distress, pessimism and other related affects that, if assessed in isolation, cannot easily be delineated from the emotional states universally experienced by all human beings when faced with life's adversities. However, depressed mood differs in some aspects that would justify considering it not only as quantitatively more intense than the normal emotional response but also as a qualitatively distinct state that qualifies as a psychopathological symptom.

The main differentiating features of the depressed mood from the non-morbid emotional reaction of sadness are as follows. The intensity and the depth of the pain become so unbearable that often the death wish provides a comforting remedy. The sadness and the associated feelings pervade all domains of personal life and impact on the individual's social performance. The depressed mood lasts long enough to be felt as an unalterable affective state. It may occur spontaneously but, even if it has been triggered by a life event, it evolves autonomously, dissociated from that event, and resists being changed through reasoning or encouragement. It is associated with cognitive and somatic symptoms (guilt, self-reproach, suicidal thoughts and a variety of unpleasant and painful bodily sensations) that are not commonly encountered in non-depressed mood states.

Anhedonia — Loss of Interest

Anhedonia and loss of interest are symptoms closely associated with the depressed mood, varying in intensity along with the feeling of sadness. Patients are unable to express emotions, even their own psychic pain. They are unable to draw pleasure from previously enjoyable activities or to preserve their interests and affections. In severe cases they disregard and abandon most of the things they valued in life. Yet to a great extent they retain insight of their own inability to experience and express normal emotions and this intensifies their suffering.

Cognitive Disturbances

Difficulty in concentrating, negative thoughts, low self-esteem and self-confidence, hopelessness, self-depreciation and self-reproach, a sense of worthlessness and sinfulness, negative outlook on the world and suicidal thoughts are some of the most common cognitive features accompanying the depressed person's state of feeling. If these thoughts are many, persistent and not amenable to change by reason, they are regarded as delusions and qualify for the diagnosis of mood-congruent (delusional-psychotic) depression. When thoughts are discordant with the depressed mood, and delusions of persecution, thought insertion, thought broadcasting and other similar delusions predominate, then mood-incongruent (delusional-psychotic) depression is diagnosed. Whether these cognitive disturbances result in depressed mood, as the cognitive theorists view it, or they are the derivatives of the depressed mood state, is still a debatable issue of limited interest to the practicing physician.

Psychomotor Disturbances

Psychomotor disturbances have the advantage of being readily observed and even objectively measured. They include, on the one hand, agitation (hyperactivity) and on the other, retardation (hypoactivity). Although agitation, usually accompanied by anxiety, irritability and restlessness, is a common symptom of depression, it lacks specificity. In contrast, retardation, manifested as slowing of bodily movements, mask-like facial expression, lengthening of reaction time to stimuli, increased speech paucity and, at its extreme, as an inability to move or to be mentally and emotionally activated (stupor), is considered a core symptom of depression. Their presence is currently being used as a diagnostic symptom of the melancholic type of depression in DSM-IV and the severe depression with somatic symptoms in ICD-10.

Vegetative Symptoms

Vegetative symptoms constitute the most biologically rooted clinical features of depressive disorders and are commonly used as reliable indicators of severity (severe depression with somatic symptoms in ICD-10 and melancholia in DSM-IV). They are manifested as profound disturbances in eating (anorexia and weight loss, or the reverse, bulimia and weight gain), in sleep (insomnia and/or hypersomnia), in sexual function (decreased sexual desire or in a minority of cases the reverse), loss of vitality, motivation, energy and capacity to respond positively to pleasant events. Additionally, concomitant bodily sensations, usually diffuse pains, and complaints of fatigue and physical discomfort are reported. Disturbances of biorhythms are frequent and are considered as characteristic features of melancholia. They are mainly manifested in sleep patterns, predominantly with early morning awakening.

Anxiety Symptoms

Although anxiety symptoms are essential for the diagnosis of anxiety disorders, they are so frequently encountered in depression that they should also be considered as an integral part of its clinical picture, particularly at the primary care settings. In ICD-10, the admixture of anxiety and depressive symptoms is listed as a distinct category under the term "mixed anxiety and depressive disorders".

Subtypes of DE/MD

The main criteria for subtyping DE/MD are basically quantitative (by symptom number, duration and content specifiers). The following are subtypes which are included in the current two major diagnostic systems and are considered as fulfilling, to a varying degree, reliability and validity criteria requirements.

Melancholia (Depression with Somatic Symptoms)

This subtype is listed as melancholia in DSM-IV and as severe depressive episode with somatic symptoms in ICD-10. Melancholia is the oldest diagnostic term used in psychiatry and is characterized by vegetative disturbances and other clinical features that indicate a profound dysfunction of neurobiological mechanisms [7, 8, 10, 43]. The main features of its clinical identity include psychomotor retardation or agitation, late insomnia, loss of weight and appetite, anhedonia (lack of reactivity to pleasurable stimuli), diurnal variation of mood and libido disturbances. The question is still raised, however, whether this cluster of symptoms identifies a separate clinical entity discrete from the other subtypes of MD or if it should be considered as a variant of MD different only on severity measures, as inferred in the ICD-10 classification [27, 44].

DSM-IV includes as a distinguishing feature of melancholia a depressed mood state that has a "distinct quality". It is felt as such by the melancholic patient and not by non-melancholic or bereaved individuals. The "distinct quality" notion is, however, challenged as lacking validity, and it has been proposed that it should be deleted until its specificity for this depressive subtype is established [45].

Support for the distinction of this subtype may derive from reports in the literature indicating its stronger association with neurobiological markers such as the response to the dexamethasone suppression test (DST) [46] and the latency of rapid eye movement (REM) sleep [47]. In a recent study, in which the question of diagnostic validity of melancholic MD was explored in a population-based sample of female twins, it was concluded that it is a valid subtype of MD with distinct clinical features and a particularly higher familial liability to depressive illness. However, from a genetic perspective, the difference is considered as quantitative (melancholia being more severe) but not qualitative [48].

Depression with Psychotic Symptoms

This subtype of depression is listed as severe episode with psychotic symptoms in ICD-10 and major depression with psychotic features (mood-congruent and mood-incongruent) in DSM-IV. It is also commonly cited in the literature as psychotic or delusional depression. On the basis of its presenting symptoms, it was found in the ECA study to cover 14% of all major depressions, representing their most severe form [49].

Clinically this subtype is identified by the presence of delusions in conjunction with psychomotor disturbances, vegetative symptoms and occasional hallucinations. Depending on the delusional content, distinction is made between mood-congruent and mood-incongruent forms.

It has long been a controversial issue and is still debated whether delusions and other psychotic features in depression denote a qualitatively distinct psychopathological entity or merely manifest a greater severity of the depressive disorder continuum [50].

Demographic and clinical characteristics (phenomenology, course and prognosis), family history, treatment response and neurobiological markers have been used as variables to validate the diagnostic autonomy of delusional from non-delusional depression [3, 10, 49–51]. Findings derived from the community survey of the ECA study indicated that delusional depression is different on a number of variables from other subtypes of MD, and the differences are not accounted for by demographic factors, symptom profile and severity [48]. The majority of studies have failed to substantiate a clear and significant difference in many other variables [51, 52]. Some authors reported higher association of delusional depression with a number of neurobiological markers (lower levels of serum dopamine-β-hydroxylase (DBH) and cerebrospinal fluid (CSF) 3-methoxy-4-hydroxyphenylglycol (MHPG); higher cortisol non-suppression to DST and higher hospitalization rates) [53]. Whereas it may still be argued that the reported differences are at best state indicators of greater severity rather than distinguishing nosological markers [50], it should be noted that premorbid vulnerability factors for delusional-psychotic depression have been identified [54] and that the homogeneity of type and content of delusions from episode to episode has been reported by independent authors. These finding may to a certain degree validate the categorization of delusional depression as a distinct subtype of major depression and warrant further investigations [5, 7, 10, 55, 56].

The mood-incongruent psychotic major depression is still debated with regard to its proper nosological placement. It may be close to schizoaffective disorder as defined by Research Diagnostic Criteria (RDC), but it differs from it in many other respects and particularly in premorbid social adjustment variables. It seems that mood incongruent major depression has a boundary problem and represents a largely heterogeneous clinical condition consisting of different cases which resemble cases of other categories (major depression, schizoaffective bipolar delusional states and even paranoid schizophrenia with affective component) qualifying for placement in either or in both the mood and delusional disorders [57].

Atypical Depression

The specifying criteria for atypical depression, according to DSM-IV, are basically the reverse vegetative-somatic symptoms most commonly encountered in typical melancholia (i.e. hypersomnia instead of insomnia, hyperphagia and weight gain instead of anorexia and weight loss), while the mood is responsive to actual or potential positive events. Excessive sensitivity to rejection is also listed as a criterion. The symptoms have to predominate in the past recent 2 weeks of an episode of major depression or during the past 2 years of dysthymia. Although the validity of atypical depression has been frequently challenged in the past [58], a recent review assessing published studies on the subject and applying Kendell's criteria for clinical validity concluded that atypical depression complies with two out of six validation criteria, the clinical description and the differential treatment response, monoamine oxidase inhibitors being more effective than tricyclics [59].

Recurrent Brief Depression (RBD)

According to ICD-10, to make the diagnosis of RBD, depression should have occurred about once a month over the past year, and each episode should have lasted less than 2 weeks (typically 2–3 days with complete recovery), not having occurred only in relation to menstrual cycle and otherwise fulfilling the symptom criteria for a mild, moderate or severe depressive episode. The risk for manic episode is low and thus it may not fall into the rapid-cycling form of bipolar disorder [2, 60, 61].

It has still to be clarified whether RBD represents a discrete form of depressive disorder or one of the clinical variants of recurrent depressive episodes. It is highly comorbid with anxiety disorders and its lifetime prevalence in the community is reported to be as high as 10% [60].

Dysthymia

Dysthymia was introduced as a new diagnostic category of mood disorder by DSM-III and was established in subsequent editions of the DSM and in ICD-10. It includes several depressive conditions that share chronicity as a common characteristic but otherwise are rather heterogeneous with regard to their clinical presentation, neurobiological correlates and treatment response [8, 10, 62, 63]. Most of the patients currently subsumed under the term dysthymia were described in the past as having "depressive neurosis", "depressive personality", and "characterological depression". The patients assigned to this category do not fulfill the criteria for recurrent depression, but in addition to depressive mood need to have at least two of the following: poor appetite or overeating, insomnia or hypersomnia, low energy, low self-esteem, poor concentration, inability to decide and hopelessness. The symptoms have to last for at least 2 years, usually without remissions or with occasional free intervals of a short duration (of a few days or weeks). The patients, most of the time, present themselves as moody, sad, tired and anhedonic, with feelings of inadequacy, but also often as demanding and complaining, self-denigrating and at the same time reproachful to others. As a consequence, dysthymics are not particularly sociable and their relationships are neither stable nor empathetic.

In most cases, it is hard to define the correct time of onset of the disorder. The patients themselves feel that it is a lifelong condition, embedded in their existence since childhood. Although it may be diagnosed in late life, the early onset is typical of dysthymia and for some authors the term should be preserved only for cases with an early onset, either as a distinct condition or as a chronic subthreshold mood or even a temperamental state [64–66]. If MD precedes or co-occurs during the 2 or more years of dysthymic symptomatology the diagnosis, according to DSM-IV, should be MD only. If, however, MD is superimposed on dysthymia after its 2 years duration, both conditions are diagnosed separately (as dual diagnosis) and according to some authors the term "double depression" should be used [67].

TABLE 1.3   Dysthymia according to ICD-10

Criteria
- At least 2 years of constant or constantly recurring depressed mood
- Intervening periods of normal mood rarely last for longer than a few weeks; no episodes of hypomania
- None, or very few, of the individual episodes of depression within the 2-year period should be sufficiently severe or long-lasting to meet the criteria for recurrent mild depressive disorder
- During at least some of the periods of depression, at least three of the symptoms listed below should be present

Symptoms
- Reduced energy or activity
- Insomnia
- Loss of self-confidence and feelings of inadequacy
- Difficulty in concentrating
- Frequent tearfulness
- Loss of interest in or enjoyment of sex and other pleasurable activities
- Feeling of hopelessness or despair
- A perceived inability to cope with the routine responsibilities of everyday life
- Pessimism about the future or brooding over the past
- Social withdrawal
- Reduced talkativeness

Cyclothymia

Cyclothymia is characterized by persistent instability of mood and involves symptoms of depression and elation, which are insufficient in severity and pervasiveness to meet the full criteria of either manic or depressive episodes. They pursue a chronic course for at least 2 years with or without normothymic intervals, which if present—according to DSM-IV—should not exceed the 2-month duration [5]. During the periods of depression, in addition to depressed mood, at least three of the ICD-10 symptoms for depressive episode should be present (see Table 1.2) [2, 3]. Mood swings as a rule start in late teenage. Cyclothymia is a condition not easily recognizable and if it does not develop to a major mood psychopathology, and especially bipolar disorder, usually does not attract medical attention. However, it impairs social and occupational functioning to a degree that depends on the intensity and the rate of change of the symptoms in each particular individual. It is not clinically distinguished from cycloid or cyclothymic personality disorders [68]. When mood instability pervades the whole of personal behaviour, the ensuing chaotic life style closely resembles the clinical presentation of a borderline personality disorder.

Cyclothymia, as a distinct entity separate from MD, does not correspond to Schneider's concept, which was synonymous to bipolar disorder. The current concept, although still ill-defined, brings it closer to a subaffective chronic state of mood fluctuations that is linked to personality disorders [29].

Other Depressive Types

Seasonal Depression

Seasonal depression is characterized by recurrent depressive episodes in temporal relationship with a particular period of the year (regular onset in fall or winter and offset usually in the spring). Full remission from depression (or change to mania or hypomania) in the spring or somewhat later, and the seasonal depressive episodes outnumbering the lifetime major depressive episodes without seasonal pattern are two of the qualifying criteria for inclusion in this disorder [69, 70].

Subsyndromal Depressive Symptoms (SSD)

Neither ICD-10 nor DSM-IV make any reference to SSD as a separate subtype of depressive disorder. Whereas there are no established criteria for their syndromal definition, recent studies have shown that they are a clinical entity, identifiable in general population surveys and frequently seen in primary care settings [65]. This entity involves a cluster of symptoms that do not differ from those of the MD but do not meet the full criteria of a depressive "case". The symptoms are fewer than formally required, are not severe enough and vary over time. Nevertheless, although subthreshold, the symptoms have a disabling impact on the individual, seriously impairing his mental, occupational and psychosocial functioning. They may precede or follow MD and not infrequently they fill the intervals between the episodes [66, 71].

Although falling short of full-fledged depression, SSD are very close to the mild depressive episode of ICD-10 and to many other conditions which in the past were known as "neurotic" or "characterological". It has been reported [64] that subthreshold depression does not significantly differ in terms of sleep parameters, family history and follow-up course from threshold depressive conditions, with the exception of the major (severe) depressive episode with psychotic features [66]. On the basis of these observations, it has been postulated that SSD and the minor depression disorders appear on a symptomatic continuum, with the other subtypes of syndromal depressive illness representing an alternative form or different symptomatic phase of the same parent illness [65].

Premenstrual Syndrome (PMS)

It is still debated whether symptoms which occur during the last week of luteal phase and remit a few days after menses constitute a distinct syndrome or are either part of or superimposed on other depressive and mental disorders. DSM-IV [5, 10] lists the premenstrual syndrome among those that may be a focus of attention, while ICD-10 [2, 3] does not attach syndromal significance to premenstrual symptoms.

Epidemiological studies yield prevalence rates of 80% for mild to moderate and 3–8% for severe premenstrual symptoms [72]. Among the many symptoms, the most frequent are depressed mood, anxiety, irritability, mood lability, tiredness, sleep and eating disturbances, and difficulty in concentrating.

The PMS has first to be differentiated from the minor and mild emotional, behavioral and somatic manifestations accompanying or forming part of the normal biological function of menstruation, which should not be labeled as psychopathological unless they are so severe and disabling that they meet the criteria of a syndrome. Cross-sectionally the premenstrual symptoms closely resemble symptoms of major depression and dysthymia. Differential diagnosis lies mainly on symptom duration and on premenstrual history. Other conditions to be considered in differential diagnosis are bipolar disorder, substance abuse, gynecological and endocrine disorders.

In a recent study to validate the PMS and to explore its phenomeno-logical and familial relationship with major depression, it was concluded that premenstrual symptoms are substantially heritable, but the associated genetic and environmental factors are not closely related to lifetime major depression [73].

Depression and Menopause

The prevalence of depressive disorders does not seem to increase during menopause [74]. However, further investigation may be needed [75]. Negative beliefs about menopause and experiencing a longer than usual menopause are associated with an increased risk of developing a depressive disorder.

Depressive Personality Disorder (DPD)

As already mentioned, Hippocrates had observed a particular type of temper-ament or "crasis", the melancholic, associated with the secretion of black bile from the liver. Galen elaborated on this personality type further in his treatise of four types of temperament or "crasis". Kraepelin, and later Kretschmer, early in this century, also recognized a distinct "depressive" temperament prone to developing depression. An excellent phenomenological analysis of the melancholic temperament was attempted by Tellenbach in his mono-graph *Melancholie* [76]. DPD was represented in the first two editions of DSM, but it was omitted from both DSM-III and DSM-III-R. In ICD-10 it is not distinguished from dysthymia [2, 3]. The interest of clinical researchers in affective temperamental disorders did not cease and amid controversy DPD was readmitted in Appendix B of DSM-IV as a putative disorder for further study [7, 29, 77]. DPD is defined in DSM-IV as a pervasive pattern of depres-sive cognitions and behaviors beginning by early adulthood and fulfilling five or more of seven criteria (variants of depressed mood, low self-esteem, self-criticism, pessimism, negativistic and critical attitude toward others, guilt feelings), the minor to negligible contribution of somatic symptoms being a differentiating feature from dysthymia [5, 10].

The relationship of DPD with depressive disorders and particularly with dysthymia, with which it shares chronicity and early life onset as well as a number of common presenting symptoms, is the subject of ongoing clinical research and vigorous debates.

In support of validation of DPD as a distinct, stable personality type qualifying for a personality disorder status are results from a recent study which showed that although it can be comorbid with dysthymia and MD it can also occur in their absence (83% of the cases did not have early onset dysthymia and 60% did not have current MD). Moreover, in a 1-year follow-up, DPD proved to be a relatively stable condition [78].

Postnatal Depressive Disorders

These disorders present in three forms. The first is a transient anxiety-depressive state known as postpartum blues that occurs a few days after delivery, peaks within 10 days and subsides usually within 3 weeks after delivery. About half of the mothers experience the blues in various degrees [4, 10, 79]. The symptoms are mild, not necessitating medical attention. Characteristic symptoms include mild depressive mood, crying, fatigue. The second form occurs in almost 10–15% of mothers [80], as a rule within the first month after delivery. The symptoms do not essentially differ from the moderate and severe non-psychotic DE/MD. They have a disrupting and long-term effect on the personal and family life of the mother. The third, known as postpartum depression with psychotic features, occurs in about one out of 1000 mothers. In this form of postnatal depression, the first month after delivery is characterized, in addition to DE/MD symptomatology, by psychotic features among which are delusional thoughts, mainly concerning the newborn, in association with severe crying spells, guilt feelings, suicidal ideation and occasionally with hallucinatory experiences [5, 79]. Differential diagnosis is necessary from thyroid dysfunction and drug-induced syndromes.

ASSOCIATION WITH AND DIFFERENTIAL DIAGNOSIS FROM NORMAL SADNESS AND OTHER MENTAL DISORDERS

Normal Sadness

Depressed mood as an essential ingredient of pathological (morbid) depression has its equivalent in the emotional response of practically all normal individuals when faced with losses, rejections and the adversities and vicissitudes of life. Sadness, disappointment, downness, gloominess, discouragement, unhappiness, and even despair, are universal human experiences: how different are these normal emotions from the clinically meaningful mood changes of a depressed patient? Is there a line demarcating the normal from abnormal feelings, or are the boundaries between the two blurred and practically non-existent? The dimensionalists view the normal and depressed mood as variations in intensity and duration rather than as distinctly delineated, qualitatively different conditions. This is reflected in the operational criteria for depressive disorders, in both ICD-10 and DSM-IV. A minimum intensity (measured by the number of symptoms) and minimum duration of symptoms are required to differentiate normal from abnormal mood states.

The impact of depressed mood on social functioning, adopted by DSM-IV as an additional criterion, may not be quantitatively as valid as the other two criteria, since socio-cultural variables seem to interfere on the level of the individual's interpersonal relations and social functioning. The quantitative approach is also reflected in the widely applied depression measuring scales [81–83]. The qualitative approach, on the other hand, that views the depressed mood as distinct from normal sadness with a different experiential content, may be difficult to validate, since subjective feeling states can only partially be communicated and objectively assessed.

The closeness of normal sadness to the depressed mood may explain why so often depressed patients do not seek help until their condition deteriorates and becomes unbearable. This also explains why depressives are not easily recognized as suffering patients by their family members and friends. The patients' complaints about their painful feelings are often interpreted by others as an excessive, but still normal distress, that they themselves had already experienced in their lives.

In severe depression, it may not be difficult to delineate normal from abnormal mood states. In addition to the mood disturbances, the distinguishing features commonly cited in the literature include impairments of body functioning and vegetative symptoms (sleep, eating and sex disturbances), disinterest and lack of desire for performing the usual and expected social roles, suicidal ideation and, in severe forms, mood-congruent delusions [1]. In mild forms of depression, such symptoms are absent and recognition of mood disturbances requires particular attention and diagnostic skills. The following are useful guidelines.

In contrast with normal sadness, the depressed mood: (a) may not be associated with a real adverse event, and if losses are reported, they are grossly exaggerated, anticipated or imagined; (b) is extremely painful, persistent and pervasive, resisting all attempts to change by encouragement or reasoning; (c) is commonly associated with worthlessness, low self-esteem, and sustained self-depreciation; (d) frequently escalates with time and impacts on interpersonal relations and daily functioning; (e) is associated with guilt feeling and death wishes; (f) involves, if severe enough, somatic-vegetative symptoms and delusional ideation; (g) is more frequently than in normal sadness associated with rhythm disturbances and hormonal dysregulation.

On theoretical grounds, the ethological paradigms and Bowlby's attachment theory may be invoked to support the qualitative distinction between normal and abnormal affects. It is postulated that depression as a normal emotion serves an adaptational function, signaling danger and alerting the individual and the fellow members of the group to meet it. In depressed patients the adaptational qualities of the affect as a signaling and protective psychological mechanism are apparently degraded [1].

Worth mentioning are the theoretical approaches on the distinguishing features between normal sadness, mourning and morbid depressed mood developed by the psychoanalytic school that still follows Abraham's and Freud's original psychodynamic formulations [84]. The German phenomeno-logical school also contributed to the analysis of human emotions and their pathological variants and has best been represented on the subject of depression by Tellenbach's work on melancholia [76].

In the past few years an attempt has been made to explore the neural substrate of those emotions of normal individuals which from the evolutionary perspective are considered primary, serving survival needs and adaptational functions. In this respect the positron emission tomography (PET) studies are relevant. In one of the first PET studies [85] it was reported that induced sadness evoked bilateral activation of the inferior orbito-frontal cortex. In another study [86] it was shown that sadness and happiness involve different neuronal networks. Finally, in a more recent study, it was shown that in human emotions several brain regions are involved, but it is possible to identify regions that distinguish between positive and negative emotions [87]. It is understood that at this stage it is premature to rely on neuroimaging technology for differentiating normal from abnormal emotions (sadness from depressed mood). Nevertheless, such findings may be used as the experimental ground for exploring the boundaries between normal and abnormal affective states.

Bereavement

Bereavement is generally considered a normal psychological reaction to loss (death) of a loved one and involves a number of symptoms that are also experienced by depressed patients. The differential features of a normal grief and clinical depression concern the number and the severity of the symptoms (being as a rule fewer and milder in the former) as well as their duration (in bereavement, they decline in 2-months and should not last for more than 6 months). The process of grieving following death includes bewilderment and "numbness" (as immediate reactions), preoccupation with the loved one, an urge to look back and inability to look forward, low mood, restlessness, occasional despair, striving to recapture the image of the lost one, disturbed sleep, loss of interest, lack of concentration and mild guilt feelings [9]. According to DSM-IV, if the depression-like picture is still present after 2 months and some symptoms not typical for "normal" grief (inappropriate guilt, preoccupation with worthlessness, psychomotor slowing and hallucinatory experiences) are added, a depressive disorder should be considered [5, 10].

Undoubtedly, bereavement is a highly stressful event and its contributing role in triggering a depressive disorder should not be overlooked in clinical practice. High rates of MD following bereavement, ranging from 20% up to over half of the cases 1 month after the loss and progressively decreasing in subsequent months, have been reported by several authors [88]. It was also reported that 50% of all widows and widowers meet the MD criteria during the first year of bereavement [8, 9].

Equal significance should, however, be given to post-bereavement subsyndromal depression, consisting of milder and fewer depressive symptoms which nonetheless seriously affect the overall adjustment of the individual and are good predictors of an increased risk for future major depressive episodes [88].

Increased risk factors for post-bereavement depression are the traumatic circumstances surrounding the death of the loved one as well as ambivalent and dependent or interdependent attachment to the deceased person, and insecure attachment to parents in childhood (particularly learned fear and learned helplessness) [90].

Anxiety and Panic

The close association of depression with anxiety has long been recognized by clinicians and clinical investigators and has initiated the vigorous and persistent dispute between the "splitters" and the "lumpers", that is, between those viewing depression and anxiety as two separate categorical entities and those advocating the unitary hypothesis considering both as dimensions of a single underlying disorder.

The intimate relationship between depression and anxiety is best reflected in the overlap of depressive and anxiety items in the most widely used scales for measuring severity of the two disorders [134]. The extent to which depression overlaps or co-occurs with anxiety has been amply demonstrated in three major epidemiological studies: the ECA study [37, 38], the US National Comorbidity Survey [39], and the WHO Study on Psychological Disorders in Primary Health Care [41, 42]. According to the US National Comorbidity Study results, the majority (61.8%) of the respondents with a lifetime history of MD had at least one other DSM-III-R disorder before the onset of depression and in only 26% depression was not preceded or overlapped by any other disorder. The 12-month comorbidity has also shown 51.8% of depressed patients to have anxiety disorders. The calculated odds ratios (qualifying the relative risk of an outcome between two exposure groups) in the study have shown considerable variability across sites but strong association of lifetime MD and specific anxiety disorders (generalized anxiety, panic, agoraphobia and social phobia) [39]. The WHO study, although methodologically close but not identical to the ECA and the US National Comorbidity studies, yielded grossly similar results on depression-anxiety comorbidity [41]. In nearly half of the cases, depression and anxiety appeared at the same time. It was also found that with an increasing number of depressive symptoms there was an increasing number of anxiety symptoms. In a recent study in which the results of an International Task Force on Affective and Anxiety Comorbidity were reported, it was found that panic followed by social phobia was more strongly associated with depression.

The overall evidence leaves no doubt that co-occurrence of depression and anxiety is the rule rather than the exception, particularly in primary care settings.

Schizophrenia

Depressive symptoms during the psychotic phase of schizophrenia, although present, may not be detected due to the "masking" effect of the more pronounced and overt psychotic symptoms. They are more evident and easily recognized when they either precede or follow the psychotic phase [4, 8]. When they precede the onset of psychotic symptoms, they are often misdiagnosed as a true depressive episode [91]. A thorough psychiatric examination as well as a close follow-up are recommended where the family history and the presence of atypical symptoms raise the suspicion that the depressive symptoms are actually the prodromal signs of an oncoming psychotic episode. The frequent occurrence of a pre-psychotic depressive phase has been variously conceptualized, but the predominant view is that it is an integral part of the psychotic process rather than a discrete non-psychotic condition that initiates the psychotic psychopathology [92].

Is not clear whether the depressive symptomatology that appears after the remission of florid psychotic symptoms in a percentage of patients represents a true depression or a mixture of symptoms, some residual of the remitted psychosis (especially with negative symptoms), some related to post-psychotic adjustment difficulties and others to neuroleptic medication. The issue is controversial, but is of relevance to clinical practice, since false-positive and false-negative diagnosis may lead to wrong treatment choices. Post-psychotic depression has been adopted as a separate psychopathological entity in ICD-10 [2, 3].

Somatization Disorder

All types of somatic (physical) symptomatology listed in ICD-10 and DSM-IV as somatization disorder, somatoform disorder, undifferentiated somatoform disorder, hypochondriacal disorder, and which share as a common denom-inator the presence of somatic (bodily) complaints and symptoms in the absence of a physical illness and not resulting from the direct effect of drug abuse or medication, bear a strong association with both depression and anxiety.

Depending on the individual patients' characteristics and their social and cultural backgrounds, the bodily symptoms vary in number and type, but commonly include bodily diffuse or ill-located pains and aches, chest pressures as well as visceral symptoms related to the function of internal organs. All symptoms are usually vague, unstable and inexplicable by the results of the physical and laboratory examinations. The presence of depressed mood is not infrequently masked by the somatizing patient; however, it is rarely missed by an experienced clinical interviewer.

Adjustment Disorder (AD)

One of the subtypes of AD is the one with depressed mood. The main features of AD, that is the development of significant emotional or behavioral response to an identified psychological stress, are presented in association with predominant depressive symptoms (crying spells, hopelessness and distress). To qualify as AD the symptoms should appear in less than 3 months following the psychosocial stressor. This subtype, like AD in general, has to be distinguished from post-traumatic stress disorder (PTSD), which, however, is a response to an exceptionally severe and threatening traumatic event that results in several long-lasting adverse effects on the patient's mental health and social functioning.

Post-traumatic Stress Disorder (PTSD)

The differentiating features of this condition are the intense and/or protracted response to a stressful event or situation of an exceptionally threatening or catastrophic nature. A qualifying criterion is that the onset of the symptoms should occur within the 6-month time frame following the stressful event. Typical symptoms include hyperarousal, episodes of reliving the traumatic experience, detachment, "numbness", maladaptive coping responses and excessive use of alcohol and drugs [93]. A recent study, in which the ability of experienced clinicians to differentiate PTSD from MD and generalized anxiety disorder (GAD) was applied as a validating criterion, has shown that the clinicians readily distinguished PTSD from the other two disorders [94].

ASSOCIATION WITH AND DIFFERENTIAL DIAGNOSIS FROM MEDICAL ILLNESSES

Prevalence rates of depressive disorders among patients suffering from a medical illness are considerable, from 22% to 33% [95], while it has been estimated that in the primary health setting the median prevalence rate for depressive disorders is more than 10% [40].

It may be difficult to distinguish a primary from a secondary depression occurring during or as a consequence of a physical disease or as a side effect of various prescribed drugs. The mode of onset (acute), the symptomatology (atypical for depression), the resistance to previous antidepressant treatment and the positive laboratory findings for a non-depressive disorder should always be considered in order not to miss a physical illness underlying or occurring with depression [4, 8, 9, 34].

Depression in Neurological Illness

Epilepsy

As many as 20% of patients with temporal lobe epilepsy become moderately or severely depressed [96] and this percentage is greatly increased (up to 62%) in patients with medically intractable complex partial seizures [34, 95]. Interictal depression is the most common. In general it is moderate to severe, with a variety of symptoms including severe anxiety, obsessions, aggressiveness, delusional and hallucinatory experiences [97, 98, 99].

Post-stroke

Depression is the most common post-stroke psychiatric condition. Predictors include left anterior brain lesions and a previous history of psychiatric and/or cerebrovascular disorder [99].

Parkinson's Disease

An association between Parkinson's disease (PD) and depression is now well established, and about half of PD patients with depressive disorders satisfy criteria for major depression, while slightly less than half qualify for dysthymia [95, 99]. Recognized risk factors include female gender, bradykinesia, gait instability and earlier age of onset of PD.

Multiple Sclerosis

Until recently, euphoria was thought to be a cardinal symptom of multiple sclerosis but there is now general agreement that depressive disorder is the most common affective disturbance in patients and it can coexist with the first even undiagnosed signs of the illness [99].

Degenerative Brain Disease

Depression is the most frequent psychiatric disorder associated with Huntington's disease and can occur in up to 38% of patients. Suicide and deliberate self-harm are reported to occur commonly and depressive symptoms can appear before neurological signs [100].

Alzheimer's Disease

The association of Alzheimer's disease and depression will be dealt with more extensively in a separate chapter of this book.

Depression in Cardiovascular Illness

Depressed patients are at significantly increased risk of developing ischemic heart disease and/or hypertension, and the converse is also true [101–103]. High rates of comorbidity between cardiovascular disease and depression are cited in the literature and pose serious diagnostic difficulties. Post-myocardial infarction patients present full-blown depression in about 16–22% of cases. Bodily complaints associated with depressive mood, such as chest pain and palpitations, may lead to a misdiagnosis of heart disease [104].

Depression in Cancer Illness

The diagnosis of depression in a cancer presents a challenge. There is a considerable overlap of cancer and depressive symptoms (loss of appetite, weight loss, insomnia, loss of interest and loss of energy) [105]. Also, cancer chemotherapeutics have been associated with depressive symptoms. The cancer patient with a depressive disorder is likely to be preoccupied with the illness, to develop feelings of worthlessness and guilt, with reliable differentiating symptoms from the normal emotional reaction to the cancerous disease. Recurrent thoughts of suicide are common in cancer patients but not as intense as in severe depression. Risk factors for depressive disorder in cancer include young age, female gender, active symptoms of the disease, presence of uncontrolled pain, history of mood disorder and social isolation [95].

Depression in Endocrine Disorders

Hypothyroidism

Patients with overt, mild or subclinical hypothyroidism present more commonly with cognitive impairment and depression. Depression has been estimated to occur in 40% of such patients. Psychiatric symptoms typically begin with mental slowing, followed by a decline in short-term memory, progressive dysphoria, affective lability and emotional withdrawal. Symptoms such as insomnia, decreased self-esteem and worthlessness are reported to be more common in major depressive disorder [95]. When compared to individuals with normal thyroid function, patients with subclinical hypothyroidism have been found in one study to have a significantly higher frequency of lifetime depression, suggesting that subclinical hypothyroidism may lower the threshold for the occurrence of depression [106]. Since most depressives are not hypothyroid, there is no necessity for a routine checking of thyroid function, unless they are under lithium prophylactic treatment. Thyroid screening should be obtained in patients with treatment refractory depression, as hypothyroidism may contribute to this condition [107]. The relationship of thyroid function and depression is reflected in the thyroid-stimulating hormone (TSH) response to thyrotropin-releasing hormone (TRH) (see neurobiological tests).

Hyperthyroidism

Although the most prevalent psychiatric manifestations in hyperthyroidism are anxiety disorders [107], an atypical presentation of hyperthyroidism with apathy and psychomotor retardation (apathetic hyperthyroidism) has been observed and it can be mistaken for depressive disorder [108]. It appears more frequently in elderly patients and is reported to be less responsive to antidepressive medications.

Hyperparathyroidism

Depressed mood, lethargy, mental slowness, decreased attention and memory may present as the initial signs of hyperparathyroidism. Depressed or anxious mood is present in as many as one quarter of cases. The relationship between symptom severity and serum calcium levels is still controversial.

Cushing's Syndrome

Depressive disorders are found in over half the cases of patients with Cushing's syndrome. Irritability, depressed mood, fatigue, decreased libido, anxiety, poor memory or concentration and agitation are the most frequently seen symptoms. Suicidal ideation is not uncommon, and it is reported that up to 10% of these patients may make a suicidal attempt. Manic or hypomanic symptoms are seen occasionally during steroid treatment.

Psychotic symptoms such as delusions and hallucinations occur only rarely. When the syndrome occurs secondary to other causes, depressive symptoms are far more common. It appears that a depressive mood secondary to Cushing's syndrome is intermittent rather than chronic and irritability is reported to be heightened beyond what is typically found in major depression [107, 109]. The onset of the affective symptoms has been reported to occur both preceding and following the onset of the medical signs and symptoms of Cushing's disease. Depressive symptoms subside following successful treatment of the endocrine disorder. Several symptoms are not dependent on cortisol plasma levels [109, 110].

Depression in Metabolic Disorders

Addison's Disease

Chronic adrenocortical insufficiency typically presents with depressed mood, irritability, apathy, withdrawal, fatigue, and weakness. Concentration may be weak and insomnia may occur. Almost all patients lose their appetite and lose some weight. A depressive episode of gradual onset may be very difficult to distinguish from chronic adrenocortical insufficiency and a relative prominence of weakness and fatigue may alert one to an adrenal cause [95, 109].

Diabetes Mellitus

Depression in patients with diabetes is common, with prevalence rates ranging from 8.5 to 27.3% in controlled studies. The mechanisms (serum glucose levels, cerebrovascular conglucation or psychological stress related to the chronicity of the condition) which account for the high comorbidity rates have to be determined [111].

Medication-induced Depression

Whilst the various aspects of depressive disorders and medical illnesses are considered, the depressogenic effect of some prescribed medications in clinical practice must not be forgotten. Strong associations or a cause–effect relationship have been established for a relatively small number of drugs (Table 1.4). The effects of other medications on mood are more likely to be at the level of depressive symptoms rather than depressive disorders [95].

Although some early studies suggested an association between depressive disorders and the use of oral contraceptives, this does not seem to hold true in recent controlled double-blind studies [112, 113].

TABLE 1.4 Depressogenic medications

Definite effect	Possible effect
Reserpine	Alpha-methyldopa
Withdrawal from amphetamines	Beta-blockers
Phenobarbital	Oral contraceptives
Steroids	Clomiphene
	Tamoxifene
	Cimetidine
	Acetazolamide

It has been observed that low cholesterol levels, caused either by diet or by drugs, are associated with increased rates of death due to suicide or violence [114–116]. The most plausible explanation is that lowered cholesterol levels result in decreased serotoninergic activity in the brain [116]. Nonetheless, this very interesting observation warrants further investigation.

Alcohol and Drugs

Alcoholism and Depression

The association between alcoholism and depression has long been documented in both clinical and epidemiological studies. The frequency of occurrence of secondary MD in hospitalized alcoholics ranges between 8 and 53% in different studies using different assessment procedures on different patient samples. An association — although not as strong — was also documented in community surveys [117].

Drug abuse/dependence and Depression

Symptoms of anxiety and depression frequently appear during the intoxication and withdrawal phases of drug dependence and in that case they are considered as part of the "substance abuse induced disorder" (with predominant anxiety or depression symptoms). Symptoms meeting the full criteria of depressive disorder, however, are encountered in drug dependants while they are free from both the direct drug effect and withdrawal symptoms. According to a number of recent studies in which structured interviews were used and operational diagnostic criteria were applied, co-occurrence of depression and drug abuse is much higher than expected in the general population. The rates vary somewhat across studies in different sites, but the overall figures of lifetime and recent prevalence of the two conditions confirm their close association [117–120]. The subthreshold depressive symptomatology was shown to have an equal or even higher impact than

MD on a number of indices including number of suicidal attempts and psychiatric hospitalizations [120].

The question as to which of the two conditions precedes the other and might have a causative influence on the other is still open. Clinical and epidemiological retrospective studies have shown that there is about an even distribution of MD prior to and following the onset of drug use [118, 120]. This finding lends support to the hypothesis that in a percentage of drug addicts the use of drugs is part of their self-medication behavior to combat depression.

RECOGNITION AND DIAGNOSTIC PROCEDURES

Steps to Diagnosing Depressive Disorders — Conducting the Interview

1. Make the patients feel relaxed and give them enough time to expand their thoughts. Interview them by listening first to their complaints, and then, by asking open-ended questions, try to elicit additional symptoms and clarify the meaning and the severity of those already reported. Questions should address all areas of the patient's physical and mental health as well as his or her occupational and social functioning.

2. If complaints and symptoms raise the suspicion of a depressive syndrome, focus specifically on such symptoms as depressed mood, loss of energy, sleep and eating disorders, tiredness, inexplicable somatic complaints (vague diffuse pains, backaches, dizziness) self-depreciation, impaired social functioning and concomitant others that may meet the symptom operational criteria for a depressive disorder. Avoid direct and inappropriate questions such are "Are you depressed?", but pay attention also to symptoms of depression manifest in the patient's appearance and movements. Try to gain the patient's trust by showing concern for his emotional distress. It is important that physicians acknowledge the patient's emotion at critical moments during the interview. Do not undervalue patients' distress nor argue against the rationale of their symptoms. Instead be understanding and supportive of all their complaints including their physical symptoms.

3. If symptom operational criteria for a depressive episode are met, proceed with obtaining the patient's reliable family and past personal history (time of onset of current episode, past and current health problems) and before reaching ICD-10 or DSM-IV diagnosis of depressive disorder consider — and exclude — the possibility: (a) that the clinical picture may be induced by a physical illness or another mental illness, by medication

or substance use; and (b) that manic or submanic episodes have occurred in the past, and the current depressive episode is part of a bipolar disorder.

4. If the diagnosis of depressive disorder is reached, before designating the clinical condition as major depression (DSM-IV) or depressive episode (ICD-10) or their respective subtypes, the following have mainly to be considered: (a) bereavement (closely associated with the death of a loved person and lasting for less than 2 months); (b) dysthymia (depressive symptomatology mild to moderate and lasting for more than 2 years); (c) adjustment disorder (depressive mood frequently mixed with anxiety in response to identifiable severe psychosocial stressors usually disrupting occupational and social functioning); (d) subthreshold depressive syndrome (the number and severity of symptom criteria are not met to qualify for major depression but are associated with occupational and emotional health impairment).

5. If only single and sporadic core symptoms of depression are detected which are insufficient to define depression, do not dismiss them — put them on record and watch their course closely.

Obstacles in the Recognition of Depression

Many studies have shown that over half of the patients with depression seeking medical care in primary health facilities were not diagnosed as such and were either misdiagnosed as suffering from a physical illness or were considered as complainers about medically insignificant psychological problems [40].

The symptoms initially presented to the physician, especially at the primary care setting, are not usually the ones defined as operational criteria for diagnosis in either the ICD-10 or the DSM-IV classification systems. In fact, somatic presentation of depressive disorder is common and early in the 1970s "masked depression" was the term to designate an underlying clinical depression covered by somatic complaints. More than half of the depressed patients in the WHO International Study presented with somatic complaints from different organ systems [121]. The most common presenting somatic complaints are inexplicable, vague and diffuse bodily pains and sensations, sleep disturbance, dizziness, muscular tension, fatigue, anorexia and gastrointestinal disturbances. The frequency and intensity of "masking" somatic symptoms depend on the patient's personal characteristics, the physician's attitude and the setting's characteristics.

Most likely to present with somatic symptoms are depressed patients who lack psychological insight, are reluctant or unable to express their emotions verbally, are elderly, poorly educated and feel ashamed to acknowledge psychological problems.

A frequent source of non-recognition or misdiagnosis of depression in the primary care setting is the presence of a comorbid to depression physical illness. The symptoms of one condition often overlap with the other, particularly when somatic manifestations prevail in the clinical presentation of depression. The physician's tendency on these occasions is to overlook the depressive symptoms, considering them as a normal and appropriate psychological reaction to the patient's awareness of his physical ill-health. This is more frequently the case with elderly patients. Such an attitude on the part of the physician is generally attributed to lack of time for a thorough insightful and empathetic interview of the patient on the one hand, and to inadequate educational background in psychiatry during his or her medical training on the other. The physician's personality attribute, reflected in resistance to dealing with the psychological aspects of the patient's problem, should also be considered [122].

Tacit collusion is a term [9] that has been used to illustrate the patient's and the physician's attitudes as contributing factors to poor recognition rates of depression in the primary care settings. It is a condition which is realized when on the one hand, the depressed patient is hesitant or unable to express his or her feelings and prefers to gain the physician's considerate attention by presenting his or her physical complaints, and on the other hand, the physician feels more comfortable talking of and looking for somatic symptoms.

Depression, as already mentioned, co-occurs, precedes or follows other mental disorders and physical illnesses. The terms comorbid, secondary and complicated may be used in such cases, because in the majority of cases temporal and clinical characteristics are not strongly discerned factors.

Diagnostic Instruments

Structured and semi-structured instruments aim at screening for psychiatric disorders and making clinical diagnosis more accurate and objective. They are based on preformed key questions pertinent to a specific topic or to the whole of the patient's psychopathology and are designed to be thorough and reproducible. They also have to provide for scoring the information obtained. Although useful, they should be considered as supplementary to, and not a substitute for, the clinical interview. Three categories of instruments are currently used in psychiatry: (a) screening instruments for detecting the presence of psychiatric disorders; (b) diagnostic instruments used to supplement or even to replace the clinical diagnostic interview;

(c) severity measurement scales used to assess severity of previously diagnosed conditions.

General Screening Instruments

The GHQ (General Health Questionnaire) is used in two stages, the first including a self-reporting questionnaire on general health, well-being and coping, and the second a clinical interview schedule for diagnosis according to WHO ICD [123], to be administered by a physician.

General Diagnostic Instruments

The CIDI (Composite International Diagnostic Interview) was produced jointly by WHO and ADAMHA (US Alcohol, Drug Abuse and Mental Health Administration) and is designed to enable the user (trained interviewer, not clinician) to arrive at a diagnosis according to both ICD-10 and DSM-III-R criteria [124].

The PSE (Present State Examination) is a semi-structured interview designed for use only by clinicians [125]. A computer program derived from PSE (CATEGO) has been developed to facilitate diagnosis. A short version of PSE has also been developed to be used as a screening diagnostic instrument in population studies.

The SCAN (Schedules for Clinical Assessment in Neuropsychiatry) is a semi-structured interview based on PSE, and is also the product of a WHO–ADAMHA collaborative study. It was primarily designed for use by clinicians, particularly psychiatrists, but may also be used by other well-trained mental health professionals [126].

The SCID (Structured Clinical Interview for DSM-IIIR) was developed along with DSM-IIIR after having been field-tested, to facilitate diagnosis by clinicians according to DSM operational criteria. The clinician makes the judgment as to whether each criterion is met and whether all criteria taken together validate the clinical diagnosis [127].

Specific Instruments for Depression Screening

The CES-D (Center for Epidemiological Studies—Depressive Scale) is a self-reporting 20-item scale intended mainly for epidemiological research in general population surveys [128]. It was developed to detect and measure depressive symptomatology in the community, has been used widely all over the world, and has contributed greatly to depression "case identification" in the community [129]. Indicatively, between 1993 and 1995, it was used in 120 published studies, second only to the Beck Depression Inventory [130]. It is validated but still presents with some shortcomings which, as recently reported, can be improved by applying special analytic methods [131].

Specific Instruments for the Diagnosis of Depression

The SADD (Standardized Assessment of Depressive Disorders) records in a standardized fashion the findings from clinical assessments of patient with depressive disorders [121].

The SADS (Schedule for Affective Disorders and Schizophrenia) is highly structured and detailed and therefore time-consuming, but scores very highly on reliability. It is mainly used in research, but a later version, the SADS-C, assessing only current psychopathology, may be used more widely even for screening purposes in population studies [132].

Specific Instruments for Measuring the Severity of Depression

The depression rating scales were developed around the 1960s mainly to objectively and accurately measure the changes brought about by the then rapidly growing psychopharmacotherapy. Assessment of severity is made by the number and intensity of the symptoms. The instruments have to be specific, valid, sensitive and reliable.

There are two kinds of rating scales: the observer- and the self-reporting. The former are more objective, including items observable in behavior that the patient may not be able to rate. The latter are more appropriate in measuring the patients' experiences and their own perception about themselves. We will include for comment those that have a long history behind them and are adequately validated.

The HAM-D (Hamilton Rating Scale for Depression) is the most widely used observer-reporting scale all over the world, particularly in clinical trials. It requires special observation skills. It is biologically oriented, and somatic symptoms weigh preferentially on the total score. Nonetheless, it rates highly for anxiety symptoms [81, 133].

The BDI (Beck Depression Inventory) is a self-rating scale that detects and rates preferentially cognitive aspects of depression with emphasis on self-esteem. It has been widely and successfully tested for validity [82].

The MADRS (Montgomery–Åsberg Depression Rating Scale) is one of the most user-friendly observer-rating scales. It includes a selected small number of items, considered to be the core and most commonly encountered depressive symptoms in clinical practice. It scores less high than HAM-D on somatic items and its specificity for depression is well established and validated [83, 134, 135].

Biological Tests and Correlates

Currently no biological findings that could be used as reliable diagnostic markers for depression are available. The potential areas from which such markers might be derived and substantially contribute to diagnosing clinical groups of depression with different etiologies are molecular genetics, neuroimaging, neuroendocrinology and sleep studies. Despite the absence of such markers of diagnostic value in clinical practice, it is worth including in this chapter research findings which presently may only have a varying degree of association with groups of depressives, but may signal exciting discoveries in the near future.

Neuroendocrine Tests

The hypothalamic–pituitary–adrenocortical axis.   The DST was the first, and is to date the most studied, putative biological marker in research on depressive disorders. In 1968 Carroll *et al* [136] showed that while depressed, patients fail to suppress plasma cortisol. This led Carroll to claim that a positive DST is a specific laboratory test for melancholia or severe forms of depression [46]. Subsequent studies confirmed the high specificity vs. normal or non-psychiatric controls (91%–93%) but not vs. dysthymic and other severe or acute psychiatric disorders as well as vs. apparently healthy individuals who had experienced a recent stressful event [137]. Moreover, high and low cortisol suppressors were found not to differ in depressive symptoms among participants in population studies [138]. However, cortisol secretion was found to be related to temperament dimensions [139]. A recent meta-analysis to determine the significance of differences in non-suppression of cortisol across studies, indicated a highly significant probability that a greater rate of cortisol non-suppression occurs in psychotic depression (64% in psychotics and 41% in non-psychotic patients) and the authors concluded that, among patients with major depression, those with psychotic depression constitute a subtype that is most closely associated with non-suppression of cortisol on the DST [53]. In another study the RDC "endogenous/non-endogenous" dichotomy was validated by the DST [161]. Interestingly, an enhanced negative feedback inhibition manifested by an exaggerated cortisol response to dexamethasone was observed in patients with post-traumatic stress disorder [140].

The adrenocorticotrophic hormone (ACTH) response to corticotropin releasing factor (CRF) is also a focus of investigation. There is accumulating evidence that the increased hypothalamic-pituitary drive reported in depression is primarily mediated by hypersecretion of CRF [141]. In some studies, patients with major depression show increased levels of CSF CRF as compared to matched controls or patients with schizophrenia [142, 143]. The elevation appears to be state-dependent, as CSF CRF levels normalize upon successful treatment. Studies utilizing challenge tests indicate that many depressed patients display a blunted ACTH response to exogenous CRF administration as compared to matched controls, and in at least one study this seems to be observed also in healthy subjects with a familial loading for affective disorders [142, 144]. In one study [145], the sensitivity of the DST/corticotropin-releasing hormone (CRH) test for MD was found to be about 80% greatly exceeding that of the standard DST (1–2 mg of dexamethasone), which has been reported to average about 44% in a meta-analysis of the literature data. Since CRF is considered as one of the primary mediators of stress responses, anxiety and fear, it is not surprising that increased CRF and blunted response to ACTH have been observed in stressful anxiety-ridden conditions [140].

The hypothalamic–pituitary–thyroid axis. Concerning the hypothalamic–pituitary–thyroid axis, depressed patients have been reported to have: (a) alterations in TSH response to the TRH; (b) an abnormally high rate of antithyroid antibodies; and (c) elevated CSF TRH concentrations. Consistently, a subgroup of depressive patients (about 30% or more) have a decreased response of TSH, to TRH and a variable prolactin (PRL) response [146, 147]. The blunted response persists in some patients after recovery and is not connected with cortisol levels or DST response. Both T4 and TSH response to TRH is reported to relate to the treatment outcome of depressed patients [148]. The significance of the pituitary–thyroid axis abnormalities in depression, however, still remains unclear.

The hypothalamic–pituitary–growth hormone system. The release of growth hormone (GH) from the anterior pituitary is regulated by hypothalamic peptides, especially GH-releasing hormone (GHRH) and somatostatin, which in turn are controlled by the classic neurotransmitters and insulin-like growth factor-1. Blunted GH response has been reported following administration of insulin, L-dopa, d-amphetamine, clonidine and GHRH, but the findings are equivocal [149]. The blunted GH secretion to clonidine is not only observed in depression and panic attacks, but also in GAD and social phobia. However, the abnormality is not observed in schizophrenia or obsessive-compulsive disorder (OCD). On the other hand, some investigators have observed no difference between depressed patients and controls in the clonidine/GH or GHRH/GH challenges [149, 150]. In a recent study, an enhanced GH release in response to pyridostigmine (PYD) in subjects with major depression (sensitivity 63%), but not inpatients with schizophrenia, alcohol dependence and panic, was reported [151]. Studies on GH nocturnal secretion in depressed patients yielded conflicting results. A marked decrease in depressed patients was observed in some studies [152], while in others secretion did not differ between patients and controls [153].

Serotonin (5-HT) tests. The implication of serotonin (5-HT) in depression is based on many findings from a variety of sources, including the beneficial effects of 5-HT reuptake inhibitors on depressive symptomatology. A number of studies used a variety of 5-HT releasing agents, mainly fenfluramine, as a challenge drug in order to probe the 5-HT functional state in the brain. The response of 5-HT receptors to the 5-HT releasing agents is measured by PRL, ACTH and cortisol secretion from the pituitary. The results of fenfluramine studies are thus far inconsistent. Negative results were reported by some investigators [154] and positive results by others [155, 156]. In a recent study in which strict control measures were applied, results were consistent with a blunted fenfluramine response. Moreover, the study indicated that the clinical recovery from depression is not associated with normalization of serotoninergic function [157].

Sleep Studies

Decreased sleep continuity, diminished slow wave sleep, altered distribution of REM sleep, and most notably, short latency to the first REM sleep period as well as lengthening of the duration of the first REM period, were frequently observed in patients with major depression disorders, particularly of the "endogenous" severe subtype [47, 158]. Claims of specificity of this aberrant sleep pattern were not substantiated, since a similar pattern has been observed in other psychiatric disorders, although not as frequently as in depressed patients, even in those with subthreshold symptomatology [64]. Whether sleep pattern abnormalities, wherever they occur, are trait or state markers is still an open question. Some sleep complaints seem to change following therapeutic interventions and others do not [159]. A recent study indicated that short REM latency and slow wave sleep latency are familial, and polysomnographic abnormalities may precede the clinical manifestation of depression and could be useful in identifying individuals at highest risk for the disorder [160].

A strategy of interest is the utilization of more than one test in order to enhance sensitivity. A recent study compared three laboratory measures in a combined in- and outpatient sample of depressed patients [161]. DST nonsuppression occurred in 46% of patients with endogenous major depression, in 15% with non-endogenous major depression, and in 56% with bipolar, depressed phase disorder. A blunted TRH-TSH response occurred in 25% of patients with endogenous major depression, 10% with non-endogenous major depression, and 44% with bipolar, depressed phase disorder. Reduced

REM latency was found in 65% of endogenous major depression, in 34% of non-endogenous major depressions, and in 53% of bipolar, depressed phase disorders. When the endogenous major depression and bipolar, depressed phase groups were combined, 28% had no laboratory abnormality, whereas 8% evidenced all three. The study suggested among other things that: (a) endogenous/non-endogenous unipolar groups are distinguished by all three laboratory tests; and (b) sensitivity is greatest and specificity is lowest for REM latency, followed by the DST and the TRH test.

Neuroimaging Studies

Neuroimaging technology is increasingly used in psychiatry in an attempt to correlate clinical manifestations with neuroanatomical and neurophysiological findings. The clinical applications of the new methods of the magnetic resonance imaging (MRI), PET, single photon emission computed tomography (SPECT) and functional MRI (FMRI) has provided exciting opportunities for exploring the neurobiological mechanisms underlying the mental disorders. A number of structural imaging studies in depressed patients revealed a variety of brain alterations in specific regions, the most common being atrophy and deep white-matter lesions in areas of the basal ganglia and prefrontal cortex. Although some of the findings indicate the presence of brain atrophy in patients with late-onset depression, the pattern of volumetric changes in these patients differs markedly from that observed in patients with primary degenerative dementia [162].

Late-life depression is associated with increased subcortical white-matter hyperintensities. There is some evidence that they are associated with a poorer response to acute treatment and with poor outcome in elderly depressed subjects [163].

MRI studies have also provided substantial evidence for state-dependent adrenal gland enlargement (40–70%) occurring during an episode of major depression [164]. Such an enlargement should not mislead the physician into diagnosing Cushing's syndrome, in which the enlargement is of greater magnitude and there are other associated laboratory and clinical features which differentiate it from depression.

Functional brain imaging techniques which permit non-invasive probing of the brain are powerful and sensitive research tools for elucidating the pathophysiology of depressive disorders. The application of these techniques in depression research has produced several studies of resting cerebral blood flow (CBF) and glucose metabolism in subjects imaged during various phases of illness and treatment, as well as during sleep [165]. In the majority of studies, decreased anterior paralimbic and cortical activity was noted: it is reported in a review article that there were 36 studies between

1984 and 1995 comparing CBF and metabolism in "primary" depression and, despite differences in techniques and methods employed, they provided evidence of prefrontal cortical deficits. Twenty-seven studies, including 419 patients, reported prefrontal decrease, while seven studies, including only 57 patients, reported increase. The magnetic resonance spectroscopy study (MRS) has only recently been applied and, although interesting findings in mood disorders have been reported, these still have to be replicated [166].

A recent PET study reported the localization of an area of abnormal decreased activity in the prefrontal cortex ventral to the genu of the corpus callosum in both familial bipolar and unipolar depressives. The differences were irrespective of mood state and persisted during antidepressant treatment. The decreased activity was attributed to the corresponding reduction in cortical volume as measured by MRI [167, 168].

SUMMARY

Consistent Evidence

Despite advances, the diagnosis of depression lacks a solid scientific foundation and still remains a symptom-based clinical exercise.

The clinical application of operationalized diagnostic criteria has resulted in the delineation of phenomenologically more homogeneous groups and has substantially improved the diagnostic reliability, but not to a satisfactory level [10, 22, 24, 26, 28, 29, 32, 170]. Validity, however, remains meagre, relying mainly on descriptive discriminant methods. There are no pathognomonic symptoms or empirically validated cut-off scores that would cut depressive psychopathology into its natural parts. Furthermore, there are no external validating criteria, such as specific biological markers, that can be used for categorical distinctions.

As a consequence, extensive clinical and epidemiological research employing a progressively more sophisticated methodology has attempted in the past years to fill the information gap. Out of the many findings, the following seem to be consolidated and acquire particular significance by introducing new perspectives in the understanding of depressive disorders.

The boundaries drawn by the use of operational criteria between depressive and adjacent disorders are blurred by overlapping symptoms. This is reflected in the structure of the currently available measuring instruments, in which a number of common items for anxiety and depression are included and greatly influence the diagnosis and severity of both these conditions [127, 134]. It is also reflected in the high cross-sectional and lifetime comorbidity of depression with anxiety, alcohol and drug abuse disorders as well as with a number of physical illnesses. The comorbidity rates with anxiety have been shown to increase as a function of severity of depressive symptomatology [25, 31, 35, 41]. In the great majority of cases, MD and depressive disorders in general are preceded by other non-depressive mental disorders or by physical illnesses. The long-term course of MD varies in symptom profile, symptom level, and symptom duration and frequently alternates with the other types of depression, dysthymic disorder, minor or subthreshold depression and, in particular, brief recurrent depression [63–66].

Due to the above and to other patient- and physician-related factors, depression is commonly underdiagnosed and/or misdiagnosed, particularly in primary health care settings [40, 95, 122].

Incomplete Evidence

Whether the distinction of normal sadness and unhappiness from a depressive mood is quantitative or qualitative remains an unresolved issue, particularly if a distinction has to be made between severe reactions of sadness and despair to vicissitudes of life on the one hand and mild but clinically significant depression on the other [7, 8, 88, 89]. The recent findings from functional brain imaging, showing brain activity correlates of transient sadness should they be compared to patients' responses during depressive phases, might eventually provide a valid distinction between normal and pathological emotions [86, 87].

The concept of dysthymia as a distinct type of depression, different from MD, although formally established by both the current diagnostic systems, remains controversial. Dysthymia is highly comorbid with MD and as a rule precedes it by varying intervals. Furthermore, familial psychiatric history does not clearly delineate dysthymia from MD. In addition to quantitative differences (fewer symptoms and longer duration), qualitative differences in symptom content have been invoked to support the descriptive validity of the MD–dysthymia distinction. The evidence that mood and cognitive symptoms are more characteristic of dysthymia, and psychomotor and somatic symptoms more characteristic of MD, remains uncertain, in view of the fact that a longitudinal change of symptoms is the rule rather than the exception in both conditions. Moreover, even duration may not be a solid discriminating criterion, since MD itself varies in duration, not infrequently having a protracted course, and dysthymia is allowed by the formal diagnostic criteria to have up to 2 months symptom-free intervals. More importantly, reliability of clinical information is questionable when it is based upon cross-sectional retrospective subjective reporting. The recently introduced specifiers of dysthymia, that is the "early" and the "late" onset dysthymia, with presumably distinct clinical features, one being more "pure", more linked to character and more stable over time and the other being more volatile, with more somatic symptoms and more likely to progress towards MD, may restrict the heterogeneity of this condition, yet the clinical relevance of this distinction in terms of prevention and treatment has to be further documented by longitudinal naturalistic studies [4, 25, 62, 63, 67, 169].

Recurrent brief depression and minor depression are the two other depressive types whose distinction from MD has to be further validated [60, 61]. Their boundaries within the diagnostic frame of depressive disorders are fuzzy. Their association with MD and dysthymia is close and, apart from their quantitative differences in the number of symptoms for minor depression and in the episode duration for brief recurrent depression, they share with MD and dysthymia several other features [30, 31, 169]. Moreover, they frequently alternate with each other and with MD and dysthymia. Symptoms of minor depression usually precede the onset of MD and dysthymia, and whether they represent the prodromal phase of these conditions is a subject to be further investigated.

Several lines of evidence exist that support the subtyping of MD into the clinical forms of melancholia and psychotic-delusional depression. Their demarcation from the other subtypes is mainly based on their distinctive clinical features, but is supported by their comparatively stronger association with a number of laboratory findings indicating brain function disturbances [27, 44, 45, 49, 50, 53, 56].

In general, the association of depressive disorders with a number of biological variables is as yet neither necessary nor sufficient to reify the clinical diagnosis. More specifically, a hormonal dysregulation manifested by a variety of neuroendocrine tests (DST, CRF, TRH, etc.) has been found to be closely associated with depression. However, according to the majority of studies, the level of sensitivity and specificity is a state-dependent measure of the severity rather than of the diagnostic type of depression [136, 149].

REM sleep polysomnographic abnormalities are consistently observed in MD, but claims of their specificity have not been substantiated, since, as subsequent studies have shown, they are also seen in subsyndromal affective and other mental disorders [47, 158].

Recent systematic genetic studies have confirmed that there is a positive familial homologous psychiatric history in a high percentage of depressed patients. However, association and linkage studies have not as yet identified a gene locus specific for depression. The consensus is that the depressive disorders are a genetically heterogeneous group.

Promising neuroimaging findings have recently appeared suggesting specific brain regional functional abnormalities in depressed patients. Further studies are, however, needed to replicate these findings and establish their relevance to clinical manifestations [166, 168].

Areas Still Open to Research

The etiology and pathogenesis of depression is the major issue to be addressed by future research in order to achieve a valid scientifically based diagnosis of depression. Until this is accomplished, we have to rely on the increased sophistication of our clinical strategies for the formulation of more objective and clinically relevant diagnostic criteria. One of the main dilemmas that researchers have to face in the immediate future is whether to continue splitting depression into more and more diagnostic groups, by increasing the number of exclusion criteria and adding more and more specifiers, or to bring the groups together and view them as a single entity varying over time on symptom pattern, level of severity, functional impairment and treatment demands [7, 25, 30, 32].

Linked with this dilemma is the validation of melancholic temperament (recently coded as depressive personality) as a separate entity, distinct from early onset dysthymia, predisposing to clinical depression. An even more challenging problem open to research is the effect — in the reverse direction — of depressive symptomatology on depressive character formation [29, 77, 78].

In conclusion, we need to be reminded that what we are measuring and classifying are not individual patients, but symptoms, clusters of symptoms, syndromes and, at best, illnesses, none of them being material objects, but concepts. The ultimate goal of the clinical investigator is to reach a diagnostic characterization that goes beyond the descriptive level and provides construct validity that will not only increase the diagnostic confidence, but will also ensure an empirically-based explanatory scheme. The clinician should be aware that the operational criteria, by themselves or supplemented by structured instruments and biological concomitants, cannot capture the experiential uniqueness of the persons, and that it is this uniqueness that he is bound to communicate with, in order to understand and effectively treat them.

The physician is not treating diagnoses. He is treating symptoms and ultimately the person who suffers from them. Diagnosis is a useful exercise to the extent that it infers meaningful clinical distinctions, informs the practitioner of the patient's past psychiatric and familial history and helps him to predict the clinical course and the response to treatment.

REFERENCES

1. Klerman G. (1980) Overview of affective disorders. In *Comprehensive Textbook of Psychiatry*, 3rd edn, vol. 2 (Eds H.I. Kaplan, A.H. Freedman, B.J. Sadock), pp. 1305–1319, Williams & Wilkins, Baltimore.

2. World Health Organization (1992) *Classification of Mental and Behavioural Disorders: Clinical Descriptions and Diagnostic Guidelines*, World Health Organization, Geneva.
3. World Health Organization (1993) *Classification of Mental and Behavioural Disorders: Diagnostic Criteria for Research*, World Health Organization, Geneva.
4. Kendell R.E. (1993) Mood (affective) disorders. In *Companion to Psychiatric Studies*, 5th edn (Eds R.E. Kendell, A.K. Zealley), pp. 427–457, Churchill Livingstone, London.
5. American Psychiatric Association (1994) *Diagnostic and Statistical Manual of Mental Disorders*, 4th edn, American Psychiatric Association, Washington, DC.
6. Hippius H., Stefánis C.N. (1994) *Research in Mood Disorders*, Hogrefe and Huber, Bern.
7. Akiskal H.S. (1995) Mood disorders: clinical features. In *Comprehensive Textbook of Psychiatry*, 6th edn (Eds H.I. Kaplan, B.J. Sadock), Williams & Wilkins, Baltimore.
8. Gelder M., Gath D., Mayou R., Cowen P. (1996) *Oxford Textbook of Psychiatry*, 3rd edn, Oxford University Press, New York.
9. World Psychiatric Association/International Committee for Prevention and Treatment of Depression (1997) *Educational Programme on Depressive Disorders, Module I, Overview and Fundamental Aspects, Core Booklet*, NCM Publishers, New York.
10. Kaplan H.I., Sadock B.J. (1998) *Synopsis of Psychiatry, Behavioral Sciences/Clinical Psychiatry*, 8th edn, Williams & Wilkins, Baltimore.
11. Kiloh L.G., Garside R.F. (1963) The independence of neurotic depression and endogenous depression. *Br. J. Psychiatry*, **109**: 451–463.
12. Mendels J., Cochrane C. (1968) The nosology of depression: the endogenous-reactive concept. *Am. J. Psychiatry*, **124**: 1–11.
13. Paykel E.S., Prussof B.A., Klerman G.L. (1971) The endogenous-neurotic continuum in depression: rater independence and factor distributions. *J. Psychiatr. Res.*, **8**: 73–90.
14. Roth M., Mountjoy C.Q. (1980) Anxiety states and their relationship to depressive disorder. In *Handbook of Affective Disorders* (Ed. E.S. Paykel), Churchill Livingstone, London.
15. Eysenck H.J. (1970) The classification of depressive illness. *Br. J. Psychiatry*, **117**: 241–250.
16. Kendell R.E. (1973) Psychiatric diagnoses: A study of how they are made. *Br. J. Psychiatry*, **122**: 437–445.
17. Brown G., Ni Bhrolchain M., Harris T. (1979) Psychotic and neurotic depression. *J. Affect. Disord.*, **1**: 195–211.
18. Feighner J.P., Robins E., Guze S.B., Woodruff R.A., Jr., Winokur G., Munoz R. (1972) Diagnostic criteria for use in psychiatric research. *Arch. Gen. Psychiatry*, **26**: 57–63.
19. Feinberg M., Carroll B.J. (1982) Separation of subtypes of depression using discriminant analysis. I: Separation of unipolar endogenous depression from nonendogenous depression. *Br. J. Psychiatry*, **140**: 384–391.
20. Akiskal H.S., McKinney W.T., Jr. (1973) Depressive disorders: towards a unified hypothesis. *Science*, **182**: 20–29.
21. Coryell W., Gaffney G., Burkhardt P.E. (1982) DSM-III melancholia and the primary-secondary distinction: a comparison of concurrent validity by means of the dexamethasone suppression test. *Am. J. Psychiatry*, **139**: 120–122.

22. Spitzer R., Williams J.B.W. (1985) Classification of mental disorders. In *Comprehensive Textbook of Psychiatry*, 4th edn, vol. 1 (Eds H. Kaplan, B. Sadock), pp. 583–598, Williams & Wilkins, Baltimore.

23. Andreasen N.C., Scheftner W., Reich T., Hirschfeld R.M., Endicott J., Keller M.B. (1986) The validation of the concept of endogenous depression: a family study approach. *Arch. Gen. Psychiatry*, **43**: 246–251.

24. Cloninger C.R. (1989) Establishment of diagnostic validity in psychiatric illness: Robins & Guze's method revised. In *Validity of Psychiatric Diagnosis* (Eds L.N. Robins, J. Barrett), pp. 9–18, Raven Press, New York.

25. Farmer A., McGuffin P. (1989) The classification of the depressions: contemporary confusion revisited. *Br. J. Psychiatry*, **155**: 437–443.

26. Robins L.N., Barrett J. (Eds) (1989) *Validity of Psychiatric Diagnosis*, Raven Press, New York.

27. Zimmerman M., Coryell W., Pfohl B. (1986) Melancholic subtyping: a qualitative distinction? *Am. J. Psychiatry*, **143**: 98–100.

28. Tsuang D.W., Winokur G. (1992) Testing the validity of the neurotic depression concept. *J. Nerv. Ment. Dis.*, **180**: 446–450.

29. Akiskal H.S. (1994) Temperament, personality and depression. In *Research in Mood Disorders* (Eds H. Hippius, C.N. Stefanis), pp. 45–60, Hogrefe and Huber, Bern.

30. Judd L.L. (1997) Pleomorphic expressions of unipolar depressive disease: summary on the 1996 CINP President's Workshop. *J. Affect. Disord.*, **45**: 109–116.

31. Kessler R.C., Zhao S., Blazer D.G., Swartz M. (1997) Prevalence, correlates, and course of minor depression and major depression in the National Comorbidity Survey. *J. Affect. Disord.*, **45**: 19–30.

32. Kendler K.S., Gardner C.O. (1998) Boundaries of major depression: an evaluation of DSM-IV criteria. *Am. J. Psychiatry*, **155**: 172–177.

33. Wittchen H.U. (1996) Critical issues in the evaluation of comorbidity of psychiatric disorders. *Br. J. Psychiatry*, **168**: 9–16.

34. Winokur G., Black D.W., Nasrallah A. (1988) Depressions secondary to other psychiatric disorders and medical illness. *Am. J. Psychiatry*, **145**: 233–237.

35. Winokur G. (1990) The concept of secondary depression and its relationship to comorbidity. *Psychiatr. Clin. North Am.*, **13**: 567–583.

36. Mezzich J.E., Ahn C.W., Fabrega H., Pilkonis P.A. (1990) Patterns of psychiatric comorbidity in a large population presenting for care. In *Comorbidity of Mood and Anxiety Disorders* (Eds J.D. Maser, C.R. Cloninger), pp. 189–204, American Psychiatric Press, Washington, DC.

37. Regier D.A., Burke J.D., Burke K.C. (1990) Comorbidity of affective and anxiety disorders in the NIMH Epidemiologic Catchment Area Program. In *Comorbidity of Mood and Anxiety Disorders* (Eds J.D. Maser, C.R. Cloninger), pp. 113–122, American Psychiatric Press, Washington, DC.

38. Regier D.A., Farmer M.E., Rae D.S., Locke B.Z., Keith S.J., Goodwin F.K. (1990) Comorbidity of mental disorders with alcohol and other drug abuse. Results from the Epidemiologic Catchment Area (ECA) Study. *JAMA*, **264**: 2511–2518.

39. Kessler R.C., Nelson C.B., McGonagle K.A., Liu J., Swartz M., Blazer D.G. (1996) Comorbidity of DSM-III-R major depressive disorder in the general population: results from the US National Comorbidity Survey. *Br. J. Psychiatry*, **168**: 17–30.

40. Ustun T.B., Sartorius N. (Eds) (1995) *Mental Illness in General Health Practice: An International Study*, Wiley, Chichester.

41. Sartorius N., Ustun T.B., Lecrubier Y., Wittchen H.U. (1996) Depression co-morbid with anxiety: results from the WHO study on Psychological Disorders in Primary Health Care. *Br. J. Psychiatry*, **168**: 38–43.
42. Sartorius N., Kaelber C.T., Cooper J.E., Roper M.T., Rae D.S., Gulbinat W., Ustun T.B., Regier D.A. (1993) Progress toward achieving a common language in psychiatry: results from the field trial of the clinical guidelines accompanying the WHO classification of mental and behavioral disorders in ICD-10. *Arch. Gen. Psychiatry*, **50**: 115–124.
43. Zimmerman M., Black D.W., Coryell W. (1989) Diagnostic criteria for melancholia. The comparative validity of DSM-III and DSM-III-R. *Arch. Gen. Psychiatry*, **46**: 361–368.
44. Schotte C.K.W., Maes M., Cluydts R., Cosyns P. (1997) Cluster analytic validation of the DSM melancholic depression. The threshold model: integration of quantitative and qualitative distinctions between unipolar depressive subtypes. *Psychiatry Res.*, **71**: 181–195.
45. Parker G., Roussos J., Eyers K., Wilhelm K., Mitchell P., Hadzi-Pavlovic D. (1997) How distinct is "distinct quality" of mood? *Psychol. Med.*, **27**: 445–453.
46. Carroll B.J., Feinberg M., Greden J.F., Tarika J., Albala A.A., Haskett R.F., James N.W., Kronfol Z., Lohr N., Steiner M. *et al* (1981) A specific laboratory test for the diagnosis of melancholia. *Arch. Gen. Psychiatry*, **38**: 15–22.
47. Berger M., Riemann D. (1993) REM sleep in depression — an overview. *Sleep Res.*, **2**: 211–223.
48. Kendler K.S. (1997) The diagnostic validity of melancholic major depression in a population-based sample of female twins. *Arch. Gen. Psychiatry*, **54**: 299–304.
49. Johnson J., Horwarth E., Weissman M.M. (1991) The validity of major depression with psychotic features based on a community study. *Arch. Gen. Psychiatry*, **48**: 1075–1081.
50. Maj M., Pirozzi R., Di Caprio E.L. (1990) Major depression with mood-congruent psychotic features: a distinct diagnostic entity or a more severe subtype of depression? *Acta Psychiatr. Scand.*, **82**: 439–444.
51. Glassman A.H., Roose S.P. (1981) Delusional depression. *Arch. Gen. Psychiatry*, **38**: 424–427.
52. Lykouras L., Vassilopoulos D., Voulgari A., Stefanis C., Malliaras D. (1986) Delusional depression: further evidence for genetic contribution. *Psychiatr. Res.*, **21**: 277–283.
53. Nelson J.C., Davis J.M. (1997) DST studies in psychotic depression: a meta-analysis. *Am. J. Psychiatry*, **154**: 1497–1503.
54. Sands J.R., Harrow M. (1995) Vulnerability to psychosis in unipolar major depression: is premorbid functioning involved? *Am. J. Psychiatry*, **152**: 1009–1015.
55. Lykouras L., Malliaras D., Christodoulou G.N., Papakostas Y., Voulgari A., Tzonou A., Stefanis C. (1986) Delusional depression: phenomenology and response to treatment. *Acta Psychiatr. Scand.*, **73**: 324–329.
56. Coryell W., Winokur G., Shea T., Maser J.D., Endicott J., Akiskal H.S. (1994) The long-term stability of depressive subtypes. *Am. J. Psychiatry*, **151**: 199–204.
57. Maj M., Starace F., Pirozzi R. (1991) A family study of DSM-III-R schizoaffective disorder, depressive type, compared with schizophrenia and psychotic and nonpsychotic major depression. *Am. J. Psychiatry*, **148**: 612–616.
58. Paykel E.S., Parker R.R., Rowan P.R., Rao B.M., Taylor C.N. (1983) Nosology and atypical depression. *Psychol. Med.*, **13**: 131–139.
59. Larn R.W., Stewart J.N. (1996) The validity of atypical depression in DSM-IV. *Compr. Psychiatry*, **37**: 375–383.

60. Angst J., Merikangas K., Scheidegger P., Wicki W. (1990) Recurrent brief depression: a new subtype of affective disorder. *J. Affect. Disord.*, **19**: 87–98.

61. Angst J. (1994) Recurrent brief depression. In *Research in Mood Disorders* (Eds H. Hippius, C. Stefanis), pp. 18–30, Hogrefe & Huber, Bern.

62. Kocsis J.H., Markowitz J.C., Prien R.F. (1990) Comorbidity of dysthymic disorder. In *Comorbidity of Mood and Anxiety Disorders* (Eds J.D. Maser, C.R. Cloninger), pp. 317–330, American Psychiatric Press, Washington, DC.

63. Akiskal H.S. (1994) Dysthymia: clinical and external validity. *Acta Psychiatr. Scand.*, **383**: 19–23.

64. Akiskal H.S., Judd L.L., Gillin J.C., Lemmi H. (1997) Subthreshold depressions: clinical and polysomnographic validation of dysthymic, residual and masked forms. *J. Affect. Disord.*, **45**: 53–63.

65. Judd L.L. (1997) The clinical course of unipolar major depressive disorders. *Arch. Gen. Psychiatry*, **54**: 989–991.

66. Judd L.L., Akiskal H.S., Maser J.D., Zeller P.J., Endicott J., Coryell W., Paulus M.P., Kunovac J.L., Leon A.C., Mueller T.I. *et al* (1998) A prospective 12-year study of subsyndromal and syndromal depressive symptoms in unipolar major depressive disorders. *Arch. Gen. Psychiatry*, **55**: 694–700.

67. Keller M.B., Shapiro R.W. (1982) "Double depression": superimposition of acute depressive episodes on chronic depressive disorders. *Am. J. Psychiatry*, **139**: 438–442.

68. Brieger P., Marneros A. (1997) Was ist cyclothymia? *Nervenarzt.*, **68**: 531–544.

69. Rosenthal N.E., Sack D.A., Gillin J.C., Lewy A.J., Goodwin F.K., Davenport Y., Mueller P.S., Newsome D.A., Wehr T.A. (1984) Seasonal affective disorder. A description of the syndrome and preliminary findings with light therapy. *Arch. Gen. Psychiatry*, **41**: 72–80.

70. Schwartz P.J., Brown C., Wehr T.A., Rosenthal N.E. (1996) Winter seasonal affective disorder: a follow-up study of the first 59 patients of the National Institute of Mental Health Seasonal Studies Program. *Am. J. Psychiatry*, **153**: 1028–1036.

71. Judd L.L., Rapaport M.H., Paulus M.P., Brown J.L. (1994) Subsyndromal symptomatic depression (SSD): a new mood disorder? *J. Clin. Psychiatry*, **55**: 18–28.

72. Pearlstein T., Stone A.B. (1998) Premenstrual syndrome. *Psychiatr. Clin. North Am.*, **21**: 577–590.

73. Kendler S.K., Karkowski L.M., Corey L.A., Neale M.C. (1998) Longitudinal population-based twin study of retrospectively reported premenstrual symptoms and lifetime major depression. *Am. J. Psychiatry*, **155**: 1234–1240.

74. Hunter M.S. (1996) Depression and the menopause. *Br. Med. J.*, **313**: 1217–1218.

75. Schmidt P.J., Rubinow D.R. (1991) Menopause-related affective disorders: a justification for further study. *Am. J. Psychiatry*, **148**: 844–852.

76. Tellenbach H. (1976) *Melancholie*, Springer, Berlin.

77. Hirschfeld R.M., Holzer C.E. (1994) Depressive personality disorder: clinical implications. *J. Clin. Psychiatry*, **55** (Suppl.): 10–17.

78. Phillips K.A., Gundeson J.G., Triebwasser J., Kimble C.R., Faedda G., Lyoo I.K., Renn J. (1998) Reliability and validity of depressive personality disorder. *Am. J. Psychiatry*, **155**: 1044–1048.

79. Kumar R., Robson K.M. (1984) A prospective study on emotional disorders in childbearing women. *Br. J. Psychiatry*, **29**: 250–264.

80. O'Hara M.W., Swain A.M. (1996) Rates and risk of postpartum depression: a meta-analysis. *Int. Rev. Psychiatry*, **8**: 37–54.

81. Hamilton M. (1960) A rating scale for depression. *J. Neurol. Neurosurg. Psychiatry*, **23**: 56–62.
82. Beck A.T., Ward C.H., Mendelson M., Mock J., Erbaugh J. (1961) An inventory for measuring depression. *Arch. Gen. Psychiatry*, **4**: 561–585.
83. Montgomery S.A., Åsberg M. (1979) A new depression scale designed to be sensitive to change. *Br. J. Psychiatry*, **134**: 382–389.
84. Freud S. (1957) *Mourning and Melancholia*, Hogarth Press, London.
85. Pardo J.V., Pardo P.J., Raichle M.E. (1993) Neural correlates of self-induced dysphoria. *Am. J. Psychiatry*, **150**: 713–719.
86. George M.S., Ketter T.A., Parekh P.I., Horwitz B., Herscovitch P., Post R.M. (1995) Brain activity during transient sadness and happiness in healthy women. *Am. J. Psychiatry*, **152**: 341–351.
87. Lane R.D., Reiman E.M., Ahern G.L., Scheartz G.E., Davidson R.J. (1997) Neuroanatomical correlates of happiness, sadness and disgust. *Am. J. Psychiatry*, **154**: 926–933.
88. Zisook S., Paulus M., Shuchter S.R., Judd L.L. (1997) The many faces of depression following spousal bereavement. *J. Affect. Disord.*, **45**: 85–95.
89. Clayton P.J. (1979) The sequelae and nonsequelae of conjugal bereavement. *Am. J. Psychiatry*, **136**: 1530–1534.
90. Parkes C.M. (1998) Coping with loss: bereavement in adult life. *Br. Med. J.*, **316**: 856–859.
91. Green M.F., Nuechterlein K.H., Ventura J., Mintz J. (1990) The temporal relationship between depressive and psychotic symptoms in recent-onset schizophrenia. *Am. J. Psychiatry*, **147**: 179–182.
92. Roy A., Thompson R., Kennedy S. (1983) Depression in chronic schizophrenia. *Br. J. Psychiatry*, **142**: 465–470.
93. Davidson J.R.T., Foa F.A. (1992) *Post-Traumatic Stress Disorder: DSM-IV and Beyond*, American Psychiatric Press, Washington, DC.
94. Keane T.M., Taylor K.L., Penk W.E. (1997) Differentiating post-traumatic stress disorder (PTSD) from major depression (MDD) and generalized anxiety disorder (GAD). *J. Anxiety Disord.*, **11**: 317–328.
95. World Psychiatric Association/International Committee for Diagnosis and Treatment of Depression (1998) *Educational Programme on Depressive Disorders, Module II, Depressive Disorders in Physical Illness, part I: 2*, NCM Publisher, New York.
96. Currie S., Heathfield K.W., Henson R.A., Scott D.F. (1971) Clinical source and prognosis of temporal lobe epilepsy: a survey of 666 patients. *Brain*, **94**: 173–190.
97. Mendez M.F., Cummings J.L., Benson D.F. (1986) Depression in epilepsy: significance and phenomenology. *Arch. Neurol.*, **43**: 766–770.
98. Robertson M.M., Trimble M.R., Townsend H.R.A. (1987) The phenomenology of depression in epilepsy. *Epilepsia*, **28**: 364–372.
99. Robertson M.M. (1997) Depression in neurological disorders. In *Depression and Physical Illness* (Eds M.M. Robertson, C.L.E. Katona), pp. 305–340, Wiley, Chichester.
100. O'Shea B. (1997) A review of Huntington's disease. *Int. J. Psychiatry Clin. Pract.*, **1**: 135–140.
101. Cunningham L.A. (1994) Depression in the medically ill: choosing an antidepressant. *J. Clin. Psychiatry*, **55A**: 90–100.
102. Lane R.M., Sweeney M., Henry J.A. (1994) Pharmacotherapy of the depressed patient with cardiovascular and/or cerebrovascular illness. *Br. J. Gen. Pract.*, **48**: 256–262.

103. Shapiro P.A., Lidagoster L., Glassman A.H. (1997) Depression and heart disease. *Psychiatr. Ann.*, **27**: 347–352.
104. Barsky A.J. (1992) Palpitations, cardiac awareness, and panic disorders. *Am. J. Med.*, **92**: 315–345.
105. Spiegel D. (1996) Cancer and depression. *Br. J. Psychiatry*, **30**: 109–116.
106. Haggerty J.J. Jr, Garbutt J.C., Evans D.L., Golden R.N., Pedersen C., Simon J.S., Nemeroff C.B. (1990) Subclinical hypothyroidism: a review of neuropsychiatric aspects. *Int. J. Psychiatry Med.*, **20**: 193–208.
107. Hendricks V., Altshuler L., Whybrow P. (1998) Psychoneuroendocrinology of mood disorders. The hypothalamic–pituitary–thyroid axis. *Psychiatr. Clin. North. Am.*, **21**: 277–292.
108. Lahey F.H. (1931) Apathetic hyperthyroidism. *Ann. Surg.*, **93**: 1026–1036.
109. Fava G.A. (1994) Affective disorders and endocrine disease: new insights from psychosomatic studies. *Psychosomatics*, **35**: 341–353.
110. Hudson J.I., Hudson M.S., Griffing G.T., Melby J.C., Pope H.G., Jr (1987) Phenomenology and family history of affective disorder in Cushing's disease. *Am. J. Psychiatry*, **144**: 951–953.
111. Popkin M.K., Callies A.L., Lentz R.D., Colon E.A., Sutherland D.E. (1988) Prevalence of major depression, simple phobia, and other psychiatric disorders in patients with long-standing type I diabetes mellitus. *Arch. Gen. Psychiatry*, **45**: 64–68.
112. Long T.D., Kathol R.G. (1993) Critical review of data supporting affective disorder caused by nonpsychotropic medication. *Ann. Clin. Psychiatry*, **5**: 259–270.
113. Patten S.B., Love E.J. (1993) Can drugs cause depression? A review of the evidence. *J. Psychiatry Neurosci.*, **19**: 92–102.
114. Muldoon M.F., Manuck S.B., Mathews K.A. (1990) Lowering cholesterol concentration and mortality: a quantitative review of primary prevention trials. *Br. Med. J.*, **301**: 309–314.
115. Law M.R., Thompson S.G., Wald N.J. (1994) Assessing possible hazards of reducing serum cholesterol. *Br. Med. J.*, **308**: 373–379.
116. Golier J.A., Marzuk P.M., Leon A.C., Weiner C., Tardiff K. (1995) Low serum cholesterol level and attempted suicide. *Am. J. Psychiatry*, **152**: 419–423.
117. Merikangas K.R., Angst J., Eaton W., Canino G., Rubio-Stipec M., Wacker H., Wittchen H.U., Andrade L., Essau C., Whitaker A. *et al* (1996) Comorbidity and boundaries of affective disorders with anxiety disorders and substance misuse: results of an international task force. *Br. J. Psychiatry*, **30**: 58–67.
118. Ross H.E., Glaser F.B., Germanson T. (1988) The prevalence of psychiatric disorders in patients with alcohol and other drug problems. *Arch. Gen. Psychiatry*, **45**: 1023–1031.
119. Mirin S.M., Weiss R.D. (1991) Psychiatric comorbidity in drug and alcohol addiction. In *Comprehensive Handbook of Drug and Alcohol Addiction* (Ed. N. Miller), pp. 641–661, Dekker, New York.
120. Kokkevi A., Stefanis C. (1995) Drug abuse and psychiatric comorbidity. *Compr. Psychiatry*, **36**: 329–337.
121. Sartorius N., Davidian H., Ernberg G., Fenton F.R., Fujü I., Gastpar M., Gulbinat W., Jablensky A., Kielholz P., Lehmann H.E. *et al* (1983) *Depressive Disorders in Different Cultures*, World Health Organization, Geneva.
122. Rost K., Smith G.R., Matthews D.B., Guise, B. (1994) The deliberate misdiagnosis of major depression in primary care. *Arch. Fam. Med.*, **3**: 333–337.
123. Goldberg D.P. (1972) *The Detection of Psychiatric Illness by Questionnaire: a Technique for the Identification and Assessment of Nonpsychotic Psychiatric Illness*, Oxford University Press, London.

124. World Health Organization (1990) *Composite International Diagnostic Interview (CIDI)*, World Health Organization, Geneva.
125. Wing J.K., Cooper J.E., Sartorius N. (1974) *Measurement and Classification of Psychiatric Symptoms*, Cambridge University Press, Cambridge.
126. World Health Organization (1992) *Glossary: Differential Definitions of SCAN Items and Commentary on the SCAN Text*, World Health Organization, Geneva.
127. Spitzer R.L., Williams J.B., Gibbon M., First M.B. (1992) The Structured Clinical Interview for DSM-III-R (SCID). I: History, rationale, and description. *Arch. Gen. Psychiatry*, **49**: 624–629.
128. Radloff L.S. (1971) The CES-D Scale: a self-report depression scale for research in the general population. *Appl. Psychol. Meas.*, **1**: 385–407.
129. Madianos M.G., Tomaras V., Kapsali A., Vaidakis N., Vlachonicolis J., Stefanis C.N. (1988) Psychiatric case identification in two Athenian communities: estimation of the probable prevalence. *Acta Psychiatr. Scand.*, **78**: 24–31.
130. Okun A., Stein R.E., Bauman L.J., Silver E.J. (1996) Content validity of the Psychiatric Symptom Index, CES-Depression Scale, and State-Trait Anxiety Inventory from the perspective of DSM-IV. *Psychol. Rep.*, **79**: 1059–1069.
131. Furukawa T., Hirai T., Kitamura T., Takahashi K. (1997) Application of the Center for Epidemiologic Studies Depression Scale among first-visit psychiatric patients: a new approach to improve its performance. *J. Affect. Disord.*, **46**: 1–13.
132. Endicott J., Spitzer R.L. (1978) A diagnostic interview: the Schedule for Affective Disorders and Schizophrenia. *Arch. Gen. Psychiatry*, **35**: 837–844.
133. Paykel E.S. (1990) Use of the Hamilton Depression Scale in general practice. *Psychopharmacol. Ser.*, **9**: 40–47.
134. Montgomery S.A. (1990) *Anxiety and Depression*, Wrightson Biomedical Publications, London.
135. Davidson J., Turnbull C.D., Strickland R., Miller R., Graves K. (1986) The Montgomery–Åsberg Depression Scale: reliability and validity. *Acta Psychiatr. Scand.*, **73**: 544–548.
136. Carroll B.J., Martin F.I., Davis B. (1968) Pituitary-adrenal function in depression. *Lancet*, **556**: 1373–1374.
137. Baumgartner A., Graf K.J., Kurten I. (1986) Serial dexamethasone suppression tests in psychiatric illness: Part II. A study in major depressive disorder. *Psychiatry Res.*, **18**: 25–43.
138. Hallstrom T., Samuelsson S., Balldin J., Walinder J., Bengtsson C., Nystrom E., Andersch B., Lindstedt G., Lundberg P.A. (1983) Abnormal dexamethasone suppression test in normal females. *Br. J. Psychiatry*, **142**: 489–497.
139. Joyce P.R., Mulder R.T., Cloninger C.R. (1994) Temperament and hypercortisolemia in depression. *Am. J. Psychiatry*, **151**: 195–198.
140. Yehuda R. (1998) Psychoneuroendocrinology of post-traumatic stress disorder. *Psychiatr. Clin. North Am.*, **21**: 359–379.
141. Gold P.W., Chrousos G., Kellner C., Post R., Roy A., Augerinos P., Schulte H., Oldfield E., Loriaux D.L. (1984) Psychiatric implications of basic and clinical studies with corticotropin releasing factor. *Am. J. Psychiatry*, **141**: 619–627.
142. Nemeroff C.B. (1996) The corticotropin-releasing factor (CRF) hypothesis of depression: new findings and new directions. *Mol. Psychiatry*, **1**: 336.
143. Butler P.D., Nemeroff C.B. (1990) Corticotropin-releasing factor as a possible cause of comorbidity in anxiety and depressive disorders. In *Comorbidity of Mood and Anxiety Disorders* (Eds J.D. Maser, C.R. Cloninger), pp. 413–438, American Psychiatric Press, Washington, DC.

144. Maes M.H.I., De Puyter M., Suy E. (1987) Prediction of subtype and severity of depression by means of dexamethasone suppression test. L-tryptophan: competing amino acid ratio and MHPG flow. *Biol. Psychiatry*, **22**: 177–188.

145. Heuser I., Yassouridis A., Holsboer (1994) The combined dexamethasone/CRH test: a refined test for psychiatric disorders. *J. Psychiatr. Res.*, **28**: 341–356.

146. Loosen P.T., Prange A.J. Jr (1982) Serum thyrotropin response to thyrotropin-releasing hormone in psychiatric patients: a review. *Am. J. Psychiatry*, **139**: 405–416.

147. Loosen P.T. (1985) The TRH-induced TSH response in psychiatric patients: a possible neuroendocrine marker. *Psychoneuroendocrinology*, **10**: 237–260.

148. Sullivan P.F., Wilson D.A., Mulder R.T., Joyce P.R. (1997) The hypothalamic–pituitary–thyroid axis in major depression. *Acta Psychiatr. Scand.*, **95**: 370–378.

149. Skare S.S., Dysken M.W., Billington C.J. (1994) A review of GHRH stimulation test in psychiatry. *Biol. Psychiatry*, **36**: 249–265.

150. Gann H., Riemann D., Stoll S., Berger M., Muller W.E. (1995) Growth hormone response to growth hormone-releasing hormone and clonidine in depression. *Biol. Psychiatry*, **38**: 325–329.

151. Cooney J.M., Lucey J.V., O'Keane V., Dinan T.G. (1997) Specificity of the pyri-dostigmine/growth hormone challenge in the diagnosis of depression. *Biol. Psychiatry*, **42**: 827–833.

152. Sakkas P.N., Soldatos, C.R., Bergiannaki J.D., Paparrigopoulos T.J., Stefanis C.N. (1998) Growth hormone secretion during sleep in male depressed patients. *Progr. Neuro-Psychopharmacol. Biol. Psychiat.*, **22**: 467–483.

153. Mendlewicz J., Linkowski P., Kerkhofs M., Desmedt D., Goldstein J., Copin-schi G., Van Cauter E. (1985) Diurnal hypersecretion of growth hormone in depression. *J. Clin. Endocrinol. Metab.*, **60**: 505–512.

154. Asnis G.M., Eisenberg J., van Praag H.M., Lemus C.Z., Friedman J.M., Miller A.H. (1988) The neuroendocrine response to fenfluramine in depressives and normal controls. *Biol. Psychiatry*, **24**: 117–120.

155. Lopez-Ibor J.J., Jr, Saiz Ruiz J., Iglesias M. (1988) The fenfluramine challenge test in the affective spectrum: a possible marker of endogenicity and severity. *Pharmacopsychiatry*, **21**: 9–14.

156. Mann J.J., McBride P.A., Malone K.M., DeMeo M., Keilp J. (1995) Blunted sero-tonergic responsivity in depressed inpatients. *Neuropsychopharmacology*, **13**: 53–64.

157. Flory J.D., Mann J.J., Manuck S.B., Muldoon M.F. (1998) Recovery from major depression is not associated with normalization of serotonergic function. *Biol. Psychiatry*, **43**: 320–326.

158. Benca R.M., Obermeyer W.H., Thisted R.A., Gillin J.C. (1992) Sleep and psychi-atric disorders: a meta-analysis. *Arch. Gen. Psychiatry*, **49**: 651–668.

159. Thase M.E., Howland R.H., Friedman E.S. (1998) Treating antidepressant non-responders with augmentation strategies: an overview. *J. Clin. Psychiatry*, **59**: 5–15.

160. Giles D.E., Kupfer D.J., Rush A.J., Roffwarg H.P. (1998) Controlled comparison of electrophysiological sleep in families of probands with unipolar depression. *Am. J. Psychiatry*, **155**: 192–199.

161. Rush A.J., Giles D.E., Schlesser M.A., Orsulak P.J., Weissenburger J.E., Fulton C.L., Fairchild C.J., Roffwarg H.P. (1997) Dexamethasone response, thyrotropin-releasing hormone stimulation, rapid eye movement latency and subtypes of depression. *Biol. Psychiatry*, **41**: 915–928.

162. Dougherty D., Rauch S.L. (1997) Neuroimaging and neurobiological models of depression. *Harvard Rev. Psychiatry*, **5**: 138–159.

163. Simpson S., Baldwin R.C., Jackson A., Burns A.S. (1998) Is subcortical disease associated with a poor response to antidepressants? Neurological, neuropsychological, and neuroradiological findings in late-life depression. *Psychol. Med.,* **28**: 1015–1026.
164. Rubin R.T., Phillips J.J., Sadow T.F., McCracken J.T. (1995) Adrenal gland volume in major depression: increase during the depressive episode and decrease with successful treatment. *Arch. Gen. Psychiatry,* **52**: 213–218.
165. Ho A.P., Gillin J.C., Buchsbaum M.S., Wu J.C., Abel L., Bunney W.E., Jr. (1996) Brain glucose metabolism during non-rapid eye movement sleep in major depression. A positron emission tomography study. *Arch. Gen. Psychiatry,* **53**: 645–652.
166. Keller T.A., George M.S., Kimbrell T.A., Benson B.E., Post R.M. (1996) Functional brain imaging, limbic function and affective disorders. *Neuroscientist,* **2**: 55–65.
167. Drevets W.C., Price J.L., Simpson J.R., Jr., Todd R.D., Reich T., Vannier M., Raichle M.E. (1997) Subgenual prefrontal cortex abnormalities in mood disorders. *Nature,* **386**: 824–827.
168. Drevets W.C. (1998) Functional neuroimaging studies of depression: the anatomy of melancholia. *Ann. Rev. Med.,* **49**: 341–361.
169. Keller M.B., Klein D.N., Hirschfeld R.M.A., Kocsis J.H., McCullough J.P., Miller I., First M.B., Holzer C.-P. III, Keitner G.I., Marin D.B. *et al* (1995) Results of the DSM-IV Mood Disorders Field Trial. *Am. J. Psychiatry,* **152**: 843–849.
170. Holzer C.P. III, Nguyen H.T., Hirschfeld R.M.A. (1996) Reliability of diagnosis in mood disorders. *Psychiatr. Clin. North Am.,* **19**: 73–84.

Commentaries

1.1
Much Diversity, Many Categories, No Entities
Robert E. Kendell[1]

Their prevalence and chronicity, and the extensive suffering and disability they produce, make depressive disorders one of the most important of all human illnesses. Clinical depression is indeed, as Stefanis and Stefanis observe in their opening paragraph, "a medically significant condition", but it is far more than that. The Global Burden of Disease Study (conducted by the Harvard School of Public Health for the World Health Organization — WHO — and the World Bank) has shown that the burden it imposes on individuals and societies throughout the world greatly exceeds that of most other illnesses. Using "disability adjusted life years" (DALYs) as the index of burden, unipolar major depression was, worldwide, the fourth most important of all causes of disability and premature death, ahead of ischaemic heart disease, cardiovascular disease, tuberculosis and AIDS. And in the industrial world it ranked second only to ischaemic heart disease, even though, in accordance with ICD-9 conventions, suicide was assessed separately [1].

Stefanis and Stefanis' authoritative and comprehensive description of contemporary classifications of depressive disorders illustrates very clearly both the unity and the diversity of depressive syndromes. All of them are characterized by the presence of a core group of symptoms consisting of a depressed mood, reduced energy and capacity for enjoyment, lowered self-esteem, impaired concentration, disturbances of appetite, sleep and libido, and a pessimistic view of the world and the future. Although none of the individual elements of this cluster of symptoms is invariably present, the syndrome occurs in every culture and in many different clinical contexts, and forms the basis of what WHO's ICD-10 calls a "depressive episode" and the American Psychiatric Association's DSM-IV calls "major depression". Stefanis and Stefanis argue that "depressio sine depressione" does not exist, that "the depressed mood is always there, it only needs to be elicited", and that the decision by both WHO and the APA not to make depression of mood

[1] Royal College of Psychiatrists, 17 Belgrave Square, London SW1X 8PG, UK

an essential feature of the syndrome is "unexplainable". The explanation is surely that mood is a subjective experience, and that only the individual concerned is entitled to make statements about it. A patient who persistently denies that he or she feels sad, or miserable, or low, cannot be contradicted. Yet every experienced psychiatrist has seen patients who look miserable, possess most of the other symptoms of the depressive syndrome, and persistently deny feeling sad or miserable. Whether this represents denial in a psychoanalytic sense or simply an idiosyncratic understanding of the terms used to denote a dysthymic mood, is immaterial. What matters is that in other important respects, particularly treatment response and outcome, "depressio sine depressione" behaves like ordinary depression with depression. It therefore seems preferable to accept the reality of "depressio sine depressione" rather than to assume that a psychiatrist is better able to make confident statements about someone else's mood than the individual himself.

Despite the ubiquity of the core symptoms of the depressive syndrome, those symptoms may vary greatly in severity and chronicity, and may coexist with a wide range of other psychiatric symptoms. And as this variation in symptomatology is associated with substantial differences in associated disability, in treatment response and in prognosis, we are forced to distinguish several different types of depressive disorder — the multiple ICD-10 and DSM-IV categories set out in Stefanis and Stefanis' Table 1.1. Unfortunately, none of these categories appears to be clearly demarcated from its neighbours. They merge into one another and the boundaries between them are in several cases explicitly arbitrary. Nor do we have evidence of boundaries or "points of rarity" [2] between the depressive syndrome (ICD-10's depressive episode or DSM-IV's major depression) and either normal sadness or the symptoms of bereavement; between depressions and anxiety states; or between psychotic depressions and schizophrenia. As recent large-scale population-based surveys have shown, whatever putative boundary one examines, the variation in symptomatology is continuous, and so far neither discriminant functions, twin and family studies, neuroendocrine tests or neuroimaging have come to our rescue.

In the 1960s and 1970s there were fierce controversies between psychiatrists who were convinced that there were distinct types of depression, which it was crucially important to distinguish, and others, of whom I confess I was one, who argued that there were no natural boundaries, no entities, and that variation in symptomatology was therefore better portrayed by dimensions than by categories. As Stefanis and Stefanis say, most of the heat of that controversy has now dissipated and an uneasy compromise has been reached. We still use a categorical classification, but accept, ever more explicitly, that the boundaries between our categories are imposed by ourselves, and that despite many attempts we have failed to identify discontinuities or "points of rarity" in nature.

This failure should influence the assumptions we make about the aetiology of depressive disorders. The evidence of family, twin and adoption studies tells us that genetic factors play a major role. We have also identified several important environmental risk factors, including the lack of a stable relationship with a parental figure during childhood, stressful events of various kinds, and a lack of social support. It seems likely that multiple genes, each individually of relatively small effect, provide the genetic substrate of depressive disorders, and that some of these genes are risk factors for other psychiatric disorders as well. Different combinations of these genes, interacting with a variety of different environmental risk factors, acting at different stages of life probably underlie the rich complexity of depressive disorders and explain our inability to distinguish one kind of depression from another. It is likely, too, that we will be unable to develop a classification of depressive disorders that is demonstrably superior to our present classifications until we have identified these genes and are beginning to understand how their products interact with the various environmental risk factors.

REFERENCES

1. Murray C.J.L., Lopez A.D. (1997) Global mortality, disability, and the contribution of risk factors: Global Burden of Disease Study. *Lancet*, **349**: 1436–1442.
2. Kendell R.E., Brockington I.F. (1980) The identification of disease entities and the relationship between schizophrenic and affective psychoses. *Br. J. Psychiatry*, **137**: 324–331.

1.2

Categorical and Dimensional Perspectives of Depression

Jules Angst[1]

Stefanis and Stefanis' paper on the diagnoses of depressive disorders stimulates some thoughts on the current development of diagnostic classification in general, and diagnoses of depression in particular. The development of psychiatric classification over the past 20 years has been very fruitful, as a consequence of the introduction by DSM-III of a more descriptive operationalized approach with specified diagnostic criteria. Nonetheless, some redundant survivals of a problematic *etiological classification* of depressive syndromes have remained, which is precisely what modern classification

[1] *Zurich University Psychiatric Hospital, Lenggstrasse 31, 8029 Zurich, Switzerland*

sought to avoid. A first example is "adjustment disorders in response to psychosocial stressors" with depressed mood and with mixed anxiety and depressed mood under the diagnostic threshold of an Axis I mood disorder. In a multiaxial perspective, a psychosocial stressor would clearly belong to Axis IV, and depressive symptoms as subdiagnostic depression to Axis I. A second example is bereavement (again following a psychosocial stressor), where a 2-month criterion is totally arbitrary for the distinction between "normal" and "pathological". The point I would like to make is that both categories are undesirable survivals even if they are built on plausible hypotheses of causation.

A similar problem dealt with by Stefanis and Stefanis is the *distinction between primary and secondary*, which also implies a causal connection, usually defined by the often very uncertain sequence of the occurrence of the two syndromes or disorders. An example is "medication-induced depression" without the evidence of controlled trials that the incidence is more frequent than expected by chance. The same is true for the consequence of somatic disorders (somatic depression), where we would need to prove, for instance, by epidemiological or case control studies that co-occurrence is significantly higher than expected by chance.

These examples raise the question of a causal relationship, which is extremely difficult to prove. Unproven assumptions are at odds with the philosophy of modern classification. A large representative population survey on comorbidity carried out prospectively over many years could provide the answers to many of these questions. The National Comorbidity Survey of Kessler and colleagues [1], with its planned follow-up, is just such a promising development. Cross-sectional investigations are insufficient in face of memory artifacts, especially in depression.

An even more serious problem is the unjustified creation of *artificial new disorders* based on the uncritical assumption that subgroups of depression represent truly distinct categories. One example is dysthymia as a form of chronic mild depression. We can observe chronic severe depression and chronic mild depression. Why should chronic mild depression be any other disorder than mild (minor) depression? Or indeed the reverse: why is chronic major depression not a different disorder from major depression? So far there is no proof that dysthymia or recurrent brief depression exist as separate depressive entities. A consequence of this categorical approach is diagnostic groups such as "double depression" or "triple depression". I support the subdivision of depression according to criteria of severity, course and recurrence, but without the assumption of true heterogeneity. From a descriptive point of view, we are dealing with dimensional criteria of severity (from mild through moderate to severe and psychotic), of length (from brief spells of a few days to episodes lasting weeks, months or years) and frequency (single, few recurrent or multiple manifestations up to rapid cycling). It is to be hoped that future development will find an even more descriptive approach simplifying the classification by avoiding the creation of artificial new disorders.

A much more complicated and difficult problem is *psychiatric comorbidity*, defined as the association of two or more psychiatric "disorders". The association rarely represents a truly separate disorder, as is the case with the association of mania with depression in bipolar illness. But even in this case we cannot be sure of being correct. Other examples are the association of depression with anxiety, neurasthenia or hypochondria. Developmental studies of childhood and adolescence show that early anxiety may precede not only anxiety disorders but also depression, and it is common knowledge that depression is highly associated with symptoms of anxiety; indeed, ICD-10 created a diagnostic category of mixed anxiety and depressive disorders.

In addition, there is ample empirical evidence supporting a unidimensional approach for depression [2] and a bidimensional one for anxiety and depression [3, 4], suggestions which have not been taken seriously enough in our nosology. The real obstacle is our inability to simultaneously think categorically and dimensionally; both ways are equally justified and useful. It is to be expected that with better measurements of depression we will approach a dimensional view even closer. The latter would consist not only of two-dimensional analyses of the association between depression and anxiety, or three-dimensional constructs between depression, mania and anxiety, but include, in principle, all psychiatric syndromes (obsessive-compulsive, phobic, paranoid, etc.). We are as yet a long way from such an empirically founded multidimensional space, in which an individual can be located as a point and described by a number of precise dimensional characteristics. The *multidimensional view* would give new insights into "comorbidity" and would allow us to describe the development of an individual patient's psychiatric syndromes over a lifetime as a path in a multidimensional space. This change of perspective would be paradigmatic; it could be a goal for the next millennium.

In summary, this commentary is intended as a constructive contribution, identifying unresolved problems and formulating hopes for a better future.

REFERENCES

1. Kessler R.C. (1994) The National Comorbidity Survey of the United States. *Int. Rev. Psychiatry*, **6**: 365–376.
2. Kendell R.E. (1975) *The Role of Diagnosis in Psychiatry*, Blackwell, Oxford.
3. Goldberg D., Bridges K., Duncan-Jones P., Grayson D. (1987) Dimensions of neuroses seen in primary care settings. *Psychol. Med.*, **17**: 461–471.
4. Goldberg D., Huxley P. (1992) *Common Mental Disorders*, Tavistock/Routledge, London.

1.3
Models of Classification of Depressive Disorders
Pierre Pichot[1]

Stefanis and Stefanis' description of depressive disorders according to the present state of knowledge raises, among other things, a basic issue: the model or models best suited for their classification. As pointed out by Stefanis and Stefanis, two models exist, the categorical and the dimensional. The purpose of both is to condense the available information as accurately as possible. In the categorical model, mutually exclusive classes are defined by specific patterns of characteristics (usually symptoms). The attribution of each subject to a given class is based on the fact that the pattern presented is closer to the pattern defining that class than to any of the other patterns. The model condenses the information by substituting this attribution to a detailed description of the characteristics of the individual. Although many patterns have been constituted on a priori grounds, in a "true" class the co-occurrence of the elements constituting the pattern must have a higher frequency in the population than if their distributions were independent. The pattern, if the elements are symptoms, is a syndrome. If the syndrome is a "true" class, it implies the existence of a common pathogenic mechanism, but may result from one or several causes. If the cause is known, the term "disease" is usually substituted. The attribution of a subject is the diagnostic procedure, the diagnosis comprising in one word a description of all the subject's characteristics. Opposed to this categorical model, traditionally used in medicine, which condenses the information by regrouping subjects, the dimensional model aims at the same result by regrouping the characteristics. On the basis of their covariation in the population, one or several dimensions are determined, the number of dimensions being in any case much smaller than the number of characteristics. Each characteristic contributes a specific weight (saturation) to the definition of each dimension. If a single dimension is used — for example a depressive one — each subject is specified by his or her position along this dimension; in the case of a multidimensional model, by his or her coordinates in the space determined by the dimensions. Thus, if one uses the two dimensions "depression" and "anxiety", a given patient can be described as "high in depression" and "low in anxiety" or, eventually, by a more precise quantitative specification of his position (his dimensional profile). Use of the dimensional model is traditional in psychology (hence the fact that most psychiatric rating scales, derived from psychological techniques, provide dimensional measures), but has only recently been introduced into psychiatry (descriptions of schizophrenic symptomatology and of personality disorders). Statistical methods (factor

[1]24 rue des Fossés-Saint-Jacques, F-75005, Paris, France

analysis and cluster analysis) are available to empirically derive dimensional and categorical models from the observed facts but cluster analysis is still rarely used, the description of categorical patterns usually being based on "clinical experience". Leaving aside the depressions with known aetiology ("due to a medical condition"), the classification of the depressive states has almost always used the two models simultaneously. As early as 1851, J.P. Falret, giving the first description of bipolar disorder, affirmed that it was, because of the existence of manic and depressive phases in the same subject, a "natural form" or, in modern terms, a "true" class according to the categorical model. But he thought that the other depressions could not be classified according to the same model. After Kraepelin's synthesis, psychiatry has again tended to dichotomize the depressive states, giving way to a classification which found its most typical expression in the work of Kurt Schneider, but which in fact dominated the scene until 1980. A special type of depression was described. Possibly — but not always — associated with mania, it constituted a well-defined class according to the categorical model. It presented a specific pattern of symptoms, the main element being the "vital" character of the depressive feeling experienced, radically different from "normal" sadness. It was hypothesized that this class of depression had endogenous causes. The remaining depressive states were in fact described according to the dimensional model. They were just quantitative variations resulting either from a deviation of personality (depressive personality) or from an interplay between personality and stresses (reactive and neurotic depressions). In both cases a continuity existed between the pathological state and normality, typical of the dimensional model and not compatible with the categorical one. By introducing a purely descriptive atheoretical approach, DSM-III repudiated this dichotomy. Although affirming its adhesion to the categorical model, it has practically destroyed the central categorical concept of endogenous depression, because one of its criteria was a hypothetical aetiological nature, and it has not even taken into consideration one of its most typical symptomatic elements, the "vital" character of the depressive feeling, because of its low interrater reliability. However, when considering the chapter on mood disorders in DSM-IV, one cannot escape the impression of a return to the dual perspective. Bipolar disorder constitutes, as proposed by Falret, the core category, a "true" class. The depressive disorders which do not belong to it are then classified according to a descriptive bidimensional model, the dimensions being related to the intensity and the evolutive mode. Although, for example, dysthymia is presented as a class, its definition is basically dimensional: low depressive intensity, chronic evolution.

The present classification of depressive states should not be criticized due to the coexistence of the two models. A similar situation exists in other branches of medicine. The symptomatology associated with increased body temperature or with raised blood pressure can be conceptualized according to the dimensional model. But one can also describe as "true" classes, in the categorical perspective, specific syndromes or diseases in which increased body temperature or raised blood pressure are elements of the specific symptomatic pattern. The danger lies in the temptation to use a single model, even if it does not apply to all known facts. The often criticized progressive multiplication of diagnostic categories in successive editions of the DSM is obviously the result of the — at least formal — absolute adhesion to the categorical model. A purely dimensional description of depressive states, such as the one proposed for schizophrenic symptomatology, would be more economical, but probably insufficient to provide a comprehensive classification. The choice of the most adequate model — or models — remains a basic issue.

1.4
Flaws of Current Diagnosis of Depression
Herman M. van Praag[1]

Stefanis and Stefanis provide an excellent survey of current depression diagnosis. Equally, it clearly reveals what I see as the failings of that system, which I will briefly discuss.

Syndromal vagueness. One and the same diagnostic construct covers a variety of syndromes. The reason is that, for a particular diagnosis, a fixed set of symptoms is not required, just the presence of x out of a list of y symptoms, no matter which ones. Moreover, lists of symptoms to choose from for the various diagnoses often overlap considerably. For instance, only two symptoms differentiate between major depression and dysthymia.

Consequently, if one studies, for example, the biological determinants, the epidemiology or the pharmacotherapy of major depression or dysthymia, it is totally unclear which syndrome has actually been scrutinized. Current diagnostic practices treat depression as if symptomatological differences were irrelevant, but obviously they are not [1].

Aetiological prudery. The DSM system does not include an aetiological axis. The factor psychogenesis in particular is neglected. This factor comprises two components: personality frailties and life events. More often than not, mental (Axis I) disorders are accompanied by personality (Axis II) disorders

[1]*Department of Psychiatry and Neuropsychology, Maastricht University, PO Box 616, 6200 MD Maastricht, The Netherlands*

and preceded by life events. Both are in fact registered, but no statement or hypothesis is required about their mutual relationship. Such a formulation, however, is of crucial importance. For example, if Axis II diagnoses and corresponding life events are considered to be causally related to the Axis I disorder, research, particularly biological research, should shift its focus from the Axis I to the Axis II disorder, and treatment efforts should at the very least include the Axis II disorders.

Horizontalism. Symptoms are grouped horizontally as if they all had the same diagnostic valency. However, they most probably have not. In all likelihood some symptoms are the direct consequence of the neurobiological substrate underlying the mental disorder, while others are its derivatives. The first type, the primary symptoms, should be the focus of biological and psychopharmacological research.

That this statement is not a pure chimera, is demonstrated by the concept of stressor-precipitated, cortisol-induced, serotonin-related, anxiety/aggression-driven depression (SeCA depression), a diagnostic concept representing a "verticalized" symptom structure [2]. Disorders in anxiety and aggression regulation are considered to be the primary symptoms, and related to certain disturbances in the serotonin system. They are both the precursor symptoms and the key symptoms that *might* trigger disturbances in mood regulation, which then would lead to the development of a depressive syndrome.

Lack of a third diagnostic tier. Today's diagnoses provide (1) a categorical rubric and (2) a characterization of the presenting symptomatology, albeit one that is profoundly inexact. What is lacking is a third tier, the one I have called the functional tier [3]. At that level the prevailing syndrome, or syndromes, is dissected into its component parts, that is the psychological dysfunctions the psychiatric disorder is composed of. For a number of reasons this third diagnostic tier is of fundamental importance to psychiatry:

1. Psychological dysfunctions are more easily measured than syndromes or nosological entities. Many of them can be assessed in a quantitative manner, such as disturbances in information processing, memory, movement, level of initiative and concentration. The domain of emotions is not (yet) accessible to quantitative measurement but it can be assessed in a much more refined way than is presently the case [4, 5].
2. Functional analysis provides insight into which components of the psychological apparatus are dysfunctioning and which are functioning within normal limits, while nosological and syndromal diagnoses do not, or only to a very limited extent.
3. So far biological disturbances correlate much better with dysfunctioning psychological domains than with syndromes or nosological entities. A

case in point is the serotonergic dysfunctions ascertained in depression. They appear not to be correlated with a particular syndromal or noso-logical depression type, but with disorders in aggression and anxiety regulation, across diagnoses.

Functional psychopathology could become to psychiatry what physiology has been for medicine: the discipline providing an understanding of what the deflections are in the psychological apparatus leading to a mental disorder.

Preoccupation with nosology. Mental pathology is considered to be subdividable into discrete disorders, each characterized by a particular symptomatology, course, outcome and causation and each separable from the other. Nosological systems are rigid and inflexible. If an abnormal mental state does not meet the preconceived criteria no diagnosis is possible. Nosological systems thus boost the creation of new diagnostic categories.

A typical case in point is the group of mood disorders. In clinical practice and in research the main DSM-certified categories, major depression and dysthymia, do not suffice and therefore a great many new entities have been added. They are now being studied each in their own right. Examples are such categories as minor depression, subsyndromal depression, recurrent brief depression, subaffective personality disorder and mixed anxiety depression disorder [6–9].

Such categories are often introduced without very many validating studies; yet they are being considered as if they were valid entities. The study of undervalidated concepts runs a considerable risk of yielding invalid results that are hard to reproduce.

"Nosologo-mania", as I have called the avalanche of new diagnoses with the introduction of and following the third edition of the DSM [10], magnifies the problems of comorbidity. Most psychiatric patients seem to suffer from a host of mental disorders. Two to three Axis I diagnoses and the same number of Axis II diagnoses are the rule rather than the exception. The more diagnoses available the greater the number per patient will be.

Comorbidity is a true crux of psychiatric research. As an illustration: one studies a patient with depression, biologically, pharmacologically, epidemio-logically or otherwise. A finding is made, but the patient happens to suffer in addition from one or two other Axis I and three additional Axis II diagnoses. What is the behavioural correlate of the finding: the depression or one of the other diagnoses or components of these diagnoses? Answers are generally not available. Most often the question is ignored. This situation is a true invalidator of psychiatric research [11].

In psychiatry validation research should take precedence above any other type of research. Moreover, the nosological doctrine should be put to the test and critically examined as to its utility in psychiatry. Can mental pathology really be systematized in discrete "packages" in which symptomatology, clinical course, outcome and causation are interconnected in a predictable way? Or is the nosological doctrine to which psychiatry since Kraepelin has firmly committed itself a fiction and a hindrance to progress? Alternative disease models should be studied and, as I have proposed elsewhere, I consider the reaction form model to be a serious competitor [12]. The nosological doctrine is too debatable to be unquestioningly accepted.

In conclusion, accurate diagnosis is the very bedrock of psychiatric research. The current diagnostic process shows serious flaws and undermines the validity of psychiatric research. In years to come we should strive towards the following changes and additions:

1. Refined syndromal analysis.
2. The addition of a statement or hypothesis regarding the relationship between the Axis I disorder and the complex Axis II disorder/traumatic life events/stress.
3. (Research) efforts to rank psychopathological symptoms vertically instead of horizontally.
4. The addition of a third (so-called functional) tier to the diagnostic process.
5. Rigorous validation of existing (DSM-accepted) diagnostic categories and the utmost reserve in official acceptance of new diagnostic constructs.
6. Critical analysis of the applicability of the nosological classification principle for mental disorders and testing of the heuristic value of alternative disease models, particularly the reaction form model.

Thus, research psychopathologists can expect a demanding but fascinating task in the next century.

REFERENCES

1. Van Praag H.M. (1998) Inflationary tendencies in judging the yield of depression research. *Neuropsychobiology*, **37**: 130–141.
2. Van Praag H.M. (1996) Faulty cortisol/serotonin interplay. Psychopathological and biological characterisation of a new hypothetical depression subtype (SeCA depression). *Psychiatry Res.*, **65**: 143–157.
3. Van Praag H.M. (1990) Two-tier diagnosing in psychiatry. *Psychiatry Res.*, **34**: 1–11.
4. Plutchik R., Kellerman H. (1989) *The Measurement of Emotions*, vol. 4, Academic Press, New York.
5. de Vries M.W. (1992) *The Experience of Psychopathology: Investigating Mental Disorders in their Natural Settings*, Cambridge University Press, Cambridge.
6. Sherbourne C.D., Wells K.B., Hays R.D., Rogers W., Burnam M.A., Judd L.L. (1994) Subthreshold depression and depressive disorder: clinical characteristics of general medical and mental health specialty outpatients. *Am. J. Psychiatry*, **151**: 1777–1784.
7. Judd L.L., Akiskal H.S., Paulus M.P. (1997) The role and clinical significance of subsyndromal depressive symptoms (SSD) in unipolar major depressive disorder. *J. Affect. Disord.*, **45**: 5–18.

8. Angst J., Merikangas K.R., Scheidegger P., Wicki W. (1990) Recurrent brief depression: a new subtype of affective disorder. *J. Affect. Disord.*, **19**: 37–38.
9. Herpertz S., Steinmeyer E.M., Sass H. (1998) On the conceptualisation of sub-affective personality disorders. *Eur. Psychiatry*, **13**: 9–17.
10. Van Praag H.M. (1995) Concerns about depression. *Eur. Psychiatry*, **10**: 269–275.
11. Van Praag H.M. (1996) Comorbidity (psycho-)analyzed. *Br. J. Psychiatry*, **168**: 129–134.
12. Van Praag H.M. (1997) Over the mainstream: diagnostic requirements for biological psychiatric research. *Psychiatry Res.*, **72**: 201–212.

1.5
Approaches to Diagnosing Depression, and the Reciprocal Relationship to Depression Research

Robert J. Boland[1] and Martin B. Keller[1]

Stefanis and Stefanis' discussion on diagnosing seems, at first, straight-forward. Yet this discussion relies on many years of development and controversy critical to the current system of nomenclature. Furthermore, this has effected the design of randomized clinical trials.

As the authors point out, "depression" is both a disease, and part of human experience. The controversies in distinguishing the two are often viewed by researchers and clinicians as contesting medical versus psychoso-cial approaches. These, in turn, derive from "mind–body" debates. The medical model takes a categorical approach, with clear boundaries between "normal" and "diseased." The psychosocial model imagines a continuum, with subjective boundaries between the normal and abnormal.

This mind–body tension can be more philosophic than scientific. Both approaches have their strengths and pitfalls. Applying the medical model to depression runs the risk of overgeneralization; the psychosocial approach risks vagueness—it becomes difficult to say what is, and what is not a "case." This problem became apparent in the 1950s, when the American Psychiatric Association attempted to evaluate psychiatric therapies. The members, however, concluded that such an evaluation would be meaningless without standardized approaches to diagnosis [1].

Much of the impetus for change resulted from the close association between nosology and neuroscience. The improved somatic treatments for depression (c. 1960–70) created a desire for better diagnostic specificity, to learn who would best benefit from new treatments. Diagnostic vagueness would clearly hold back such research.

[1]*Department of Psychiatry and Human Behavior, Brown University, Butler Hospital, 345 Blackstone Blvd., Providence, RI 02906, USA*

In response, several groups began developing empirical approaches to psychiatric diagnosis. This included reliability research at the New York State Psychiatric Institute, and validity research at Washington University in St Louis. These two movements helped form the National Institutes of Mental Health Collaborative Depression Study (CDS). Important instruments developed by this group included the Research Diagnostic Criteria (RDC), which was the immediate forerunner of DSM-III.

The results have been explosive. The major advances in our knowledge of depression have resulted from changes in how we diagnose mood disorders as much as from advances in biomedical technology.

An example of this can be seen in results from the CDS. Using the RDC, we have learned about the natural course of depression. In the CDS, 70% of the patients recovered from their index episode of depression within the first year. However, for those patients not recovered within the first year, the majority still had not recovered after 5 years [2]. This group made up 12% of the entire sample of depressed patients. After 10 years, 7% were still chronically depressed [3], and 6% had not recovered by 15 years. Thus, the longer a subject was depressed, the less likely he was to recover.

The CDS also found a high rate of recurrence: up to 40% by 2 years, 60% after 5 years, 75% after 10 years, and 87% after 15 years [4]. This suggests that, in contrast to rates of recovery (which level off after 5–10 years), individuals continue to be at a high risk for recurrence, even after 10 years. Such a finding was unanticipated.

Studies such as this have changed the way we view depression — rather than as an acute event, depression is recognized as a potentially chronic illness. A practical result of this change has been the addition of longitudinal course modifiers to DSM-IV. Thus, research also reciprocally affects diagnosis.

Improved diagnosis has also allowed for a better understanding of depressive subgroups. For example, the concept of double depression was only possible when we could reliably distinguish major depression from dysthymia, and the two from seemingly similar conditions, such as major depression with incomplete remission. Keller and colleagues found that patients with double depression recovered more rapidly from episodes of major depression than those with major depression alone [5]. However, this recovery is not to a state of "normalcy," but to one of dysthymia. Relapse is also more frequent in patients with double depression than in those with major depression alone. Such relationships are only understandable with better diagnostic criteria.

Improved diagnostic techniques have shed light on more than pharmacotherapy. Standardized diagnosis, along with better instruments for measuring stress and psychosocial functioning, has helped investigators to show the efficacy of psychosocial treatments, such as cognitive-behavioral therapy. As such, we are now potentially able to ease the previous mind–body tensions, and simultaneously to consider the role and importance of neurobiological and environmental factors in depression, and bridge our conceptual "mind–body" gap. Ultimately, better diagnosis should help us abolish this archaic notion, much as we eliminated "organic mood disorders" from DSM-IV. Thus, nosology and neuroscience will continue to influence each other.

REFERENCES

1. Wilson M. (1993) DSM-III and the transformation of American psychiatry: a history. *Am. J. Psychiatry*, **150**: 399–410.
2. Keller M.B., Lavori P.W., Mueller T.I., Endicott J., Coryell W., Hirschfeld R.M.A., Shea T. (1992) Time to recovery, chronicity, and levels of psychopathology in major depression: a 5 year prospective follow-up of 431 subjects. *Arch. Gen. Psychiatry*, **49**: 809–816.
3. Mueller T.I., Keller M.B., Leon A.C., Solomon D.A., Shea M.T., Coryell W., Endicott J. (1996) Recovery after five years of unremitting major depressive disorder. *Arch. Gen. Psychiatry*, **53**: 794–799.
4. Lavori P.W., Keller M.B., Scheftner W., Fawcett J., Coryell W. (1994) Recurrence after recovery in unipolar major depressive disorder: an observational follow-up study of clinical predictors and somatic treatment as a mediating factor. *Int. J. Methods Psychiatr. Res.*, **4**: 211–229.
5. Keller M.B., Lavori P.W., Endicott J., Coryell W., Klerman G.L. (1983) "Double depression": two-year follow-up. *Am. J. Psychiatry*, **140**: 689–694.

1.6

The Practical Importance of Temporal Sequencing and Secondary Depression

William Coryell[1]

Nearly all of the controversy concerning the classification of depressive disorders reduces to three major issues, each of which Stefanis and Stefanis discuss in some detail. The first concerns the point at which dysphoria and associated cognitive and vegetative changes become pathological and the second, the boundary between depressive disorders and other, nonaffective disorders. Some consensus to both of these issues is prerequisite to progress in the third area, the increase of within-group homogeneity through subtyping.

Clear resolution of the first issue is unlikely, however. The examples of hypertension and obesity remind us that many thresholds used to define given illnesses are, by necessity, arbitrary and shifting and that there are few variables with which to empirically fix them. Kendler *et al* [1] took a

[1]*Department of Psychiatry, University of Iowa, Psychiatry Research/Medical Education Building, Iowa City, IA 52242, USA*

particularly powerful approach to this question and showed that the heritability of major depressive disorder (MDD) among female twins rose steadily with the "index of caseness." This index, derived elsewhere as a correlate of the consistency with which subjects remembered lifetime episodes [2], incorporated severity, persistence and resulting disability. The relationship yielded no breakpoint and so recommended no threshold to separate the less from the more heritable conditions. This is more of a concern to researchers searching for genetic linkage than to clinicians, however. The same variables which correlate with heritability are also strongly associated with the likelihood that an individual will seek treatment for an episode of MDD [3].

Of greater clinical relevance are the boundaries between depressive disorders and those nonaffective illnesses which seem so often to coexist with them. Here circumstances are complicated by the fact that the clinical phenomena which define many of these other illnesses may also arise as epiphenomena of depressive episodes. When they appear as such, though, they do not connote the presence of an additional illness. For example, panic attacks, when confined to depressive episodes, are not associated with increases in risks for panic disorder among family members [4] nor do such panic attacks predict the later development of panic symptoms outside of depressive episodes [5]. Obsessions and compulsions which appear only within depressive episodes are rarely followed by obsessions and compulsions during periods of euthymia [5] and, similarly, delusions do not portend an eventual, chronic psychosis unless they have occurred outside of depressive episodes [6].

As Stefanis and Stefanis noted, much of the effort to increase homogeneity through subclassification has focused on distinctions between MDD with and without melancholia and between primary and secondary depression. The latter rose from medical tradition and the observation that depressive syndromes seemed to complicate various psychiatric disorders at much higher than chance rates. A recent longitudinal study of a large, nonclinical sample, showed, for example, that a history of any major nonaffective disorder increased the risk for onset of MDD in the ensuing 6 years by three- to four-fold [7].

Though many investigators have failed to find useful differences between primary and secondary depression, a great number have. Findings which are both replicated and practical include the greater likelihood that patients with secondary depression will express suicidal behavior or ideas, will remain symptomatic after hospitalizations, electroconvulsive therapy and antidepressant therapy, and will relapse after recovery (reviewed in [8]).

Efforts to validate this distinction with biological measures have yielded inconsistent results. Some, particularly those using the dexamethasone suppression test, have been very supportive but others have not. Whether the clinician accepts the distinction between primary and secondary depression as any more, or less, valid and useful than the officially recognized separation of melancholic and nonmelancholic MDD, careful attention to the possibility that a nonaffective disorder underlies a given case of MDD is extremely important. In this writer's long experience as attending on a University Hospital inpatient unit, the most common factor in the chaotic courses and apparent treatment resistance preceding admission has been the failure to recognize other illnesses underlying depressive symptoms.

Just what these illnesses are should do much to shape the clinician's management of specific patients. For instance, because persistent alcohol abuse markedly reduces the likelihood of recovery from MDD [9], the clinician must first detect alcoholism and then direct treatment efforts at the achievement of abstinence, often in the face of the patient's efforts to maintain treatment focus on depressive symptoms instead. Patients with borderline personality disorder are often inappropriately treated for psychotic features when they report intracranial voices, and for rapid cycling bipolar illness when they display mood lability, irritability and reckless behavior. Tricyclic antidepressants are unlikely to be helpful and benzodiazepines may markedly worsen affairs. These patients often improve when the focus of treatment is shifted away from the pharmacological management of depressive symptoms and toward the patient's own control over impulsiveness and anger.

Other illnesses likely to shape the course of depressive symptoms and effectiveness of treatment include stimulant or opiate dependence, somatization disorder, obsessive-compulsive disorder, antisocial personality disorder and anorexia nervosa. While a careful history, and the interview of informants, will often uncover important, pre-existing conditions, the following should increase suspicion that another disorder underlies the depressive symptoms for which the patient is seeking help. The inability to clearly identify an episode onset is foremost among these. A simple question as to when the patient last experienced two or more months without depressive symptoms will reveal a chronic mood disorder in many patients. Even if further investigation reveals no additional underlying disorder, knowledge that symptoms are longstanding has powerful prognostic significance. In a similar vein, the tendency of a patient to view depressive symptoms as characteristic of his or her normal self is much more likely if the depression is secondary. Another useful though rarely described feature of secondary depressive syndrome is the tendency of individual depressive symptoms to abate and reappear erratically, in poor temporal concordance with other symptoms.

Careful attention to whether other disorders do or do not coexist with a depressive syndrome will make further subtyping of that syndrome more meaningful. Reports of hallucinations are much less likely to indicate a psychotic depression when a patient meets criteria for somatization disorder; knowledge of ongoing stimulant abuse will put reverse vegetative symptoms in a different light; and an agitated depression will be managed differently when extensive benzodiazepine dependence, and the likelihood of a withdrawal state, is appreciated. In summary, the awareness that MDD is best viewed as a syndrome of many possible etiologies will promote effective clinical management regardless of flux in official classification systems.

REFERENCES

1. Kendler L.S., Neale M.C., Kessler R.C., Heath A.C., Eaves L.J. (1993) The lifetime history of major depression in women. *Arch. Gen. Psychiatry*, **50**: 863–870.
2. Rice J.P., Rochberg N., Endicott J., Lavori P.W., Miller C. (1992) Stability of psychiatric diagnoses. *Arch. Gen. Psychiatry*, **49**: 824–830.
3. Coryell W., Endicott J., Winokur G., Akiskal H., Solomon D., Leon A., Mueller T., Shea T. (1995) Characteristics and significance of untreated major depressive disorder. *Am. J. Psychiatry*, **152**: 1124–1129.
4. Coryell W., Endicott J., Andreasen N., Keller M., Clayton P., Hirschfeld R., Scheftner W., Winokur G. (1988) Depression and panic attacks: the significance of overlap as reflected in follow-up and family study data. *Am. J. Psychiatry*, **145**: 293–300.
5. Coryell W., Endicott J., Winokur G. (1992) Anxiety syndromes as epiphenomena of primary major depression: outcome and familial psychopathology. *Am. J. Psychiatry*, **149**: 100–109.
6. Coryell W., Keller M., Lavori P., Endicott J. (1990) Affective syndromes, psychotic features and prognosis I. Depression. *Arch. Gen. Psychiatry*, **47**: 651–657.
7. Coryell W., Endicott J., Keller M. (1992) Major depression in a non-clinical sample: Demographic and clinical risk factors for first onset. *Arch. Gen. Psychiatry*, **49**: 117–125.
8. Coryell W. (1988) Secondary depression. In *Psychiatry* (Eds R. Michels, J. Cavenar, A. Cooper, S.B. Guze, L.L. Judd, G. Klerman, A. Solnit), pp. 1–9, Lippincott, Philadelphia.
9. Mueller T.I., Lavori P.W., Keller M.B., Swartz A., Warshaw M., Hasin D., Coryell W., Endicott J., Rich J., Akiskal H. (1994) Prognostic effect of the variable course of alcoholism on the 10-year course of depression. *Am. J. Psychiatry*, **151**: 701–706.

1.7

Depression: the Complexity of its Interface with Soft Bipolarity

Hagop S. Akiskal[1]

The last two decades have witnessed a great deal of research effort to provide the clinician with reliable and valid approaches to diagnosis of this protean illness, known from at least Hippocratic times. Much of this effort pertains to patients who consult a psychiatrist. Despite the notable

[1] *International Mood Center, University of California at San Diego, La Jolla, CA 92093-0603, USA*

progress made, especially the attempt to subtype the illness with respect to differential treatment options, there is still a great deal of uncertainty about how different subtypes of mood disorder are related to one another. My commentary to Stefanis and Stefanis' masterful review will focus on recent provocative developments about the bipolar border of major depressive disorder.

Of all the classificatory schemas for affective disorders, the unipolar–bipolar distinction is the one that has the broadest consensus among both researchers and clinicians. Stefanis and Stefanis wisely avoid the term "unipolar." This caution is justified in as much as an increasing body of research data has indicated the existence of a prevalent group of soft bipolar disorders that occupy an intermediary position between the two poles. Bipolar II, which is the prototype of soft bipolarity, has affinity to classic manic depressive illness from a familial standpoint, but in some respects resembles unipolar patients, especially from the point of view of anxiety comorbidity. Unlike unipolars, these patients tend to cycle with antidepressants, hence the need for mood stabilizers. Their treatment is often a nightmare, because treatments for anxiety disorders tend to destabilize the course of these patients, and mood stabilizers may not always bring about the necessary stabilization. Indeed, matters are complicated, because these patients are temperamentally disinclined to any attempts to bring stabilization to their habitual way of existing! Thus, a classification that ignores the temperamental substrates of the special depressions and affective states from which patients with bipolar II suffer, will not do justice to the therapeutic options available to these patients. In brief, as proposed by us, many unipolar depressions (up to 50%) may have to be reclassified under the rubric of pseudo-unipolar [1–3]. History of spontaneous hypomania is not always easily obtained. In many patients, the bipolar nature of the depression is made manifest for the first time during pharmacotherapy with antidepressants; although the latter are not officially classified as bipolar, much of the evidence favors their inclusion within a soft bipolar spectrum.

A recent study from Johns Hopkins [4] has shown that bipolar II with a history of anxiety attacks might be a specific genetic form of affective illness. Our research indicates that temperamental cyclothymia — measured as traits of mood lability — represents the best longitudinal marker for this disorder and should be incorporated into the diagnostic approach to these patients. One of these studies was conducted as part of the National Institute of Mental Health prospective study of depression [5], where this temperament was the best predictor of the bipolar II outcome of patients who were, at entry, unipolar. Another study, as part of the French multicenter EPIDEP study, found that the best diagnostic correlate of bipolar II was temperamental cyclothymia [3]; moreover, patient- and physician-rated cyclothymia were highly correlated. This raises the possibility of developing a simple paper-and-pencil test for screening depression with the possibility of subtyping it along soft bipolar lines. This is very important, not only in psychiatry, where many of these patients fail repeated antidepressant trials, but also in primary care, where this subtype is more prevalent than previously thought [6]. Indeed, all so-called anxious depressions should be examined for the possibility of a soft bipolar disorder; I am proposing that temperamental measures might be the best approach in this much-needed precision.

Bipolar II patients with cyclothymic temperamental background may exhibit a tempestuous life, often have a creative bent, but may also exhibit socially undesirable behaviors because of their impulsivity. To complicate matters, a more severe version of bipolar II disorder may manifest as borderline personality. These patients will often require low-dose neuroleptics in the long term, but will probably do best on anticonvulsants. Atypical depression with reverse vegetative signs shares many of the characteristics of bipolar II with borderline features. The overlap may be as high as 70% [7].

The main point of this commentary is that many clinical subtypes in the official classifications in existence seem to be separating disorders that may have the same or overlapping diatheses. Soft bipolarity spans atypical depression, panic and social phobic disorders, bipolar II, cyclothymic and borderline personality disorders. I submit that when molecular genetics delineates the fundamental substrates of these disorders, many phenotypes currently listed as distinct disorders will probably come to be viewed as variants of a related group of affective and temperamental dispositions.

REFERENCES

1. Akiskal H.S., Mallya G. (1987) Criteria for the "soft" bipolar spectrum. *Psychopharmacol. Bull.*, **23**: 68–73.
2. Akiskal H.S. (1996) The prevalent clinical spectrum of bipolar disorders: beyond DSM-IV. *J. Clin. Psychopharmacol.*, **16** (Suppl. 1): 4s–14s.
3. Hantouche E.G., Akiskal H.S., Lancrenon S., Allilaire J.-F., Sechter D., Azorin J.-M., Bourgeois M., Fraud J.-P., Châtenet-Duchêne L. (1998) Systematic clinical methodology for validating bipolar-II disorder. *J. Affect. Disord.*, **50**: 163–173.
4. MacKinnon D.F., Xu J., McMahon F.J., Simpson S.G., Stine O.C., McInnis M.G., DePaulo J.R. (1998) Bipolar disorder and panic disorder in families. *Am. J. Psychiatry*, **155**: 829–831.
5. Akiskal H.S., Maser J.D., Zeller P., Endicott J., Coryell W., Keller M., Warshaw M., Clayton P., Goodwin F.K. (1995) Switching from "unipolar" to bipolar II. *Arch. Gen. Psychiatry*, **52**: 114–123.
6. Manning J.S., Haykal R.F., Connor P.D., Akiskal H.S. (1997) On the nature of depressive and anxious states in a family practice setting. *Compr. Psychiatry*, **38**: 102–108.
7. Perugi G., Akiskal H.S., Lattanzi L., Cecconi D., Mastrocinque C., Patronelli A., Vignoli S., Bemi E. (1998) The high prevalence of soft bipolar (II) features in atypical depression. *Compr. Psychiatry*, **39**: 63–71.

1.8
Contextualizing the Diagnosis of Depression

Juan E. Mezzich[1] and Miguel R. Jorge[2]

We cannot but admire the clear and erudite review of the diagnosis and classification of depression offered by Stefanis and Stefanis, drawing on Costas Stefanis' refined clinical investigational skills and on his international experience as a leader of the World Psychiatric Association. After presenting a masterful analysis of the literature on the nosology of depression, Stefanis and Stefanis conclude that the clinician should be aware that operational criteria by themselves or supplemented by structured instruments and associated biological features cannot capture the experiential uniqueness of the person and it is this uniqueness that he is bound to consider in order to understand and treat effectively.

This commentary responds to Stefanis and Stefanis' plea for attention to the particularities and complexity of the depressive patient by briefly discussing ways to contextualize the diagnosis of depression. We do this by outlining critical aspects and levels of a comprehensive diagnostic model that succinctly describes the clinical condition of the person experiencing depressive disorders and that articulates the evaluational perspectives required to accomplish the diagnostic task validly and competently.

First to be recognized is the nosological complexity of depression. This makes it compelling to attend to the variety of forms to be depressed specified in the Tenth Revision of the *International Classification of Diseases and Health Related Problems* (ICD-10) [1] and its local versions or annotations such as DSM-IV [2], the *Chinese Classification of Mental Disorders*, 2nd edition, revised (CCMD-2-R) [3], and the *Third Cuban Glossary of Psychiatry* (GC-3) [4]. The nosological map covers psychotic and non-psychotic depressive disorders, episodic and persistent conditions, severe and milder cases. This nosology also includes organic and substance-induced depressive disorders as well as adjustment disorders with depressed mood.

This quick review reveals that the nosological matrix of depression is bio-psychosocial and that both etiological and morphological factors decisively inform the classification of depressive disorders. This is neither accidental nor restricted to mental disorders. In fact, from its inauguration in 1893 to its current Tenth Revision, the ICD displays the participation of both causation and form as a key classificatory principle. This speaks of a fundamental nosological complexity throughout the range of human illness that is to be

[1]*Division of Psychiatric Epidemiology and International Center for Mental Health, Mount Sinai School of Medicine of the City University of New York, Fifth Avenue and 100th Street, Box 1093, New York, NY 10029-6574, USA*
[2]*Clinical Psychiatry Section, Paulista School of Medicine, Federal University of Sao Paulo, 740 Botucatu, Sao Paulo 04023-900, Brazil*

recognized and taken into account for both diagnostic understanding and clinical action [5].

A second level of contextualization refers to the systematic description of the patient's entire clinical condition. This requires stratified attention to the possibility and even the likelihood that several disorders (mental and non-mental) may be found in the same individual. This brings up the problematic issue of "comorbidity", which confronts us with the dilemma between clearcut morbid plurality and the different faces (e.g. anxious and depressive) of one morbid condition.

This contextualization also requires attention to the level of adaptive functioning (or, alternatively, disabilities) of the depressed individual, a point illustrated by the interest attracted by the emerging second edition of the World Health Organization's (WHO) *International Classification of Impairments, Disabilities and Handicaps*. Careful assessment of functioning is important to verify the presence and severity of illness (and to guard against the trivialization of clinical assessment and care) as well as to guide the planning and evaluation of acute treatment and rehabilitation.

Furthermore, the absence or presence and levels of psychosocial stressors and supports can have an important role in the development and course of depression. Also to be considered is the appraisal of quality of life, a multidimensional and pre-eminently subjective concept that may range from physical well-being to spiritual fulfillment.

Through the use of pertinent scales and typologies, a multiaxial formulation may offer an encompassing and standardized appraisal of the key parameters of a depressed patient's condition. Implementation of a multiaxial schema may enhance communication and sharing of professional experience across town and across the world.

To complement and round up the standardized description furnished by a multiaxial formulation, one may want to consider an appraisal that pointedly looks at the particularities of the depressed person. Given the intricacy of the required informational task, a descriptive statement using all the resources of natural language seems advisable. Furthermore, the perspectives of the clinician and of the patient (and his/her family) as well as the articulation and resolution of these potentially discrepant perspectives need to be obtained.

An idiographic formulation along these lines is in fact a key component (in addition to a standardized multiaxial formulation) of the comprehensive diagnostic model underlying the International Guidelines for Diagnostic Assessment (IGDA) being prepared by the Section on Classification and Diagnostic Assessment of the World Psychiatric Association.

The above levels or components of a more comprehensive diagnostic approach [6] seem to offer jointly not only a more valid understanding of the patient's condition and the bases for more effective treatment and prognosis, but to incorporate an ethical dimension in diagnosis and clinical care by orienting these processes and tasks towards the promotion of health and quality of life as understood and planned collaboratively by patient and clinician.

REFERENCES

1. World Health Organization (1992) Tenth Revision of the *International Classification of Diseases and Related Health Problems* (ICD-10), World Health Organization, Geneva.
2. American Psychiatric Association (1994) *Diagnostic and Statistical Manual of Mental Disorders*, 4th edn (DSM-IV), American Psychiatric Association, Washington, DC.
3. Chinese Medical Association (1995) *Chinese Classification of Mental Disorders*, 2nd edn, revised (CCMD-2-R), Dong Nan University Press, Nanjing.
4. Otero A.A. (Ed.) (1998) *Tercer Glosario Cubano de Psiquiatria*, Hospital Psiquiátrico de La Habana, La Habana.
5. Mezzich J.E., Jorge M.R. (1993) Psychiatric nosology: achievements and challenges. In *International Review of Psychiatry* (Eds J.A. Costa e Silva, C.C. Nadelson), pp. 5–11, American Psychiatric Press, Washington, DC.
6. Mezzich J.E., Otero A.A., Lee S. (1999) International psychiatric diagnosis. In *Comprehensive Textbook of Psychiatry*, 7th edn (Eds H.I. Kaplan, B.J. Sadock), Williams & Wilkins, Baltimore.

1.9
Age, Loss and the Diagnostic Boundaries of Depression
Sidney Zisook[1]

Stefanis and Stefanis' comprehensive review covers all the major areas and many of the key controversies regarding the diagnoses of depressive disorders. In this commentary, I will expand or highlight additional diagnostic issues in two areas: life cycle considerations and bereavement.

The ICD-10 and DSM-IV operationalize diagnostic criteria for major depression that are particularly pertinent to young and mid-life adults, but may be less helpful for the diagnosis of individuals at the extremes of age. In older children and adolescents, for example, depression may not present with the classical symptoms of dysphoria or anhedonia. Instead, irritability, behavioral changes, social withdrawal, a change in school performance, an excursion into alcohol or other drugs, and vague somatic complaints may be the predominant manifestations [1]. Furthermore, when dysthymia or major depression occurs for the first time in adolescence, it often is the forerunner of a chronic or recurring illness that continues into adulthood, and may be

[1]*Department of Psychiatry, University of California, San Diego, 9500 Gilman Drive, La Jolla, CA 92093-0603, USA*

more likely than major depression beginning later in life to become a bipolar disorder [2].

Depression in late life shares many features with depression beginning in adolescence. As with the latter, such depressions tend to present with irritability, behavioral changes, withdrawal, and somatic symptoms rather than with dysphoria [3]. In addition, complaints of cognitive decline are quite common, sometimes, as Stefanis and Stefanis report, blurring the distinction between mood and cognitive disorders. As in adolescence, depressions in late life may be more recognizable by relatives or caregivers than by the patients themselves. Finally, in both adolescent and late life depressions, each episode is more likely to be a part of a continuum throughout one's life than a single episode. When depression occurs for the first time in late life, it is not infrequently closely associated with general medical and neurological problems, structural brain abnormalities and chronicity [4]. Many of these patients have vascular depression, characterized by greater overall cognitive impairment than patients with nonvascular depression, more impaired fluency and naming, more retardation, less agitation and insight, and fewer guilt feelings [5].

According to DSM-IV, if a major depressive syndrome begins after the death of a loved one it is not considered a major depressive episode until at least 2 months following the death; instead, it should be classified as "bereavement." DSM-IV does make allowances for very severe major depressive syndromes accompanied by feelings of worthlessness, psychomotor retardation and suicidal ideation being considered depressive episodes even within 2 months, but it rules out other, milder forms. Yet, recent data suggest these depressive syndromes, so called "bereavement," have all the clinical characteristics of other major depressive episodes. They are more common in individuals with past or family histories of major depression, tend to be chronic and/or recurrent, interfere with social and occupational functioning, are associated with impaired immunologic function, disrupt the resolution of grief and may be associated with ongoing adjustment difficulties [6].

Furthermore, bereavement stands *alone* as a life event capable of negating the diagnosis of major depression. Thus, for example, depression following divorce, financial ruin, or the destruction of one's home is depression. Why should depression following this one life event, loss of a loved one, be any different? Finally, depression is the *only* disorder negated by loss. If a bereaved individual develops recurrent panic attacks and associated worries after a death, the diagnosis of panic disorder is made (like depression, anxiety disorders also may be precipitated by loss); or if severe, crushing, left-sided chest pain occurs, no cardiologist would call it "bereavement" rather than what it really is. Thus, it might be argued that "bereavement," a throwback to the outworn notion of "reactive" depression, should be eliminated from DSM-V.

That bereavement and depression have symptoms in common, such as sadness and poor sleep, cannot be contested. But the same can be said for depression and generalized anxiety disorder (initial insomnia and poor concentration), depression and old age (poor sleep, poor appetite), depression and cancer (fatigue and thoughts of death), and on and on. In none of these cases, including grief, does the overlap mean a challenging differential diagnosis should not be made, and in each case, a prompt and accurate diagnosis of major depression can be literally life-saving.

REFERENCES

1. Birmaher B., Ryan N.D., Williamson D.E., Brent D.A., Kaufman J., Dahl R.E., Perel J., Nelson B. (1996) Childhood and adolescent depression: a review of the past 10 years. Part 1. *J. Am. Acad. Child Adolesc. Psychiatry*, **35**: 1427–1439.
2. Kovacs M., Akiskal H.S., Gatsonis C., Parrone P.L. (1994) Childhood-onset dysthymic disorder: clinical features and prospective naturalistic outcome. *Arch. Gen. Psychiatry*, **51**: 365–374.
3. Zisook S., Downs N. (1998) Diagnosis and treatment of depression in late life. *J. Clin. Psychiatry*, **59**: 80–91.
4. Krishnan K.R.R. (1993) Neuroanatomic substrates of depression in the elderly. *J. Geriatr. Psychiatr Neurol.*, **6**: 39–58.
5. Alexopoulos G.S., Meyers B.S., Young R.C., Kakuma T., Silbersweig D., Charlson M. (1997) Clinically defined vascular depression. *Am. J. Psychiatry*, **154**: 562–565.
6. Zisook S., Shuchter S.R. (1993) Uncomplicated bereavement. *J. Clin. Psychiatry*, **54**: 365–372.

1.10

Depression Among Elderly and Postpartum Women

Paul S.F. Yip[1] and Dominic T.S. Lee[2]

In this commentary on Stefanis and Stefanis' review of depression we should like to make comments on two specific topics: (1) the prevalence and the recognition of depression among the elderly and its relationship with suicide; (2) depression among childbearing women.

Suicide risk is high among depressed people [1]. Stefanis and Stefanis have highlighted the problems of non-recognition or misdiagnosis of depression at the primary care setting. This is particularly common in the presence of a comorbid physical illness or if the physician has a tendency to overlook depressive symptoms. The situation is particularly applicable to the Chinese

[1] *Department of Statistics and Actuarial Science, University of Hong Kong, Pokfulam, Hong Kong*
[2] *Department of Psychiatry, Chinese University of Hong Kong, Shatin, Hong Kong*

elderly population. Hong Kong has one of the highest suicide rates among the elderly in the world. For example, the recent suicide rate was 50 per 100 000 among elderly aged 75 or above, about four times above the population average [2].

In a recent study, we found that 80% of the elderly (60 or over) who committed suicide had severe or terminal illness and 24% had a history of psychiatric treatment [3]. The chronic illnesses were strongly related to the presence of depression among the suicide cases. Seeking treatment from psychiatrists to deal with psychological problems is the exception rather than the norm in Hong Kong. Also, elderly people tend to conceptualize mental health problems as physical and this is especially true for the Chinese. It is important for physicians at the primary care setting to recognize the clues of depression and to provide a proper counselling service when the elderly seek medical treatment, in view of the high risk of their committing suicide. It was found that 40% of the suicide cases had consulted a doctor about their physical illness within a month before committing suicide [3]. Physicians have to be better trained in diagnosis and more alert about the high risk of suicide among the sick elderly. At the very least physicians should warn family members about the possibilities and make appropriate referral for the patients. It is encouraging to see that more emphasis on doctor and patient communication is included in the medical education curriculum in Hong Kong, such that the mental state of patients (including depression) stands a better chance of being diagnosed and recognized by physicians. It is suggested that the low rate of recognition and inadequate treatment of mental disorders, especially depression, could be one of the reasons explaining the high suicide rate in the elderly Chinese community [4]. However, the prevalence of drug and alcohol abuse among elderly suicide deaths in Hong Kong was less than their Western counterparts [3].

Next, we should also like to supplement information on postpartum depression. The occurrence of depression in the postpartum period has attracted much attention and research. Postnatal depression affects 10–15% of women in the early months of postpartum [5]. Apart from causing suffering and distress to the mother at a time of anticipated joy, postnatal depression undermines marital relationships and adversely affects the cognitive and emotional development of the baby [6]. Despite the potential deleterious consequences of postnatal depression and the opportunity for repeated clinical contacts in the postpartum period, research shows that as many as 90% of postnatal depressions are undiagnosed and untreated.

In some countries, systematic screening programmes have been implemented to improve the detection of postnatal depression. Self-report questionnaires, such as the Edinburgh Postnatal Depression Scale (EPDS), can be administered during the postpartum follow-up visits to identity individuals who have significant depressive symptomatology and hence deserve further assessments [7, 8].

It is generally forgotten that as much as one third of postnatal depression has onset in pregnancy and hence the term "postnatal depression" is, strictly speaking, a misnomer, which potentially misleads clinical attention away from the antepartum period. Unless we remember that "postnatal depression" is actually "perinatal depression" and a significant proportion of the so-called "postnatal depression" actually begins in pregnancy, the opportunities to detect depression antepartum will remain forgotten. For this reason, it is perhaps better to refer to depression occurring in the postpartum period as "perinatal depression."

REFERENCES

1. Harris E.C., Barraclough B. (1997) Suicide as an outcome for mental disorder. *Br. J. Psychiatry*, **170**: 205–228.
2. Yip P.S.F., Chi I., Yu K.K. (1998) An epidemiological profile of elderly suicides in Hong Kong. *Int. Geriatr. Psychiatry*, **13**: 631–637.
3. Chi I., Yip P.S.F., Yu K.K. (1997) Elderly suicides in Hong Kong. *Befrienders International*, 1–62, Hong Kong.
4. Yip P.S.F., Callanan C., Yuen H.K. (1999) Urban/rural and gender differentials in suicide rates: East and West. *J. Affect. Disord.*, **57**: 99–106.
5. O'Hara M.W., Swain A.M. (1996) Rates and risk of postpartum depression — a meta-analysis. *Int. Rev. Psychiatry*, **8**: 37–54.
6. Cooper P.J., Murray L. (1998) Fortnightly review. Postnatal depression. *Br. Med. J.*, **316**: 1884–1886.
7. Cox J.L., Holden J.M., Sagovsky R. (1987) Detection of postnatal depression: development of the 10-item Edinburgh Postnatal Depression Scale. *Br. J. Psychiatry*, **150**: 782–786.
8. Lee D.T.S., Yip S.K., Chiu H.F.K., Chan K.P.M., Chau I.O.L., Leung C.M., Chung T.K.H. (1998) Detecting postnatal depression in Chinese. *Br. J. Psychiatry*, **172**: 433–437.

1.11
Self-rating Depression Scales: Some Methodological Issues

Toshinori Kitamura[1]

As Stefanis and Stefanis have succinctly noted, depression is a clinical condition with multiple manifestations, multiple subcategories, and possibly multiple aetiologies. Self-report scales of depression are useful tools for shedding light on these complexities of the disorder both in research and practice. Stefanis and Stefanis have listed, among many others, a few very

[1]*National Institute of Mental Health, National Center of Neurology and Psychiatry, 1-7-3 Kohnodai, Ichikawa, Chiba, 272-0827, Japan*

well-known and established instruments to measure depression. These scales can reliably screen cases of depression and measure the severity of the condition. They are cheap and less time-consuming and therefore are suitable for epidemiological studies. They are provided with predetermined questions so that comparison is easy even between different cultures. However, they are not necessarily without shortcomings.

An important but much neglected issue of self-rating scales is their reduced validity after repeated use. Self-rating scales are often used to measure the temporal change of the condition. Kitamura et al [1] administered Zung's Self-Rating Depression Scale (SDS) [2] to the same women twice during pregnancy and twice after childbirth. The SDS validity was measured in terms of sensitivity and specificity using operationalized diagnoses made by psychiatrists. The SDS sufficiently identified cases of depressive disorders on the first occasion (the first trimester) but subsequently lost its validity. In the same sample, the scores of the General Health Questionnaire (GHQ) [3] lost significant differences between those women with and those without minor psychiatric morbidity [4]. This was due to the fact that the GHQ score decreased among the suffering women while the score of the non-suffering women did not change. In the literature, we have found ample reports of "improvement" of questionnaire scores from the first test to the retest. This was found in measures of neurotic symptoms [5], anxiety [6], depression [7], and adjustment [8]. Reduced validity of a self-report when used repeatedly is to be overcome in future studies.

Another methodological issue of self-report scales is the contrast between positive and negative wordings of a questionnaire. The "usually" answer to the question "Did you sleep well recently?" is equivalent to the "never" or "rarely" answer to the question "Do you have difficulty sleeping recently?" However, the impact that these two questions have on the cognition of the subject may be different.

For example, the Center for Epidemiologic Studies Depression Scale (CES-D) [9], a widely used self-rating measure of depression, contains four positive affect items. Iwata et al reported that the Japanese responses to these positive items were less affirmative than American responses [10]. They suggested that the Japanese were more likely to suppress the expression of positive affect. Therefore, they revised the CES-D so that all the positive items were rewritten into negative wording. Japanese psychiatric patients with dysphoric mood-related symptoms were compared with matched controls in terms of responses to the original CES-D items and the negatively revised items. Whereas there were no significant differences between the patient and control groups in the scores of the positive items, significant differences appeared in the scores of the negatively revised items. Furthermore, the internal consistency of the scale improved after the original positive items were converted into the negative items [11]. These findings suggest that: (1) questions must be worded carefully; and (2) international and transcultural comparison using a self-rating scale needs adjustment not only in the cut-off point of the total score but also in the item-by-item comparison.

REFERENCES

1. Kitamura T., Shima S., Sugawara M., Toda M.A. (1994) Temporal variation of validity of self-rating questionnaires: repeated use of the General Health Questionnaire and Zung's Self-rating Depression Scale among women during antenatal and postnatal periods. *Acta Psychiatr. Scand.*, **90**: 446–450.
2. Zung W.K. (1965) A self-rating depression scale. *Arch. Gen. Psychiatry*, **12**: 63–70.
3. Goldberg D.P. (1972) *The Detection of Psychiatric Illness by Questionnaire: A Technique for the Identification and Assessment of Non-psychotic Psychiatric Illness*, Oxford University Press, Oxford.
4. Kitamura T., Toda M.A., Shima S., Sugawara M. (1994) Validity of the repeated GHQ among pregnant women: a study in a Japanese general hospital. *Int. J. Psychiatr. Med.*, **24**: 149–156.
5. Jorm A.F., Duncan-Jones P., Scott R. (1989) An analysis of the retest artefact in longitudinal studies of psychiatric symptoms and personality. *Psychol. Med.*, **19**: 487–493.
6. Knowles E.S., Coker C.C., Scott R.A., Neville J.W. (1996) Measurement-induced improvement in anxiety: mean shifts with repeated assessment. *J. Pers. Soc. Psychol.*, **71**: 352–363.
7. Nolen-Hoeksema, S., Seligman M.E., Girgus J.S. (1992) Predictors and consequences of childhood depressive symptoms: a 5-year longitudinal study. *J. Abnorm. Psychol.*, **101**: 405–422.
8. Popham S.M., Holden R.R. (1991) Psychometric properties of MMPI factor scales. *Person. Individ. Diffs.*, **12**: 513–517.
9. Radloff L.S. (1977) The CES-D scale: a self-report depression scale for research in the general population. *Appl. Psychol. Measure.*, **1**: 385–401.
10. Iwata N., Roberts C.R., Kawakami N. (1995) Japan–US comparison of responses to depression scale items among adult workers. *Psychiatry Res.*, **58**: 237–245.
11. Iwata N., Umesue M., Egashira K., Hiro H., Mizoue T., Mishima N., Nagata S. (1998) Can positive affect items be used to assess depressive disorders in the Japanese population? *Psychol. Med.*, **28**: 153–158.

1.12
Underdiagnosis of Depression: Its Impact on the Community

Ahmed Okasha[1]

The proper diagnosis of depression is of paramount importance, not only because of the high prevalence of this condition in different patient

[1] Institute of Psychiatry, Ain Shams University, 3 Shawarby Street, Kasr El Nil, Cairo, Egypt

populations, but also because it is associated with poor physical and social functioning and significant impairment of everyday activities as well as an increased number of disability days.

Mental disorders present a greater burden globally than cerebrovascular and heart disease combined. Mental health problems account for more than 8% of the disability-adjusted life years lost [1]. It is estimated that depressive disorders produce more than 17% of disability associated with mental health problems worldwide. It is predicted that in the year 2020 depressive disorders will be the second cause of disability amongst all medical disorders. The comprehensive review by Stefanis and Stefanis emphasizes the meaning and definition of the word depression. It can be a mood state of sadness common to all humans, or a complaint (symptom) which is prevalent in several psychiatric and medical disorders, as well as a syndrome or a disorder defined by specific criteria listed in ICD-10 and DSM-IV. The common mistake in the methodology of many studies is the misdifferentiation between depression as a normal human mood, depressive symptoms and depressive disorder. This may lead to different results concerning prevalence, sex ratio, risk factors, and response to treatment.

Psychiatrists are aware that more than 80% of depressed patients are treated by general practitioners or traditional healers and, in some studies, specialists treat fewer than 5% of all patients with depressive disorders [2]. Several studies confirm that primary care physicians do not make the diagnosis of depressive disorders in more than half of patients who satisfy the criteria for depressive disorder. The obstacles to recognition and diagnosis are: (1) the stigma associated with diagnosis; (2) presentation with somatic symptoms that mask the depression; (3) lack of training in diagnosing depressive disorders.

There is no medical disorder which can impair the quality of life more than depression. There was a belief that depression is more frequent in developed than in developing countries, in urban areas more than in the rural, among the rich more than in the poor. These assumptions are wrong and many studies showed their invalidity. In an epidemiological study conducted in Egypt, the prevalence of depressive disorders in the rural region was 19.7%, whilst in the urban areas it was 11.4%. Adjustment disorder was the most common category of depression in rural people, while dysthymic disorder was the most frequent in urban dwellers [3]. What is usually met with in daily clinical practice is a medical or a psychiatric comorbidity. Recognition of this comorbidity has been facilitated by the introduction of multiaxial classifications in ICD-10 and DSM-IV. This requires a thorough knowledge of interactions between psychotropic and other drugs. Recognizing depression associated with medical disorders will improve the quality of life of the patient in spite of the persistence of medical disorder. Results of various studies show that depressive disorders occur in 22–33% of hospitalized patients [4], in 38% of those with cancer [5], in 47% of those with stroke [6], in 45% of those with myocardial infarction (7), and in 39% of those with Parkinson's disease [8]. Thus, underrecognizing, underdiagnosing and undertreating depressive disorder is an ethical issue facing the medical profession.

The ICD-10 diagnostic criteria for research contain 10 items, in contrast to the 9 DSM-IV items (loss of self-esteem is separate from inappropriate guilt), in diagnosing major depressive disorder. ICD-10 provides separate criteria sets for each level of severity of a depressive episode: a threshold of 4 out of 10 symptoms defines mild, 6 out of 10 defines moderate, and 8 out of 10 defines severe. Furthermore, the diagnostic algorithm differs by requiring that there be at least 2 of the following 3 symptoms — depressed mood, loss of interest and decreased energy — for mild and moderate depressive episodes and all of them for severe depressive episodes. ICD-10 episodes with psychotic features exclude Schneider's first rank symptoms and bizarre delusions. The ICD-10 criteria for research specify that there should be a period of at least 2 months free from significant mood symptoms between mood episodes, whereas DSM-IV criteria indicate an interval of at least 2 consecutive months in which full criteria for a major depressive episode are not met. The American Psychiatric Association has produced a crossover between the ICD-10 and DSM-IV, called the international version with ICD-10 codes, which facilitates the diagnosis with the two systems.

The proper diagnosis of depression will lead to better management, which is cost-effective, reducing the burden of disability and improving the quality of life of millions of people. Awareness of primary care physicians, families, patients and the general public in the detection of depressive disorders is the pathway to a better life.

REFERENCES

1. World Bank (1993) *World Development Report*, Oxford University Press, New York.
2. Madianos M.G., Stefanis C.N. (1992) Changes in the prevalence of symptoms of depression and depression across Greece. *Soc. Psychiatry Psychiatr. Epidemiol.*, **27**: 211–219.
3. Okasha A., Abdel Hakeem R. (1988) Prevalence of depressive disorder in a sample of rural and urban Egyptian communities. *Egyp. J. Psychiatry*, **11**: 167–181.
4. Katon W., Sullivan M.D. (1990) Depression and chronic medical illness. *J. Clin. Psychiatry*, **51** (Suppl.): 3–11.
5. Bukberg J., Penman D., Holland J.C. (1984) Depression in hospitalized cancer patients. *Psychosom. Med.*, **46**: 199–212.
6. Robinson R.G., Starr L.B., Kubos K.L., Price T.R. (1983) A two-year longitudinal study of post-stroke mood disorders: findings during the initial evaluation. *Stroke*, **14**: 736–741.

7. Schleifer S.J., Macari-Hinson M.M., Coyle D.A., Slater W.R., Kahn M., Gorlin R., Zucker H.D. (1989) The nature and course of depression following myocardial infarction. *Arch. Intern. Med.*, **149**: 1785–1789.
8. Mayeux R., Stern Y., Cote L., Williams J.B. (1984) Altered serotonin metabolism in depressed patients with Parkinson's disease. *Neurology*, **34**: 642–646.

1.13

Limited Options on Diagnosing Depression

Santosh K. Chaturvedi[1]

The diagnosis of depression has remained unsatisfactory and the limited options force one to compromise on what is available and attempt to revise it periodically. As pointed out in Stefanis and Stefanis' review, one difficulty is with the term "depression" itself. This term is used in the general day-to-day conversations on any subject and is commonly misinterpreted. "Depression" sounds so simplistic that lay people feel they are as cognizant about this disorder as the treating physician or psychiatrist. An alternative, scientific term is needed to indicate that the disorder being diagnosed and treated is not a simple or common "sadness," but a specific morbid disorder which requires careful management.

The lack of knowledge about the specific etiological factors has complicated the issue of diagnosis and treatment. Till now, the diagnosis has been based on counting the number of symptoms, and the treatment has been symptomatic. The diagnosis also takes into account the duration of symptoms. Since one has to wait for the minimum period of 2 weeks to arrive at a diagnosis of major depression, and for a period of 2 years for a diagnosis of dysthymia, the person has to suffer during this period, and there is no scope for early intervention. If one noticed features of depression for a day or two and intervened successfully to relieve depression, the skepticism and doubt about the diagnosis would linger. What is so special about 14 days? On day 13 it is not depression, on day 15 it can be diagnosed as depression! In most physical diseases, the treatment begins the moment the first symptoms are noticed.

Somatic symptoms add to further confusion. The *International Classification of Diseases* (ICD-10) classifies some types of depressive disorders as those with somatic symptoms. Here somatic symptoms refer to loss of interest, psychomotor retardation, marked loss of appetite, loss of weight, diurnal variation, early morning awakening, and loss of libido. In many psychiatric centers, somatic symptoms imply headache, chronic pain, fatigue, lethargy and a number of other bodily symptoms which are termed "somatic."

[1]*National Institute of Mental Health and Neurosciences, Bangalore 560 029, India*

Thus, this category of ICD-10 adds further to the prevailing confusion in diagnosing and subtyping depressive disorders. Whereas a depressed patient with a number of bodily or somatic symptoms without vegetative symptoms will receive a diagnosis of depression without somatic symptoms, another depressed patient without the bodily or physical symptoms is likely to receive a diagnosis of depression with somatic symptoms if the vegetative features are noted.

The presence of somatic symptoms further complicates diagnosing depressive disorders in patients with medical illnesses such as cancer or those who are elderly [1, 2]. It may be difficult to discern whether the somatic symptoms are due to depression or to the underlying medical or physical disease [3]. Some methods have been used effectively to overcome this difficulty, such as revising the number of criteria to be fulfilled [4], or substituting some of the somatic symptoms with non-somatic ones [2]. The Hospital Anxiety and Depression Scale (HADS) has proved to be an effective scale to detect depression and assess its severity in patients with medical or physical illnesses, since it contains mainly cognitive and affective symptoms of depression and anxiety [5].

REFERENCES

1. Holland J.C. (1986) Managing depression in the patient with cancer. *Clin. Oncologist*, **1**: 11–13.
2. Rapp S.R., Vrana S. (1989) Substituting nonsomatic for somatic symptoms in the diagnosis of depression in elderly male medical patients. *Am. J. Psychiatry*, **146**: 1197–2000.
3. Chaturvedi S.K., Maguire P. (1998) Persistent somatization in cancer: a follow up study. *J. Psychosom. Res.*, **45**: 249–256.
4. Endicott J. (1984) Measurement of depression in patients with cancer. *Cancer*, **53** (Suppl.): 2243–2247.
5. Zigmond A.S., Snaith R.P. (1983) The Hospital Anxiety and Depression Scale. *Acta Psychiatr. Scand.*, **67**: 361–370.

1.14

Diagnosis of Depressive Disorders: Taxonomical Systems and Clinical Practice

Angel A. Otero Ojeda[1]

The lack of etiological knowledge and accurate markers to conceptualize and identify the so-called depressive disorders (DD) has brought about a rather arbitrary formulation of the diagnosis of these disorders.

[1] *Department of Psychiatry, University of Havana, Cuba*

Even though the definition of depression has been always eluded in contemporary taxonomic systems until ICD-9, it has been implicit that a collapse of the patient's affectivity and vitality lies at the basis of its clinical expression.

Clinicians, assessing the current picture in the light of the patient's past-current existential environment, were the ones entitled to diagnose depression and to select the adequate subcategory, according to its current manifestations, background, and the (hypothetical) predominant mechanism of production (endogenous dysfunction, current exogenous factors, or morbid intrapsychic mechanisms and affective needs). This caused subjectivism and a low level of diagnostic concordance, creating a taxonomic structure based, in the best cases, on neither confirmed nor universally accepted hypotheses, and on ambiguous, incomplete, contaminated and partial truths suggested by a non-standardized practice of psychiatry.

Current diagnostic systems standardize diagnoses through objective guidelines, which are considered an interim solution until the discovery of biological markers [1]. These systems, although being recognized as an indispensable step to guide research on DD, have been criticized for the following reasons:

1. Being designed to diagnose diseases or disorders (rather than patients) and for research, they ignore many of the biopsychosocial aspects as well as hypotheses and assertions of relative (probabilistic) or partial validity which are indispensable in guiding medical actions (in actual patients) and in mental health settings.
2. They lose, for the sake of objectivity, the contextual-integral assessment of the patient, who is confined to his objective-generalizable symptoms.
3. They pay insufficient attention to cultural and age-related factors, reflecting the way of expressing depression of average young adults from a northwestern society. Variations imposed by age and culture to DD are recorded elsewhere, therefore being out of diagnosis.
4. Being designed to diagnose a diseased subject at the secondary level of care, they are not appropriate to meet the needs of a contemporary psychiatry that changes its epicenter towards mental health community care.

Fewer than half of the depressed patients attending health care services (HCS) are adequately diagnosed. Figures several-fold higher of depressed subjects do not attend or have no access to HCS. Approaching such a situation requires a change of strategy for HCS; training general practitioners and other professionals in these services on diagnosing depression is necessary but is not enough. Working teams need to be expanded by the inclusion of active community members who are not traditionally integrated in the HCS (mental health multipliers), and to be provided with diagnostic instruments appropriate for identifying not only disorders, but also "people at risk" and social dysfunctions.

Our research [2] confirms that the underdiagnosis of depression by general practitioners is associated with: (1) insufficient knowledge of the concept, atypical manifestations and frequency of depression; (2) use of interviews excessively centered on somatic aspects; (3) lack of appropriate diagnostic instruments; and (4) regarding depressive manifestations as natural consequences of somatic diseases or life events.

The diagnostic results improved significantly when general practitioners were provided with appropriate interviewing techniques and diagnostic instruments, such as the ICD-10 primary care version and the Tetradimensional Structural Questionnaire (CET-DE) [3].

REFERENCES

1. Fábregas H. (1996) Cultural and historical foundations of psychiatric diagnosis. In *Culture and Psychiatric Diagnosis* (Eds J.E. Mezzich, A. Kleinman, H. Fábregas, D.L. Parrón), pp. 3–14, American Psychiatric Press, Washington, DC.
2. Otero Ojeda A.A. (1997) Prevención secundaria de la depresión (diagnóstico precoz). In *Nuevas Aportaciones sobre la Depresión* (Ed. F. Alonso-Fernández), pp. 95–108, Edikamed, Barcelona.
3. Alonso-Fernández F. (1995) *CET-DE, Cuestionario Estructural Tetradimensional para la Depresión*, Tea, Madrid.

1.15
The Identification of Diagnostic Subtypes of Depressive Disorders
Nikolai Kornetov[1]

The clinical core of the modern diagnosis of depressive disorders (DD) is the "depressive episode" (DE) or "major depression" (MD), which can occur as a single episode or be recurrent. DE is presented descriptively in ICD-10, whereas MD is defined by operational criteria in DSM-IV. These diagnostic categories are comparable, and include depression with or without psychotic symptoms, with or without catatonic features, and with or without somatic (melancholic) symptoms. Other subtypes of depression include subsyndromal symptomatic depression [1] and specific conditions limited mostly by temporal frameworks: recurrent brief depression, dysthymia, cyclothymia, seasonal depression, premenstrual dysphoric disorders, postpartum and menopausal depressions, and so on.

[1]*Mental Health Research Institute of RAMSci, Department of Affective Disorders, 634014 Tomsk, Russia*

An advantage of typological DD grouping is impartiality concerning various hypotheses and theories of their origin. Previous quasi-etiological dichotomies of DD into endogenous and psychogenic, psychotic and neurotic, created diagnostic "niches", which hampered the integration of psychiatry within general care. At the same time, it is necessary to take into account that patients with DE/MD often present a family history of affective disorders, melancholic symptoms, psychomotor retardation, circadian and circannual rhythm changes, and show more substantial neurobiological alterations. On the other hand, minor depressive types are more often associated with precipitating psychosocial stressors, and have a less frequent family history of DD and tendency to recurrence.

An ambiguity of current classifications is the use of the term "bereavement". First, a situation of loss is often observed in major depressive episodes; second, depressive symptoms when a loss has occurred are sometimes prolonged and may develop into dysthymia; third, there is an increase in vulnerability to illness and mortality for the first 2 years after a significant loss [2–3].

In our department we conducted studies involving 217 inpatients with DD occurring after a significant loss. These studies revealed several psychobiological changes in neuroendocrine and immune systems: hypothalamic-pituitary axis (HPA) activation, increase of plasma concentration of beta-endorphin, reduction of thyroid secretion and significantly increased levels of thyrotropic hormone; decreased levels of insulin; an imbalance of cellular and humoral immunity. These changes were observed in patients with depressive disturbances of various degrees of severity: 73.7% of the cases did not meet the criteria for a depressive adaptive reaction according to duration and severity. In 120 inpatients (females) having experienced the loss of a parent (21.7%), a spouse (42.5%) or a child (35.8%), the criteria were fulfilled for DE in 33.3% of cases, for bereavement in 35.0% of cases, and for subsyndromal depression with unstable neurovegetative symptoms in 31.7% of cases. In 40% of patients dysthymia was diagnosed catamnestically. Clinical-biological aspects of stress-induced depressions require further attention.

Clinical observations show that in the presence of significant loss there is frequently a reinforcement of morning dysphoria and terminal insomnia. However, such states are only similar to circadian mood fluctuations. In reality, they represent "pseudo-circadian" symptoms, the cause of which comprises frequent nightmares associated with loss of the loved one, encountering him in dreams, or the presence of hypnopompic hallucinations when waking up in the morning. These clinical facts are confirmed by ethnographic data in the analysis of funeral rites among Slavs and the experiences of widows (our own investigations).

In fact, the co-occurrence of multiple genetic, constitutional and neurobiological risk factors with personality, psychodynamic and social-environmental factors of varying specificity is a clinical reality in DD. Their interactions produce DD and give them their unique clinical polymorphism. At the same time, clinical manifestations of DD have to be considered within distinguished diagnostic subtypes unless something is changed in the modern classification of depressive disorders. Initially, this approach seems to be syndromological. However, this is no more than a myth. Kraepelin [4], in the first page of the section of his textbook devoted to manic-depressive insanity, wrote the following: "it is probable that a lot of subforms will be created later or completely separate small groups will begin to detach themselves. If this should happen, so the same symptoms which up to date used to move into the foreground will serve as the standard". It is likely that the founder of psychiatric nosology was not wrong in his prediction, and that the DD subtype differentiation will continue.

REFERENCES

1. Judd L.L., Akiskal H.S., Paulus M.P. (1997) The role and clinical significance of subsyndromal depressive symptoms (SSD) in unipolar major depressive disorder. *J. Affect. Disord.*, **45**: 5–17.
2. Kornetov N.A. (1993) *Psychogenic Depression*, University Press, Tomsk.
3. Biondi M., Picardi A. (1996) Clinical and biological aspects of bereavement and loss-induced depression: a reappraisal. *Psychother. Psychosom.*, **65**: 229–245.
4. Kraepelin E. (1993) *Psychiatrie*, 8th edn, Abel, Leipzig.

2

Pharmacological Treatment of Depressive Disorders: A Review

Per Bech

Frederiksborg General Hospital, Hillerød, Denmark

INTRODUCTION

The term "antidepressants" was introduced in the 1950s, based on evidence that imipramine reduced the symptoms of moderate to severe depression without being a psychostimulant or a "happy pill". The development of the first generation of antidepressants was based on either the chemical tricyclic structure of imipramine (the various tricyclic antidepressants, TCAs) or the mechanism of action (e.g. monoamino-oxidase inhibitors, MAOIs). Some of the new-generation antidepressants have been developed strictly on the basis of their mechanism of action (e.g. selective serotonin reuptake inhibitors, SSRIs, or selective noradrenaline reuptake inhibitors, NARIs), whereas this is only in part the case for other drugs (e.g. trazodone, nefazodone, mianserin or mirtazapine).

Antidepressants vs. Psychostimulants

Most patients suffering from depressive illness feel that they have some kind of "psychological stress". On the other hand, a certain degree of anxiety and depression is to be expected and is perhaps even desirable among members of a modern society that provides them with many schedules for their daily life. This was discussed by Hinkle [1] when summarizing the concept of stress after 50 years.

The most common complaints by persons seeking psychotherapy seem to be stress-related symptoms such as anxiety and depression [2]. The chemical substances often used as "anti-stress medication" are alcohol and related psychoactive substances. However, these have the obvious disadvantage

Depressive Disorders, Second Edition. Edited by Mario Maj and Norman Sartorius.
© 2002 John Wiley & Sons Ltd.

of impairing ability to carry out the many activities of modern daily life. As emphasized by Hinkle, only tobacco provides a feeling of well-being without creating drunkenness. However, both alcohol and tobacco create dependency, and tobacco has the other great disadvantage of causing cancer or myocardial infarction.

One of the best textbooks in clinical psychiatry from the early 1950s [3] recommends ECT (electroconvulsive therapy) for severely depressed patients hospitalized for their illness, and a combination of barbiturates and amphetamine for milder forms of depressive illness. In 1955 Skottowe [4] even recommended opium for moderate degrees of depression. It is against this background that the work done by Kuhn [5] on the effect of imipramine should be assessed. Kuhn showed that the effect of imipramine was antidepressive rather than antipsychotic, to some extent similar to ECT. The response was not immediate but had a delayed onset [6].

The evidence of the antidepressive effect of imipramine was described by Kuhn [6] with the sole aid of clinical observations. There was no Hamilton Depression Scale (HAM-D, [7]) and no computer with which to establish statistical evidence, such as effect size or odds ratio test when compared to a placebo. Kuhn's clinical descriptions of the efficacy of imipramine in moderate to severe depression have withstood the test of time.

However, after Kuhn's first observations of depressed patients in 1956, more than 3 years passed before imipramine was marketed. Resistance to the term "antidepressant drugs" came both from psychiatrists, who considered depression as nothing but a reactive or "psychic" illness (i.e. time and place but not drugs could be curative), and from the drug manufacturing company, that was afraid that imipramine might turn out to be an amphetamine [8]. However, Kuhn had already shown that imipramine was not a psychostimulant.

As discussed by Healy [8], it was probably the evidence of the therapeutic activity of another drug, iproniazid, that finally pushed the marketing of imipramine as an antidepressant. At the beginning of the 1950s, Selzer and Lurie [9] showed that the antitubercular drug isoniazid had what they called an antidepressive effect. Another antitubercular drug, iproniazid, was also shown to have this effect, which the authors referred to as a "psychic energizing" effect [10]. At that time it was assumed that iproniazid but not isoniazid was an MAOI. However, as stated by Sitsen [11] isoniazid is a reversible inhibitor of monoamine-oxidase type A (RIMA), like moclobemide, whereas iproniazid is an irreversible and unselective MAOI, like phenelzine (Table 2.1).

While Kuhn was convinced that imipramine was an antidepressant, Loomer et al [10] were convinced that iproniazid was a psychic energizer rather than an antidepressant. However, today both classes of drugs are considered as antidepressants, although the clinical profile is somewhat different.

TABLE 2.1   Classification of antidepressants by mode of action

Monoamine-oxidase inhibitors (MAOIs)	*Original*	*Most used*
Unselective MAOIs	Iproniazid	Phenelzine
Selective reversible inhibitors of monoamine-oxidase type A (RIMA)	Isoniazid	Moclobemide
Monoamine reuptake inhibitors	*Unselective*	*Selective*
More serotonin than noradrenaline	Clomipramine	Venlafaxine
More noradrenaline than serotonin	Imipramine	Desipramine
	Amitriptyline	Nortriptyline
Selective serotonin reuptake inhibitors (SSRIs)		Citalopram
		Fluoxetine
		Fluvoxamine
		Paroxetine
		Sertraline
Selective noradrenaline reuptake inhibitors (NARIs)		Reboxetine
Serotonin receptor modulators (SRMs)	*Original*	*Most used*
With serotonin reuptake inhibition	Trazodone	Nefazodone
With alpha-2 adrenoreceptor inhibition	Mianserin	Mirtazapine

Chemical Structure vs. Mechanisms of Action

The antidepressive action of iproniazid was from the very first trials ascribed to monoamine-oxidase inhibition, and its successors, such as phenelzine and isocarboxazide, were introduced as MAOIs. Imipramine, however, was not an MAOI and its antidepressive action was assumed to be through its chemical structure. Thus, amitriptyline was developed from the tricyclic structure of imipramine. The two drugs differ only in regard to one nitrogen atom.

TCAs are monoamine reuptake inhibitors, that is they inhibit the reuptake of both serotonin and noradrenaline in the brain synapses (Table 2.1). Clomipramine is more a serotonin than a noradrenaline reuptake inhibitor [12]. Desipramine and nortriptyline are metabolites of imipramine and amitriptyline, respectively, and are rather selective noradrenaline reuptake inhibitors.

The tetracyclic antidepressant maprotiline is a noradrenaline reuptake inhibitor, whereas other tetracyclic antidepressants, such as mianserin and mirtazapine, are neither MAOIs nor monoamine reuptake inhibitors. They are, among other modes of action, serotonin 2A (5HT-2A) receptor antagonists and alpha-2-blockers [13]. By blocking alpha-2 autoreceptors, mirtazapine stimulates the serotonergic neurotransmission. Thus, mirtazapine and nefazodone have both a 5HT-2A inhibition and serotonergic neurotransmission stimulating activity, although the latter effect is achieved by different pathways [14]. This class of antidepressants is called serotonin receptor modulators (SRMs) [15], although mirtazapine also has an effect on noradrenaline [14].

The SSRIs seem to act on 5HT-1A receptors ("serotonin 1A agonists") [14]. Nefazodone is both a 5HT-2A antagonist and a weak 5HT-1A agonist [14]. The NARIs in Table 2.1 are represented by reboxetine.

There are many other drugs on the market in various countries besides those shown in Table 2.1. However, in the following discussion the focus will mostly be on those antidepressants that are included in the table.

THE CLINICAL TARGET SYNDROME

With the release of the evidence-based classification system DSM-III [16], the diagnosis of major depression became the target syndrome for antidepressants. Clinical research with symptom rating scales such as the HAM-D from 1960 to 1980 had shown that around ten symptoms are often sufficient to reflect the syndrome of acute depressive states [17]. The clinical syndrome of depression described by Kuhn included the same depression-specific symptoms as the HAM-D, as well as the nine symptoms of depression to be considered for the diagnosis of major depression in DSM-III (Table 2.2).

Both DSM-IV [18] and ICD-10 [19] are in accordance with the DSM-III diagnosis of major depression (Table 2.2). It has been argued that the current editions of DSM and ICD are essentially attempts to standardize the Kraepelin categories [20], which also applies to Kuhn's and Hamilton's syndromes of depression. Table 2.3 shows the concordance between Kuhn, Hamilton and DSM-IV/ICD-10 for the clinical target syndrome for antidepressants: major depressive episode [21, 22].

Severity and Duration of Major Depressive Episode (MDE)

Severity of symptoms in an episode of major depression is a key dimension [23]. DSM-IV and ICD-10, as well as the HAM-D, use the term "psychotic depression" to mean the most severe degree of the depressive syndrome accompanied by either delusions or hallucinations. A major depressive episode (MDE), therefore, may be with or without psychotic features. Furthermore, the psychotic features can be either mood-congruent (i.e. severe degree of such symptoms as guilt or hypochondriasis) or mood-incongruent (i.e. independent of the depression symptoms).

A major depressive episode may be with or without melancholia. The terms "melancholic" as used in DSM-IV and "somatic" as used in ICD-10

TABLE 2.2 Imipramine-responsive symptoms, DSM-IV major depression symptoms, and the Hamilton depression symptoms

Symptoms responsive to imipramine (according to Kuhn, [5])	DSM-IV syndrome profile of major depression	Hamilton's Depression Scale (HAM-D-17) *Depression factor (HAM-D-6)
Lack of vitality	Psychomotor retardation	Retardation*
	Fatigue or loss of energy	Somatic feelings, general*
	Diminished ability to concentrate	
Decreased social ability	Diminished interest in social activity	Work and interests*
Anxiety	Psychomotor agitation	Anxiety, psychic*
		Anxiety, somatic
		Psychomotor agitation
Depressive affect	Depressed mood	Depressed mood*
	Feelings of worthlessness or guilt	Guilt feelings*
	Suicide ideas or plans	Suicidal impulses
Somatic or vegetative symptoms	Insomnia	Insomnia (initial, middle, late)
	Decreased appetite, weight loss	Decreased appetite, weight loss
		Hypochondriasis, sexual disturbances, loss of insight

TABLE 2.3 Relationship between the DSM-IV/ICD-10 categories of major depression and the total severity score on HAM-D-17

DSM-IV/ICD-10 categories of Major Depressive Episode (MDE)	HAM-D-17 Total scores
MDE with psychotic features	30 or higher
MDE with melancholic features	25–29
MDE without melancholic features	18 –24
Less than major depression:	
—probably major depression	
—dysthymia	13–17
—mixed anxiety-depression	

refer to the classical concept of endogenous depression, characterized by a "distinct quality" of depressed mood (i.e. depressed mood is experienced as distinctly different from the kind of feeling experienced after the death of a loved one), early morning awakening, regular worsening of depression in the morning, marked psychomotor retardation or agitation, significant anorexia or weight loss, and excessive or inappropriate guilt.

Patients with MDE without psychotic features typically have a score range of 18–29 on the HAM-D, while patients with psychotic features have a score of 30 or more [21] (see Table 2.3). The randomized clinical trials with antidepressants performed after 1976 have used inclusion scores of 18 or more on the HAM-D [24, 25].

Most trials with second-generation antidepressants have excluded patients with bipolar disorder. Therefore, the evidence shows their antidepressive effect on major depression, single or recurrent. The antidepressant buproprion has not been included in this review, because as a reuptake inhibitor of noradrenaline and dopamine its major indication is bipolar depression.

The duration of an MDE has a rather large dispersion, from less than 1 month to around 2 years, typically from 6 to 12 months. Kuhn showed that in some patients who had responded to imipramine the treatment should be continuous for 2 years.

Dysthymia and Minor Depression

Table 2.3 includes the diagnosis of dysthymia among the categories of less than major depression. Patients with dysthymia in accordance with both DSM-IV and ICD-10 have a chronic depression, that is a duration of symptoms of at least 2 years. The symptomatology is fluctuating, but the severity of depression is typically between 13 and 17 on HAM-D, as shown in Table 2.3. Dysthymia equals the DSM-II diagnosis of depressive neurosis in that it is a state of chronic, but mild depression.

The depressive symptoms in dysthymia and major depression are thus covered by the HAM-D. Angst [26] has shown that dysthymia is often superimposed by episodes of major depression (double depression). Most pure dysthymia is seen in the elderly.

Table 2.3 also includes probable major depression (or minor depression) as a category of less than major depression. Minor depression means an episode of depression with a score between 13 and 17 on the HAM-D of non-chronic nature, that is with a duration of less than 2 years.

Symptom Profile: Sedative vs. Activating Antidepressants

Factor-analytic studies with the HAM-D [25] have shown that the first factor is a severity one whereas the second factor is a bipolar one, measuring anxiety vs. retardation. As discussed elsewhere [21], the Kielholz classification system for antidepressants includes a sedative-anxiolytic vs. an activating profile.

The SRMs, especially mianserin and mirtazapine whose action is also anti-histaminergic, are sedative-anxiolytic drugs. This is reflected in the use of reference drugs when evaluating the antidepressive effects of new drugs in patients with major depression. Thus, mirtazapine has typically been compared to amitriptyline, whereas the SSRIs and moclobemide typically have been compared to imipramine, and reboxetine to imipramine or desipramine.

TREATMENT OF AN EPISODE OF MAJOR DEPRESSION

Figure 2.1 shows the terminology of response, remission, relapse, and recovery as introduced by Frank *et al* [27] and Kupfer [28]. With reference to HAM-D, a response is defined as at least a 50% reduction of the pre-treatment score, and a full remission as a score of 7 or less. According to the European guidelines for antidepressants [29], the treatment of an episode of major depression covers both a short- and a medium-term period. The short-term treatment Kupfer [28] calls the acute therapy of depression. The duration of the acute therapy is typically 6–8 weeks; the response will typically occur after 4 weeks of therapy and full remission after 8 weeks. However, as shown by Stassen and Angst [30], a 20–25% reduction of HAM-D will typically occur after 2 weeks of therapy (early improvement, Figure 2.1).

The medium-term treatment typically lasts 6–12 months (Figure 2.1). If the full remission after 8 weeks is sustained after the end of the treatment,

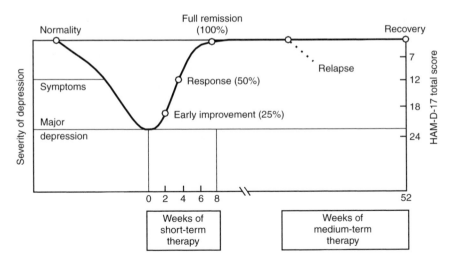

FIGURE 2.1 Terminology of the treatment of a major depressive episode of which the short-term treatment is 8 weeks and the medium-term trial period is 44 weeks
Source: modified from Kupfer, 1991 [28]

the patient has then recovered (i.e. has returned to the state of health prior to the episode of major depression). The medium-term treatment is called relapse prevention therapy because the depressive symptoms will develop again if the treatment is stopped during this period, and is referred to by Frank *et al* [27] as continuation therapy.

Long-term treatment is an interepisodic treatment to prevent the recurrence of new episodes of major depression. It is a prophylactic or maintenance therapy according to Frank *et al* [27].

EVIDENCE OF CLINICAL EFFECT OF FIRST-GENERATION ANTIDEPRESSANTS

Evidence-based medicine refers to the outcome of randomized clinical trials (RCTs). Evidence means empirical documentation. The use of placebo tablets when evaluating the effect of pharmacological treatment in randomized controlled trials was introduced in medicine at a time when the first-generation antidepressants had already been found to be effective in open trials. At that time, in the late 1950s or early 1960s, ECT was the only effective reference treatment.

The first review that selectively included RCTs for measuring efficacy of first-generation antidepressants was published by Morris and Beck [31]. All RCTs were pertinent to short-term treatment. Morris and Beck noticed many intertrial differences, for example in the diagnostic assessment of depression, in definition of response, in the nature of control treatment, and in the statistical analysis. In the following, short-term trials have been classified according to the setting in which they were conducted: inpatients vs. outpatients. The first trial conducted in the setting of general practice (GP) was published in 1970 [32]. As with the second-generation antidepressants, a very limited number of trials have been performed in the GP setting, although this is the setting from which more than 80% of the prescriptions come. The term superior or inferior as outcome of an RCT in the following means that the difference between two forms of treatment under investigation is of statistical significance.

Comparison to ECT

In a series of clinical trials with HAM-D and global ratings in the early 1960s, Robin *et al* in England found that ECT was superior to imipramine in severely depressed inpatients and that imipramine was superior to phenelzine in moderately depressed patients [33–35].

In a more comprehensive British study [36], which was a multicenter trial, it was confirmed that ECT was superior to imipramine, while imipramine was found superior to placebo, contrary to phenelzine.

Most patients with psychotic depression do not respond even to high-dose TCAs. However, combination therapy with neuroleptics such as perphenazine seems to be useful [37].

Comparison to Placebo

Table 2.4 shows the antidepressive effect of MAOIs (phenelzine is the most investigated one) and TCAs (imipramine most thoroughly investigated, followed by amitriptyline). While Table 2.4 contains most of the RCTs for the medium- and long-term treatment, only a few RCTs have been included for short-term treatment, about which several meta-analyses are available [31, 56–60].

Concerning phenelzine, Paykel [38] reported that it was inferior to TCAs in hospitalized patients and that it was no better than placebo. However, in depressed outpatients phenelzine was found superior to placebo in short-term treatment [40]. As shown in Table 2.4, phenelzine was better than placebo in relapse prevention as well as in recurrence prevention trials [40]. In medium-term relapse prevention trials it was found that phenelzine was superior to placebo, while nortriptyline was no better [39]. The dose of phenelzine in short- as well as medium- and long-term treatment was between 45 and 90 mg daily.

As a non-selective MAOI, phenelzine provokes a so-called "cheese reaction", that is a tyramine-related hypertensive crisis. The dietary restriction of foods containing tyramine is considered too problematic for family doctors and for at least 75% of psychiatrists [61].

Concerning imipramine, Table 2.4 shows most of the RCTs in the medium- and long-term treatment. The most elegant of the RCTs is the one performed by Frank et al [46], in which plasma levels of imipramine have been monitored. It was shown that the dose which had proven effective in the short-term treatment should also be used in medium- and long-term treatment. In the medium-term study performed by Mindham et al [44] imipramine was not found superior to placebo, probably because of the low dose. The trial by Seager and Bird [43] was a post-ECT study. There was a high frequency of relapse after ECT (around 50%) and imipramine was found significantly better than placebo.

The first RCT in a GP setting was carried out by Porter in 1970 [32]. He found that imipramine after 2 weeks of treatment had a response rate of 64%, while placebo had a response rate of 58%. The difference was statistically not significant, emphasizing the rather high placebo response in general practice.

Placebo-controlled amitriptyline trials are few in hospitalized patients. The examples shown in Table 2.4 for the outpatient studies are from the

TABLE 2.4 Randomized controlled trials of first-generation antidepressants compared to placebo in major depression

Classes of antidepressants	Short-term		Medium-term ≤12 months	Long-term ≥24 months
	Inpatients	Outpatients		
Monoamine oxidase inhibitors (MAOIs)				
Phenelzine (dose 45–90 mg daily)	*not superior* MRC, 1965 [36]	*superior* Paykel, 1979 [38]	*superior* Georgotas et al, 1989 [39]	*superior* Robinson et al, 1991 [40]
Monoamine reuptake inhibitors (TCAs)				
Imipramine (dose 150–300 mg daily)	*superior* Kenning et al, 1960 [41] MRC, 1965 [36]	*superior* Ball and Kiloh, 1959 [42] *not superior* Porter, 1970 [32]	*superior* Seager and Bird, 1962 [43] Mindham et al, 1973 [44]a	*superior* Prien et al, 1973 [45] Frank et al, 1990 [46] Kupfer et al, 1992 [47] Frank et al, 1993 [48]
Amitriptyline (dose 150–300 mg daily)	*superior* Rees and Davis, 1965 [49]a Garry and Leonard [50]	*superior* Paykel et al, 1988 [51]	*superior* Mindham et al, 1973 [44]a Klerman et al, 1974 [52] Coppen et al, 1978 [53] Stein et al, 1980 [54]	*superior* Glen et al, 1984 [55]a

aTrial with major methodological drawbacks.

well-performed trial by Paykel *et al* [51] in the setting of family doctors. Most antidepressants are prescribed by the family doctor, but the number of trials is very limited. Paykel *et al* [51] showed that amitriptyline was superior to placebo both in the group of patients with pre-treatment HAM-D scores between 18 and 24 (corresponding to major depression, Table 2.3, and illustrated in Figure 2.1) and with pre-treatment HAM-D scores between 13 and 17 (corresponding to probably major depression). In patients with lower pre-treatment HAM-D scores, placebo was equal to amitriptyline.

The very comprehensive overview by Smith *et al* [56], comparing TCAs with placebo in the setting of psychiatric care (inpatients or outpatients), showed a response advantage of 15–20% in favour of TCAs. Thus, the response rate was 64% for TCAs and 45% for placebo, which is similar to the rates found by the British multicenter study [36]. This is in agreement with other meta-analyses comparing TCAs with placebo [57–59].

The duration of RCTs with first-generation antidepressants was typically 4–5 weeks in the short-term evaluation against placebo. In terms of HAM-D, the results were traditionally illustrated as shown in Figure 2.2. Thus, before treatment the HAM-D score was typically around 25, and after 4–5 weeks of treatment it was around 10 in the active therapy group (TCAs) and around 15 in the placebo group [60]. This difference of 5 points on HAM-D at endpoint (i.e. after 5 weeks of treatment) between TCAs and placebo is still accepted as a clinically significant difference. It equals the 15–20% advantage of TCAs over placebo in short-term trials when response to treatment is measured as a 50% reduction of HAM-D from pre-treatment to endpoint.

Part of the placebo effect in short-term trials has been explained by Hamilton [62] as the therapeutic contrast effect. The treating doctor is often

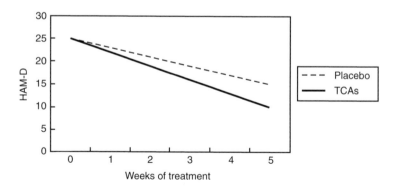

FIGURE 2.2   The short-term outcome in terms of HAM-D scores in placebo-controlled trials with TCAs. Notice that at endpoint (5 weeks of treatment) the difference between TCAs and placebo is 5 points on the HAM-D. This has been accepted as a clinically significant difference
Source: modified from Bech, 1978 [60]

in doubt on how to rate some of the items on HAM-D. The doctor will tend to give the patient a higher score at the beginning of treatment and a lower score at the end on such "doubtful" items. Hamilton estimated that up to 6 points of the placebo improvement is due to this therapeutic contrast effect.

Within the TCAs, amitriptyline was considered a sedative-anxiolytic antidepressant, whereas imipramine was considered to be an activating antidepressant (e.g. [63]). The study by Hordern *et al* [63] is one of the few trials in which the age of the patients has been associated with antidepressive response. However, in so far as the patients' age in the study ranges from 18 to 70 years, this study is typical for the other RCTs with first-generation antidepressants. Hordern *et al* subdivided their patients into "young" (18–49 years), "middle-aged" (50–59 years) and "elderly" (60–70 years). They found no difference in antidepressive response between the three groups. On the HAM-D, the only difference in symptom profile was that the elderly patients scored higher on the item agitation, which was confirmed by Stage [64]. Hordern's study also included a 6-month medium-term trial in which amitriptyline was shown to be superior to imipramine.

The review by Gerson *et al* [24] shows that RCTs with antidepressants in "aging" patients have been conducted with patients between 55 and 70 years of age rather than with patients between 70 and 85. Gerson *et al* found very few trials with aging patients in which imipramine, amitriptyline, and phenelzine had been investigated, but all RCTs with these antidepressants showed that the active drug was superior to placebo. The results summarized in Table 2.4 are in agreement with the conclusions by Morris and Beck [31], namely that the TCAs are more effective than placebo; in no trial was placebo found more effective than TCAs. In outpatients also phenelzine is more effective than placebo. Finally, Morris and Beck showed that in the depressive episode lithium is no better than placebo.

EVIDENCE OF CLINICAL EFFECT OF NEW-GENERATION ANTIDEPRESSANTS

With the introduction of the new generation of antidepressants in the 1980s, the RCTs became more sophisticated. Thus, the DSM-III diagnosis of major depression became more and more accepted and the HAM-D was used in more than 90% of the trials.

Such methodological standardization has facilitated the use of meta-analyses, which are a statistical tool to provide an objective summary of the various RCTs. This method takes into consideration the size of the RCTs with a weighting to attach more importance to larger trials. However, one problem with meta-analyses is the publication bias, that is negative results may not have been published. Another problem is that many trials only include data of patients who have completed at least 2 weeks of treatment (protocol analysis), although the clinically most meaningful analysis is to include all randomized patients (intention-to-treat analysis). One of the few examples of a meta-analysis including both published and unpublished trials with an intention-to-treat analysis is the citalopram vs. amitriptyline study by Bech and Cialdella [65].

The use of other clinician-administered rating scales than HAM-D, such as the Montgomery–Åsberg Scale (MADRS [66]) has not improved the RCTs but rather made the prospective meta-analyses more difficult [67], because it is often difficult to see which scale had been used as the primary outcome scale.

Among the meta-analyses on published RCTs comparing SSRIs with TCAs in short-term treatment, the most appropriate was made by Anderson and Tomenson in 1994 [68], whereas the most appropriate meta-analysis on the medium- and long-term treatment with antidepressants has been made by Loonen and Zwanikken [69]. The latter review concludes that in continuation therapy (medium-term treatment) the antidepressant treatment at the end of the treatment period should be discontinued very gradually in order to evaluate relapsing symptoms. Withdrawal reactions after abrupt discontinuation of SSRIs can induce a syndrome of dizziness, paraesthesia, and headache [70].

The new-generation antidepressants have been approved by the regulators on the basis of short-term trials against placebo. In general, the new drugs have not been found superior to the first-generation drugs in the short-term treatment, but they have been found safer. Only post-marketing trials have focused on the patient's own assessment of outcome — referred to as quality of life [71]. The number of trials evaluating medium- or long-term outcome has been rather limited.

Second-generation Antidepressants vs. Placebo

Table 2.5 shows examples of the placebo-controlled trials evaluating short-term treatment, and all RCTs evaluating medium- and long-term treatment.

Among the new generation of antidepressants, only moclobemide has been included from the MAOIs. From the class of monoamine reuptake inhibitors, venlafaxine and the SSRIs have been included. Although rather selective, desipramine and nortriptyline are first-generation antidepressants. On the other hand, reboxetine is so new that there are no published medium- or long-term trials.

TABLE 2.5 Randomized controlled trials of second-generation antidepressants compared to placebo in major depression

	Short-term		Medium-term (≤12 months)	Long-term (≥24 months)
	Inpatients	Outpatients		
Reversible inhibitors of monoamine-oxidase type A (RIMA)				
Moclobemide	Angst et al., 1993 [72] Lecrubier and Guelfi, 1990 [73]	Stabl et al., 1989 [74]		
Selective serotonin and noradrenaline reuptake inhibitors (SNRIs)				
Venlafaxine	Guelfi et al., 1995 [75]	Rudolph et al., 1998 [76]	Entsuah et al., 1996 [77]	
Selective serotonin reuptake inhibitors (SSRIs)				
	Feighner et al., 1989 [78] (fluvoxamine)	Feighner and Overo, 1999 [79] (citalopram) Greenberg et al., 1994 [80] (fluoxetine) Anderson and Tomenson, 1994 [68] (all SSRIs)	Doogan and Caillard, 1992 [81] (sertraline) Montgomery and Dunbar, 1993 [82] (paroxetine) Montgomery et al., 1993 [83] (citalopram) Robert and Montgomery, 1995 [84] (citalopram) Reimherr et al., 1998 [85] (fluoxetine) Montgomery et al., 1988 [86] (fluoxetine)	Terra and Montgomery, 1998 [87] (fluvoxamine) Wade et al., 1998 [88] (citalopram)
Serotonin receptor modulators (SRMs)				
Nefazodone	Feighner et al., 1998 [89]	Mendels et al., 1995 [90]	Anton et al., 1994 [91]	
Mirtazapine	Vartiainen and Leinonen, 1994 [92] Khan, 1995 [93]	Bech and Zivkov, 1998 [94]	Montgomery et al., 1998 [95]	

Bupropion was introduced in the US in 1989, but was temporarily removed from the American market because of an unacceptable occurrence of seizures. It was reintroduced with clearer guidelines for its prescription, and since 1997 a sustained release preparation has secured a more gradual dosage. In contrast to the SSRIs, bupropion is only rarely associated with sexual complaints, and as its main indication is bipolar depression it has not been included in Table 2.5. From the class of SRMs, nefazodone and mirtazapine have been included.

Nefazodone was introduced in 1995 and has a structural relationship to trazodone, which has been on the US market since 1981. A review of the antidepressive effect of trazodone by Schatzberg et al [96] showed it to be as effective as amitriptyline or imipramine in inpatients as well as out-patients. However, in Europe trazodone was found inferior to amitriptyline in hospitalized patients [97].

Mirtazapine has recently been introduced both in the US and Europe and has a structural relationship to mianserin, which has been on the European market over two decades and whose EEG profile was shown by Itil et al [98] to be similar to amitriptyline. The antidepressive effect of mianserin has been shown to be inferior to that of amitriptyline in severe endogenous depression [99]. In the GP setting, however, mianserin was found superior to placebo, with an onset of action after 2 weeks [100]. In long-term treatment it was found inferior to lithium [53].

Table 2.5 shows that placebo-controlled trials to evaluate the medium- and long-term effects of moclobemide in major depression are lacking. The short-term study by Angst et al [72] includes both in patients and outpatients. However, the clearest advantage of moclobemide over placebo was seen in patients with a pre-treatment HAM-D score of 28 or higher.

The class of SSRIs includes five drugs: citalopram, fluoxetine, fluvox-amine, paroxetine, and sertraline, while the class of dual reuptake inhibitors, the SNRIs (selective serotonin and noradrenaline reuptake inhibitors) only includes venlafaxine.

At low doses, that is below 150 mg daily, venlafaxine predominantly inhibits the reuptake of serotonin and should in principle be acting as an SSRI. At higher doses, especially around 300 mg, the reuptake inhibition of noradrenaline is significant. In the study by Rudolph et al [76], the increase of the dosage in a range from 75 to 375 mg was associated with a greater anti-depressive effect. In contrast to the SSRIs, venlafaxine shows a dose–response relationship [101] which in some trials has also been reported for TCAs, for example imipramine [102]. The dose for venlafaxine in the medium-term, relapse prevention trial was around 175 mg daily. In the short-term treatment of hospitalized patients with major depression, a venlafaxine dose of around 300 mg is needed, while the continuation dose might be around 175 mg daily, indicating that reuptake inhibition of serotonin is important for relapse prevention.

The placebo-controlled trials with SSRIs, as shown in Table 2.5, support the hypothesis that they are useful for relapse prevention (five trials showing superiority to placebo) and for recurrence prevention (two trials showing superiority to placebo). The dose used in the medium- and long-term trials of the different SSRIs is similar to the dose effective in short-term trials. The most appropriate dose for fluvoxamine in the short-term treatment of major depression is 100 mg daily, as shown by Bech [21], and this is also the dose of fluvoxamine in the long-term study by Terra and Montgomery [87].

The SRMs nefazodone and mirtazapine were both superior to placebo in the medium-term relapse prevention trials, in a dose similar to that found effective in short-term trials. However, the two mirtazapine trials with inpatients (Table 2.5) showed only a marginal drug advantage over placebo.

Second-generation vs. First-generation Antidepressants in Major Depression

In general, very few RCTs have been carried out to evaluate the relative effects of second-generation vs. first-generation antidepressants in medium-term treatment (Table 2.6). Moclobemide has a much safer profile than phenelzine or isocarboxazide; in particular, it has no "cheese reaction". However, compared to phenelzine or isocarboxazide, moclobemide seems to be less effective in atypical depression [106]. In atypical depression, anxiety is often the predominant feature, including states of phobias (see, e.g., [133]). Controlled studies in patients with social phobia have shown that both phenelzine [134] and moclobemide [135] are effective. The moclobemide dose in the latter trial was 600 mg daily. However, Noyes et al [136] have not been able to confirm the effect of moclobemide in social phobia when compared to placebo. Even a moclobemide dose of 900 mg daily showed no superiority to placebo. In the trials shown in Table 2.6, which indicate that moclobemide is inferior to clomipramine in major depression, a dose less than 600 mg daily was administered.

In elderly depressed patients (60–80 years of age), moclobemide has been found equal to maprotiline and mianserin [137]. In a meta-analysis, Angst and Stabl [138] showed that moclobemide was as effective as TCAs in younger and elderly patients, using 65 as the cut-off age. However, it was found inferior to nortriptyline in patients with major depression in the age range 60–90 years [105]. Finally, in the general practice setting, Kragh-Sørensen et al [107] showed that moclobemide was equal to clomipramine, whereas Beaumont et al [108] had found it inferior to dothiepin (a TCA), though only marginally.

TABLE 2.6 Randomized controlled trials of second-generation vs. first-generation antidepressants in major depression

	Short-term treatment			Medium-term continuation treatment
	Inpatients	Outpatients	GP patients	
Reversible inhibitors of monoamine-oxidase type A (RIMA)				
Moclobemide	*vs. clomipramine* equal: Guelfi et al., 1992 [103] inferior: DUAG, 1993 [104] inferior: Nair et al., 1995 [105]	*vs. clomipramine* inferior: Larsen et al., 1991 [106]	*vs. clomipramine* equal: Kragh-Sørensen et al., 1995 [107] *vs. dothiepin* inferior: Beaumont et al., 1993 [108]	
Selective serotonin and noradrenaline reuptake inhibitors (SNRIs)				
Venlafaxine	*vs. imipramine* superior: Benkert et al., 1996 [109]	*vs. imipramine* equal: Morton et al., 1995 [110]	*vs. imipramine* superior: Lecrubier et al., 1997 [111]	*vs. imipramine* equal: Burnett and Dinan, 1998 [112]
Selective serotonin reuptake inhibitors (SSRIs)				
Paroxetine	*vs. imipramine* equal: Nielsen et al., 1991 [113] *vs. clomipramine* inferior: DUAG, 1990 [114] *vs. amitriptyline* inferior: Anderson, 1998 [115]	*vs. imipramine* equal: Øhrberg et al., 1992 [116] *vs. clomipramine* equal: Samuelian and Hackett, 1998 [117]	*vs. amitriptyline* equal: Christiansen et al., 1996 [118]	*vs. imipramine* superior: Lauritzen et al., 1996 [119]
Citalopram	*vs. clomipramine* inferior: DUAG, 1986 [120] *vs. maprotiline* equal: Timmermann et al., 1987 [121]	*vs. amitriptyline* equal: Bech and Cialdella, 1992 [65]	*vs. imipramine* equal: Fuglum et al., 1996 [122]	

continues overleaf

TABLE 2.6 (*continued*)

	Short-term treatment			Medium-term continuation treatment
	Inpatients	Outpatients	GP patients	
Fluoxetine and fluvoxamine	*vs. TCAs* *equal*: Anderson, 1998 [115]	*vs. TCAs* *equal*: Bech, 1989 [67] Stokes and Holtz, 1997 [123]	*vs. dothiepin* *equal*: Corne and Hall, 1989 [124]	
Sertraline	*vs. amitriptyline* *equal*: Hegerl et al, 1997 [125]	*vs. amitriptyline* *equal*: Reimherr et al, 1990 [126]	*vs. clomipramine* *equal*: Moon et al, 1994 [127]	
Serotonin receptor modulators (SRMs)				
Nefazodone	*vs. imipramine* *equal*: Marcus and Mendels, 1996 [128]	*vs. imipramine* *equal*: Rickels et al, 1994 [129]		*vs. imipramine* *equal*: Anton et al, 1994 [91]
Mirtazapine	*vs. amitriptyline* *equal*: Zivkov and de Jongh,1995 [130] *vs. clomipramine* *equal*: Rickels et al, 1995 [131] *vs. imipramine* *inferior*: Bruijn et al, 1996 [132]	*vs. amitriptyline* *equal*: Bech, 2001 [94]		*vs. amitriptyline* *superior*: Montgomery et al, 1998 [95]

Venlafaxine has been found to have an earlier onset of action than imipramine in patients hospitalized for major depression when the venlafaxine dose was escalated over 5 days, resulting in a daily dose of 375 mg [109]. The imipramine dose was only 200 mg daily, that is lower than the 300 mg recommended by Simpson et al [102].

The SSRIs have been shown to differ from TCAs in severely depressed inpatients [115]. No clear dose–response relationship has been found for the SSRIs. Still, one of the most comprehensive fixed-dose studies with SSRIs [79] found that only a dosage of 40 or 60 mg daily of citalopram was superior to placebo on HAM-D. However, dosages of 10 and 20 mg daily were superior to placebo on the depressive core symptoms on the HAM-D, that is the depression factor HAM-D-6 (see Table 2.2), which has also been found valid in meta-analyses of mirtazapine against placebo [94]. In other words, there is a rather flat dose–response curve for the SSRIs.

Among the TCAs, amitriptyline and to some extent clomipramine, but not imipramine, seemed to be superior to SSRIs in hospitalized patients with major depression. However, when the Danish University Antidepressant Group (DUAG) study [120] was reanalysed by using a 50% reduction of HAM-D as outcome [122], 69% of the patients had responded to clomipramine and 58% to citalopram. This difference was not statistically significant.

In the medium-term relapse prevention therapy, paroxetine was found superior to imipramine [119]. Table 2.4 shows that Seager and Bird [43], but not Mindham et al [44], found imipramine to be superior to placebo in relapse prevention. The study by Seager and Bird was a post-ECT trial, like the study by Lauritzen et al from 1996 [119], which showed that patients treated with paroxetine had a 12% relapse rate over 6 months, whereas imipramine had a 30% relapse rate. One trial has compared nefazodone with TCAs in the short-term treatment of hospitalized patients with major depression, while three trials compared mirtazapine to TCAs. No differences were found in these trials, apart from the study by Bruijn et al [132], in which mirtazapine was found inferior to imipramine. In that trial the imipramine dose was optimal by blood level determinations, while the optimal effective dose for mirtazapine in hospitalized patients is unknown. However, the amitriptyline dose in the medium-term trial by Montgomery et al [95] was suboptimal (140 mg daily) which might explain the superiority of mirtazapine (30 mg daily) in that study.

The new selective noradrenaline reuptake inhibitor reboxetine has been evaluated against desipramine in hospitalized patients with major depression [139] and against imipramine in outpatients with major depression [140]. In both trials reboxetine was found equal to the TCAs. However, in the latter study, reboxetine was superior to imipramine when HAM-D was used, and equal when the assessment was made by the MADRS.

Other Second-generation Antidepressants vs. Fluoxetine in Major Depression

Available RCTs comparing other second-generation antidepressants with fluoxetine have usually found no difference in terms of efficacy. However, venlafaxine has been found to be superior to fluoxetine in two trials (Table 2.7). An inpatient trial by Clerc et al [145] compared 200 mg venlafaxine with 40 mg fluoxetine daily, and the difference between the two drugs was significant when measured on HAM-D after 4 weeks of treatment.

Moreover, mirtazapine has been found to be marginally superior to fluoxetine in the study by Wheatley et al [156]. Outpatients as well as inpatients were included in this study. The difference between mirtazapine and fluoxetine was statistically significant after 3 and 4 weeks of treatment, but only marginal at endpoint.

TREATMENT OF DYSTHYMIA AND MINOR DEPRESSION

In a recent review on antidepressant efficacy in the treatment of dysthymia [157], it was concluded that many methodological problems are still unresolved in the clinical trials for reliably distinguishing between pure dysthymia and double depression. Among the trials in which HAM-D has been used with a separation of the diagnostic subgroups and with imipramine and placebo as references, it has been shown that moclobemide [158] and sertraline [159] were similar to imipramine and superior to placebo. However, more reliable and valid trials are needed. Furthermore, very few trials have evaluated the long-term outcome of antidepressants in dysthymia [160, 161].

There have been very few RCTs to evaluate the various antidepressants in minor depression or probable major depression. The most important trials have been carried out by Paykel et al [51] showing in the setting of general practice that amitriptyline was superior to placebo. In recent trials it has been shown that paroxetine equals maprotiline [162] and that citalopram equals imipramine [122].

ADVERSE DRUG REACTIONS

While the antidepressive efficacy of the first- and second-generation antidepressants is assessable in terms of response and remission on the HAM-D, no internationally accepted scale for measuring the adverse reaction profile of the different antidepressants has been developed. By adverse drug reactions in this context we mean pharmacological, dose-related reactions, not the idiosyncratic or allergic types.

TABLE 2.7 Randomized controlled trials of second-generation antidepressants vs. fluoxetine in major depression

	Short-term treatment			Medium-term
	Inpatients	Outpatients	GP patients	
Reversible inhibitors of monoamine-oxidase type A (RIMA)				
Moclobemide	equal Gattaz et al., 1995 [141]	equal Lönnqvist et al., 1994 [142] equal Williams et al., 1993 [143] equal Geerts et al., 1994 [144]		
Selective serotonin and noradrenaline reuptake inhibitors (SNRIs)				
Venlafaxine	superior Clerc et al., 1994 [145]	superior Dierick et al., 1996 [146]	equal Tylee et al., 1997 [147]	
Selective serotonin reuptake inhibitors (SSRIs)	vs. paroxetine: equal Tignol, 1993 [148]	vs. paroxetine: equal Geretsegger et al., 1994 [149] vs. sertraline: equal Bennie et al., 1995 [150]	vs. citalopram: equal Patris et al., 1996 [151]	vs. sertraline: equal van Moffaert, 1995 [152]
Serotonin receptor modulators (SRMs)				
Nefazodone		equal Aguglia et al., 1993 [153] Gillin et al., 1997 [154] Rush et al., 1998 [155]		
Mirtazapine		marginally superior Wheatley et al., 1998 [156]		

Compared to the first-generation MAOIs moclobemide is a very safe drug, for example without any "cheese effect" and it is also safe when used in anaesthesia [163].

When Kuhn demonstrated the antidepressive effect of imipramine, he observed no major side effects. However, he later reported [164] that imipramine, after it had been marketed in 1958, was associated with a number of side effects when used at therapeutic doses in less severely depressed outpatients. Imipramine and the other TCAs have anticholinergic (dry mouth, constipation, urinary retention, somnolence, blurred vision), antihistaminic (fatigue, somnolence, weight gain) or antiadrenergic (postural hypotension and dizziness) side effects, which are common within the therapeutic antidepressive dosage. These side effects of the TCAs have particular relevance in older patients [165]. In overdose TCAs have a high lethality risk because of their cardiovascular (quinidine-like) effect. The SSRIs show such side effects as nausea, headache, tremor, increased perspiration, and sexual dysfunction.

When comparing TCAs and SSRIs in meta-analyses based on RCTs in short-term treatment, the discontinuation rates due to side effects in the two classes of antidepressants are the focus of attention. Montgomery and Kasper [166] showed, in their meta-analysis including 67 trials, that the discontinuation rate due to side effects was 14% in patients treated with the SSRIs and 19% in those treated with the TCAs. The difference, although not great, is statistically significant. In a recent meta-analysis by Hotopf et al [167], it was confirmed that fewer patients on SSRIs discontinued treatment because of side effects. However, when the TCAs were subdivided into "old" (imipramine and amitriptyline) and "newer" (nortriptyline and desipramine), the difference in discontinuation rates between SSRIs and TCAs was only statistically significant in relation to the "old" TCAs.

In a meta-analysis of adverse drug reactions in short-term trials with citalopram against amitriptyline, the greatest difference at endpoint concerned dry mouth, whose frequency was 27% in the amitriptyline group vs. 3% in the citalopram group [65].

Another side effect of TCAs in medium- or long-term treatment is weight gain. Paykel et al [168] showed that, in medium-term treatment with amitriptyline, the mean weight increase was around 3 Kg, with a tendency to an increased weight of 5% per year. In the 8-week study by Christiansen et al [118] comparing paroxetine with amitriptyline, a significant weight increase was seen only in the amitriptyline-treated patients. Of the second-generation antidepressants, mianserin and mirtazapine also have weight gain as a side effect.

In trials measuring behavioral toxicity in connection with cognitive and psychomotor function, for example car-driving, it has been shown that TCAs induce more impairments than SSRIs [169]. Toxicity in overdose has been compared in some studies, although such data obviously are retrospective in nature. Cassidy and Henry [170] showed that amitriptyline and imipramine had higher mortality than clomipramine, while mortality with mianserin was rather low. The overdose toxicity of SSRIs seems very low or absent [171]. However, fatal cases of overdoses with SSRIs plus moclobemide, or clomipramine plus moclobemide, have been reported [172].

The first-generation antidepressants—both MAOIs and TCAs—have been associated with sexual dysfunction, including decreased sexual interest, erection failure, impaired ejaculation and impaired orgasm [173]. Although phenelzine induces more sexual dysfunction than imipramine [174], moclobemide induces far fewer complaints [175].

All SSRIs can induce sexual dysfunction. Baldwin and Birtwistle [173] have reviewed fluoxetine, showing that from the first reports in 1985 until 1995 the percentage of sexual dysfunction increased from 5 to 30%, probably because of a greater awareness of this side effect. Neither nefazodone nor mianserin or mirtazapine have been associated with sexual dysfunction.

The evaluation of social functioning has not been systematically performed in medium-term trials. In a short-term trial of 8 weeks, reboxetine compared to fluoxetine showed no difference in outcome measured on HAM-D, but it was superior on the Social Adaptation Self-evaluation Scale (SASS) [176]. As discussed elsewhere [177] quality of life assessments in medium- or long-term trials with antidepressants are important.

COMBINATIONS BETWEEN ANTIDEPRESSANTS

The synergistic benefits of serotonin and noradrenaline reuptake inhibitors in the acute treatment of major depression were first noticed by Nelson *et al* in 1991 [178], in an open trial in which fluoxetine and desipramine were combined. In this trial fluoxetine raised the blood levels of desipramine.

The combination of phenelzine or isocarboxazide with amitriptyline is safe [179], while combinations of MAOIs with clomipramine or SSRIs or venlafaxine can have a fatal outcome. The combination of mianserin with isocarboxazide is safe [180].

Lithium augmentation trials are those in which lithium is added to an antidepressant after 3–6 weeks in a short-term trial in non-responders. In a placebo-controlled trial with amitriptyline, de Montigny *et al* [181] showed a response rate of 100% in the amitriptyline-treated vs. only 20% in the placebo-treated patients. In patients treated with fluoxetine [182] lithium augmentation showed superiority to placebo augmentation, with a response rate of 52 vs. 25%. Lithium augmentation with venlafaxine in an open study by Hoencamp *et al* [183] showed a reduction on HAM-D but not a response [112].

The combination of pindolol, a serotonin autoreceptor antagonist, with SSRIs has induced a rapid onset of action in some trials, but not in others [184]. Augmentation with mianserin in fluoxetine-resistant patients with major depression is superior to continuation with fluoxetine alone [185], which is in agreement with the study by Dam *et al* [186].

Augmentation with buspirone, a partial 5HT-1A agonist, in therapy-resistant depressed patients has also been suggested [187, 188]. In mild degrees but not severe forms of depression buspirone might itself have an antidepressive effect [189]. One double-blind placebo-controlled trial with buspirone has been carried out in patients resistant to SSRIs [190]. However, a high placebo response was operating.

Augmentation as well as combination therapy have, of course, pharmacokinetic implications. Thus, although the various SSRIs are rather similar in their antidepressive effect, there are many pharmacokinetic differences among them. Although all SSRIs inhibit CYP 2D6, paroxetine and fluoxetine are the most potent [191]. Therefore, paroxetine and fluoxetine have the potential for causing serious drug–drug interactions with some CYP 2D6 substrates. For example, desipramine is a CYP 2D6 substrate, which is why the blood level of desipramine raises when combined with fluoxetine, as found by Nelson *et al* [178]. Fluvoxamine is a very potent inhibitor of CYP 1A2, and several TCAs (amitriptyline, imipramine, and clomipramine) are CYP 1A2 substrates. The doses of these TCAs should be reduced by at least 50% when combined with fluvoxamine.

When combination therapy has been suggested, for example the use of mianserin with phenelzine or isocarboxazide, and mianserin or mirtazapine with fluoxetine, it has, among other things, been recommended because pharmacokinetics have been considered safe.

Nefazodone is an inhibitor of CYP 3A4 particularly at a dose of 300 mg or more daily. Among the CYP 3A4 substrates are alprazolam, diazepam, and imipramine.

PROFILE OF ANTIDEPRESSANTS AND DOSAGE RECOMMENDATIONS

Most RCTs with antidepressants have focused on short-term treatment, although a substance is accepted as an antidepressant not only if it can be shown to be more effective than placebo in short-term trials, but also if it is effective in medium-term trials, corresponding to the total duration of a major depressive episode [29], typically carried out in an outpatient setting (although more than 80% of the patients with major depression are treated in the GP setting). It is also a paradox that so few trials have been carried out in the elderly between 75 and 90 years of age, as the benign safety profile of the second-generation antidepressants has special clinical relevance for this group of patients [192].

The drug–placebo advantage in short-term trials is 15–20% when measured as a 50% reduction of the HAM-D score from pre-treatment (baseline) to endpoint, which equals a global assessment of very much and much improvement. In their review of the first-generation antidepressants, Smith *et al* [56] found the 15–20% drug advantage relatively low. The short-term trials with second-generation antidepressants also have a 15–20% advantage over placebo. However, in medium-term trials, the new-generation antidepressants have a greater advantage over placebo. In fact, the SSRIs have a relapse rate below 20% in the continuation treatment, while placebo has a rate of 50%. The first-generation antidepressants have a relapse rate closer to 30 than 20%. In the short-term trials comparing first- and second-generation antidepressants, it is safety rather than antidepressive efficacy that gives the new drugs their advantage. When comparing the second-generation drugs with each other, the differences in efficacy are so small that only large trials with around 300 patients in each group are needed to show them, as discussed by Lader [193].

The advantage of second-generation antidepressants over placebo is there-fore especially to be found in continuation therapy. This aspect should have been considered by Medawar [194] when making attempts to downregulate the clinical outcome of RCTs with antidepressants. The problem of clinical vs. statistical significance of first-generation antidepressants in the short-term trials is equal to other pharmacological treatments in medicine [195]. However, Medawar's critical remarks concerning the quality of the journals in which many of the RCTs have been published might be valid, although it is not illogical that most RCTs are published in psychopharmacological jour-nals. Nevertheless, the reliability of the outcome measures in the hand of the treating psychiatrist is rarely shown and publication in general psychiatric journals might have had some balancing influence in this respect.

Table 2.8 shows the profile and dosage recommendations of first-generation antidepressants in major depression without psychotic features. In patients with major depression with psychotic features ECT is still recommended, although combination with antipsychotics in some cases is sufficient [196]. However, in the medium-term post-ECT relapse prevention period, an SSRI antidepressant should be used.

Table 2.9 shows the profile and dosage recommendations of second-generation antidepressants in major depression. Venlafaxine and the SSRIs are the best documented drugs for the treatment of a major depressive episode (short- and medium-term). The SSRIs have also been shown to be effective in the long-term therapy of recurrent major depression. In contrast, the documentation pertaining to moclobemide and reboxetine is still very limited in medium- and long-term treatment. The problem with venlafaxine

TABLE 2.8 Profile and dosage recommendations of first-generation antidepressants in major depression

Classes of antidepressants	Profile	Dosage
Monoamine-oxidase inhibitors		
Phenelzine	Outpatients in psychiatric setting with chronic-like, atypical major depression	
	Non-sedating	45–90 mg
Monoamine reuptake inhibitors		
Clomipramine	Psychiatric inpatients with severe major depression	
	Short-term	50–150 mg
	Non-sedating	
Amitriptyline	Psychiatric inpatients with severe major depression	
	Especially agitated	
	Short- and medium-term	100–300 mg
	Sedating	
Imipramine	Psychiatric outpatients with major depression	
	Short-, medium- and long-term	100–300 mg
	Non-sedating	

and the SSRIs is sexual dysfunction. Combination therapy with nefazodone or mirtazapine in this context may be recommended, but RCTs are still needed to confirm this. In combination therapy, the various antidepressants should be tested for their effect on the cytochrome 450 system in the liver; for example the SSRIs differ considerably in this respect.

It has been outside the scope of this chapter to evaluate the choice and duration of antidepressant treatment in bipolar disorders. Over 80% of treatment of major depression is carried out in the GP setting, while bipolar disorders are still mostly treated in the psychiatric practice setting.

Antidepressants with well-documented effects in major depression also seem to be effective in double depression, that is the comorbidity of dysthymia and a major depressive episode [161]. In pure dysthymia, however, RCTs are still needed for both the old and new antidepressants. The new-generation antidepressants are, because of their benign safety profile, much more applicable in the GP setting and in elderly patients than the first-generation ones.

The dosage shown in Table 2.9 is only tentative. In elderly depressed patients, the lowest dose should be used in the first weeks of treatment. All antidepressants shown in Table 2.9 are safe in overdose. The number of dose-response studies with these antidepressants is as limited as is the situation for the TCAs [102, 198]. In general, the studies with the SSRIs have shown a flat dose-response pattern [e.g., 79, 199, 200]. However, for venlafaxine a clearer linear dose-response curve seemed to emerge [76, 201],

TABLE 2.9 Profile and dosage recommendations of second-generation antidepressants in major depression

Classes of antidepressants	Profile	Dosage
Reversible inhibitors of monoamine-oxidase type A (RIMA)		
Moclobemide	Major depression in general practice	
	Short-term	300–600 mg
	Non-sedating	
Selective serotonin and noradrenaline reuptake inhibitors (SNRIs)		
Venlafaxine	Major depression in in/outpatients and general practice	
	Short-term inpatients	225–375 mg
	Short-term outpatients and	150–225 mg
	Medium-term	
	Non-sedating	
Selective serotonin reuptake inhibitors (SSRIs)		
Citalopram	Major depression outpatients/	
Fluoxetine	general practice	20–60 mg
Fluvoxamine	Non-sedating	20–40 mg
Paroxetine		50–150 mg
Sertraline		20–50 mg
		50–150 mg
Selective noradrenaline reuptake inhibitors (NARIs)		
Reboxetine	Major depression in in/outpatients	4–8 mg
	Short-term	
	Non-sedating	
Serotonin receptor modulators (SRMs)		
Nefazodone	Major depression in in/outpatients	
	Short-, medium-term	300–600 mg
	Sedating (mild)	
Mirtazapine	Major depression in in/outpatients	
	Short-, medium-term	15–45 mg
	Sedating	

and a re-analysis of the citalopram study [202], using the HAM-D6 and a specific serotonin side-effect scale to measure clinical outcome, showed a clearer dose-response pattern also for this drug. Such studies showing linear dose-response relationships are of importance in the debate of the specific clinical effects of antidepressants [203]. The relationship between response and dose-range indicated in Table 2.9 is therefore rather diffuse, perhaps even curvilinear. Although the response to antidepressants is delayed, it is important, as shown by Stassen *et al* [197], to assess an early improvement (Figure 2.2). For the individual patient it is important to know when the improvement will appear. The dosage found effective in short-term treatment is often also the effective dose in medium- or long-term therapy.

Before the advent of antidepressants, Skottowe [3] stated that ''The initial psychiatric interview is always important, but in no group of illnesses is it of greater importance as a first step in treatment than it is in the depressions. The gentle elucidation of all the symptoms is of the highest importance.

Let the patient see that the doctor is thoroughly familiar with the kind of illness that confronts him; he knows the kind of feelings and thoughts that it brings the patient. This in itself is a most reassuring step." This observation is still valid and the HAM-D interview covers the symptoms of major depression. The second step is to let the patient be informed of the choice of antidepressant with reference to the current knowledge as summarized in this chapter. It is important thereafter to inform the patient when early improvement can be expected, and when response, remission, and recovery will take place. If the chosen antidepressant is not sufficient, combination therapy should be considered as a rational pharmacotherapy based on the mode of action in regard both to the wanted antidepressive effect and to the side effects, such as nausea, agitation, sexual dysfunction or weight gain. However, combined pharmacotherapy and psychotherapy should also be considered when residual symptoms of depression appear [204]. The use of patient-related scales for general psychological well-being during therapy with antidepressants should be considered in monitoring outcome [71, 205].

SUMMARY

Consistent Evidence

In the treatment of major depression, there have been many more RCTs of the TCAs than of the MAOIs. Among the TCAs, amitriptyline, clomipramine and imipramine have been most frequently compared to the new-generation antidepressants. As sedative antidepressants, the SRMs, especially mirtazapine, have been found equal to amitriptyline. As a reuptake inhibitor of both serotonin and noradrenaline, venlafaxine has been found equal to clomipramine. The SSRIs have been found equal to imipramine, while reboxetine as a NARI has been found equal to desipramine. With a more benign side-effect profile than the TCAs, the new-generation antidepressants have been found globally superior to the TCAs, especially in medium- or long-term treatment, and in the treatment of elderly depressed patients.

In psychotic depression ECT is the most effective treatment. In atypical depression with phobia, MAOIs such as phenelzine are still of importance.

Incomplete Evidence

The efficacy of reversible inhibitors of monoamine oxidase type A (RIMA) such as moclobemide is uncertain both in major depression and in atypical depression.

The efficacy of the new-generation antidepressants in pure dysthymia is still uncertain, while in double depression (dysthymia superimposed with major depression) these antidepressants probably are effective.

In minor depression, the SSRIs seem effective, but the number of RCTs is still limited.

Areas Still Open to Research

While the SSRIs, SNRIs and SRMs are very effective in medium- and long-term treatment, RCTs evaluating reboxetine are still needed.

The new-generation antidepressants have not been found to have an earlier onset of action than the first-generation antidepressants. The use of combination or augmentation treatment should be evaluated to a greater degree, both in terms of early onset of action and in therapy-resistant depression.

In long-term treatment, side effects such as sexual disturbances and body weight gain should be more strictly evaluated. Measurement of social functioning and quality of life should be made by the use of patients' own assessment, especially in medium- and long-term treatment.

REFERENCES

1. Hinkle L.E. (1987) Stress and disease. The concept after 50 years. *Soc. Sci. Med.*, **6**: 561–566.
2. Frank J.D. (1974) *Persuasion and Healing*, Schocken, New York.
3. Skottowe I. (1953) *Clinical Psychiatry*, Eyre and Spottiswoode, London.
4. Skottowe I. (1955) Drugs in the treatment of depression. *Lancet*, **i**: 1129.
5. Kuhn R. (1957) Über die Behandlung depressiver Zustände mit einem Iminodibenzylderivat (G 22355). *Schweiz. Med. Wochenschr.*, **87**: 1135–1140.
6. Kuhn R. (1958) The treatment of depressive states with G 22355 (imipramine hydrochloride). *Am. J. Psychiatry*, **115**: 459–464.
7. Hamilton M. (1967) Development of a rating scale for primary depressive illness. *Br. J. Soc. Clin. Psychol.*, **6**: 278–296.
8. Healy D. (Ed.) (1998) *The Psychopharmacologists II*, Lippincott-Raven, Philadelphia.
9. Selzer H.M., Lurie M. (1953) Anxiety and depressive states treated with isonicotinyl (isoniazid). *Arch. Neurol.*, **70**: 217–324.
10. Loomer H.P., Saunders J.C., Kline N.S. (1957) A clinical and pharmaco-dynamic evaluation of iproniazid as a psychic energizer. *Psychiatr. Res. Rep.*, **8**: 129–141.
11. Sitsen A. (1998) Comments. In *The Psychopharmacologists II* (Ed. D. Healy), pp. 132–134, Lippincott-Raven, Philadelphia.
12. Carlsson A., Jonason J., Linqvist M. (1969) Demonstration of extraneural 5-hydroxy tryptamine accumulation in brain following membrane-pump blockade by clomipramine. *Brain Res.*, **12**: 456–460.
13. Pinder R.M. (1997) Designing a new generation of antidepressant drugs. *Acta Psychiatr. Scand.*, **96** (Suppl. 391): 7–13.
14. Stahl S.M. (1996) *Essential Psychopharmacology*, Cambridge University Press, London.
15. Freeman H.L. (1997) Advantages and limitations of the concept of antidepressant theory. *Eur. Neuropsychopharmacol.*, **7** (Suppl. 3): 315–321.
16. American Psychiatric Association (1980) *Diagnostic and Statistical Manual of Mental Disorders, 3rd edn (DSM-III)*, American Psychiatric Association, Washington, DC.

17. Bech P. (1981) Rating scales for affective disorders: Their validity and consistency. *Acta Psychiatr. Scand.*, **64** (Suppl. 295): 1–101.
18. American Psychiatric Association (1994) *Diagnostic and Statistical Manual of Mental Disorders, 4th edn (DSM-IV)*, American Psychiatric Association, Washington, DC.
19. World Health Organization (1993) *International Classification of Diseases, 10th revision*, World Health Organization, Geneva.
20. Shepherd M. (1998) Psychopharmacology: specific and non-specific. In *Psychopharmacologists II* (Ed. D. Healy) pp. 237–258, Lippincott-Raven, Philadelphia.
21. Bech P. (1993) Acute therapy of depression. *J. Clin. Psychiatry*, **54** (Suppl. 8): 18–27.
22. Bech P. (1996) *The Bech, Hamilton and Zung Scales for Mood Disorders*, 2nd edn, Springer, Berlin.
23. Goethe J.W., Fischer E.H., Wright J.S. (1993) Severity as a key concept of depression. *J. Nerv. Ment. Dis.*, **181**: 718–724.
24. Gerson S.C., Plotkin D.A., Jarvik L.F. (1988) Antidepressant drug studies 1956–1986: Empirical evidence for aging patients. *J. Clin. Psychopharmacol.*, **8**: 311–322.
25. Bech P., Coppen A. (Eds) (1990) *The Hamilton Scales*, Springer, Berlin.
26. Angst J. (1998) The prevalence of depression. In *Antidepressant therapy* (Eds M. Briley, S. Montgomery), pp. 191–212, Martin Dunitz, London.
27. Frank E., Prien R.F., Jarrett R.B. (1991) Conceptualization and rationale for consensus definitions of terms in major depression. *Arch. Gen. Psychiatry*, **48**: 851–855.
28. Kupfer D.J. (1991) Long-term treatment of depression. *J. Clin. Psychiatry*, **52** (Suppl. 5): 28–34.
29. European Community (1994) Guidelines on psychotropic drugs: Antidepressant medical products. *Eur. Neuropsychopharmacol.*, **4**: 62–65.
30. Stassen H.H., Angst J. (1998) Delayed onset of action of antidepressants: fact or fiction? *CNS Drugs*, **9**: 177–184.
31. Morris J.B., Beck A.T. (1974) The efficacy of antidepressant drugs. *Arch. Gen. Psychiatry*, **30**: 667–674.
32. Porter A.M.W. (1970) Depressive illness in a general practice. A demographic study and a controlled trial of imipramine. *Br. Med. J.*, **i**: 773–778.
33. Harris J.A., Robin A.A. (1960) A controlled trial of phenelzine in depressive reactions. *J. Ment. Sci.*, **106**: 1432–1437.
34. Robin A.A., Harris J.A. (1962) A controlled comparison of imipramine and electroplexy. *J. Ment. Sci.*, **108**: 217–220.
35. Robin A.A., Langely G.E. (1964) A controlled trial of imipramine. *Br. J. Psychiatry*, **110**: 419–422.
36. Medical Research Council (1965) Clinical trial of the treatment of depressive illness. *Br. Med. J.*, **i**: 881–886.
37. Spiker D.G., Weiss J.C., Dealy R.S. (1985) The pharmacological treatment of delusional depression. *Am. J. Psychiatry*, **142**: 430–436.
38. Paykel E.S. (1979) Predictors of treatment response. In *Psychopharmacology of Affective Disorders* (Eds E.S. Paykel, A. Coppen), pp. 193–220, Oxford University Press, Oxford.
39. Georgotas A., McCue R.E., Cooper T.B. (1989) A placebo-controlled comparison of nortriptyline and phenelzine in maintenance therapy of elderly depressed patients. *Arch. Gen. Psychiatry*, **46** (Suppl. 8): 46–51.

40. Robinson D.S., Lerfeld S.C., Bennett B. (1991) Continuation and maintenance treatment of major depression with the monoamine oxidase inhibitor phenelzine: a double-blind placebo-controlled discontinuation study. *Psychopharmacol. Bull.*, **27**: 31–39.
41. Kenning I.S., Richardson V.L., Tucker F.G. (1960) The treatment of depressive states with imipramine hydrochloride. *Can. Psychiat. Ass. J.*, **5**: 60–64.
42. Ball J.R.B., Kiloh L.G. (1959) A controlled trial of imipramine in treatment of depressive states. *Br. Med. J.*, **ii**: 1052–1055.
43. Seager C.P., Bird R.L. (1962) Imipramine with electrical treatment in depression: A controlled trial. *J. Ment. Sci.*, **108**: 704–709.
44. Mindham R.H.S., Howland C., Shepherd M. (1973) An evaluation of continuation therapy with tricyclic antidepressants in depressive illness. *Psychol. Med.*, **3**: 5–17.
45. Prien R.F., Klett C.H., Caffey E.M. (1973) Lithium carbonate and imipramine in prevention of affective episodes. *Arch. Gen. Psychiatry*, **29**: 420–425.
46. Frank E., Kupfer D.J., Perel J.M. (1990) Three year outcomes for maintenance therapies in recurrent depression. *Arch. Gen. Psychiatry*, **47**: 1093–1099.
47. Kupfer D.J., Frank E., Perel J.M., Cornes C., Mallinger A.G., Thase M.E., McEachran A.B., Grochocinsky V.J. (1992) Five year outcome for maintenance therapies in recurrent depression. *Arch. Gen. Psychiatry*, **49**: 769–773.
48. Frank E., Kupfer D.J., Perel J.M., Cornes C., Mallinger A.G., Thase M.E., McEachran A.B., Grochocinski V.J. (1993) Comparison of full-dose versus half-dose pharmacotherapy in the maintenance treatment of recurrent depression. *J. Affect. Disord.*, **27**: 139–149.
49. Rees L., Davis B. (1965) A controlled study of amitriptyline in severe depressive states. *Int. J. Neuropsychiatry*, **1**: 158–160.
50. Garry J., Leonard T.J. (1963) Trial of amitriptyline in chronic depression. *Br. J. Psychiatry*, **109**: 54–55.
51. Paykel E.S., Hollyman J.A., Freeling P., Sedgwick P. (1988). Predictors of a therapeutic benefit from amitriptyline in mild depression: a general practice placebo-controlled study. *J. Affect. Disord.*, **14**: 83–95.
52. Klerman G.E., Dimasco A., Weissman M., Prusoff B., Paykel E.S. (1974) Treatment of depression by drugs and psychotherapy. *Am. J. Psychiatry*, **131**: 186–191.
53. Coppen A., Ghose K., Rao R., Bailey J., Peet M. (1978) Mianserin and lithium in the prophylaxis of depression. *Br. J. Psychiatry*, **133**: 206–210.
54. Stein M.K., Rickels K., Weise C.C. (1980) Maintenance therapy with amitriptyline. A controlled trial. *Am. J. Psychiatry*, **137**: 370–371.
55. Glen A.I.M., Johnson A.L., Shepherd M. (1984) Continuation therapy with lithium and amitriptyline in unipolar depressive illness. A randomized, double-blind controlled trial. *Psychol. Med.*, **14**: 37–50.
56. Smith A., Traganza E., Harrison G. (1969) Studies on the effectiveness of antidepressant drugs. *Psychopharmacology* (special issue), 1–2.
57. Wechsler H., Grosser G.H., Greenblatt M. (1965) Research evaluating antidepressant medication on hospitalized patients: a survey of published reports during a five-year period. *J. Nerv. Ment. Dis.*, **141**: 231–239.
58. Bielski R.J., Friedel R.O. (1976) Prediction of tricyclic antidepressants response: A critical review. *Arch. Gen. Psychiatry*, **33**: 1479–1489.
59. The Quality Assurance Project (1983) A treatment outline for depressive disorders. *Aust. N. Zeal. J. Psychiatry*, **17**: 129–146.
60. Bech P. (1978) Depressive symptomatology and drug response. *Commun. Psychopharmacol.*, **2**: 409–418.

61. Clary C., Mandos L.A., Schweizer E. (1990) Results of a brief survey on the prescribing practices for monoamine-oxidase inhibitor antidepressants. *J. Clin. Psychiatry*, **51**: 226–229.
62. Hamilton M. (1974) General problems of psychiatric rating scales. In *Psychological Measurements in Psychopharmacology* (Ed. P. Pichot), pp. 125–138, Karger, Basel.
63. Hordern A., Burt C.G., Holt N.F., Cade J.F. (1965) *Depressive States. A Pharmacotherapeutic Study*, Charles C. Thomas, Springfield, IL.
64. Stage K.B. (1996) Differences in Symptomatology, Diagnostic Profile as well as Adverse Drug Reactions Between Younger and Elderly Depressed Patients. Thesis, Odense University, Denmark.
65. Bech P., Cialdella P. (1992) Citalopram in depression: meta-analysis of intended and unintended effects. *Int. Clin. Psychopharmacol.*, **6** (Suppl. 5): 45–54.
66. Montgomery S.A., Åsberg M. (1979) A new depression rating scale designed to be sensitive to change. *Br. J. Psychiatry*, **134**: 382–389.
67. Bech P. (1989) Clinical effects of selective serotonin reuptake inhibitors. In *Clinical Pharmacology in Psychiatry* (Eds S.G. Dahl, L.F. Gram), pp. 81–93, Springer, Berlin.
68. Anderson I.M., Tomenson B.M. (1994) The efficacy of selective serotonin reuptake inhibitors in depression: a meta-analysis of studies against tricyclic antidepressants. *J. Psychopharmacol.*, **8**: 238–249.
69. Loonen A.J.M., Zwanikken G.J. (1990) Continuation and maintenance therapy with antidepressive agents. An overview of research. *Pharm. Weekbl. (Scientific Edition)*, **12**: 128–141.
70. Stahl M.M.S., Lindquist M., Pettersson M., Edwards I.R., Sanderson J.H., Taylor N.F.A., Fletcher A.P., Schou J.S. (1997) Withdrawal reactions with selective serotonin reuptake inhibitors as reported to the WHO system. *Eur. J. Clin. Pharmacol.*, **53**: 163–169.
71. Bech P. (1995) Social aspects of treatment of depression. *Int. Clin. Psychopharmacol.*, **10** (Suppl. 1): 11–14.
72. Angst J., Scheidegger P., Stabl M. (1993) Efficacy of moclobemide in different patient groups. Results of new subscales of the Hamilton Depression Rating Scale. *Clin. Neuropharmacol.*, **16** (Suppl. 2): 55–62.
73. Lecrubier Y., Guelfi J.D. (1990) Efficacy of reversible inhibitors of monoamine oxidase A in various forms of depression. *Acta Psychiatr. Scand.*, **82** (Suppl. 1): 74–87.
74. Stabl M., Biziere K., Schmid-Burgk W. (1989) Review of comparative clinical trials: moclobemide versus tricyclic antidepressants and versus placebo in depressive states. *J. Neural Transm.*, **28** (Suppl.): 77–89.
75. Guelfi J.D., White A.C., Hackett D., Guichoix J.V. (1995) Effectiveness of venlafaxine in hospitalized patients with major depression. *J. Clin. Psychiatry*, **56**: 450–458.
76. Rudolph R.L., Fabre L., Feighner J., Rickels K. (1998) A randomised, placebo-controlled, dose–response trial of venlafaxine hydrochloride in the treatment of major depression. *J. Clin. Psychiatry*, **59**: 116–122.
77. Entsuah A.R., Rudolph R.L., Hackett D., Miska S. (1996) Efficacy of venlafaxine and placebo during long-term treatment of depression: a pooled analysis of relapse rates. *Int. Clin. Psychopharmacol.*, **11**: 137–145.
78. Feighner J.P., Boyer W.F., Meredith C.H., Hendrickson G.C. (1989) A placebo-controlled inpatient comparison of fluvoxamine maleate and imipramine in major depression. *Int. Clin. Psychopharmacol.*, **4**: 239–244.

79. Feighner J.P., Overø K. (1999) Multicenter, placebo-controlled, fixed-dose study of citalopram in moderate to severe depression. *J. Clin. Psychiatry*, **60**: 824–830.
80. Greenberg R.P., Bornstein R.F., Zborowski M.J., Fisher S., Greenberg M.D. (1994) Meta-analysis of fluoxetine outcome in treatment of depression. *J. Nerv. Ment. Dis.*, **182**, 547–551.
81. Doogan D.P., Caillard V. (1992) Sertraline in the prevention of depression. *Br. J. Psychiatry*, **160**: 217–222.
82. Montgomery S.A., Dunbar G.C. (1993) Paroxetine is better than placebo in relapse prevention and the prophylaxis of recurrent depression. *Int. Clin. Psychopharmacol.*, **8**, 181–188.
83. Montgomery S.A., Rasmussen J.G.C., Tanghøj P. (1993) A 24 week study of 20 mg citalopram, 40 mg citalopram and placebo in the prevention of relapse of major depression. *Int. Clin. Psychopharmacol.*, **8**, 181–188.
84. Robert P., Montgomery S.A. (1995) Citalopram in doses of 20 mg to 60 mg are effective in relapse prevention: a placebo-controlled 6 month study. *Int. Clin. Psychopharmacol.*, **10** (Suppl. 1): 29–35.
85. Reimherr F.W., Amsterdam J.W.D., Quitkin F.M., Rosenbaum J.F., Fava M. (1998) Optimal length of continuation therapy in depression: a prospective assessment during long-term fluoxetine treatment. *Am. J. Psychiatry*, **155**: 1247–1253.
86. Montgomery S.A., Dufour H., Brion S., Gailledreau J., Laqueille X., Ferrey G., Moron P., Parantolucenn N., Singer L., Danion J.M. *et al* (1988) The prophylactic efficacy of fluoxetine in unipolar depression. *Br. J. Psychiatry*, **153** (Suppl. 3): 69–76.
87. Terra J.L., Montgomery S.A. (1998) Fluvoxamine prevents recurrence of depression. Results of a long-term, double-blind, placebo-controlled study. *Int. Clin. Psychopharmacol.*, **13**: 55–62.
88. Hochstrasser B., Isaksen P.M., Koponen H., Lauritzen L., Mahnert F.A., Rouillon F., Wade A.G., Andersen M., Pedersen S.F., Swart J.C., *et al* (2001) Prophylactic effect of citalopram in unipolar, recurrent depression: placebo-controlled study of maintenance therapy. *Br. J. Psychiatry*, **178**: 304–310.
89. Feighner J., Targum S.D., Bennett M.E., Roberts D.L., Kensler T.T., D'Amico M.F., Hardy S.A. (1998) A double-blind, placebo-controlled trial of nefazodone in the treatment of patients hospitalized for major depression. *J. Clin. Psychiatry*, **59**: 246–253.
90. Mendels J., Reimherr F., Marcus R.N. (1995) A double-blind placebo-controlled trial of two dose ranges of nefazodone in the treatment of depressed outpatients. *J. Clin. Psychiatry*, **56** (Suppl. 6): 30–36.
91. Anton S.F., Robinson D.S., Roberts D.L., Kensler T.T., English P.A., Archibald D.G. (1994) Long-term treatment of depression with nefazodone. *Psychopharmacol. Bull.*, **30**: 165–169.
92. Vartiainen H., Leinonen E. (1994) Double-blind study of mirtazapine and placebo in hospitalized patients with major depression. *Eur. Neuropsychopharmacol.*, **4**: 145–150.
93. Khan M.C. (1995) A randomized, double-blind, placebo-controlled 5 week study of Org 3370 (mirtazapine) in major depression. *Human Psychopharmacol.*, **10** (Suppl. 2): 119–124.
94. Bech P. (2001) Meta-analysis of placebo-controlled trials with mirtazapine using the core items of the Hamilton Depression Scale as evidence of a pure antidepressive effect in the short-term treatment of major depression. *Int. J. Neuropsychopharmacol.*, **4**: 337–345.

95. Montgomery S.A., Reimitz P.E., Zivkov M. (1998) Mirtazapine versus amitriptyline in the long-term treatment of depression: a double-blind placebo-controlled study. *Int. Clin. Psychopharmacol.*, **13**: 63–73.
96. Schatzberg A.F., Dessain E., O'Niel P., Katz D.L., Cole J.O. (1987) Recent studies on selective serotonergic antidepressants: trazodone, fluoxetine, and fluvoxamine. *J. Clin. Psychopharmacol.*, **7** (Suppl. 6): 44–49.
97. Moises H.W., Kasper S., Beckmann H. (1981) Trazodone and amitriptyline in treatment of depressed inpatients. A double-blind study. *Pharmacopsychiatry*, **14**: 167–171.
98. Itil T.M., Polvan N., Hsu W. (1972) Clinical and EEG effects of GB 94, a tetracyclic antidepressant. *Curr. Ther. Res.*, **14**: 395–413.
99. Cording-Tömmel C., von Zerssen D. (1982) Mianserin and maprotiline as compared to amitriptyline in severe endogenous depression. *Pharmacopsychiatry*, **15**: 197–204.
100. Murphy J.E., Donald J.F., Molla A.L. (1976) Mianserin in the treatment of depression in general practice. *Practitioner*, **271**: 135–141.
101. Mendels J., Johnston R., Mattes J., Reisenberg R. (1993) Efficacy and safety of b.i.d. doses of venlafaxine in a dose-response study. *Psychopharmacol. Bull.*, **29**: 169–174.
102. Simpson G.M., Lee J.H., Cuculie Z. (1976) Two dosages of imipramine in hospitalized endogenous and neurotic depressions. *Arch. Gen. Psychiatry*, **33**: 1093–1102.
103. Guelfi J.D., Payan C., Fermanian J. (1992) Moclobemide versus clomipramine in endogenous depression. A double-blind randomized clinical trial. *Br. J. Psychiatry*, **160**: 519–524.
104. Danish University Antidepressant Group (DUAG) (1993) Moclobemide: a reversible MAO-A inhibitor showing weaker antidepressant effect than clomipramine in a controlled multicenter study. *J. Affect. Disord.*, **28**: 105–116.
105. Nair N.P.V., Amin M., Holm P. (1995) Moclobemide and nortriptyline in elderly depressed patients. A randomized, multicenter trial against placebo. *J. Affect. Disord.*, **33**: 1–9.
106. Larsen J.K., Gjerris A., Holm P. (1991) Moclobemide in depression: a randomized multicenter trial against isocarboxazide and clomipramine emphasizing atypical depression. *Acta Psychiatr. Scand.*, **84**: 564–570.
107. Kragh-Sørensen P., Müller B., Andersen J.V., Buch D., Stage K.B. (1995) Moclobemide versus clomipramine in depressed patients in general practice. A randomized, double-blind, parallel, multicenter study. *J. Clin. Psychopharmacol.*, **15** (Suppl. 2): 24–30.
108. Beaumont G., Gringoas M., Hobbs F.D.R. (1993) A randomized, double-blind, multi-centre, parallel-group study comparing the tolerability and efficacy of moclobemide and dothiepin hydrochloride in depressed patients in general practice. *Int. Clin Psychopharmacol.*, **7**: 159–165.
109. Benkert O., Gründer G., Wetzel H., Hackett D. (1996) A randomized double-blind comparison of a rapidly escalating dose of venlafaxine and imipramine in inpatients with major depression and melancholia. *J. Psychiatr. Res.*, **30**: 441–451.
110. Morton W.A., Sonne S.C., Verga M.A. (1995) Venlafaxine: a structurally unique and novel antidepressant. *Ann. Pharmacother.*, **29**: 387–395.
111. Lecrubier Y., Moon C.A.L., Schifano F. (1997) Efficacy of venlafaxine in depressive illness in general practice. *Acta Psychiatr. Scand.*, **95**: 485–493.

112. Burnett F.E., Dinan T.G. (1998) The clinical efficacy of venlafaxine in the treatment of depression. *Rev. Contemp. Pharmacother.*, **9**: 303–320.
113. Nielsen A.A., Morsing I., Petersen J.S., Larsen T., Møller S.E., Manniche P., Skausig O.B. (1991) Paroxetine and imipramine treatment of depressive patients in a controlled multicentre study with plasma amino acid measurements. *Acta Psychiatr. Scand.*, **84**: 233–241.
114. Danish University Antidepressant Group (DUAG) (1990) Paroxetine: a selective serotonin reuptake inhibitor showing better tolerance, but weaker antidepressant effect than clomipramine in a controlled multicenter trial. *J. Affect. Disord.*, **18**: 289–299.
115. Anderson I.M. (1998) SSRIs versus tricyclic antidepressants in depressed inpatients: a meta-analysis of efficacy and tolerability. *Depression and Anxiety*, **7** (Suppl. 1): 11–17.
116. Øhrberg S., Christiansen P.E., Severin B. (1992) Paroxetine and imipramine in the treatment of depressed patients in psychiatric practice. *Acta Psychiatr. Scand.*, **86**: 437–444.
117. Samuelian J.C., Hackett D. (1998) A randomised, double-blind, parallel group comparison of venlafaxine and clomipramine in outpatients with major depression. *J. Psychopharmacol.*, **12**: 273–278.
118. Christiansen P.E., Behncke K., Black C., Öhrström J.K., Bork-Rasmussen H., Nilsson J. (1996) Paroxetine and amitriptyline in the treatment of depression in general practice. *Acta Psychiatr. Scand.*, **93**: 158–163.
119. Lauritzen L., Odgaard K., Clemmesen L., Lunde M., Öhrström J., Black C., Bech P. (1996) Relapse prevention of paroxetine in ECT treated patients with major depression. A comparison with imipramine and placebo in medium-term continuation therapy. *Acta Psychiatr. Scand.*, **94**: 18–25.
120. Danish University Antidepressant Group (DUAG) (1986) Citalopram: clinical effect profile in comparison with clomipramine. A controlled multicenter study. *Psychopharmacology*, **90**: 131–138.
121. Timmermann L., de Beurs P., Tan B.K. (1987) A double-blind comparative clinical trial of citalopram versus maprotiline in hospitalized depressed patients. *Int. Clin. Psychopharmacol.*, **2**: 239–253.
122. Fuglum E., Rosenberg C., Damsbo N., Stage K., Lauritzen L., Bech P. (1996) Screening and treating depressed patients. A comparison of two controlled citalopram trials across treatment settings: hospitalized patients versus patients treated by their family doctors. *Acta Psychiatr. Scand.*, **94**: 18–25.
123. Stokes P.E., Holtz A. (1997) Fluoxetine tenth anniversary: the progress continues. *Clin. Ther.*, **19**: 1–86.
124. Corne S.J., Hall J.R. (1989) A double-blind comparative study of fluoxetine and dothiepine in the treatment of depression in general practice. *Int. Clin. Psychopharmacol.*, **4**: 245–254.
125. Hegerl V., Gallinat J., Möller H.J., Arato M., Janka Z. (1997) Double-blind, multicenter, comparative study of sertraline and amitriptyline in hospitalized patients with major depression. *Eur. Neuropsychopharmacol.*, **7** (Suppl. 2): 180.
126. Reimherr F.W., Chouinard G., Cohn C.K., Cole J.O., Itel T.M., LaPierre Y.D., Masco H.L., Mendels J. (1990) Antidepressant efficacy of sertraline: a double-blind, placebo- and amitriptyline-controlled multicenter comparison study in outpatients with major depression. *J. Clin. Psychiatry*, **51** (Suppl. 12): 18–27.
127. Moon C.A.L., Jago W., Wood K., Doogan D.P. (1994) A double-blind comparison of sertraline and clomipramine in the treatment of major depressive disorder and associated anxiety in general practice. *J. Psychopharmacol.*, **8**: 171–176.

128. Marcus R.M., Mendels J. (1996) Nefazodone in the treatment of severe, melancholic, and recurrent depression: results of a meta-analysis. *J. Clin. Psychiatry*, **51**: 226–229.

129. Rickels K., Schweizer E., Clary C. (1994) Nefazodone and imipramine in major depression: a placebo-controlled trial. *Br. J. Psychiatry*, **164**: 802–805.

130. Zivkov M., de Jongh G.D. (1995) Org 3770 versus amitriptyline: a 6 week, randomized, double-blind multicenter trial in hospitalized depressed. *Hum. Psychopharmacol.*, **10**: 173–180.

131. Rickels K., Robinson D.S., Schweizer E., Marcus R.N., Roberts D.L. (1995) Nefazodone: aspects of efficacy. *J. Clin. Psychiatry*, **56**: 43–46.

132. Bruijn J.A., Moleman P., Mulder P.G.H. (1996) A double-blind, fixed blood level study comparing mirtazapine with imipramine in depressed patients. *Psychopharmacology*, **127**: 231–237.

133. West E.D., Dally P.J. (1959) Effects of iproniazid in depressive syndromes. *Br. Med. J.*, **i**: 1491–1493.

134. Liebowitz M.R., Schneier F.R., Campeas R. (1992) Phenelzine vs. atenolol in social phobia: a placebo-controlled comparison. *Arch. Gen. Psychiatry*, **49**: 290–300.

135. Versiani M., Nardi A.E., Mundiom F.D., Alves A.B., Liebowitz M.R., Amrein R. (1992) Pharmacotherapy of social phobia. A controlled study with moclobemide and phenelzine. *Br. J. Psychiatry*, **161**: 353–360.

136. Noyes R., Moroz G., Davidson J.R.T. (1997) Moclobemide in social phobia: a controlled dose-response trial. *J. Clin. Psychopharmacol.*, **17**: 247–254.

137. De Vanna M., Kummer J., Agnoli A. (1990) Moclobemide compared with second-generation antidepressants in elderly people. *Acta Psychiatr. Scand.*, **82** (Suppl. 360): 64–66.

138. Angst J., Stabl M. (1992) Efficacy of moclobemide in different patient groups: a meta-analysis of studies. *Psychopharmacology*, **106**: 109–113.

139. Ban T.A., Gaszner P., Aguglia E. (1998) Clinical efficacy of reboxetine: a comparative study with desipramine, with methodological considerations. *Hum. Psychopharmacol.*, **13**: 29–39.

140. Berzewski H., van Moffaert M., Gagiano C.A. (1997) Efficacy and tolerability of reboxetine compared with imipramine in a double-blind study in patients suffering from major depressive episodes. *Eur. Neuropsychopharmacol.*, **7** (Suppl. 1): 37–47.

141. Gattaz W.F., Vogel P., Kick H., Kohnen R. (1995) Moclobemide versus fluoxetine in the treatment of inpatients with major depression. *J. Clin. Pharmacol.*, **15** (Suppl. 2): 35–40.

142. Lönnqvist J., Sintonen H., Syvälathi T. (1994) Antidepressant efficacy and quality of life in depression: a double-blind study with moclobemide and fluoxetine. *Acta Psychiatr. Scand.*, **89**: 363–369.

143. Williams R., Edwards R.A., Newburn G.M., Muller R., Menkes D.B., Segkar C. (1993) A double-blind comparison of moclobemide and fluoxetine in the treatment of depressive disorders. *Int. Clin. Psychopharmacol.*, **7**: 155–158.

144. Geerts S., Bruynooghe F., DeCuyper H., Demeuleneester F., Haazen L. (1994) Moclobemide versus fluoxetine for major depressive episodes. *Clin. Neuropharmacol.*, **17** (Suppl. 1): 50–57.

145. Clerc G.E., Ruimy P., Verdeau-Pailles J. (1994) A double-blind comparison of venlafaxine and fluoxetine in patients hospitalized for major depression and melancholia. *Int. Clin. Psychopharmacol.*, **9**: 193–243.

146. Dierick M., Ravizza L., Realini R., Martin A. (1996) A double-blind comparison of venlafaxine and fluoxetine for treatment of major depression in outpatients. *Progr. Neuro-Psychopharmacol. Biol. Psychiatry*, **20**: 57–71.

147. Tylee A., Beaumant G., Bowden M.W., Reynolds A. (1997) A double-blind, randomized, 12 week comparison study of the safety and efficacy of venlafaxine and fluoxetine in moderate to severe major depression. *Prim. Care Psychiatry*, **3**, 51–58.

148. Tignol J. (1993) A double-blind, randomized, fluoxetine-controlled multicenter study of paroxetine in the treatment of depression. *J. Clin. Psychopharmacol.*, **13** (Suppl. 2): 18–22.

149. Geretsegger C., Bohmer F., Ludwig M. (1994) Paroxetine in the elderly depressed patient: randomized comparison with fluoxetine of efficacy. Cognitive and behavioural effects. *Int. Clin. Psychopharmacol.*, **9**: 25–29.

150. Bennie E.H., Mullen J.M., Martindale J.J. (1995) A double-blind multicenter trial comparing sertraline and fluoxetine in outpatients with major depression. *J. Clin. Psychiatry*, **56**: 229–237.

151. Patris M., Bouchard J.-M., Bougerol T. (1996) Citalopram versus fluoxetine: a double-blind, controlled, multicentre, phase III trial in patients with unipolar depression treated in general practice. *Int. Clin. Psychopharmacol.*, **11**: 129–136.

152. van Moffaert M., Bartholomé F., Cosyns P. (1995) A controlled comparison of sertraline and fluoxetine in acute and continuation treatment of major depression. *Hum. Psychopharmacol.*, **10**: 393–405.

153. Aguglia E., Casacchia M., Cassano G.B. (1993) Double-blind study of the efficacy and safety of sertraline versus fluoxetine in major depression. *Int. J. Psychopharmacol.*, **8**: 197–202.

154. Gillin J.C., Rapaport M., Erman M.K., Winokur A., Albala B.J. (1997) A comparison of nefazodone and fluoxetine on mood and on objective, subjective, and clinician-rated measures of sleep in depressed patients: a double-blind, 8-week clinical trial. *J. Clin. Psychiatry*, **58**: 185–192.

155. Rush A.J., Armitage R., Gillin J.C. (1998) Comparative effects of nefazodone and fluoxetine on sleep in outpatients with major depressive disorder. *Biol. Psychiatry*, **44**: 3–14.

156. Wheatley D.P., van Moffaert M., Timmermann L., Kremer C. (1998) Mirtazapine: efficacy and tolerability in comparison with fluoxetine in patients with moderate to severe major depressive disorder. *J. Clin. Psychiatry*, **59**: 306–312.

157. Invernizzi G., Mauri M.C., Waintraub L. (1997) Antidepressant efficacy in the treatment of dysthymia. *Eur. Neuropsychopharmacol.*, **7** (Suppl. 3): 329–336.

158. Versiani M., Amrein R., Stabl M. (1997) Moclobemide and imipramine in chronic depression (dysthymia): an international double-blind, placebo-controlled trial. *Int. Clin. Psychopharmacol.*, **12**: 183–193.

159. Thase M.E., Fava M., Halbreich V., Kocsis J.H., Koran L., Davidson J., Rosenbaum J., Harrison W. (1996) A placebo-controlled, randomized clinical trial comparing sertraline and imipramine for the treatment of dysthymia. *Arch. Gen. Psychiatry*, **53**: 777–784.

160. Kocsis J.H., Friedman R.A., Markowitz J.C., Leon A.C., Miller N.L., Gniwesch L., Parides M. (1996) Maintenance therapy for chronic depression. A controlled clinical trial of desipramine. *Arch. Gen Psychiatry*, **53**: 769–774.

161. Keller M.B., Kocsis J.H., Thase M.E., Gelenberg A.J., Rush J.A. (1998) Maintenance phase efficacy of sertraline for chronic depression. A randomized controlled trial. *JAMA*, **280**: 1665–1672.

162. Szegedi A., Wetzel H., Angersbach D., Philipp M., Benkert O. (1997) Response to treatment in minor and major depression: results of a double-blind comparative study with paroxetine and maprotiline. *J. Affect. Disord.*, **45**: 167–178.

163. Blom-Peters L., Lamy M. (1993) Monoamine oxidase inhibitors and anesthesia: an updated literature review. *Acta Anaesth. Belg.*, **44**: 57–60.

164. Kuhn R. (1970) The imipramine story. In *Discoveries in Biological Psychiatry* (Eds F.J. Ayd, B. Blackwell), pp. 205–217, Lippincott, Philadelphia.

165. Katona C.L.E. (1994) *Depression in Old Age*, Wiley, Chichester.

166. Montgomery S.A., Kasper S. (1995) Comparison of compliance between serotonin reuptake inhibitors and tricyclic antidepressants: a meta-analysis. *Int. Clin. Psychopharmacol.*, **9** (Suppl. 4): 33–40.

167. Hotopf M., Hardy R., Lewis G. (1997) Discontinuation rates of SSRIs and tricyclic antidepressants: a meta-analysis and investigation of heterogeneity. *Br. J. Psychiatry*, **170**: 120–128.

168. Paykel E.S., Mueller P.S., de la Verque P.M. (1973) Amitriptyline, weight gain and carbonate craving. A side effect. *Br. J. Psychiatry*, **123**: 501–507.

169. Hindmarch I., Harrison C. (1988) Three antidepressants (amitriptyline, dothiepine, fluoxetine) with and without alcohol compared with placebo on tests of psychomotor activity related to car driving. *Hum. Psychopharmacol.*, **2**: 177–183.

170. Cassidy S., Henry J. (1987) Fatal toxicity of antidepressant drugs in overdose. *Br. Med. J.*, **295**: 1021–1024.

171. Currie D.J., Fairweather D.B., Hindmarch I. (1993) Social aspects of treating depression. In *Health Economics of Depression* (Eds B. Jönsson, J. Rosenbaum), pp. 129–139, Wiley, Chichester.

172. Neuvonen P.J., Pohjola-Sintonen S., Tacke U., Vuari E. (1993) Five fatal cases of serotonin syndrome after moclobemide-citalopram or moclobemide-clomipramine overdoses. *Lancet*, **342**: 1419.

173. Baldwin D.S., Birtwhistle J. (1998) Antidepressant drugs and sexual function: improving the recognition and management of sexual dysfunction in depressed patients. In *Antidepressant Therapy at the Dawn of the Third Millennium* (Eds M. Briley, S.A. Montgomery), pp. 231–253, Martin Dunitz, London.

174. Harrison W.M., Rabkin J.G., Ehrhardt A. (1986) Effects of antidepressant medication on sexual function: a controlled study. *J. Clin. Psychopharmacol.*, **6**: 144–149.

175. Philipp M., Kohnen R., Benkert O. (1993) A comparison study of moclobemide and doxepin in major depression with special reference to effects on sexual dysfunction. *Int. Clin. Psychopharmacol.*, **7**: 149–153.

176. Dubini A., Bosc M., Polin V. (1997) Noradrenaline-selective versus serotonin-selective antidepressant therapy: differential effects on social functioning. *J. Psychopharmacol.*, **11** (Suppl. 4): 17–23.

177. Bech P. (1997) Quality of life instruments in depression. *Eur. Psychiatry*, **12**: 194–198.

178. Nelson J.C., Mazure C.M., Bowers M.B., Jatlow P.I. (1991) A preliminary open study of the combination of fluoxetine and desipramine for rapid treatment of major depression. *Arch. Gen. Psychiatry*, **48**: 303–307.

179. Young J.P.R., Lader M., Hughes W.C. (1979) Controlled trial of imipramine, monoamine-oxidase inhibitors, and combined treatment in depressed outpatients. *Br. Med. J.*, **ii**: 1315–1317.

180. Riise I.S., Holm P. (1984) Concomitant isocarboxazide/mianserin treatment of major depressive disorder. *J. Affect. Disord.*, **6**: 175–179.

181. de Montigny C., Courmoyer G., Morisette R. (1983) Lithium carbonate addition in tricyclic antidepressant resistant unipolar depression: correlations with neurobiologic actions of tricyclic antidepressant drugs and lithium ion on the serotonin system. *Arch Gen. Psychiatry*, **40**: 1327–1334.

182. Katona C.L.E., Abou-Saleh M.T., Harrison D.A. (1995) Placebo controlled trial of lithium augmentation of fluoxetine and lofepramine. *Br. J. Psychiatry*, **166**: 80–86.

183. Hoencamp E., Haffmanns P.M.J., Dijken W.A., Huijbrechts I.P.A.M. (1997) Lithium augmentation of venlafaxine: an open controlled trial. Presented at the ECNP meeting, Vienna, 14–17 September.

184. Blier P., Bergeron R., de Montigny C. (1998) Adjunct treatments for rapid onset of action and greater efficacy in major depression. In *Antidepressant Therapy at the Dawn of the Third Millennium* (Eds M. Briley, S.A. Montgomery), pp. 279–295, Martin Dunitz, London.

185. Ferreri M., Lavergne F., Berlin I., Payan C., Puech A.J. (2001) Benefits from mianserin augmentation of fluoxetine in patients with major depression non-responders to fluoxetine alone. *Acta. Psychiatr. Scand.*, **103**: 66–72.

186. Dam J., Ryde L., Svejsø J., Lauge N., Lauritsen B., Bech P. (1998) Morning fluoxetine plus evening mianserin versus morning fluoxetine plus evening placebo in the acute treatment of major depression. *Pharmacopsychiatry*, **31**: 48–54.

187. Jacobsen F.M. (1991) Possible augmentation of antidepressant response by buspirone. *J. Clin. Psychiatry*, **52**: 217–218.

188. Joffe R.T., Schuller D.R. (1993) An open study of buspirone augmentation of serotonin reuptake inhibitors in refractory depression. *J. Clin. Psychiatry*, **54**: 269–271.

189. Robinson D.S., Rickels K., Feighner J. (1990) Clinical effects of 5-HT-1A partial agonist in depression: a composite analysis of buspirone in the treatment of depression. *J. Clin. Psychopharmacol.*, **10**: 67–76.

190. Landén M., Björling G., Ågren H., Fahlen T. (1998) A randomized, double-blind, placebo-controlled trial of buspirone in combination with an SSRI in patients with treatment-refractory depression. *J. Clin. Psychiatry*, **59**: 664–668.

191. Brøsen K., Rasmussen B.B. (1996) Selective serotonin reuptake inhibitors: pharmacokinetics and drug interactions. In *Selective Serotonin Reuptake Inhibitors*, 2nd edn (Ed. J. Feighner), pp. 87–108, Wiley, Chichester.

192. Salzman C. (1993) Pharmacological treatment of depression in the elderly. *J. Clin. Psychiatry*, **54** (Suppl. 2): 23–28.

193. Lader M. (1988) Fluoxetine efficacy versus comparative drugs: an overview. *Br. J. Psychiatry*, **153** (Suppl. 3): 51–58.

194. Medawar C. (1997) The antidepressant web. *Int. J. Risk and Safety in Medicine*, **10**: 75–126.

195. Chalmers T.C., Berrier J., Sacks H.S., Levin H., Reitman D., Nagalingam R. (1987) Meta-analysis of clinical trials as a scientific discipline. II: Replicate variability and comparison of studies that agree and disagree. *Statistics in Medicine*, **6**: 733–744.

196. Rothschild A.J., Samson J.A., Bessette M.P. (1993) Efficacy of the combination of fluoxetine and perphenazine in the treatment of psychotic depression. *J. Clin. Psychiatry*, **54**: 338–342.

197. Danish University Antidepressant Group (DUAG) (1999) Clomipramine dose-effect study in patients with depression: clinical end points and pharmacokinetics. *Clin. Pharmacol. Ther.*, **66**: 152–165.

198. Wernicke J.F., Dunlop S.R., Dornseif B.E., Zerbe R.L. (1987) Fixed-dose fluoxe-tine therapy for depression. *Psychopharmacol. Bull.*, **23**: 164–168.
199. Fabre L.F., Abuzzahab F.S., Amin M., Claghorn J.L., Mendels J., Petrie W.M., Dube S., Small J.G. (1995) Sertraline safety and efficacy in major depression: a double-blind fixed-dose comparison with placebo. *Biol. Psychiatry*, **38**: 592–602.
200. Kelsey J. (1995) Dose-response relationship with venlafaxine. *J. Clin Pharmacol.*, **16** (Suppl. 2): 215–265.
201. Bech P., Tanghøj P., Andersen H.F., Overø K. (2002) Citalopram dose-response revisited using an alternative psychometric approach to evaluate clinical effects of four fixed citalopram doses compared to placebo in patients with major depression. *Psychopharmacology*, in press.
202. Moncrieff J. (2002) The antidepressant debate. *Br. J. Psychiatry*, **180**: 195–197.
203. Stassen H.H., Delini-Stula A., Angst J. (1993) Time course of improvement under antidepressant treatment: a survival-analytic approach. *Eur. Neuropsy-chopharmacol.*, **3**: 127–135.
204. Fava G.A., Rafanelli C., Cazzaro M., Conti S., Grandi S. (1998) Well-being therapy. A novel psychotherapeutic approach for residual symptoms of affec-tive disorders. *Psychol. Med.*, **28**: 475–480.
205. Bech P., Hackett D., Pitrosky B. (2002) Assessment of venlafaxine efficacy on a derived measure of well-being in major depressive disorder and generalized anxiety disorder. Presented at the NCDEU Meeting, Boca Raton, June 10–13.

Commentaries

2.1
Antidepressants: Forty Years of Experience
Eugene S. Paykel[1]

Antidepressants of modern types have now been available for 40 years. They are well established in the pharmacopoeia, and have a longer history than many of the drugs used today elsewhere in medicine. They are products of the controlled trial era, and their efficacy has been tested in a very large number of randomized trials. The novelty has worn off. Now is a time to draw some conclusions. In this commentary I will discuss a few selected issues.

Prof. Bech correctly points out that overall efficacy of the antidepressants is limited, with a 15–20% advantage over placebo. Part of this is due to the good outcome often seen in placebo groups, which probably reflects spontaneous remission and the benefits of non-specific therapeutic elements inherent in psychiatric care, rather than being due to the placebo. The drugs themselves also have limited effects in some patients. Incomplete remission with residual symptoms and later relapse is also common [1]. It is this limited overall advantage which makes it hard to detect differences in efficacy between drugs and still mandates placebo-controlled trials for new antidepressants.

The limited effects when different studies are pooled obscure insights from more detailed examination of individual trials. Thus, in earlier years the necessity for adequate length of acute treatment was not appreciated. Few controlled trials under 4 weeks in duration show significant antidepressant effects, and 6 weeks is better, although non-significant trends may occur earlier.

A range of trials can also show the effective dose, particularly where dose-ranging trials have not been conducted. This seems particularly important for monoamine oxidase inhibitors (MAOIs). One reason for failure to find efficacy for phenelzine in some major early inpatient studies was the use of

[1] *Department of Psychiatry, University of Cambridge, Addenbrooke's Hospital, Cambridge CB2 2QQ, UK*

low doses or short treatment periods. Moclobemide, although introduced with a dose range of 150–600 mg daily, has only convincingly been shown superior to placebo at doses of 450 mg and above. Many have expressed doubts as to its efficacy. In my own clinical experience, it is a valuable and comparatively safe drug, but only at doses of 600–900 mg daily, and occasionally higher.

In an era of clinical guidelines, there is a need for good evidence as to when antidepressants are indicated, particularly in the very common milder depressions. Two studies [2, 3] have found a clear threshold of severity for tricyclics, with superiority of drug over placebo starting around a total score of 13 on the Hamilton Rating Scale for Depression. This corresponds to a little below probable major depression.

In the UK and in most countries, the majority of antidepressant prescribing is by non-psychiatrists, mostly in primary care. Even in the USA, with a highly developed specialist system, a large amount of treatment of depression is by non-psychiatrists [4].

In this setting, and also in psychiatric outpatient care, wider issues about treatment delivery become important. Prescribing practices may be suboptimal. The general public often views the use of medications for psychological problems with suspicion [5], compared with positive attitudes towards psychotherapy. Compliance with prescribed medication is often poor. In recent years, therefore, educational programmes aimed towards prescribers, such as the Götland programme, and clinical guidelines and campaigns aimed towards the general public, such as the Defeat Depression Campaign, have become important.

Pharmacological research produces new drugs: clinical trials reveal effective pharmacologies. Many years of research, during which a number of novel antidepressants have appeared promising but then been found ineffective, suggest a conclusion regarding modes of action. Forty years on, virtually all the antidepressants available today can be seen as possessing actions which potentiate neurotransmission by noradrenaline and/or serotonin.

There is a lesson here, but it is still too early to be sure what it is. Either the fundamental systems subserving mood are mediated by these neurotransmitters, or the major and very costly avenues of drug development, and the animal screening tests involved, have had to become too focused on the safer bets, at the expense of the unknown long shot.

We still need more antidepressants, to increase overall efficacy, speed of response, and particularly to reach those patients not helped by the current drugs. The best chances may still lie in drugs with novel actions. At the time of writing there is considerable interest in a new substance P antagonist, which has shown promise in an early trial, but further studies are awaited.

REFERENCES

1. Paykel E.S., Ramana R., Cooper Z., Hayhurst H., Kerr J., Barocka A. (1995) Residual symptoms after partial remission: an important outcome in depression. *Psychol. Med.*, **25**: 1171–1180.
2. Paykel E.S., Hollyman J.A., Freeling P., Sedgwick P. (1988) Predictors of therapeutic benefit from amitriptyline in mild depression: a general practice placebo-controlled trial. *J. Affect. Disord.*, **14**: 83–95.
3. Stewart J.W., McGrath P.J., Liebowitz M.R., Harrison W., Quitkin E., Rabkin J.G. (1985) Treatment outcome validation of DSM-III depressive subtypes: clinical usefulness in outpatients with mild to moderate depression. *Arch. Gen. Psychiatry*, **42**: 1148–1153.
4. Schurman R.A., Kramer P.D., Mitchell J.B. (1985) The hidden mental health network. *Arch. Gen. Psychiatry*, **42**: 89–94.
5. Paykel E.S. (1998) Book review of *The Antidepressant Era* (David Healy). *Br. J. Psychiatry*, **173**: 444.

2.2
Targeting Antidepressant Treatment: The Evidence is Weak
Chris Thompson[1]

In any therapeutic area the choice of treatment depends on three factors. First is the scientific evidence that one drug is superior to another in its efficacy or tolerability. The combination of this evidence with the current pricing regimes determines the cost-effectiveness of the different drugs. Second is the degree to which your patients are similar to the patients in the clinical trials. This will determine how much you can extrapolate from the scientific evidence to your practice. Most studies of antidepressants have been carried out on selected patients in secondary care, which creates problems for primary care workers, or those who treat a wide range of comorbid conditions alongside the depression. Third, and most important in the choice of an antidepressant for an individual patient, are the attitudes and beliefs of the patient. Most would prefer counselling, for which there is no evidence of effectiveness, and 74% think antidepressants are addictive [1]. Since depression is often a chronic illness, the patient may have had experience with antidepressants in the past and may have a preference of his own. Doctors who take the time to elicit the patients' preferences and (where the evidence allows) treat accordingly, gain outcomes. This probably has a greater effect than the detail of the choice between drugs, or even perhaps between classes of drug.

There is good consensus about some aspects of prescribing antidepressants [2, 3]. Several guidelines concur about the diagnostic indications for

[1]*University of Southampton, Royal South Hants Hospital, Brinton's Terrace, Southampton, SO14 0YG, UK*

antidepressants and the need for correct dosage and duration of treatment [4]. Treatment should be for depressive episode (ICD-10 mild, moderate or severe), in full therapeutic dose, and that dose should be continued for 4–6 months after recovery from a first episode, and for 5 years if there has been a history of recurrence. Schulberg et al [5] and Katon et al [6] in randomized controlled trials (RCTs) have shown that adequate treatment according to the US Agency for Health Care Policy and Research (AHCPR) guidelines gives a clinical outcome that is superior to the usual treatment.

The evidence is weak for clinically important differences between drugs within a class, but there clearly are significant differences between classes, particularly the selective serotonin reuptake inhibitors (SSRIs) and the tricyclics. They have different dosage schedules (tricyclics have to be titrated up to a known therapeutic dose while SSRIs can be started at a therapeutic dose). They have different side effects (tricyclics have a range of receptor blocking actions while SSRIs induce nausea and headache). They have different costs (tricyclics are much cheaper to prescribe). Finally they have different toxicities (SSRIs have a much broader therapeutic index).

Most of the other commonly used antidepressants, on the other hand, have a wide range of chemical structures, pharmacological actions, toxicities, dosing schedules and adverse effects. Only one, lofepramine, is at all commonly prescribed, having been identified as a possibly cost-effective alternative to the SSRIs, with a low toxicity in overdose and a lower burden of side effects than the tricyclics.

There is little consensus about the merits of different classes of drug as first line treatment. Meta-analyses suggest that SSRIs and tricyclics are of roughly equal efficacy when the latter are given in full dose [7, 8], but this does not necessarily indicate equal effectiveness in routine practice, for which pragmatic trials in representative patients would be required.

It is clear that major depressive disorder responds to antidepressants better than to a placebo in the short term (up to 8 weeks). Are there patients within that category who respond best or patients outside the category who also respond? In other words, how should we target treatment in clinical practice? In fact a wide range of other "neurotic disorders" also respond to the SSRIs, suggesting that careful identification of those with major depressive disorder may not be necessary. However, very few studies have adequately addressed this question in the primary care setting where most prescribing takes place. Paykel et al [9] reported that only the severity of depression predicted the differences between amitriptyline and placebo. Those with probable major depressive disorder responded but those with minor depression did not. There is clearly room for many more studies on this question, since this pivotal study was small, of short duration, used amitriptyline in a dose that is rarely used in practice, and reported only efficacy, not tolerability.

REFERENCES

1. Paykel E.S., Hollyman J.A., Freeling P., Sedgwick P. (1988) Predictors of therapeutic benefit from amitriptyline in mild depression: a general practice placebo controlled study. *J. Affect. Disord.*, **14**: 83–95.
2. Paykel E.S., Priest R.G. (1992) Recognition and management of depression in general practice. *Br. Med. J.*, **305**: 1198–1202.
3. Montgomery S.A., Henry J., McDonald G., Dinan T., Lader M., Hindmarch I., Clare A., Nutt D. (1994) Selective serotonin reuptake inhibitors: a meta-analysis of discontinuation rates. *Int. Clin. Psychopharmacol.*, **9**: 47–53.
4. Stevens L., Thompson C. (1995) Consensus statements on the treatment of depression. *Primary Care Psychiatry*, **1**: 45–46.
5. Schulberg H.C., Block M.R., Madonia M.J., Scott P., Rodriguez E., Imber S.D., Perel J., Lave J., Houck P.R., Coulehan J.L. (1996) Treating major depression in primary care practice, eight month clinical outcomes. *Arch. Gen. Psychiatry*, **53**: 913–919.
6. Katon W., Robinson P., VonKorff M., Lin E., Bush T., Ludman E., Simon G., Walker E. (1996) A multifaceted intervention to improve treatment of depression in primary care. *Arch. Gen. Psychiatry*, **53**: 924–932.
7. Song F., Freemantle N., Sheldon T.A., House A., Watson P., Long A., Mason J. (1993) Selective serotonin reuptake inhibitors: a meta-analysis of efficacy and acceptability. *Br. Med. J.*, **306**: 683–687.
8. Hotopf M., Hardy R., Lewis G. (1997) Discontinuation rates of SSRIs and tricyclic antidepressants: a meta analysis and investigation of heterogeneity. *Br. J. Psychiatry*, **170**: 120–127.
9. Paykel E.S., Hart D., Priest R.G. (1998) Changes in public attitudes to depression during the defeat depression campaign. *Br. J. Psychiatry*, **173**: 519–522.

2.3
The Selection of the Antidepressant in Clinical Practice

Sheldon H. Preskorn[1]

There are over 25 different antidepressants marketed worldwide. These agents can be grouped into eight classes as defined by their putative mechanism of action [1]. They range from agents with an apparently single mechanism of action mediating their antidepressant efficacy, such as serotonin selective reuptake inhibitors (SSRIs) (e.g. citalopram and sertraline) and norepinephrine selective reuptake inhibitors (e.g. desipramine and reboxetine) to agents with multiple mechanisms of action (e.g. amitriptyline).

Such a mechanistically based classificatory system can help the prescriber in four specific ways. First, it can be used to anticipate and understand the pharmacological effects that these drugs will produce in most patients. Second, it can facilitate the selection of a specific agent for a patient with a specific symptom cluster (e.g. insomnia and anorexia versus hypersomnia

[1]*Department of Psychiatry, University of Kansas Medical School, Wichita, KS 67214-2878, USA*

and hyperphagia). Third, it can be used to anticipate pharmacodynamically mediated drug–drug interactions. Fourth, it can aid the prescriber in selecting an alternative antidepressant for a patient who has not benefited from a trial of a first drug.

This last issue is particularly problematic since only a small percentage of patients specifically respond to any single antidepressant. Specific antidepressant response is based on clinical trial data and refers to the percentage of patients who respond on the antidepressant minus the percentage who respond on the parallel placebo control. In general, specific antidepressant response is 15–25% (e.g. 60% response rate on the antidepressant vs. 35–45% response rate on the parallel placebo arm).

For this reason, one of the most pressing needs in clinical psycho-pharmacology relative to antidepressants is what to do when the first antidepressant selected has failed to treat the patient adequately. A survey done in clinical practice found that the majority of primary care and psychiatric physicians choose one of the SSRIs as their antidepressant of first choice, presumably because of their safety and good tolerability along with adequate antidepressant efficacy. While this choice is understandable, most physicians also switch patients who have not benefited from one SSRI to a second and even a third SSRI. This pattern of drug selection does not make intuitive sense since these antidepressants appear to have the same mechanism mediating antidepressant response [2]. Yet, rigorous clinical data supporting or refuting this practice are not available.

A study is now ongoing that should help to answer this question. This study is comparing, with a double-blind, parallel prospective design, the relative efficacy of citalopram versus venlafaxine in patients who have not benefited adequately from a previous trial of an SSRI other than citalopram. The hypothesis is that treatment with venlafaxine, due to its apparent dual mechanism of action, will produce superior antidepressant efficacy in comparison to citalopram in patients who have previously not responded to serotonin uptake inhibition as a mechanism capable of mediating antidepressant response [3].

Several other double-blind crossover studies have indeed indicated that a sizable percentage of patients who do not respond to an antidepressant with one mechanism of action will respond when switched to an antidepressant with a different mechanism of action [4].

Another serious limitation for the practicing psychiatrist is the nature of patients selected for most antidepressant clinical trials which support a new drug application to drug regulatory agencies. These limitations stem from the inclusion and exclusion criteria used in such studies. These typically exclude patients with depressive episodes that have lasted more than 2 years, have not been responsive to two adequate trials of two different antidepressants, or are not severe enough to require hospitalization. Patients are also typically excluded if they have concomitant psychotic symptoms or suicidal thoughts, meet criteria for more than one psychiatric syndrome, or have abused alcohol or used illicit drugs within the past 24 months. Patients are also excluded if they are medically unstable, are on other psychotropic medications, or are on any medication which has not been given at a stable dose for at least 3 months. For these reasons, only a small percentage of patients seen by a private practice psychiatrist would actually be eligible for most clinical trials for most antidepressants. Yet, this same physician must extrapolate from results in this rarefied patient population to the patient he/she must treat in everyday practice.

Physicians, particularly psychiatrists, need more rigorous information on the effectiveness of different antidepressants in the patients that they actually treat, including effectiveness in patients who have not benefited from a previous trial of an antidepressant. The World Psychiatric Association and similar such bodies can be important advocates to encourage companies which market antidepressants to conduct studies which will aid the prescriber in selecting a given antidepressant for a specific patient situation.

REFERENCES

1. Catterson M., Preskorn S.H., Bremner J.D., Dessain E.C. (1996) Double-blind crossover study of mirtazapine, amitriptyline and placebo in patients with major depression. Presented at the 36th Annual Meeting of the American Psychiatric Association, New York, 7 May.
2. Preskorn S.H. (1999) *Outpatient Management of Depression*, 2nd edn, Professional Communications, Caddo, Oklahoma.
3. Preskorn S.H. (1998) Recent dose-effect studies regarding antidepressants. In *European Cooperation in the Field of Scientific and Technical Research* (Eds L.P. Balant, J. Benitez, S.G. Dahl, L.F. Gram, R.M. Pinder, W.Z. Potter), pp. 45–61, European Commission, Brussels.
4. Thase M.E., Rush A.J. (1995) Treatment-resistant depression. In *Psychopharmacology: The Fourth Generation of Progress* (Eds F.E. Bloom, O.J. Kupfer), pp. 1081–1097, Raven Press, New York.

2.4

Gender and Antidepressant Response

Alan F. Schatzberg[1] and Susan G. Kornstein[2]

The past decade has witnessed the rapid growth of antidepressant therapy, with a host of new antidepressants available for treating patients with

[1] *Department of Psychiatry and Behavioral Sciences, Stanford University School of Medicine, Stanford, CA 94305-5717, USA*
[2] *Department of Psychiatry, Virginia Commonwealth University, Richmond, Virginia, USA*

depressive disorders. Prof. Bech's review highlights several of these advances and concludes that the major advantages of the newer antidepressants for acute therapy lie more with their better side-effect profiles than with enhanced efficacy. This argument has been made by a number of others. Although it seems reasonable on the surface, it is at some variance with the marked public acceptance and success enjoyed by the newer agents, particularly the selective serotonin reuptake inhibitors (SSRI). These agents have been heralded by so many patients and treaters that it is hard to believe the many studies that do not support superior efficacy over the tricyclic antidepressants (TCAs).

Recent data suggest the situation is far more complex and that efficacy between older and newer agents may indeed not be equivalent in both men and women patients, particularly those with chronic major depression, major depression with dysthymia (so-called double depression), or dysthymic disorder. A recent review and meta-analysis of the TCA literature indicates that in some 15 studies that have explored gender the TCAs proved significantly more effective in men than in women [1]. This poorer efficacy in women suggests that a potentially large group of undertreated female patients existed when the SSRIs were initially introduced in the late 1980s.

In our recent collaborative study of patients with either chronic major depression or so-called "double depression," we observed a significant effect of gender on acute antidepressant response to treatment with imipramine or sertraline [2]. In this large study of 635 cases, patients were initially treated for 12 weeks with imipramine or sertraline under double-blind conditions [3]. Maximum doses were 300 mg/day and 200 mg/day for imipramine and sertraline respectively. Men responded significantly better to treatment with imipramine than they did to sertraline. In contrast, women responded significantly better to sertraline than to imipramine. Moreover, the preferential response in women to the SSRI was primarily found in premenopausal women. Postmenopausal women responded equally to both drugs — that is imipramine was relatively more effective in older than in younger women [2]. These data do indeed suggest a possible interaction between hormonal status and SSRI response.

In this study, nonresponders were crossed over to the other drug. Women who failed to respond to imipramine did well when switched over to sertraline, providing further evidence of preferential responsivity to SSRIs in chronically depressed women.

In another study of some 400 patients, Yonkers et al [6] reported that women with dysthymia significantly more often responded to sertraline than they did to imipramine or placebo. These data again suggest differential responses to TCAs vs. sertraline in chronically depressed women. In addition, Steiner et al [5], reviewing the paroxetine trials data base, reported that women responded better to paroxetine than they did to imipramine.

Many previous studies have not reported differential responses to medication based on gender. One possibility is that gender was not explored. More likely, however, is that a confluence of factors may have played a role in others not making this observation. First, for many years in the US, women of child-bearing age were routinely excluded from investigational drug trials. This situation has changed in recent years, in part due to legislation. Thus, older previous studies often included primarily postmenopausal women which would have lessened the likelihood of making such observations. Second, the findings on sertraline were derived from relatively large-scale studies (of 400 and 600 patients each). Thus, previous studies may also not have had sufficient power to detect differences. Third, the observations may be more likely to be found in chronically depressed patients, that had not been commonly studied previously. Last, this differential responsivity may not be true for all SSRIs. A meta-analysis of the possible effect for gender on fluoxetine response did not observe this effect, although menopausal status was not taken into account in this analysis [4].

Thus, recent studies indicate that the conclusions that the newer antidepressants — particularly the SSRIs — are not particularly more effective than the TCAs may be misleading. They may have potential greater efficacy in chronically depressed premenopausal women. Further studies are required to determine whether this is true of all SSRIs and whether this differential response is seen in women whose depressions are of shorter duration.

REFERENCES

1. Hamilton J.A., Grant M., Jensvold M.F. (1996) Sex and treatment of depression. In *Psychopharmacology and Women: Sex, Gender, and Hormones* (Eds M.J. Jensvold, U. Halbreich, J.A. Harvi Hon), pp. 241–260, American Psychiatric Press, Washington, DC.
2. Keller M.B., Gelenberg A.J., Hirschfeld R.M.A., Rush A.J., Thase M.E., Kocsis J.H., Markowitz J.C., Fawcett J.A., Koran L.M., Klein D.N. *et al* (1998) The treatment of chronic depression, part 2. A double-blind randomized trial of sertraline and imipramine. *J. Clin. Psychiatry*, **59**: 598–607.
3. Kornstein S.G., Schatzberg A.F., Thase M.E., Yonkers K.A., McCullough J.P., Keitner G.I., Gelenberg A.J., Davis S.M., Harrison W.M., Keller M.B. (1999) Gender differences in treatment response to sertraline versus imipramine in chronic depression. Submitted for publication.
4. Lewis-Hall F.C., Wilson M.G., Tepner R.G. (1997) Fluoxetine vs. tricyclic antidepressants in women with major depressive disorder. *J. Women's Health*, **6**: 337–343.
5. Steiner M., Wheadon D.E., Kreider M.S., Bushwell W.D. (1993) Antidepressant response to paroxetine by gender. Presented at the APA Meeting, San Francisco, 22–27 May.
6. Yonkers K.A., Rush A.J., Kornstein S.G., Halbreich U., Pearlstein T., Stone A. (1995) Gender differences in the response to pharmacotherapy among early onset dysthymics. Presented at the ACNP Meeting, San Juan, PR, 11–15 December.

2.5
Validity of Atypical Depression: Evidence Provided by Pharmacological Dissection
Frederic M. Quitkin[1]

The focus of this commentary is atypical depression, a recently recognized depressive subtype with heuristic and clinical implications. Recently reported data add support to the hypothesis that atypical depression is a categorically distinct subtype of depression. Evidence supporting the validity of a depressive subgroup with reversed vegetative symptoms was first proposed by the Columbia group [1–6]. This work focused on the increased responsivity of atypical depressives to monoamine oxidase inhibitors (MAOIs) compared to tricyclic antidepressants (TCAs). This led to the inclusion of atypical depression as a parenthetical modifier in DSM-IV [7].

Subsequently, in a prospective epidemiological study of female twins, Kendler *et al* [8] also supported a categorical distinction for atypical depressives. They used latent class analysis and identified three depressive subtypes—mild typical, atypical, and severe typical depression. Subjects with atypical depression were characterized by reversed vegetative depressive symptoms (overeating and oversleeping). These groups differed on many validating criteria, supporting a categorical distinction.

The Columbia group has done a series of studies comparing placebo, imipramine and phenelzine in atypical depressives [1–5]. A patient was considered to be an atypical depressive if he met DSM-III criteria for major depressive disorder or dysthymia and had two of four associated features. The associated features are overeating, oversleeping, pathological rejection sensitivity and leaden paralysis (feeling one's limbs are weighted down). In a series of four studies, atypical depressives had a superior response on phenelzine compared to imipramine and placebo [5]. Since no other prospective study had demonstrated the superiority of an MAOI to a TCA, these studies support the validity of atypical depression as a distinct depressive subgroup.

Adherents to a dimensional view attribute observed differences in depressive subtypes to severity. If atypical depression were mild melancholia, a robust TCA response would be expected. Our work supported a categorical distinction between severe typical (melancholic) and atypical depression since the poor TCA response of the latter is inconsistent with a dimensional view. Could other factors interfere with these patients' ability to benefit from drug treatment? Chronicity or maladaptive character traits (superimposed on mild melancholia) did not seem to preclude TCA responsivity and explain

_____

[1] *New York State Psychiatric Institute, 722 West 168th Street, New York 10032, USA*

the low TCA improvement rate, because the high MAOI improvement rate is consistent with a drug-responsive group. Because the 44% TCA response rate was observed in 147 subjects with atypical depression, the confidence limits (95% confidence interval, 35–54) are narrow and a good approximation of what exists in the population. A preliminary family study also supports the distinction between atypical depression and melancholia [6]. Most prior discussion of the binary, versus the unitary, view of depression focused on patients with psychotic and melancholic symptoms, that is, are mood congruent delusions sufficient for inclusion in a particular categorical type? [9]. Of particular interest is that these current studies offer a nosological distinction of patients formerly considered in the neurotic pole of the distribution, where categorical difference seemed unlikely.

In summary, the salient aspects of the subtypes defined by Kendler *et al*, using latent class analysis (in a female population sample of twins), are strikingly similar to the subtypes that we have identified using psychopharmacologic dissection (in male and female treatment seekers). The similar outcome in men and women in our studies suggests the findings by Kendler *et al* in women may also be applicable to men. The work of Kendler *et al* adds further support to including atypical as a parenthetical modifier of major depression in DSM-IV. Both sets of data support the possibility of categorically distinct subtypes.

Although phenelzine, a non-selective MAOI, was clearly demonstrated to have a beneficial response in this patient group, because of side effects its widespread use is unlikely. Unfortunately, at present there are no controlled studies demonstrating a robust response of one of the second generation drugs in this patient group.

REFERENCES

1. Quitkin F.M., Stewart J.S., McGrath P.J., Liebowitz M.R., Harrison W.M., Tricamo E., Klein D.F., Rabkin J.G., Markowitz J.S., Wager S.G. (1988) Phenelzine versus imipramine in the treatment of probable atypical depression: defining syndrome boundaries of selective MAOI responders. *Am. J. Psychiatry*, **145**: 306–311.
2. Quitkin F.M., McGrath P.J., Stewart J.W., Harrison W., Wager S.G., Nunes E., Rabkin J.G., Tricamo E., Markowitz J., Klein D.F. (1989) Phenelzine and imipramine in mood reactive depressives: further delineation of the syndrome of atypical depression. *Arch. Gen. Psychiatry*, **46**: 787–793.
3. Quitkin F.M., McGrath P.J., Stewart J.W., Harrison W., Tricamo E., Wager S.G., Ocepek-Welikson K., Nunes E., Rabkin J.G., Klein D.F. (1990) Atypical depression, panic attacks, and response to imipramine and phenelzine: a replication. *Arch. Gen. Psychiatry*, **47**: 935–941.
4. Quitkin F.M., Harrison W., Stewart J.W., McGrath P.J., Tricamo E., Ocepek-Welikson K., Rabkin J.G., Wager S.G., Nunes E., Klein D.F. (1991) Response to phenelzine and imipramine in placebo non-responders with atypical depression: a new application of the crossover design. *Arch. Gen. Psychiatry*, **48**: 319–323.

5. Quitkin F.M., Stewart J.W., McGrath P.J., Tricamo E., Rabkin J.G., Ocepek-Welikson K., Nunes E., Harrison W., Klein D.F. (1993) Columbia atypical depression. A subgroup of depressives with better response to MAOI than to tricyclic antidepressants or placebo. *Br. J. Psychiatry* **163** (Suppl. 21): 30–34.
6. Stewart J.S., McGrath P.J., Rabkin J.G., Quitkin F.M. (1993) Atypical depression: a valid clinical entity? *Psychiatr. Clin. N. Am.*, **16**: 479–495.
7. American Psychiatric Association (1994) *Diagnostic and Statistical Manual of Mental Disorders*, 4th edn, American Psychiatric Association, Washington, DC.
8. Kendler K.S., Eaves L.J., Walters E.E., Neale M.C., Heath A.C., Kessler R.C. (1996) The identification and validation of distinct depressive syndromes in a population-based sample of female twins. *Arch. Gen. Psychiatry*, **53**: 391–399.
9. Glassman A., Kantor S., Shostak M. (1975) Depressions, delusions and drug response. *Am. J. Psychiatry*, **132**: 716–719.

2.6
Increasing Our Understanding of the Working Mechanism of Antidepressants

Johan A. den Boer[1]

During the last two decades, a number of different research strategies, including investigations in postmortem tissue, neuroendocrine studies, and neuroimaging studies, have refined our understanding of the underlying biological correlates of depression. During the same period a large number of agents with different pharmacological profiles have been developed which exert antidepressant actions.

Antidepressants play a major role in the treatment of major depression. Per Bech has described the developments in antidepressant therapy in a lucid and comprehensive way. The clinician will find this chapter a useful update of differences between older and second generation antidepressants in terms of clinical efficacy, side-effect profile and safety. It is interesting to see that the pendulum swings from broad-spectrum pharmacological profiles to high degrees of selectivity and recently, with the introduction of dual action antidepressants, back to a broader pharmacological profile with a reduced propensity for disabling side effects such as impotence and toxicity at higher dosages. There is, mainly due to the publication of recent meta-analyses, an ongoing debate concerning the differential efficacy of dual action versus selective monoamine reuptake inhibitors. The recently introduced dual action antidepressants venlafaxine and mirtazapine in particular have been compared to SSRIs. It is of great interest to see that both venlafaxine and mirtazapine were found to be more efficacious compared to fluoxetine [1, 2]. More recently,

[1] *State University Groningen, PO Box 30001, 9700 RB Groningen, The Netherlands*

mirtazapine has been studied in two double-blind comparative trials versus paroxetine and citalopram. Compared with citalopram, mirtazapine showed a significantly greater improvement in depressive symptoms on three efficacy measures at week 2 of treatment. Compared with paroxetine, mirtazapine was significantly better only at week 1. More patients were responding to treatment with mirtazapine than to paroxetine at all time points, and the difference reached statistical significance at weeks of 1 and 4. In both studies patients on mirtazapine had fewer SSRI-associated side effects such as headaches, nausea and sweating. In addition, no differences were observed between the drugs in the number of patients experiencing somnolence [3].

What is rather surprising is that data on the other dual action antidepressant milnacipran have not been included in Bech's review, whereas milnacipran has been studied in several well-designed studies and has been marketed in Portugal and France. Milnacipran also has proven superior to SSRIs in some, but not all studies, and was found to be ineffective in therapy-resistant depression [4].

A topic which has received considerable attention at many recent international conferences and is also touched upon in Bech's review, is the degree to which augmentation strategies using pindolol as add-on to treatment with SSRIs may enhance the onset of antidepressant response in patients suffering from major depression. The idea behind this strategy is that 5-HT release induced by SSRIs is augmented by co-administration of a $5-HT_{1A}$ autoreceptor antagonist. Several studies using different SSRIs such as fluoxetine, paroxetine and citalopram have in the meantime been published indicating (although it is not unequivocal) that pindolol addition may indeed in some (as yet undefined) patients improve the latency and efficacy of SSRIs. It has been suggested that the large variability in the treatment response seen in these studies reflects $5-HT_{1A}$ genetic polymorphism [5], allelic variants of the 5-HT transporter [6] or factors related to differences in patients' characteristics [7, 8]. Interestingly, a recent study failed to find any efficacy of pindolol addition to fluvoxamine in panic disorder patients [9]. This might hint at differences between major depression and panic disorder at the level of the $5-HT_{1A}$ receptor.

REFERENCES

1. Clerc G.E., Ruimy P., Verdeau-Pailes J. (1994) A double-blind comparison of venlafaxine and fluoxetine in patients hospitalized for major depression and melancholia. *Int. Clin. Psychopharmacol.*, **9**: 139–143.
2. Wheatley D.P., Van Moffaert M., Timmerman L., Kremer C. (1998) Mirtazapine: efficacy and tolerability in comparison with fluoxetine in patients with moderate to severe major depressive disorder. *J. Clin. Psychiatry*, **59**: 306–312.
3. Kasper S. (1997) Efficacy of antidepressants in the treatment of severe depression: the place of mitazapine. *J. Clin. Psychopharmacol.*, **17**: 195–285.

4. Steen A., den Boer J.A. (1997) A double-blind six months comparative study of milnacipran and clomipramine in major depressive disorder. *Int. Clin. Psychophar-macol.*, **12**: 269–281.
5. Isaac M.T., Tome M.B. (1997) Selective serotonin reuptake inhibitors plus pindolol (letter). *Lancet*, **350**: 288–289.
6. Artigas F. (1997) Potential rapid onset: mechanisms of action. *Eur. Neuropsy-chopharmacol.*, **7** (Suppl. 2): S100–S101.
7. Tome M.B., Cloninger C.R., Watson J.P., Isaac M.T. (1997) Serotonergic autore-ceptor blockade in the reduction of antidepressant latency: personality variables and response to paroxetine and pindolol. *J. Affect. Disord.*, **44**: 101–109.
8. den Boer J.A., Slaap B.R., Bosker F.J. (1998) Biological aspects of anxiety disor-ders and depression. In *SSRIs in Depression and Anxiety* (Eds S.A. Montgomery, J.A. Den Boer), pp. 23–80, Wiley, Chichester.
9. Van Vliet I.M., Westenberg H.G.M., den Boer J.A. (1998) Pindolol does not augment the panicolytic effects of fluvoxamine in panic disorder patients. Submitted for publication.

2.7

Are the First Generation Monoamine Reuptake Inhibitors Still Needed in the Treatment of Major Depressive Episode?

Annette Gjerris[1]

With the toxicity and side effects of tricyclic antidepressants (TCAs) and monoamine oxidase inhibitors (MAOIs) in mind, I think that most patients and psychiatrists would prefer to stop using these drugs. However, what is myth, what is reality and what is a matter of interpretation of data when it comes to evaluation of the efficacy of the new generation of antidepressants? Per Bech, through a very comprehensive review of the literature, enables the reader to evaluate results from a large number of randomized clinical trials (RCTs) and against this background to try to answer the question put forward in the title of this commentary.

One controversial point is whether it is meaningful to distinguish between efficacy in the treatment of inpatients and outpatients, when they are all classified as suffering from a major depressive episode (MDE). In other words, are the two groups clinically similar or are we dealing with two different groups although they fulfil the same inclusion criteria except for status with regard to hospitalization? Bech demonstrates that the key issue of major depression is the severity of the depression. Thus, it appears that subjects treated in an outpatient setting primarily comprise patients with MDE without melancholic features, with a score on the Hamilton Rating

[1]*Department of Psychiatry, Gentofte University Hospital, Niels Andersensvej 65, 2900 Hellerup, Denmark*

scale for Depression, 17-item version (HAM-D 17) of 18–24, whereas patients treated in an inpatient setting primarily comprise the group of patients with MDE with melancholic or psychotic features HAM-D 17 = 25 or higher). With this in mind, it seems easier to understand the results showing that in 6 out of 15 randomized clinical trials TCAs are found more effective than SSRIs in the treatment of MDE in inpatients.

The benefits of the second generation antidepressants compared with the first generation ones with regard to toxicity and side effects are obvious, although, as stated by Prof. Bech, a number of the new drugs do have some of the same side effects connected with the first generation drugs, such as weight gain, sexual dysfunction and sedation. Thus, while first and second generation antidepressants are apparently comparable with regard to efficacy in treatment of *outpatients* with major depression, the groups do differ from each other to some extent with regard to side effects and definitely with regard to toxicity.

Combination therapies may be dangerous and surprisingly little is known about drug interactions. Very little documentation is required by the regulatory authorities about this issue when the applications for registrations are evaluated. Psychiatrists are often very creative when a patient does not respond satisfactorily to the treatment given, and therefore feel tempted to turn to "add-on treatment". It is, therefore, recommended that the regulatory authorities in the future pay much more attention to the matter of drug interaction. Furthermore, it should be stressed that recommendations of combination therapies in therapy-resistant depressed patients are often based on studies comprising rather small numbers of patients. When it comes to combinations between second generation antidepressants, no systematic data from research programmes seem to be available.

The review by Bech is extremely useful, and I fully agree with him on most of the conclusions given. However, when it comes to replacement of TCAs with second generation antidepressants, I still think that convincing data are missing, showing the efficacy of SSRIs in the treatment of severe MDE, maybe defined by HAM-D = 25 or higher or by the presence of somatic or psychotic features.

With regard to the second generation antidepressants, I would reserve the SSRIs as well as the other drugs to the short-term treatment of outpatients or patients with a Hamilton score below 25 without somatic or psychotic features. The SSRIs seem furthermore to be useful for medium-term therapy and for prevention of recurrences. Concerning venlafaxine, it seems in many ways to be equivalent to the SSRIs, and to be useful in medium-term treatment as well. Reboxetine and nefazadone still need to show their efficacy outside the acute treatment.

In other words, second generation antidepressants may appear to be proper alternatives to the classic antidepressants in the treatment of moderate MDE in outpatients, and in the prevention of relapses or recurrences. However, it is still to be proven whether this goes for all second generation antidepressants or only for subgroups and whether they are as potent as the classic drugs.

2.8
Antidepressants in Broader Context
Cyril Höschl[1]

The whole psychosocial context of mental disorders significantly changed after the introduction of psychopharmacology [1, 2] into clinical practice in the middle of this century. In parallel with increasing knowledge of the pharmacodynamics of major psychotropic drugs, attempts to find an alternative treatment and/or explanation of psychotropic effectiveness have continued. New non-pharmacological therapeutic modalities have been shown to be effective, for example cognitive-behavioral [3, 4] and light [5] therapy. The social situation of psychiatric patients in many countries changed hand in hand with the increased emphasis on human rights in the 1970s. Thus, in psychopharmacotherapy, the emphasis was moved from efficacy onto safety. This is also reflected in evidence-based summaries of the efficacy and safety of older vs. newer drugs.

There is currently a trend to transform custodial psychiatric care toward more community-based service. This also necessitates developing drugs with higher compliance and safety. On the other hand, the need for treatment of pharmacoresistant depression has become more important in inpatient facilities. The change of one antidepressant for another, their combination or augmentation with lithium, with thyroid hormones (for review see [6]), with pindolol [7] or with other drugs (e.g. buspirone [8]) has been recommended to overcome resistance. In bipolar depression, calcium channel blockers have also been studied (for review, see [9]). Verapamil has been superior to placebo in the treatment of mania in a double-blind study, but failed in the treatment of depressive episode [10]. Serious attempts to develop practically useful treatment guidelines have recently been made [11].

Besides antidepressants, anticonvulsants [12], herbal remedies (*Hypericum perforatum* [13]), acupuncture, exercise, sleep deprivation, and other complementary therapies have also been successfully used in the treatment of depression, although the evidence of efficacy is rather scarce [14]. Despite the "monoaminergic dogma," there are still other pharmacological approaches to target depression. Dysregulation of the

_____
[1]*Prague Psychiatric Center, Ústavní 91, 181 03 Prague 8-Bohnice, Czech Republic*

hypothalamo–pituitary–adrenocortical axis resulting in hypercortisolemia is characteristic of major depression [15]. This observation led to attempts to treat depression with either other steroids or with glucocorticoid inhibitors such as metyrapone (for review see [16]). These treatments, however, have not been routinely adopted.

In the search for distinct mechanisms of antidepressant activity, a significant breakthrough has been achieved recently (for a review and new research see [17]). It has been demonstrated that substance P-preferring neurokinin-1 (NK_1) receptors are highly expressed in brain regions that are critical for the regulation of affective behavior. Higher concentrations of substance P were found in the cerebrospinal fluid of depressed patients. Established antidepressant drugs cause down-regulation of substance P biosynthesis. Substance P antagonists inhibit vocalizations evoked in guinea pig pups by transient maternal separation. Furthermore, the substance P antagonist MK-869 is an efficacious and well-tolerated antidepressant in patients with major depressive disorder. As substance P antagonists do not significantly interfere with monoaminergic metabolism, a novel mechanism of antidepressant activity is being postulated. The possibility that alterations in substance P or NK_1 receptors are primarily involved in the pathogenesis of depression requires further investigation.

Advances in molecular biology have also shed a new light on mechanisms of activity of established antidepressants. Long-term treatment with antidepressants results in sustained activation of intracellular signal transduction pathways. Activation of protein-kinase A and its translocation into the nucleus leads to higher expression and activity of cAMP-response element binding protein (CREB), which seems to be a common post-receptor place of action of antidepressants. These changes are in relation to higher expression of brain derived neurotropic factor (BDNF). Up-regulation of neurotropic factors increases the activity and survival of neurons in several brain regions and plays an important role in synaptic remodulation [18].

It is stimulating to read of current achievements in psychopharmacology, its perspectives and practical implications, in the larger context of recent progress in neuroscience.

REFERENCES

1. Delay J., Bernitzer P. (1952) Le traitment des psychoses par une méthode neuroleptique dérivée de l'hibernothérapie. In *Congres de Médecins Alienistes et Neurologistes de France* (Ed. P.C. Ossa), pp. 497–502, Masson, Paris.
2. Deniker P. (1983) Discovery of the clinical use of neuroleptics. In *Discoveries in Pharmacology, vol. 1, Psycho- and Neuro-Pharmacology* (Eds M.J. Parnham, J. Bruinvels), pp. 163–180, Elsevier, Amsterdam.
3. Lewinsohn P.M., Clarke G.N., Hops H., Andrews J. (1990) Cognitive-behavioral treatment for depressed adolescents. *Behav. Ther.*, **21**: 385–401.

4.   Lidren D.M., Watkins P.L., Gould R.A., Clum G.A., Asterino M., Tulloch H.L. (1994) A comparison of bibliotherapy and group therapy in the treatment of panic disorder. *J. Consult. Clin. Psychol.*, **62**: 865–869.
5.   Sack R.L., Lewy A.J., White D.M., Singer C.M., Fireman M.J., Vandiver R.(1990) Morning vs evening light treatment for winter depression. Evidence that the therapeutic effects of light are mediated by circadian phase shifts. *Arch. Gen. Psychiatry*, **47**: 343–351.
6.   Cadieux R.J. (1998) Practical management of treatment-resistant depression. *Am. Fam. Physician*, **58**: 2059–2062.
7.   Blier P., Bergeron R., de Montigny C. (1998) Adjunct treatments for rapid onset of action and greater efficacy in major depression. In *Antidepressant Therapy at the Dawn of the Third Millennium* (Eds M. Briley, S.A. Montgomery), pp. 279–295, Dunitz, London.
8.   Jacobsen F.M. (1991) Possible augmentation of antidepressant response by buspirone. *J. Clin. Psychiatry*, **52**: 217–218.
9.   Höschl C. (1991) Do calcium antagonists have a place in the treatment of mood disorders? *Drugs*, **42**: 721–729.
10. Höschl C., Kožený J. (1989) Verapamil in affective disorders: a double-blind, controlled study. *Biol. Psychiatry*, **25**: 128–140.
11. Goodwin G.M., Nolen W.A. (1997) Treatment of bipolar depressive mood disorders: algorithms for pharmacotherapy. *Int. J. Psychiatry Clin. Practice*, **1**: S9–S12.
12. Dunn R.T., Frye M.S., Kimbrell T.A., Denicoff K.D., Leverich G.S., Post R.M. (1998) The efficacy and use of anticonvulsants in mood disorders. *Clin. Neuropharmacol.*, **21**: 215–235.
13. Rey J.M., Walter G. (1998) *Hypericum perforatum* (St John's wort) in depression: pest or blessing? *Med. J. Aust.*, **169**: 583–586.
14. Ernst E., Rand J.I., Stevinson C. (1998) Complementary therapies for depression: an overview. *Arch. Gen. Psychiatry*, **55**: 1026–1032.
15. Carroll B.J. (1982) The dexamethasone suppression test for melancholia. *Br. J. Psychiatry*, **140**: 292–304.
16. Murphy B.E. (1997) Antiglucocorticoid therapies in major depression: a review. *Psychoneuroendocrinology*, **22**: S125–S132.
17. Kramer M.S., Cutler N., Feighner J., Shrivastava R., Carman J., Sramek J.J., Reines S.A., Liu G., Snavely D., Wyatt-Knowles E. *et al* (1998) Distinct mechanism for antidepressant activity by blockade of central substance P receptors. *Science*, **281**: 1640–1645.
18. Duman R.S., Heninger G.R., Nestler E.J. (1997) A molecular and cellular theory of depression. *Arch. Gen. Psychiatry*, **54**: 597–606.

2.9

Antidepressants for Better Quality of Life

Siegfried Kasper[1]

Antidepressant pharmacotherapy revolutionized treatment in both unipolar and bipolar depression. Whereas the first antidepressants were found by

[1]*Department of General Psychiatry, University of Vienna, Währinger Gürtel 18–20, A-1090 Vienna, Austria*

chance, their successful usage stimulated further basic research programs with the aim of finding more specifically acting antidepressants with a distinct mechanism of action. Together with non-pharmacological, biologically based antidepressant treatment modalities, such as electroconvulsive treatment, therapeutic sleep deprivation, light therapy and transcranial magnetic stimulation, a line of antidepressant treatment modalities emerged for the benefit of our patients (see [1] for a review).

Whereas first generation antidepressants (tricyclics and MAO inhibitors) were associated with burdensome side effects, the class of selective serotonin reuptake inhibitors (SSRIs) first exhibited a favourable side-effect profile, which opened the way for effective pharmacotherapy for the necessary long-term treatment in depression (see [2] for a review). Since depression should be considered as a lifelong disorder, in the same way as hypertension or diabetes mellitus, the SSRIs revolutionized treatment, in the sense that antidepressants could be used in the necessary dosage for long-term treatment. Contrastingly, patients were not willing to take first generation antidepressants in the right dosage for much longer than the acute phase and therefore exposed themselves to a higher risk of relapse. Fortunately the same successful strategy, a favourable side-effect profile, has been followed for the antidepressants introduced after the SSRIs.

Newer antidepressants are often described with short abbreviations related to their pharmacodynamic properties (RIMA = reversible inhibitors of monoamine oxidase A; NaSSA = nonadrenaline serotonin specific antidepressants; SNRIs = serotonin noradrenaline reuptake inhibitors; NRI = noradrenaline reuptake inhibitors; DAS = dual serotonergic antidepressants). Of course, these abbreviations are used by the pharmaceutical industry for marketing purposes, but they also help the clinician to understand the efficacy and most importantly the side-effect profile. For instance, it is on a very practical everyday level necessary to know that the combination of two SSRIs does not make any sense, since the same mechanism of action is involved. Contrastingly, the combination of an SSRI with a noradrenergic reuptake inhibitor makes sense for the clinician, since a better efficacy can be expected in certain patient groups. Furthermore, pharmacokinetic properties which make it necessary to know the interaction profile are more and more considered in everyday clinical practice, in order to avoid troublesome side effects. Taking together the long-term perspective of depressive illness, and the pharmacodynamic and pharmacokinetic properties of the antidepressants considered to be beneficial for our patients, it is evident that the choice of medication should be "side-effect guided" on the basis of individual assessment of our patients.

Whereas psychiatrists 20–30 years ago did not really have a documented rationale for pharmacotherapy of depression, there is now solid evidence of biological disturbances in depression. However, these documented disturbances do not rule out the fact that acute or chronic life events are substantial factors at the beginning or during the course of depression. The necessity of combining a pharmacotherapeutic with a psychotherapeutic approach is therefore evident in order to maximize the treatment outcome. The question then emerges which sort of psychotherapy should be used, since such a range of pharmacotherapeutic modalities are available. The first and probably the best psychotherapy in the sense of supportive psychotherapy is to know about the nature of the disorder in the acute and long-term perspective and the possible influences of life events and pharmacotherapy. This seems to be so obvious, but its complexity and the necessity of integrating new research findings into each therapist's own level of experience are often underestimated. The best antidepressant, whatsoever it might be, does not work in the necessary long-term perspective if this integrative viewpoint is forgotten or considered to be of lower priority.

REFERENCES

1. Kasper S., Neumeister A. (1998) Non-pharmacological treatments for depression—focus on sleep deprivation and light therapy. In *Antidepressant Therapy at the Dawn of the Third Millennium* (Eds M. Briley, S. Montgomery), pp. 255–278, Dunitz, London.
2. Kasper S. (1993) The rationale for long-term antidepressant therapy. *Int. Clin. Psychopharmacol.*, **8**: 225–235.

2.10

Would Rational Polypharmacy Improve Quality of Life?

Santosh K. Chaturvedi[1]

A number of the antidepressants reviewed by Prof. Bech, especially the newer ones, are not available in India, and possibly many other countries. This in effect means that the majority of depressed patients in the world are treated using traditional tricyclic antidepressants (TCAs) and perhaps a couple of selective serotonin reuptake inhibitors (SSRIs). Treatment of depressed patients in India is usually accomplished using TCAs such as imipramine or amitriptyline in general, dothiepin or doxepin for those with cardiac or physical problems, and SSRIs such as fluoxetine and sertraline. Other antidepressants used sometimes include amoxapine, mianserin, trazodone, amineptine and tianeptine. The review is silent on these latter

[1]*National Institute of Mental Health and Neurosciences, Bangalore 560 029, India*

drugs. A number of antidepressants currently popular in the West, such as nefazodone, bupropion, venlafaxine, moclobemide, maprotiline, citalopram, fluvoxamine, lofepramine and paroxetine, are not yet available for Indian psychiatrists to treat their depressed patients. Mirtazapine is currently undergoing a trial. Electroconvulsive therapy (ECT) is still a popular, safe and cost-effective method available for treatment of those with severe depression, or depression with psychotic symptoms.

Bech's review also indicates that most studies have focused on adult males; there are few studies on the elderly (75 years and over) and studies on women are conspicuous by their lack. This is a strange situation, since major depression is at least twice as common in women than in men, and, to treat depressed women, guidelines provided by trials done on men are used! There are no studies to indicate that data obtained on men can be generalized safely to women.

The evidence provided by the review confirms the general view held by most practising psychiatrists that, by and large, most antidepressants are equally effective, but their safety and side-effect profiles differ. The choice of the antidepressant would therefore depend on three factors. Firstly, the cost factor: the cheapest TCAs are imipramine and amitriptyline. Fluoxetine preparations were expensive until some months back, after which the prices crashed because of the price war among the pharmaceutical companies. Secondly, the availability factor: as mentioned above, a number of the newer antidepressants are not yet available. Thirdly, the choice depends on the side-effect profile, as emphasized by the review. Keeping these three factors in mind, the first line of treatment is using TCAs in those who cannot afford the other drugs, and fluoxetine in those who can afford it. For milder depressions, and those with anxiety symptoms, alprazolam is still quite popular, especially among general practitioners.

Another lacuna which becomes obvious is the lack of studies on quality of life (QOL) of patients on antidepressant medications. QOL may be compromised by adverse drug reactions such as weight gain, nausea, constipation, sexual dysfunction, agitation, orthostatic hypotension, dry mouth and other anti-cholinergic side effects.

Bech's review also underscores information on the clinical predictors of response to antidepressants, that is, who will and who will not respond to a given antidepressant drug. What is now known is that several clinical features of depression are not particularly helpful in making this distinction, and these have fallen out of diagnostic utility in the 1990s. They include biological — non-biological, endogenous — reactive, melancholic — neurotic, acute — chronic, familial — non-familial and others [1].

Another important issue in the treatment of depression is related to the severity of depression. Though most studies reviewed have focused on depression of at least moderate severity or those with a high score on the

Hamilton Depression Scale, patients with mild depression, or those with subthreshold symptoms or syndrome, and those with a duration shorter than 2 weeks (necessary for making a diagnosis of depressive disorder) also suffer unnecessarily and have a poor QOL. There is a need to study these groups of patients as well.

To sum up, there is a need for more studies or trials on the elderly, on women, medium- and long-term treatment, fixed dose vs. variable doses, combination of TCAs and SSRIs, or combination with other psychotropics. Whereas the search is on for new products which are safe and effective, the focus obviously is on the QOL of the patients, and whether this might be achieved with rational polypharmacy, using a combination of available products, needs to be addressed.

REFERENCE

1. Stahl S.M. (1998) *Essential Psychopharmacology. Neuroscientific Basis and Clinical Applications*, Cambridge University Press, Cambridge.

2.11
Compliance Issues and the Efficacy of Antidepressants

Koen Demyttenaere[1]

The depressive condition, with its cognitive deficit, helplessness, poor motivation and withdrawal, leads to forgetfulness and passive non-compliance. Disturbing beliefs about antidepressants often result in active non-compliance: you only take antidepressants when you feel depressed and not when you feel better; you need to give your body some rest from antidepressants once in a while or otherwise you become dependent on the medication; you feel you are being controlled by these drugs, and so on [1]. Such passive and active non-compliance makes 50% of depressed patients prematurely discontinue treatment within 10 weeks [2].

The fact that compliance problems are often overlooked when discussing treatment with antidepressant drugs is probably due to several causes. Firstly, measuring compliance is difficult: simple methods are not accurate and accurate methods are not simple. Self-reporting, diaries and pill counts are unreliable: in a study comparing self-reporting with electronic monitoring [3], it was shown that 67% of patients overestimated their compliance; in another study [4], diaries, pill counts and electronic monitoring gave a

[1]*University Hospitals Gasthuisberg, Department of Psychiatry, Herestraat 49, B-3000 Leuven, Belgium*

compliance rate of respectively 94.1, 91.5 and 78.5%. Given the prevalence of the use of pill counts as the predominant tool on which researchers depend to document compliance with study drugs, it can be suggested that this practice should be re-evaluated. Blood sampling is not a solution, since compliance is lower on days further away from clinic visits than on days just before or just after clinic visits [5]. Secondly, doctors are particularly inaccurate in predicting the level of compliance in their patients: a recent study investigating compliance with antidepressant drugs in general practice demonstrated that 32% of the patients dropped out within 6 weeks and in 63% of cases this was unknown to their doctor [2]. Doctors are usually quite convinced that "their" patients demonstrate a high fidelity to "their" treatment and the topic is not addressed.

On the other hand, compliance issues have become a major promotional strategy in the pharmaceutical industry, where the whole problem of non-compliance is most often reduced to differences in side-effect profiles. We demonstrated earlier that male sex, severe adverse events and younger age significantly predicted the risk of becoming a dropout within the first 5 weeks of treatment, but afterwards, adverse events were no longer predictive. Adverse events were also not predictive for another compliance measure, that is the number of days with a correct intake [6].

The clinical importance of compliance and non-compliance is obvious. Taking longer drug holidays can result in discontinuation symptoms, particularly with antidepressants with a shorter half-life [7–9]. Taking extra doses of antidepressants can result in an increased incidence of adverse events again threatening compliance. The most important clinical aspect of non-compliance during the acute, continuation or maintenance phase is impaired efficacy: non-response, (pseudo)resistance and (pseudo)loss of efficacy. The return of depressive symptoms during maintenance antidepressant treatment (full-dose treatment and not lithium alone) occurs in 9–33% of patients [10]: possible explanations for this "perplexing clinical problem" suggested in Bech's review are loss of placebo effect, pharmacologic tolerance, increase in disease severity, change in disease pathogenesis, the accumulation of a detrimental metabolite, unrecognized rapid cycling, and prophylactic inefficacy. The possibility of impaired compliance was not mentioned. In another study [11], 83% of patients who relapsed on fluoxetine 20 mg/day did respond to an increase in dose up to 40 mg/day: the authors "believe that patients may develop tolerance to SSRIs through poorly understood mechanisms". Again the possibility that relapse was due to irregular pill intake (skipping of doses) and subsequent response to at least a higher pill intake (at least one pill per day) was not mentioned.

In conclusion, non-compliance seems to be the rule rather than the exception and side effects are only a partial explanation for this human behaviour. Addressing the cognitions and representations on the nature of the depressive illness, of the aetiology and of taking psychotropics within a confident doctor–patient relationship is probably the most effective compliance-enhancing strategy.

REFERENCES

1. Demyttenaere K. (1997) Compliance during treatment with antidepressants. *J. Affect. Disord.*, **43**: 27–39.
2. Maddox J.C., Levi M., Thompson C. (1994) The compliance with antidepressants in general practice. *J. Psychopharmacol.*, **8**: 48–53.
3. Straka R.J., Fish J.T., Benson S.R., Suh J.T. (1997) Patient self-reporting of compliance does not correspond with electronic monitoring: an evaluation using isosorbide dinitrate as a model drug. *Pharmacotherapy*, **17**: 126–132.
4. Matsui D., Hermann C., Klein J., Berkovitch M., Olivieri N., Koren G. (1994) Critical comparison of novel and existing methods of compliance assessment during a clinical trial of an oral iron chelator. *J. Clin. Pharmacol.*, **34**: 944–949.
5. Cramer J.A., Scheyer R.D., Mattson R.H. (1990) Compliance declines between clinic visits. *Arch. Intern. Med.*, **150**: 1509–1510.
6. Demyttenaere K., Van Ganse E., Gregoire J., Gaens E., Mesters P. (1998) Compliance in depressed patients treated with fluoxetine or amitriptyline. *Int. Clin. Psychopharmacol.*, **13**: 11–17.
7. Dilsaver S.C. (1994) Withdrawal phenomena associated with antidepressant and antipsychotic agents. *Drug Safety*, **10**: 103–114.
8. Coupland N.J., Bell C.J., Potokar J.P. (1996) Serotonin reuptake inhibitor withdrawal. *J. Clin. Psychopharmacol.*, **16**: 356–362.
9. Rosenbaum J.F. (1998) Selective serotonin reuptake inhibitor discontinuation syndrome: a randomized clinical trial. *Biol. Psychiatry*, **44**: 78–87.
10. Byrne S.E., Rothschild A.J. (1998) Loss of antidepressant efficacy during maintenance therapy: possible mechanisms and treatments. *J. Clin. Psychiatry*, **59**: 279–288.
11. Fava M., Rappe S.M., Pava J.A., Nierenberg A.A., Alpert J.E., Rosenbaum J.F. (1995) Relapse in patients on long-term fluoxetine treatment: response to increased fluoxetine dose. *J. Clin. Psychiatry*, **56**: 52–55.

2.12
The Parallel Need for Medicine-based Evidence
David S. Baldwin[1]

We live in an era of "evidence-based medicine". As most psychiatrists know, this starts by asking clear clinical questions; when considering treatment, it continues by becoming familiar with the results of randomized controlled

[1]*Department of Psychiatry, University of Southampton, Royal South Hants Hospital, Brinton's Terrace, Southampton, SO14 0YG, UK*

trials (RCTs) identified by systematic literature review (whenever possible coupled with meta-analysis of the findings); and concludes by applying this knowledge to the clinical conundrum that caused the question to be asked. But is this process in itself sufficient to produce meaningful decisions when treating individual depressed patients [1]?

Prof. Bech provides a characteristically clear and comprehensive review of the pharmacological treatment of depression, derived mainly from the findings of RCTs. I believe there are many other sources of evidence that are required to guide practice when treating depressed patients. Of course, RCTs are essential for establishing the relative efficacy and tolerability of antidepressants. However, it seems to me that the patients recruited into RCTs are a highly selective sample, unrepresentative of the total population of depressed patients seen by psychiatrists, and certainly dissimilar from the patients seen by general practitioners.

RCTs have other problems. By reporting group mean differences in treatment response, much potentially useful clinical data is lost: it would be helpful to identify patients who did especially well with one treatment, or notably poorly with another, so that individual treatment decisions could be "tailored" more effectively. Finally, the lack of a generally accepted rating scale for estimating the side-effect burden precludes accurate comparison of the tolerability of differing antidepressant drugs.

Typically, depressed patients are excluded from participating in pharmacological treatment studies through having the "wrong" kind of depression; by the presence of psychotic symptoms or high suicide risk; when there has been a poor response to previous treatment; by coexisting physical illness, mental or personality disorder; or when there is a need for concomitant medication.

In the Mood Disorders Service in Southampton, these factors together exclude the majority of patients from potentially participating in psychopharmacological treatment studies. For example, most have not derived any lasting benefit from two previous antidepressant treatments, even before referral. We see many patients with bipolar depression, "double" depression, seasonal affective disorder or recurrent brief depression; and psychological comorbidity and physical ill-health appear to be the rule. Put simply, the results of most RCTs do not apply to our clinical population.

So, the findings of RCTs are not enough. What about systematic reviews? The value of systematic reviews and meta-analytic techniques is limited by differences in trial design that can interfere with meaningful comparison of the results of treatment studies; without quality control, by the inclusion of poorly designed trials that may obscure the results from studies of good methodology; and sometimes by publication bias, that reduces the likelihood of "negative" studies making a timely appearance in scientific journals. Most investigators have been involved in treatment studies that have yet to see the light of day, five years after closure.

As such, other forms of clinical evidence also need to be examined, when considering the likely value of treatment. As noted by Prof. Bech, the antidepressant effects of imipramine were established through the detailed observations by Roland Kuhn in a sample of only 40 patients. These other sources could therefore include the reports of extensive case series of depressed patients treated openly in standard clinical practice, but followed systematically [2].

When considering the side effects of treatment, case series reveal valuable information: who would have anticipated that selective serotonin reuptake inhibitors (SSRIs) could cause treatment-emergent sexual dysfunction so frequently? [3]. We should also harness the insights offered by patient self-help organisations, such as Depression Alliance, which regularly surveys its membership, on the effectiveness and acceptability of old and new antidepressant treatments. By tapping these additional sources of information, traditional measures of clinical response would be complemented by patient-based data on recovery of social and occupational function, and improvement in quality of life.

Other potential sources include the analysis of prescribing patterns in primary care, which repeatedly demonstrate that older tricyclic antidepressants are used at subtherapeutic doses [4]; and through post-marketing surveillance, such as the prescription-event monitoring service conducted in parts of the United Kingdom, which demonstrates significant differences in the side-effect profiles of SSRIs, not apparent in clinical trials [5]. In addition, pharmacoeconomic evaluations of naturalistic practice reveal complex and often surprising findings [6].

Before concluding, a series of questions might be pertinent. Why are so few pharmacological studies conducted in primary care, the arena in which the vast majority of depressed patients are seen? Why is it that inclusion and exclusion criteria for studies in patients with bipolar depression are so narrow, that recruitment is so arduous, and the resulting "evidence base" so limited? Why has it been so difficult to develop a widely used side-effect rating scale? Why are patient-rated measures used less often than observer rating scales, and why are the findings of these patient measures reported even less frequently?

Depression is a common and often disabling condition, for which many pharmacological and psychological treatments are available. It is also notoriously undertreated. If we are going to treat more patients, and for longer, then it is imperative to consider all the potential sources of clinical information when making decisions with our patients. We need "medicine-based evidence", too!

REFERENCES

1. Black N. (1996) Why we need observational studies to evaluate the effectiveness of health care. *Br. Med. J.*, **312**: 1215–1218.
2. Baldwin D.S., Hawley C.J., Szabadi E., Burgess J., Thomson J., Bullock R., Lagnado M. (1998) Reboxetine in the treatment of depression: early clinical experience in the UK. *Int. J. Psychiatr. Clin. Pract.*, **2**: 195–201.
3. Baldwin D.S., Birtwistle J. (1998) Antidepressant drugs and sexual function: improving the recognition and management of sexual dysfunction in depressed patients. In *Antidepressant Therapy at the Dawn of the Third Millennium* (Eds M. Briley, S.A. Montgomery), pp. 231–253, Dunitz, London.
4. Baldwin D.S., Kempe D., Priest R.G. (1996) The Defeat Depression Campaign: interim results and future directions. *Int. J. Meth. Psychiatr. Res.*, **6**: S21–S26.
5. Price J.S., Waller P.C., Wood S.M., Mackay A.V.P. (1996) A comparison of the post-marketing safety of four selective serotonin reuptake inhibitors including the investigation of symptoms occurring on withdrawal. *Br. J. Clin. Pharmacol.*, **42**: 757–763.
6. Treglia M., Neslusan C.A., Dunn R.L. (1999) Fluoxetine and dothiepin therapy in primary care and heath resource utilisation: evidence from the United Kingdom. *Int. J. Psychiatr. Clin. Pract.* (in press).

2.13

What is a Lot of Antidepressants for so Few Criteria of Choice?

Frédéric Rouillon[1]

There are three levels of choice in the treatment of a depressive episode: (1) whether to use or not to use an antidepressant; (2) to select the appropriate antidepressant; (3) to choose other therapeutic strategies in the event of drug resistance.

As regards the first level, as underlined in Prof. Bech's paper, the drug advantage over placebo is relatively low (15–20%) in short-term trials, both for first and for second generation antidepressants. Around 50% of depressed patients in fact have a good response to placebo. Thus it may be reasonable to treat some depressions without drugs. Unfortunately, it is difficult to know which patients will have a clear benefit with antidepressants or with psychotherapy.

Concerning the second level of choice, the great majority of double-blind studies comparing two antidepressants did not find statistical differences in efficacy. Therefore, it is difficult to make the best choice of first line prescription. Except in the case of contraindications of some products, psychiatrists have only empirical knowledge to choose between a tricyclic antidepressant (TCA), a selective serotonin reuptake inhibitor (SSRI), a

[1]*Department of Psychiatry, Hospital A. Chenevier, 40 rue de Mesly, 94000 Creteil, France*

monoamine oxidase inhibitor (MAOI) or another class of drug. We usually rely on clinical subtypes of depression (presence of agitation or retardation, severity, atypical depression, presence of impulsivity, and so on), or on the response to an antidepressant in a previous episode, or on the benefit/risk ratio. But none of these criteria has been scientifically established. Even the conclusions of meta-analyses of studies comparing TCAs and SSRIs did not clarify the advantages of one class over the other. Double-blind studies generally compare efficacy and tolerance between groups, but rarely try to identify predictive factors of response. Thus there is no scientific basis on which to make a good choice for a patient according to his socio-demographic, clinical or biological characteristics.

In the event of drug resistance, a new choice has to be made. After a prescription has proved unsuccessful, at an appropriate dosage and with a sufficient treatment duration, the antidepressant must be changed. Good clinical practices recommend choosing a product of another class. But the validity of this strategy has never been clearly proved. After two or three failures, other treatments can be proposed: augmentation treatment (e.g. lithium adjunction) or electroconvulsive therapy, or cognitive psychotherapy, or hormonal association, or sleep deprivation, or light-therapy. But there are no convincing data on which to build up a decisional model to hierarchize the choices.

After Kraepelin, we know that the mean duration of a depressive episode is more or less 6 months. Therefore the maintenance treatment must be as long as the natural length of depression. After an acute phase of 2 months, treatment aimed at preventing relapse must last 6 months.

Recurrent depressive disorders can be treated by long-term use of antidepressants. Double-blind studies of antidepressants versus placebo report a recurrence rate of 20% with active drugs and of 40–50% with placebo. Some patients benefit from being treated with antidepressants and others stay in remission without pharmacological treatment. Therefore it would be very useful to be able to identify patients with high risk of recurrence to distinguish those who would really benefit from taking antidepressants for a long time. Moreover, one question remains unclear: "How long should treatment last?" Double-blind prophylactic studies generally last 2 years. After this period the physician and the patient might wish to discuss the pros and cons of a trial without medication.

In conclusion, antidepressants were introduced 45 years ago, and around 50 products have been and/or are being marketed. Nevertheless, despite numerous studies, it is surprising that the choice of antidepressant is still more empirical than rational. Moreover, not every clinician can be equally familiar with the wide variety of treatments which are available for depressed patients. Therefore psychiatrists and general practitioners need clear recommendations to make the best choice for each patient. Moreover, they must know the criteria of severity and frequency of recurrent depression which are needed to continue the antidepressive treatment for a prolonged period of time, or in some cases indefinitely.

2.14

Depression and its Treatment: a General Health Problem

Ahmed Okasha[1]

Depressive disorders are amongst the most common health problems in any community. They are usually underrecognized, underdiagnosed and undertreated.

The selective serotonin reuptake inhibitors (SSRIs) are actually not selective, as they act on the six subtypes of serotonin receptors. Although they may have the same efficacy in treating depressive disorders, however, the diversity of their chemical structure may imply different clinical profiles, side effects and targeted symptoms. It seems that most clinicians agree with Per Bech that acute treatment of depression requires a period of 6–8 weeks, although we observed a reduction of Hamilton Rating Scale score by 20–25% in 2 weeks. The continuation treatment (relapse prevention) should be maintained for 6–12 months, preferably with the same therapeutic dose. This may limit the use of tricyclics (TCAs) or other antidepressants, as non-compliance will be evident because of the side effects. The maintenance therapy (recurrence prevention) can be for many years, depending on certain recognized criteria.

In particular, long-term maintenance treatment is recommended for: (1) patients who have experienced three or more episodes of depressive disorder; (2) those who have had two episodes of major depressive plus one of the following: family history of bipolar disorder or recurrent major depression; history of recurrence within 1 year after previously effective medication was discontinued; early onset (before the age of 20) of the first episode; sudden, severe or life-threatening episodes in the past 3 years. The presence of residual symptoms without full remission indicates a strong tendency for relapse and medication should be continued.

I believe that response of psychotic depression to antidepressants (ADs) is more or less like a placebo response, while its response to neuroleptics (NLs) is about 40%. However, the combination of ADs and NLs may reach 60%, while electroconvulsive therapy (ECT) has the best response, of 80–90%. It is clear in Bech's discussion that although 80% of depressed patients go to general practitioners, the majority will have mild or moderate depressions, as shown by their response to imipramine (64%) and placebo

[1] *Institute of Psychiatry, Ain Shams University, 3 Shawarby Street, Kasr El Nil, Cairo, Egypt*

(58%) with a non-significant difference [1], although it seems that the doses were subtherapeutic and the duration was only 2 weeks.

There is no scientific evidence that the new ADs are superior to older ones in treating depressive disorders, but they may have another clinical spectrum in diverse psychiatric disorders. However, there is evidence that they are safer and subsequently allow a better quality of life, which is the actual measure for health and the sense of well-being. Unfortunately, the number of trials for medium- and long-term outcome using the new ADs has been rather limited. It seems that bupropion is more used and available in the USA than in other countries, especially developing ones. It is recommended for bipolar depression, because there is less possibility of manic shifts, apart from fewer side effects than other new ADs. Low doses of venlafaxine, that is 150 mg/day, will act as a SSRI, while in doses of 300 mg/day it can be a noradrenaline reuptake inhibitor, thus it has this quality of dose–response relationship, in contrast to SSRIs.

The discontinuation of ADs and the occurrence of withdrawal symptoms is part of our daily clinical practice. It was observed that 14% of patients on SSRIs will discontinue the drug because of side effects, as compared to 19% on TCAs, but the latter produce more cognitive and psychomotor impairment [2]. Sexual dysfunction occurs frequently with SSRIs (20–25%), and less with TCAs (12–15%), while it is less than 1% with trazodone, moclobemide, venlafaxine, nefazodone and mirtazapine [3].

Prof. Bech draws the useful conclusion that venlafaxine can replace clomipramine, and mirtazapine can replace amitriptyline. The role of cyto-chome enzymes is worth mentioning, since the dose of amitriptyline, imipramine and clomipramine should be reduced by 50% if we use fluvox-amine, because of the inhibition of CYP IA2, and the same applies to desipramine used in association with paroxetine and fluoxetine because of the inhibition of CYP 2D6.

It seems that venlafaxine and SSRIs are the best-documented group of drugs for the short- and medium-term treatment of a major depressive disorder. The SSRIs have also been shown to be effective in the long-term therapy of recurrent major depression. The problem with these two drugs is sexual dysfunction. Combination therapy of nefazodone or mirtazapine in this context may be recommended, but research controlled trials are still needed.

In the future, our choice of an AD or a combination of ADs will be based on thorough knowledge of the mode of action, drug–drug interactions and the influence of cytochrome enzymes, and the profile of side effects. A rational pharmacotherapy is to be abreast of evidence-based scientific approaches.

We should be aware, when training physicians in the management of depressive disorders, that the majority of unipolar depressives will be seen by general practitioners, while most bipolars will be seen by psychiatrists.

The recent population-based studies of TCA use make it clear that suboptimal use is the norm rather than the exception. The study of Isomesta *et al* [4] found that 71% of prescriptions of TCAs were below 75 mg daily. In contrast, virtually 100% of patients treated with SSRIs receive an effective dose [5]. There seems to be little point in stubbornly clinging to treatments which, despite their familiarity, are used ineffectively and subtherapeutically. This may lead to increased risk of chronic depression, suicide and lesser quality of life [6]. The continued use of TCAs as firstline treatment for depression must be called into question.

REFERENCES

1. Porter A.M.W. (1970) Depressive illness in a general practice. A demographic study and a controlled trial of imipramine. *Br. Med. J.*, **1**: 773–778.
2. Montgomery S.A., Kasper S. (1995) Comparison of compliance between serotonin reuptake inhibitors and tricyclic antidepressants: a meta-analysis. *Int. Clin. Psychopharmacol.*, **9** (Suppl. 4): 33–40.
3. Baldwin D.S., Birtwhistle J. (1998) Antidepressant drugs and sexual function: improving the recognition and management of sexual dysfunction in depressed patients. In *Antidepressant Therapy at the Dawn of the Third Millennium* (Eds M. Briley, S.A. Montgomery) pp. 231–253, Dunitz, London.
4. Isometsa E., Seppala I., Henriksson M., Kekki P., Lonnquist J. (1998) Inadequate dosaging in general practice of tricyclic vs. other antidepressants for depression. *Acta Psychiatr. Scand.*, **98**: 451–454.
5. Bingefors K., Isacson D., von Knorring L. (1997) Antidepressant dose patterns in Swedish clinical practice. *Int. Clin. Psychopharmacol.*, **25**: 771–778.
6. Donoghue J.M. (1998) Sub-optimal use of tricyclic antidepressants in clinical care. *Acta Psychiatr. Scand.*, **98**: 429–431.

2.15
Antidepressant Drugs: The Indian Experience
R. Srinivasa Murthy[1]

The Indian experience with antidepressants, in terms of indications, effectiveness, duration of treatment, long-term outcome, is very limited. Currently, only a limited number of tricyclic antidepressants are available (imipramine, amitriptyline, clomipramine, doxepin, nortriptyline, trimipramine and dothiepin) [1]. The other drugs that are available are trazodone, mianserin, tianepine, amineptine, and among selective serotonin reuptake inhibitors (SSRIs), fluoxetine. In addition, lithium is available. Other

[1]*National Institute of Mental Health, Department of Psychiatry and Neuroscience, Post Bag 2900, Bangalore 56002-9, India*

drugs mentioned in the table in Prof. Bech's review are not available. In view of this, our experience, until about 5 years ago, was largely with the tricyclic antidepressants.

In terms of evidence for the clinical effect of the antidepressants, all the studies done in India have been limited to short-term efficacy. These studies have been mostly for purposes of registration and have not covered periods longer than 4–6 weeks. Though professionals have suggested that trials should last at least 12 weeks, such studies are not available. There are no clinical trials evaluating medium- or long-term outcome with any of the drugs.

Another area of great importance is the utility of antidepressants at the primary health care level. Though the majority of patients are treated by primary care doctors, because of the limited mental health manpower no studies have been done to understand the practice as well as the effectiveness of antidepressants when used at the level of primary care [1]. This is especially important as recent studies have shown that depression is the most common mental disorder at the level of the community as well as the primary care settings [2,3]. Currently, in contrast to the Western reports, the use of very long-term maintenance drugs in patients with depression is limited by the lack of clinical trials as well as the unwillingness of patients to continue drugs when they are not having active symptoms. The available evidence is only in relation to lithium in bipolar disorder. There is a need for long-term studies of the value of maintenance treatment with the different antidepressants. An interesting point about the cost of the different antidepressants is that, because of current trade practices, the various drugs are all available at about the same cost. However, this will change again with the new trade agreements: the latest antidepressants may not be easily available, because of cost factors, for use in developing countries. It is for this reason that mental health professionals have to develop both evidence and experience concerning the choice of antidepressants, their dosage, the duration of treatment and its cost-effectiveness. For this purpose the systematic efforts of the Western countries will be of value.

REFERENCES

1. Gulati C.M. (1998) *Monthly Index of Medical Specialities*, **18**: 86–91.
2. Harding T.W., De Arango N., Baltazar J., Climent C.E., Ibrahim H.H.A., Ladrido-Ignacio L., Srinivasa Murthy R., Wig N.N. (1980) Mental disorders in primary health care: a study of their frequency and diagnosis in four developing countries. *Psychol. Med.*, **10**: 231–241.
3. Ustun T.B., Sartorius N. (Eds) (1995) *Mental Illness in General Health Care: An International Study*, Wiley, Chichester.

3

Psychotherapies for Depressive Disorders: A Review

A. John Rush[1] and Michael E. Thase[2]

[1]*University of Texas Southwestern Medical Center, Dallas, Tx, USA*
[2]*University of Pittsburgh Medical Center and Western Psychiatric Institute and Clinic, Pittsburgh, PA, USA*

INTRODUCTION

The Therapies

"Psychotherapy" has different objectives, including improved adherence to medication (or other disease management procedures), symptom reduction or attainment of symptom remission, reduction of disability (e.g. improved marital/occupational functioning), prevention of relapses/recurrences, or prevention or delay of the onset/progression of depressive conditions [1]. This review evaluates the evidence for efficacy and indications of psychoeducational problem-solving, interpersonal, cognitive, behavioral, marital, and psychodynamic therapies for depressive disorders in attaining these goals.

General clinical management includes explaining the diagnosis, prognosis, and treatment options. Psychoeducation may be seen as a more extensive/intensive effort at providing information about the longer-term management, including more about the benefits and side effects of treatment options. Problem-solving therapy may be viewed as an extension of clinical management or a formal therapy itself, since most clinicians help in resolving daily problems as part of general care.

Formal psychotherapies may also be used to reduce symptoms or restore function. Therapies designed to reduce symptoms acutely include interpersonal (IPT), cognitive (CT), behavioral (BT), marital (MT), and brief psychodynamic (BPD) psychotherapies. These therapies address intermediate variables (e.g. disrupted interpersonal relationships, negative automatic thinking) that theoretically account for the depressive symptoms.

Others (behavioral-marital) also focus on the disability (marital distress) as well as depressive symptoms.

Recently, therapies to address specific populations (e.g. adolescents [2]) or types of depression (e.g. [3]) have been developed. Therapies that focus largely on functional disability due to depression (e.g. rehabilitative or vocational interventions) — while often used clinically — have not been subjected to randomized controlled trials (RCTs).

Finally, whether or not full symptom remission and functional restoration is accomplished, psychotherapy may also aim at prophylaxis (e.g. changing schemas/beliefs for cognitive therapy to prevent/delay new episodes) [4]. There is growing evidence that continuation/maintenance phase therapy may help to delay relapses/recurrences [5, 6]. In sum, both the aims and types of therapy change in the course of managing depression.

The Depressions

The depressive disorders considered in this review are major depressive disorder (MDD), dysthymic disorder (DD), depression not otherwise specified (D-NOS), and depressions associated with (not physiologically caused by) general medical conditions (GMCs) as defined by the *Diagnostic and Statistical Manual of Mental Disorders*, Fourth Edition (DSM-IV [7]) or the *International Classification of Diseases*, Tenth Revision (ICD-10 [8]). D-NOS refers to a significant level of depressive symptoms that cause functional impairment/distress and do not meet criteria for DD or MDD. D-NOS symptom levels may occur autonomously, be residual of, or may herald the onset of, DD or MDD. Substantial functional disability is associated with D-NOS [9], yet we found no RCTs focused exclusively on this condition.

Finally, when depressive symptoms (e.g. DD, MDD, or D-NOS) co-occur with GMCs (e.g. myocardial infarction (MI), stroke, diabetes, etc.), a worsened prognosis of the GMC and more functional impairment is found as compared to GMCs without depression [10]. This increased morbidity, and often mortality, makes these depressions important targets for psychotherapy treatment and research.

THE EVIDENCE

This review addresses several practical questions. Does the therapy have efficacy in attaining specific goals (e.g. improved adherence, reduced symptoms, preventing recurrence)? Does it add to benefits obtained with antidepressant medications alone in attaining these goals? Which patients and which depressions preferentially benefit?

To compile efficacy studies, we conducted literature reviews by using specific key words to specify the type of therapy and type of depression, as well as searching for psychotherapies in general. This chapter relies on definitive reviews and meta-analyses by others, and on large pivotal trials to weigh the evidence.

RCTs that compare the therapy to either a waiting list (WL), a "placebo" (PLA), or another active, established treatment control give the best evidence as to efficacy — even though these trials cannot be double-blinded (a single-blind with independent evaluators is possible). While what constitutes a "placebo" for psychotherapy remains controversial, if different RCTs agree as to comparative efficacy, one is reassured. Less convincing are open, consecutive, uncontrolled case series which may suggest — but cannot conclude — there is efficacy.

Reports to determine for whom the treatment is effective rely heavily on post hoc analyses of efficacy trials to explore relationships between baseline characteristics and outcomes. While useful in generating hypotheses, this method is inconclusive without subsequent prospective trials to establish actual clinical utility (e.g. randomize patients with and without the indicator to treatment to determine the degree to which the indicator is associated with a better/worse outcome). Further, the available studies report only correlations and do not report the performance of the indicator (e.g. specificity or sensitivity) [11].

The degree to which results from research trials generalize to routine care with the same therapy is not clear [12]. Several features distinguish research studies and routine care application (e.g. manuals vs. no manuals, less comorbidly ill research populations, different therapists, different time limits, different system incentives, etc.).

While we must be cautious about generalizing from research to routine care, we must not disregard the value of evidence to inform practice. Consequently, policy-makers, system administrators, and purchasers of care cannot either totally ignore or exclusively rely upon research evidence. For example, several forms of therapy are in common use (e.g. process groups, Gestalt, or experiential therapies), yet they have not been evaluated formally for efficacy. They may or may not be quite effective. On the other hand, in most cases, patients/families are *likely* best served initially by treatments with established efficacy/safety before pursuing less well-documented approaches.

CLINICAL MANAGEMENT/PSYCHOEDUCATION

Medication Adherence

Basco and Rush [13] reviewed the evidence for the efficacy of patient education for patients with mood disorders. Several positive RCTs found that informed vs. noninformed patients with MDD evidenced greater medication adherence.

Most studies [14–25] have found that patient education was associated with greater medication compliance, using various methods to define compliance (e.g. patient self-report, medication blood levels, discontinuation from treatment, and appointment attendance). One RCT ($n = 120$) compared informational nonspecific groups and no information groups [26]. Both information groups had greater compliance than the no information group, suggesting that time with patients *and* information improve adherence. That patient education also increases knowledge [27] and improves attitudes toward illness or treatment has been found repeatedly, even at 5-month follow-up independent of diagnosis [e.g. 28, 29].

In sum, largely consistent evidence indicates that educating patients about the nature of the illness, treatment options, medication side effects, and expected outcome, increases knowledge, improves attitudes, and enhances medication adherence.

Bibliotherapy (BBT)

BBT provides psychoeducation in a practical, time-efficient manner. Both clinically and statistically significantly more improvements in symptom severity were found with cognitive BBT than with WL. These gains were maintained at 3-month follow-up [30]. Treatment involved reading the book *Feeling Good* [31], and emphasized a self-help approach to treating depression with minimal staff involvement. The effect was large in that the Hamilton Rating Scale for Depression (HAM-D) [32, 33] score decreased from 20.2 to 9.6 for BBT as compared to 19.6 to 19.0 for controls. Two previous trials of BBT also report significant benefits [34, 35]. Individuals in these studies, however, were recruited by media announcements, suffered milder (i.e. 21-item HAM-D score ≥ 10) forms of depression, were not formally evaluated for either Axis I or Axis II disorders, and could be taking medication during the trial. While this evidence does not recommend BBT alone for self-identified, more severely ill patients, it does suggest BBT helps in milder depressions and consequently may be a useful part of general clinical management.

Problem-solving Therapy (PST)

One can consider PST as clinical management, because most depressed patients ask for and are given brief counselling by primary care (PC) practitioners. PST has been evaluated in PC settings. Catalan *et al* [36] randomly allocated patients with major affective disorder to brief problem-solving and counselling or to routine medication treatment by general practitioners (GPs). At end of treatment and 6-month follow-up, the PST group had improved as much as the medication-treated group. A recent study compared a GP-provided PST, amitriptyline (AMI), and PLA delivered to PC patients with MDD. AMI and PST were equally effective and superior to PLA [37].

Arean *et al* [38] randomly assigned 75 patients with MDD over age 55 who scored ≥18 on the HAM-D and ≥20 on the Beck Depression Inventory (BDI) [4] to one of three conditions: social problem-solving (PST) [39], reminiscence therapy (RemT), or WL. PST and RemT (provided in 12 weekly group sessions) significantly reduced depressive symptoms compared to WL. PST participants experienced slightly less depression than those in RemT. More PST than RemT participants were classified as improved or remitted at post-treatment and at 3-month follow-up. Most WL patients (90%) still met criteria for MDD at the end of treatment compared to 70% for RemT and 39% for PST. These findings are consistent with other trials of PST in nonelderly and older adults [40–42].

In summary, PST appears effective in several trials of PC patients. Whether PST adds to medication benefits is not known.

Stress Management for Depression with GMCs

McEwen and Stellar [43] related stress and disease processes to provide a theoretical basis for using psychological interventions to treat those with GMCs and ongoing stress. When both GMCs and psychopathology co-occurred, a substantial increase in disability was found. A large epidemiological study has found that age, female gender, and less than a high school education were related to incident disability [44]. Significant age- and gender-adjusted associations were observed between incident disability and antecedent alcohol abuse and dependence (odds ratio = 2.5; 95% confidence interval (CI) = 1.5–4.2), MDD (odds ratio = 4.2; CI = 2.2–8.3), and phobia (odds ratio = 1.9; CI = 1.3–2.8). The adjusted odds ratio for the joint effect of depression and chronic GMCs on incident disability was 17.0 (CI = 6.9–41.7), which was not related to the type of chronic GMC. Thus, strategies that reduce depression or other psychopathology should reduce disability from a variety of GMCs.

In fact, patients with psychological distress and GMCs have been the focus of several studies and reviews of supportive/educational treatment [45–49]. A recent review [50] revealed that in patients with cardiovascular disease some stress management/behavior counseling programs reduce the risk of recurrent cardiovascular events [51, 52], or increase 5-year survival rates [53–55].

Frazer-Smith and Prince [54] conducted a randomized, controlled trial of stress monitoring and intervention in 453 male post-myocardial infarction (MI) patients, using the General Health Questionnaire (GHQ) [56] to monitor patients. Whenever GHQ scores rose above a critical level, patients received various stress reduction interventions. The monitored group ($n = 229$) had a greater decline in stress levels, similar rates and durations of rehospitalization, fewer cardiac deaths (4.4 vs. 8.9%), and fewer deaths from all causes (9.8 vs. 5.2%) than controls ($n = 224$). The 5-year follow-up found significant reductions in cardiac mortality (p = 0.006) and acute MI recurrences (p = 0.004) among highly stressed patients [54]. Thus, post-MI patients with high stress benefited from the monitoring/intervention program.

On the other hand, other psychosocial treatment studies [57, 58] have found no apparent benefit to patients or an even worse outcome for women compared to usual care [59]. Clearly, more studies of antidepressant psychosocial interventions in patients with various GMCs — not just cardiovascular disease — are needed to determine if they lower morbidity or mortality.

INTERPERSONAL THERAPY (IPT)

Major Depressive Disorder

IPT [60] is based on the theories of Adolf Meyer, Henry Stack Sullivan, and Frida Fromm-Reichman, that focus upon the interpersonal and familial factors in the development of psychopathology. IPT targets pathological grief, role transitions, role disputes, and interpersonal deficits. Standard IPT acute treatment includes 16–20 sessions. IPT has been adapted to depressed adolescents [61] and evaluated prospectively in depressed HIV-positive patients [62]. It has been subjected to several large acute phase RCTs in nonpsychotic outpatients with MDD in both psychiatric [63–67] and PC [68] settings. A number of reviews [12, 69–71] and meta-analyses [46, 72, 73] are available.

In prospective comparative outcome trials, Jarrett and Rush [70] found IPT to be superior to nonscheduled treatment [64], and no different from antidepressant medication [64, 65], CT [65], or PLA plus clinical management (CM) [65]. The Depression Guideline Panel [46] found IPT to provide a 52.3% response rate based on Elkin et al [65].

In Elkin et al [65], patients were randomly assigned to CT, IPT, imipramine (IMI) plus CM, or PLA plus CM, each lasting 16 weeks with experienced trained therapists conducting each treatment. The dropout rates were 23% (IPT), 32% (CBT), 33% (IMI-CM), and 40% (PLA-CM). Follow-up was conducted at 6, 12, and 18 months after completion of the acute phase [74].

The intent-to-treat (ITT) sample ($n = 239$) revealed no significant differences between therapies or between therapies and IMI-CM. Recovery was defined as a 17-item HAM-D score ≤ 6 or a BDI score ≤ 9. Using the HAM-D definition, patients with IMI-CM (42%) or IPT (43%) were significantly more likely to recover than those with PLA-CM (21%). CT (36%) was not significantly different than any other treatment cell. Using a BDI score ≤9, all cells were equal.

A secondary analysis based on baseline severity (more depressed: HAM-D score ≥20 or a Global Assessment of Functioning (GAF [7]) score ≤50) revealed no differences between the four groups for the less depressed [65]. However, better outcomes were found with IMI-CM than PLA-CM and some significant differences between IPT and PLA-CM were found for the more severely symptomatic. Patients receiving either IMI-CM or IPT were significantly more likely to recover than those in PLA-CM. Outcomes were generally intermediate between IMI-CM and IPT, and higher than PLA-CM, although none of the comparisons with CT were significant.

A more recent random regression analysis also found equivalence of all interventions for the less depressed, but better differentiated among therapies for the more depressed [75]. With HAM-D and BDI scores as outcomes, IMI-CM and IPT were equally effective for these patients; IMI-CM more effective than CT and than PLA-CM. IPT tended (p < 0.08) toward greater efficacy than PLA-CM; CT was no more effective than PLA-CM. With Global Assessment Scale (GAS [76]) scores to declare recovery, a different pattern emerged: IMI-CM was more effective than the other three interventions, which were equal. Roth et al [12] suggest that for the less-depressed, minimal support or counseling is active and effective, but IPT or IMI-CM may be preferred for the more severely depressed.

The Sheffield project compared prescriptive psychotherapy — analogous to CT — and psychodynamic-interpersonal therapy — analogous to IPT [66, 67]. We place this study among those evaluating IPT because the theoretical orientation of these therapies is very similar to IPT or CT, though the specific procedures [4, 60] were not followed exactly in either cell. Since initial symptom severity and different treatment durations were of interest, 50% were assigned to each psychotherapy, dispensed in either 8 or 16 sessions, and patients were stratified into low (BDI score of 16–20), moderate (BDI score of 21–26), or high (BDI score ≥27) baseline symptom severity (i.e. 12 cells based on symptom severity, therapy type, and treatment duration) (n = 120).

Both therapies were equally effective; each was associated with equally rapid responses. Equal results were obtained for all three baseline severity levels, although an interaction between baseline symptom severity and duration was found. Those with mild–moderate depression fared equally well in either 8 or 16 weeks. Those with severe depressions had significantly better outcomes with 16 as opposed to 8 weeks of therapy.

While acute phase outcomes revealed no benefit of 16 vs. 8 sessions for the mild-to-moderately symptomatic, justifying longer therapy only for the more severely ill, the 1-year follow-up (n = 117) found a trend favouring the maintenance of gains with 16 sessions of CT as compared to the other three treatment conditions [67]. There were no differences in outcomes or maintenance of gains between CT and IPT, and no interaction between initial symptom severity and therapy duration. Overall, patients with greater initial symptom severity had greater symptom levels during the naturalistic follow-up.

In a smaller analogous study ($n = 36$) in routine care, Barkham *et al* [77] allocated patients to the same two therapies for 8 or 16 sessions. Those with 16 sessions fared significantly better than those with 8 sessions. Post-therapy gains were similar to Shapiro *et al* [66], but at 3-month follow-up patients began to lose the gains. The severity by duration interaction previously noted [66] was not found, likely due to small sample sizes [77].

Taken together, these two studies indicate that both therapies are equally effective and equally rapid in onset of action. Also, 16, as opposed to 8, sessions are effective because longer duration appears associated with better *longer-term* outcomes in the more severely ill, and longer durations may be needed in "routine care".

Primary Care (PC)

In an RCT conducted in PC, Schulberg and colleagues [68] assigned patients with MDD to nortriptyline (NT) ($n = 91$), IPT ($n = 93$), or usual care (UC) ($n = 92$). They found by 8 months that UC patients scored 13.1 on the 17-item HAM-D compared to 9.3 for IPT and 9.0 for NT (ITT sample). With a HAM-D score ≤ 7 to define remission, 48% in NT, 46% in IPT, but only 18% of UC attained remission (ITT sample) by 8 months. Thus, both active treatments were equal and superior to UC.

Adolescents

An open trial in 14 depressed adolescents treated for 12 weeks with IPT (most with MDD) found HAM-D scores to drop from 17.8 to 2.1 by week 12, which suggests an RCT with IPT for depressed adolescents is needed [61].

Dysthymic Disorder (DD)

No RCTs of DD were found. Mason *et al* [78] described a small series ($n = 9$) of patients with dysthymia treated with IPT; 5 patients responded to time-limited treatment. Markowitz [79] subsequently described an enlarged series of 17 patients in which 11 (65%) achieved a final HAM-D score ≤ 8 by week 16.

Depression with GMCs

Markowitz *et al* [62] treated HIV-positive, depressed outpatients with 16 weeks of IPT in an RCT, comparing it to supportive therapy ($n =$ 16/group). Differential improvement for IPT was shown by mid-treatment, which persisted at termination. Specifically, end of treatment HAM-D scores had dropped from 19.8 (baseline) to 6.4 for IPT, compared to 20.7 (baseline) to 11.9 for supportive therapy. BDI scores showed similar results. These preliminary data have recently been replicated and extended to show significantly greater improvement on depressive measures in HIV-infected patients treated with IPT alone ($n = 24$) and IPT plus IMI ($n = 26$) over those treated with supportive psychotherapy alone ($n = 24$) or cognitive-behavioral therapy alone ($n = 27$) (ITT sample). Similar results were also evident in the completers only subsample [80]. Since therapy contact time was identical for these treatments, this study provides evidence of the specific effect of a particular therapy (i.e. not all psychotherapies are equal).

Indications

Several post hoc analyses with data from prospective efficacy trials [65–67] have been reported [77, 81, 82]. Sotsky *et al* [82] found that lower baseline symptom severity was associated with better response to all treatments and that six variables predicted outcome *across all treatments*: social dysfunction, cognitive dysfunction, expectation of improvement, endogenous symptoms, double depression, and duration of the index episode. The combination of lower social dysfunction and a relatively greater symptom severity predicted better response within the IPT group. Lower cognitive dysfunction was associated with better response both to CT and to IMI. Greater symptom severity, more functional impairment, and higher work dysfunction predicted better response to IMI. Atypical symptoms, including oversleeping and overeating, were associated with poorer responses to IMI-CM and significantly better responses to CT; IPT response was not affected by reverse neurovegetative features. Thus, different treatments are affecting different persons differentially. However, baseline correlates of response seemingly are insufficiently specific to be clinically useful in selecting one as opposed to another treatment for a patient.

In a separate analysis [83], personality pathology was associated with poorer responses to IPT and IMI-CM, but not CT. Similar findings were obtained in the Sheffield trial [81]. Patients with cluster C personality disorders (PD) (27/114) had greater baseline symptom severity than others, and for IPT they were still more severely ill at post-treatment and at 1-year follow-up. The presence of PD did not affect outcome for CT.

COGNITIVE THERAPY (CT)

Major Depressive Disorder (MDD)

CT (sometimes also referred to as cognitive behavioral therapy or CBT) is classically a time-limited (16–20 session, 12–16 week) directive therapy designed to reduce symptoms by countering patients' negative view of self, world, and future, and to prevent or delay relapses/recurrences by changing schemas or beliefs [4]. CT derives its model from ego-psychological, behavioral, and psychoanalytic sources. First, the rationale of treatment and steps involved in change are described. Then, early sessions focus on identifying and reality-testing negative automatic thoughts (using either cognitive or behavioral tasks). Patients learn to monitor and reevaluate their thinking for logical errors and consider alternative views. By mid-therapy, beliefs that are the basis for evaluating diverse situations are identified and challenged, shifting the focus to relapse/recurrence prevention.

CT has been subjected to several large RCTs [65, 84–86], as well as several meta-analyses [46, 87–89]. Various summary reviews [12, 90, 91] have used different criteria to include/exclude particular studies. For example, psychotherapy alone was not excluded from Steinbrueck et al [90] and Conte [91], while Dobson [87] and Nietzel and Russell [88] included only studies with outcomes assessed by the BDI. Roth et al [12] judged Robinson et al [89] as providing the most comprehensive meta-analysis, including a wide range of studies, multiple outcome domains, and more diverse forms of therapy. Robinson et al [89] reviewed 39 studies with outcomes by BDI, and evaluated clinical significance. They found that CT shifted the average patient from 2.4 standard deviations above the mean for the general population to 0.8 standard deviations above the mean (i.e. a large clinical effect).

The Depression Guideline Panel [46] meta-analysis estimated response rates based on ITT samples (not on author reports, which often rely on completer samples) to find an overall response to CT (12 trials) of 46.6%. CT was 9.4% more effective than PLA-CM, and 15.3% more effective than medication based on three studies. Jarrett and Rush [70] detailed these RCTs. CT was generally more effective than WL (8 of 10 studies), equally effective to nonspecific therapy (2 of 2 studies), more effective than behavior therapy (BT) (1 of 5 studies), equally effective to BT (4 of 5 studies), equally effective to IPT (1 study), more effective than brief psychodynamic therapy (BPD) in 2 of 4 studies and equally effective in 2 of 4 studies. CT was more effective than pharmacotherapy in 2 of 7 studies, and equally effective in 5 others. They concluded that CT exceeded the effect of WL, was usually not different from other therapies or from pharmacotherapy, with some exceptions due either to inadequate pharmacotherapy or entering less severe depressions for which pharmacotherapy is not expected to be effective.

A recent meta-analysis of 65 studies of CT for depression tried to control for potential investigator bias [92]. Even with researcher allegiance taken into account, Dobson's [87] meta-analytic results (i.e. CT was at least as effective as pharmacotherapy for depression with some evidence for its superiority taking all studies together) were upheld. Conversely, Gelder [93] noted that Dobson [87] found eight studies in which CT was at least as effective as antidepressant medication, but criticized them for lacking a PLA control—noting that CT was less effective than IMI-CM [65, 75]. He concluded that medication with CM was as effective as CT but was easier to administer.

In addition to the above reviews/meta-analyses, a number of individual trials deserve comment. The original trial [94] found CT to exceed IMI (acute treatment) for outpatients with MDD, but was rightly criticized because IMI was tapered by the end of the acute phase, and could have been subject to the "Lourdes Effect".

Two subsequent British studies found CT to be effective [84, 95]. Blackburn et al [84] engaged both hospital clinic and GP outpatients in a random assignment to CT or pharmacotherapy (doctors' choice) or the combination. For GP patients, CT was more effective than pharmacotherapy, while hospital clinic outpatients responded equally well to all three treatments; a trend favoured combined treatment. In a family practice setting, Teasdale et al [95] found that CT, when added to UC, resulted in significantly better outcomes than UC alone.

Murphy and colleagues [85] conducted an RCT in psychiatric clinic outpatients with MDD, comparing CT alone, NT alone, CT plus PLA, or CT plus NT. All treatments equally reduced symptoms acutely. CT plus NT did not exceed either treatment alone.

Elkin et al [65] compared CT, IPT, PLA, and IMI. This three-site study entered 239 moderately–severely depressed outpatients, of which 40% had been depressed <6 months. CT was no different than other treatments, including IMI-CM (ITT sample). Based on recovery (defined as a HAM-D score ≤6 or a BDI score ≤9), CT was no different than IPT, IMI-CM, or PLA-CM. Khan et al [96] have also found that antidepressant medication was equal to placebo in patients with a current episode ≤6 months.

A recent reanalysis [97] of Elkin et al [65] underscores the importance of site/treatment/severity interactions. Data revealed at one site CT did as well as IMI-CM and better than PLA-CM with the severely depressed; notably, the same site was rated as having conducted CT the best. At another site, data favored either IPT or IMI-CM over both CT and PLA-CM (the latter two being equal) [75].

While secondary analyses have found all four treatments equal in the less severely ill, for the more depressed CT did not differ from IPT or IMI-CM or PLA-CM. In a random regression analysis, Elkin et al [75] found IMI-CM more effective than CT (and than PLA-CM), and CT tended to be (p < 0.08) less effective than IPT, and no more effective than PLA-CM. While this post hoc exploratory analysis suggests that initial symptom severity is important in treatment selection, other studies have not been as confirmatory [66, 86, 98].

Hollon and colleagues [86, 98] randomly assigned 107 moderately–severely depressed outpatients (all BDI scores ≥20) to one of four treatments. In three conditions, patients received 12 weeks of acute treatment: IMI plus CM, CT, or CT plus IMI. In the fourth condition, patients received an initial 12 weeks of IMI-CM *and* an additional 12 months of IMI-CM. Experienced therapists provided 20 CT sessions over 12 weeks.

Attrition rates, while high (64/107 completed acute phase), were no different between groups. All three treatments were of equal efficacy after acute treatment (taking the two IMI-CM cells together), with a trend toward better outcomes for CT plus IMI. No differential response depending on baseline severity was found — possibly due to small samples.

Another definitive study (*n* = 120) [66] described above, randomly assigned to either an analog of CT or psychodynamic-interpersonal therapy for either 8 or 16 sessions. Therapies were equal. Baseline symptom severity was not predictive of acute response for those with mild–moderate depression, but those with more severe depressions had significantly better outcomes with 16 as opposed to 8 sessions.

Two large RCTs from Germany compared CBT with pharmacotherapy [99, 100]. The first study [101] compared CBT, AMI, and the combination (COMB), in both in- and outpatients. AMI was given (fixed dose = 150 mg/day for 8 weeks) with CM (3 times/week for 20–30 minutes) in individual sessions (*n* = 24) over 8 weeks (3 times weekly for 50–60 minutes). The CBT included *both* behavioral and cognitive techniques [102]. A naturalistic (treatments uncontrolled) 1-year follow-up was also conducted.

Patients had either MDD (80.4%) without melancholia or DD (19.6%); 116 were outpatients and 75 were inpatients. All three treatments were equally effective during acute phase, although inpatients were more severely depressed than outpatients, both at baseline and at the end of the acute phase. Using a BDI score ≤9 and a HAM-D score ≤9 to define response (a definition closer to remission than response), response rates were 30% for AMI, 33% for CBT, and 39% for COMB (inpatients), and 36% for AMI, 43% for CBT, and 53% for COMB (outpatients). Of note is that these rates seem to be based on completers only. A 1-year follow-up of patients who had received CBT alone or the COMB revealed a lower depression symptom severity than for those receiving AMI only in the acute phase.

The second RCT focused on patients with MDD *and* melancholic features (by DSM-III-R) who received AMI (150 mg/day) (*n* = 80) or COMB (AMI plus CBT in 24 sessions) (*n* = 75), as either in- or outpatients for 8 weeks [103]. Patients scored at least 20 on the BDI and the HAM-D to enter; 70% had recurrent MDD. Response (as defined above) rates (outpatients) were 55% for AMI and 75% for COMB. For inpatients, response rates were 67% (AMI) and 66% (COMB) (apparently based on completers). Both treatments were equally effective. Acute gains were retained at 1-year follow-up. Initial symptom severity was not related to outcome in either RCT.

A more recent RCT compared CT, desipramine (DMI), and applied relaxation (AR) in PC MDD outpatients [104]. DMI was given in therapeutic doses with plasma level monitoring. Both therapies (20 sessions in 16 weeks) were superior to DMI. Remission rates (final BDI score ≤9) (ITT sample) were 82% for CT, 73% for AR, and 29% for DMI.

Group CT has also been shown to be effective [105, 106]. CT treatment of geriatric patients with MDD has been the subject of several positive RCTs [107–110] (see Depression Guideline Panel [46]).

Inpatients/Severe Depression

CT has been adapted to inpatients [111, 112]. Roth *et al* [12] recently reviewed results of several trials with severely depressed patients. In an open trial of 16 unmedicated inpatients with MDD using CT alone 5 times a week for up to 4 weeks (patients averaged 13 sessions), Thase *et al* [113] found that 81% responded (defined as a 50% reduction in HAM-D score *and* a final HAM-D score ≤10).

In an expanded case series, unmedicated outpatients ($n = 110$) or inpatients ($n = 32$) received 20 sessions of CT over 20 weeks (outpatients) or over 4 weeks (inpatients) [114–116]. HAM-D scores were significantly reduced in both samples, but higher initial depression severity scores were associated with poorer response rates, an effect most marked if the initial HAM-D was ≥20.

Bowers [117] compared NT alone, relaxation in combination with NT, or CBT and NT in 30 inpatients (combined with usual hospital milieu; therapy consisted of 12 group sessions) to find, in this moderately–severely depressed group, that all groups improved, but patients receiving CBT or relaxation had significantly fewer depressive symptoms and negative cognitions than those on medication alone. Patients receiving CT were less likely to be judged depressed at discharge than any other treatment conditions. When recovery was defined (HAM-D score ≤6), 8 of 10 patients in CT compared to 1 of 10 or 2 of 10 in relaxation or medication alone, respectively, were found.

Miller and colleagues [118] treated 47 patients with standard hospital care milieu (medication plus clinical management), CT plus standard care, or social skills training plus standard care. Therapies were conducted daily while patients were hospitalized and continued weekly following discharge. All therapies led to significant gains on various measures. Patients receiving either added treatment tended to be declared responders more often at discharge, a trend that reached significance with further outpatient treatment. The differential dropout rate (41% from standard treatment, 31% from CT, and 14% from social skills) suggests caution when interpreting these results.

Primary Care (PC)

Five RCTs have been conducted in PC [37, 84, 95, 119, 120], which generally support the efficacy of CT for patients with MDD in PC settings (see [71] for a review).

Blackburn et al [84] found CT and CT combined with pharmacotherapy both superior to pharmacotherapy alone in depressed PC outpatients, although the medication response was low. Teasdale et al [95] found PC patients receiving CT improved more than those receiving UC, but by 3-months post-therapy the two groups were equal. Ross and Scott [119] found group CT superior to UC and CT patients maintained improvements at 3, 6, and 12 months later. Scott and Freeman [120] found pharmacotherapy, CT, and social work counseling superior to UC. Mynors-Wallis et al [37] found 6 sessions of PST (which approximates a portion of CT) exceeded PLA and equaled AMI in acute phase treatment.

Children/Adolescents

CT has been adapted to depressed children and adolescents [3, 121–123]. A recent systematic review [124] of six RCTs [122, 125–129] of subjects aged 8–19 revealed a higher remission rate (62%) for CT than for controls (36%), with a pooled odds ratio of 3.2 (Cl = 1.9 to 5.2). The authors note a variable quality in the trials, and a focus on less severely symptomatic patients.

Brent et al [122] applied individual CBT, systemic behavior family therapy (SBFT), or individual nondirective supportive therapy (NST) in an RCT of 107 adolescent outpatients with MDD. At treatment end, CBT was associated with a lower incidence of MDD (17.1%) than NST (42.4%), and a higher remission rate (64.7%) (absence of MDD and at least three consecutive BDI scores <9) than did SBFT (37.9%) or NST (39.4%). CBT resulted in more rapid relief in interviewer-rated depression than either other treatment.

In a controlled trial of 53 child and adolescent patients with either MDD or minor depression (8%), Wood et al [128] compared CT to RT for 5–8 treatment sessions. Treatment consisted of a cognitive component based on Beck et al [4], a social problem-solving component, and a symptom-focused component (e.g. sleep hygiene, activity scheduling). CT was more effective than relaxation on depression and overall outcome.

Other positive RCTs include Kahn and colleagues [130], Reynolds and Coates [131] and Butler et al [132]. The latter compared cognitive restructuring with role play, attention placebo, and no treatment control in fifth and sixth graders using self-reported depressive symptoms. Role playing and cognitive restructuring improved depression and related constructs compared to both control conditions.

Kahn *et al* [130] compared a CBT intervention, RT (progressive muscle relaxation), and self-monitoring intervention to WL in 68 moderately depressed middle school students. The CBT focused on acquisition of self-control, problem-solving, and social skills. The CBT and RT included 12 50-minute sessions over 6–8 weeks (group format with a single therapist). All treatments were effective at decreasing depression and increasing self-esteem at post-test and 1-month follow-up.

Vostanis *et al* [127] compared CBT with a controlled, nonfocused intervention treatment in a 2-cell RCT ($n = 28$ in each). There were no group differences (87% of CBT subjects and 75% of controls no longer had a depressive disorder) at the end of an average of 6 sessions (over 3.5 months) or at follow-up.

Dysthymic Disorder (DD)/Depression, Not Otherwise Specified (D-NOS)

Markowitz [133] reviewed seven studies (largely open trials) to find a median response rate of 41% for CT given to DD patients ([134] [$n = 5$]; [135] [$n = 12$]; [136] [$n = 6$]; [137] [$n = 10$]; and [138] [$n = 15$]).

Gonzales *et al* [139] ($n = 113$) provided 12 2-hour individual or "psycho-educational" sessions over 2 months (with 6-month follow-ups) to find more improvement with MDD (75% recovery criterion) than with chronic intermittent depression (43%) or double depression (27%).

De Jong *et al* [140] treated 30 unmedicated DD inpatients over 3 months with the combination of activities scheduling, social competence training, and cognitive restructuring, resulting in a higher response rate (60%) than with cognitive restructuring alone (30%) or WL (10%). Response was defined as a BDI score ≤ 14 or a $\geq 50\%$ reduction of pre-treatment BDI scores.

Depression with GMCs

Both cognitive and behavioral interventions have been found to improve well-being in a variety of GMCs, including cardiovascular illness, chronic pain, AIDS, cancer, and asthma [141, 142]. However, few studies use CT to reduce depression coexisting with GMCs [142]. Larcombe and Wilson [143], in a controlled study, showed CBT to improve depression in patients with multiple sclerosis. Kelly *et al* [144] demonstrated the effectiveness of group CBT and social support for depressed HIV-infected patients.

Recently, Miranda and Muñoz [145] compared a CBT prevention course to a no-intervention control in minor depression. The course was associated with greater depressive and somatic symptom reduction than controls, and symptomatic improvement was maintained at 1-year follow-up. Intervention patients missed fewer medical appointments during the year following treatment, but the number of medical visits was no different between the two groups.

Indications

Several post hoc analyses have tried to relate baseline features to response to CT. In a combined sample of 110 outpatients (20 sessions over 16 weeks) and 32 inpatients (20 sessions over 4 weeks) with MDD, treated with CT alone, nonresponse was associated with unemployment, higher pretreatment symptom severity, and abnormal sleep electroencephalograms (EEGs) [116]. Chronicity was associated with poorer outcomes in male outpatients, whereas high dysfunctional attitude scores were associated with (trend) poorer outcomes only in women. Among inpatients, male gender, diagnostic comorbidity, and elevated urinary-free cortisol levels were associated with poorer outcomes. Whether indicators of poor response to CT are predictors of good response to pharmacotherapy is unclear.

Beutler *et al* [146] compared 63 patients with MDD treated with group CT, focused expressive therapy (FET), or supportive self-directed (SSD) therapy. This study hypothesized a priori that various coping styles would relate to response. Externalizing as opposed to internalizing depressed patients improved more with CT, while internalizing patients improved more with SSD. Highly defensive patients improved more in SSD than either FET or CT; low defensive patients improved more with CT than SSD. Apparently, different patients are responding to different therapies, consistent with the notion that each therapy contains active ingredients. Whether these predictions are sufficiently predictive for clinical use is unclear.

While the National Institute of Mental Health (NIMH) trial [65, 75] found initial symptom severity predictive of differential acute response, Hollon *et al* [86] (using the same criteria) as well as others [66, 147] have found no differential effect of CT or IMI on patients defined by baseline severity (see also [148]). Craighead and colleagues [149] concluded that with too few severely ill patients, along with inconsistent results across sites/studies, baseline symptom severity was not strongly related to treatment selection (e.g. CT versus IMI-CM).

Blatt *et al* [150] reanalysed the Elkin *et al* [65] data and divided people into those with a need for approval (sociotropy) and those with high perfectionism, using the baseline Dysfunctional Attitude Scale (DAS) [151]. DAS perfectionism was consistently negatively related to outcome in all four treatments (CT, IPT, IMI, or PLA). Sotsky *et al* [82] reported that lower DAS scores predicted more favorable outcomes, especially in IMI-CM and CBT from the same study. Jacobson *et al* [152] did not find baseline DAS predictive of CT response/nonresponse in MDD. In a small study ($n = 25$), Zettle and Harring [153] did not find sociotropy or autonomy relating to outcome with CT in an individual versus group format (most patients did well on both treatments), but sample sizes may have been too small.

Blatt *et al* [154] found that the quality of the therapeutic relationship (reported by patients early in treatment) contributed significantly to the prediction of therapeutic gain, especially for the moderately perfectionistic. Jones and Pulos [155] also found the quality of the relationship significantly related to outcome for both psychodynamic therapy and CBT. Similarly, Burns and Nolen-Hoeksema [156] found that therapist empathy (rated by clients at end of treatment) was negatively associated with dropping out of CBT for depression and positively associated with outcome. Similar findings regarding the important role of therapeutic alliance have also been reported from the NIMH Treatment of Depression Collaborative Study [157].

Patience *et al* [158] evaluated the effect of personality on outcome to the four treatments in Scott and Freeman [120]. Those with a PD had slightly higher baseline HAM-D scores (19.6 vs. 16.8), and lower recovery rates (end of treatment HAM-D score <7) (47%) after 16 weeks of treatment than those without PD (67%). Those without a PD were functioning better in several domains of social functioning than those with a PD at the end of treatment, but no differences in function or symptoms were noted at 18-month follow-up. Shea *et al* [83] found that comorbid PD was predictive of poor response, except for CT. Simons and Thase [159] have also found no effect on PD or CT response ($n = 59$). Thus, as suggested, CT may be preferred for depressed people with PD [149].

Is the failure to respond to medication an indication for CT and vice versa? Few studies have directly addressed this question. Stewart *et al* [160] treated a group of patients with largely MDD or DD with 16 weekly CT sessions. The 53% nonresponders were randomly assigned to IMI (up to 300 mg/day) or PLA for 6 weeks. All five assigned to IMI responded, but none responded to PLA.

British investigators have presented data from two open trials of combined medication and CT on chronically (≥2 years) depressed inpatients who had previously failed to respond to standard antidepressants. Pharmacotherapy included phenelzine, L-tryptophan, and lithium. Barker *et al* [161] found that 11 of 20 patients randomly assigned to either pharmacotherapy alone or combined treatment with CT over 12 weeks (twice weekly for 3 weeks followed by 9 weekly sessions) responded (≥50% reduction in HAM-D). No evidence for additional benefit from CT was found. In a similar population, Scott [162] treated 8 patients with 12 weeks of a combined pharmacotherapy/CT approach (as described above) and compared them to 16 patients offered a more intensive and prolonged CBT package and pharmacotherapy. Greater symptom reductions occurred with the extensive/intensive program than with standard care.

BEHAVIORAL THERAPY (BT)

Major Depressive Disorder (MDD)

The theoretical models that underpin BT rest on learning theory (functional analysis) and/or social learning theory [163, 164]. BT aims to elevate mood by ameliorating the covarying target responses or by changing the low rate of response contingent to positive reinforcements, which, in turn, may result from reduced availability of reinforcers, skills deficit, or reduced potency.

The first step in BT is usually a functional analysis by which clinicians determine the functional relationship between behaviors and the environment. They identify antecedents and consequences that surround and presumably control specific depressive behaviors. Detailed descriptions of BT approaches include activity scheduling [165], self-control techniques [166], social skills training [167], behavioral marital therapy [168], and stress management [165]. Some variations of BT also include problem-solving [42] in this grouping. Lewinsohn et al [165] have developed a treatment manual entitled *The Coping with Depression Course*, which outlines strategies often used in BT for depressed patients. BT has been used to treat MDD and DD in adults and MDD in adolescents [123].

The Depression Guideline Panel [46] meta-analysis of BT alone revealed a 55.3% response rate (ITT sample) in 10 studies. Jarrett and Rush [70] detailed the individual studies. BT exceeded WL in 7 of 8 trials [40, 42, 169–173]. Only Usaf and Kavanaugh [174] found no difference between WL and BT, while Brown and Lewinsohn [170] found no difference between BT and nonspecific therapy, and McLean and Hakstian [175] reported no difference between BT and RT. Nonsignificant differences between CT and BT were reported by Beach and O'Leary [169], Gallagher and Thompson [176], Jacobson et al [177], Rabin et al [178] and Thompson et al [173] and BT exceeded BPD [173, 176, 179]. Miller et al [118] found no difference between BT and pharmacotherapy. Both McLean and Hakstian [175] and Steuer et al [107] found that BT reduced symptoms more than BPD based on the BDI but not on the HAM-D. One study found that BT reduced depressive symptoms less than CT, but only for depressed wives without concomitant marital discord [177].

Recently, van den Hout et al [180] reported a 12-week self-control therapy (SCT) program [166] for depressed day-treatment patients. SCT was added to UC, and 25 patients were assigned either to the combination of UC plus SCT or UC only. UC included structured group therapy, nonverbal forms of therapy, physical exercise, social skills training, and occupational therapy. Medications were also used as needed. Most patients had MDD, but some had

DD. At post-test, patients receiving SCT showed significant improvement in self-control, self-esteem, depression, depressed mood, and frequency and potential enjoyment of pleasant events compared to controls, with significant differences on 5 of 6 measures. The positive benefits were maintained at 13-week follow-up, though most group differences were no longer significant.

Adolescents

As noted above, a recent systematic review revealed six RCTs, most of which employed a behavioral-cognitive [165] or cognitive [4] approach in depressed adolescents [124]. The 62% response rate with treatment versus 36% with controls argues strongly for acute phase efficacy, though the quality of the studies was mixed. Using ITT samples, 129 of 218 remitted (no longer met criteria) vs. 75 of 82 in controls (odds ratio = 2.2; CI = 1.4–3.5).

Other reviews also found quite positive results for Lewinsohn *et al*'s [165] approach either in symptomatic outpatients or in adolescents with some symptoms or who are at risk for depression [123].

In a large, definitive trial, Clarke *et al* [181] identified 150 adolescents with some depressive symptoms (but without a formal disorder) and randomized one half to *The Coping with Depression Course* (CWDC) (15 sessions) [165]. A significant benefit was found (survival analysis) at 12-month follow-up, with 14.5% in CWDC and 25.7% in the control group developing a major affective disorder.

Depressed adolescents (58 of 66 with MDD; 8 with DD) were treated with BT, in which two forms of short-term group therapy were used: social skills training (SST) or therapeutic support group [182]. The latter was associated with significantly greater reductions in depression and increases in self-concept than SST, but differences were not present at 9 months of follow-up. Subjects were not assigned randomly; however, SST and support groups were run alternately each for 12 weeks (5 with social support groups and 5 with SST groups).

Stark *et al* [183] compared self-control, behavioral problem-solving, and WL in 29 4th–6th graders with moderate depression. Self-control consisted of self-evaluation, self-monitoring, self-reinforcement, and attribution retraining. Behavior problem-solving consisted of training to recognize and self-monitoring pleasant events. Twelve 45–50-minute group sessions were delivered over 5 weeks. At post-test, both treatment groups exceeded controls on improvements in depressive and anxious symptoms, which were maintained at 5-week follow-up.

Indications

Several investigations have tried to determine the relationship between pre-treatment symptom severity and response to BT [184–186]. Pre-treatment severity was not generally predictive of response. Kendall and Morris [187] suggested that parental involvement was critical to response for depressed adolescents, although decisive empirical evidence developed prospectively is not readily available [123].

Taylor and McLean [188] attempted to discriminate between those who recovered and sustained the recovery and those who were unremitted in a prior RCT [175] to find (regardless of treatment type) that patients with longer index episodes, those with higher pre-treatment BDI scores, and those with higher neuroticism were less likely to attain sustained full remission. Notably, gender, marital status, and family history of depression (predictors of vulnerability to depression) did not distinguish the groups. Further, no single treatment was more effective than any other based on baseline symptom severity [185].

MARITAL THERAPY (MT)

Jacobson *et al* [177] note several reasons to expect that MT (also referred to as behavioral marital therapy or BMT) is effective for depression: spouses of depressed individuals might have a facilitative effect on treatment outcome [189]; depression and marital satisfaction are inversely related [190]; disruptions in close relationships often precipitate depression [191]; marital distress predicts depressive relapse following recovery [192]; the degree to which marital satisfaction improves with therapy is inversely related to relapse [193]; a close confiding relationship with a spouse buffers otherwise depressogenic life events [194].

BMT conceptualizes depression as an interpersonal context such that both members of the marital dyad are included in therapy. The treatment program (20 sessions) has been detailed [168, 195]. Treatment initially focuses on behavioral exchange and then moves on to training in communication and problem-solving. In the latter, couples are taught to resolve conflicts around issues such as finance, sex, affection, parenting, and intimacy. The techniques and theoretical base are both cognitive and behavioral in nature. The latter include behavioral rehearsal and contingency management; cognitive techniques include reframing and other cognitive restructuring techniques. Socratic questioning and hypothesis development and testing, typical of Beck *et al*'s CT [4], are not used.

Major Depressive Disorder (MDD)

Reviews [196, 197] have revealed 17 clinical trials indicating efficacy for BMT. Jacobson *et al* [177] compared CT ($n = 20$), BMT ($n = 19$), and the combination of both BMT and CT ($n = 21$) (COMB), to reduce depression (in the wife) and enhance marital satisfaction. Based on a definition of recovery (BDI score ≤ 9), 71.4% of the distressed CT treated individuals recovered, compared to 84.6% of the nondistressed CT treated individuals. For BMT, 87.5% of the distressed individuals recovered compared to 54.5% of the nondistressed individuals. For the COMB, 37.0% of the distressed and 69.2% of the nondistressed individuals recovered.

BMT was less effective than CT for depression in maritally nondistressed couples, but for maritally distressed couples BMT and CT were equal. Only BMT had a significant positive impact on relationship satisfaction in depressed couples, whereas COMB was the only treatment to enhance marital satisfaction of nondistressed couples. Follow-ups after 6 and 12 months revealed low (0–15%) and equivalent relapse rates for all three groups [198].

Study limitations include the fact that an unknown number of subjects, initially taking antidepressant medication and who refused to discontinue, were excluded. Response rates included only completers (i.e. ITT analyses not conducted). Treatment consisted of 20 sessions of BMT or CT, but only 20 reported total sessions for COMB (i.e. 10 for CT and 10 for BMT), so COMB was half dose of each treatment.

O'Leary and Beach [199] also evaluated married couples complaining of both depression in the wife and marital discord. Random assignment to BMT, CT, or WL revealed both active treatments to be equally effective in alleviating depression. Only BMT was successful in enhancing marital satisfaction. This study suggests that BMT is effective in improving marriages, but efficacy appears related to the couples' distress levels [199].

BRIEF PSYCHODYNAMIC PSYCHOTHERAPY (BPD)

The premise of BPD is that depressive symptoms remit as patients learn new methods to cope with inner conflicts. Several different approaches to BPD include those of Malan [200, 201], Mann [202] and Wolberg [203]. Specific treatment manuals have been developed [204, 205].

Few clinical trials of BPD have been conducted on homogeneous samples of depressed individuals, perhaps because psychodynamically-oriented therapists do not view criterion-based psychiatric diagnosis as a useful way to group patients. Further, most trials that contain BPD use it as a type of nonspecific control in efficacy trials of BT or CT conducted by advocates of those two treatments.

Major Depressive Disorder (MDD)

Crits-Christoph [72] reviewed these studies, although he also included IPT trials. Both the Depression Guideline Panel [46] and Jarrett and Rush [70] found BPD to exceed WL in 1 of 1 study, and not to differ from BT in 3 of 5 studies [173, 176, 179], but to be less effective than BT in 2 of 5 studies. In a comparison of CT, BPD was equal in 2 of 4 studies [173, 176], but less effective in 2 of 4 studies [107, 206].

A recent meta-analysis of BPD [73] included citations previously reviewed and summarized [72, 207]. Two analyses [72, 73] included IPT [75, 173, 208] with BPD, and did not restrict their meta-analysis to depression. Svartberg and Stiles [207] found CBT produced a significantly larger effect size than BPD, while Anderson and Lambert [73] concluded that BPD achieved a moderate effect size relative to no treatment, a small effect size relative to minimal treatment, and no differential effect relative to other formal treatments. The effect sizes in their review were somewhat lower than Crits-Christoph [72], who used only studies that included manuals, experienced therapists trained in BPD, and specific outcome measures.

McLean and Hakstian [175], like Steuer et al [107], found BT significantly more effective than BPD in symptom reduction. However, Hersen et al [209] found no difference between BPD plus PLA and SST plus PLA in depressive symptom reduction.

The Depression Guideline Panel [46] meta-analysis (6 studies) of RCTs revealed numerically smaller response rate (34.8%) for BPD than for BT (55.3%), CT (46.6%), or IPT (52.3%). On the other hand, the Sheffield studies [66, 67] found psychodynamic-IPT (more akin to IPT) equal to CT.

Other Depressions

No RCTs of BPD for DD, D-NOS, or depression associated with GMCs were found.

Indications

Diguer and colleagues [210] found that depressed patients with a comorbid PD had more severe psychiatric disturbances at intake, at termination of BPD, and at follow-up. While patients improved and maintained their gains at follow-up, those with a comorbid PD did not improve as much as those without a PD. These findings are consistent with others [211–213]. Thus, like most other forms of therapies, comorbid PD and depression is associated with poorer acute response to BPD.

CONTINUATION/MAINTENANCE THERAPIES IN MAJOR DEPRESSIVE DISORDER (MDD)

Acute treatment is only the first phase in managing depression with medication, which must be continued to prevent a return of the episode (relapse) or new episodes (recurrences) [46]. For psychotherapy, two questions must be addressed: (1) are there enduring effects of therapy once discontinued? (2) does continuing therapy (and at what dose?) result in better outcomes than if treatment is discontinued following acute or continuation phases? Most studies to address either question have focused on MDD in adult or geriatric patients treated with either IPT or CT.

Studies of the first question provide therapy and another treatment acutely, then discontinue both and measure longer-term outcomes once each treatment is stopped (i.e. do benefits follow the end of active therapy?). These studies, however, have often been flawed by naturalistic follow-ups (i.e. further treatment is uncontrolled) in which patients may receive medication or therapy from other sources once the research treatments are discontinued.

To address the second question, randomization occurs at the end of treatment — subjects assigned either to continue or discontinue therapy. One asks whether gains made by acute treatment continue preferentially for those who continue therapy as opposed to those who do not.

Interpersonal Psychotherapy (IPT)

In the NIMH follow-up study [74], only 20% of the original sample and 24% of patients with follow-up data met criteria for recovery with no relapse in their 18-month follow-up after acute treatment with CT, IPT, PLA-CM, or IMI-CM, if it resulted in ≥8 weeks of minimal or no symptoms following end of treatment. At 6-month follow-up, *nonrelapse* rates were 30% (14 of 46) in CT, 26% (14 of 53) for IPT, 19% (9 of 48) for IMI plus CM, and 20% (10 of 51) for PLA. At 18 months, nonrelapse rates were 24, 23, 16, and 16%, respectively. While these data are based on naturalistic follow-up (treatment was uncontrolled), they suggest no differential benefit in terms of prevention of relapse/recurrence for IPT or CT over other treatments.

Maintenance IPT has been evaluated in two pivotal RCTs with recurrent MDD [6, 214]. Adult patients [6] were randomly assigned to one of five maintenance treatments: IMI, PLA, IPT plus IMI, IPT alone, and IPT plus PLA. A clear advantage for medication (whether used alone or in combination with IPT) was found. IPT alone did not differ in efficacy from IPT combined with PLA, though maintenance IPT cells exceeded PLA. This definitive study provides strong evidence for the benefit obtained with IPT and the even greater benefit obtained with IMI (whether alone or combined with IPT). It argues *against* using a combination of IMI and IPT in maintenance treatment, at least in classically recurrent depressions with full interepisode recovery.

The recent geriatric study [214] is a PLA-controlled maintenance phase RCT with 187 elderly patients with nonpsychotic MDD (average age = 67), who were initially treated acutely and then with 4 months of continuation using *both* IPT and NT. Thereafter, those successfully completing were randomly assigned to 1 of 4 maintenance treatments (monthly for 3 years): NT, PLA, IPT plus PLA, or both IPT and NT. Survival function analyses revealed that all three treatments were significantly better than PLA. Recurrence rates were 20% (CI = 4–36) for NT plus IPT; 43% (CI = 25–61) for NT; 64% (CI = 45–83) for IPT plus PLA; and 90% (CI = 79–100) for PLA. NT plus IPT was superior to IPT plus PLA; a trend (p = 0.06) favored NT plus IPT over NT alone. Patients aged 70 or older had higher and more rapid rates of recurrences than those aged 60–69.

Cognitive Therapy (CT)

Several studies have followed patients after response to acute phase CT and relapse/recurrence rates range from 0 to 50% [119, 206, 215–220].

Kovacs *et al* [217] found that relapse was lower after CT than after medication, both of which were discontinued after acute response (follow-up uncontrolled). In their 2-year follow-up, Blackburn *et al* [147] found relapse to be more frequent after CT than after medication though medication was uncontrolled, and CT was provided both acutely and 6 months following acute phase CT. Simons *et al* [218] compared CT, NT, and the combination over a 12-month follow-up, to find lower relapse rates for those receiving CT acutely than for those who did not (follow-up uncontrolled).

As noted above, Shea *et al* [74] found no differential effect for those receiving CT as compared to other treatments. Evans *et al* [98] provided 2-year post-treatment follow-up data on MDD outpatients successfully treated acutely with IMI, CT, or the COMB. Recall that half the patients initially treated with IMI alone continued the medication for the first year of follow-up, whereas the other half discontinued it at the end of acute treatment. A total of 10 patients received medication acutely without continuation treatment, 11 received medication in both acute and continuation phases, 10 received CT only acutely, and 13 received CT and IMI acutely, both of which were discontinued after acute treatment.

Patients treated with CT acutely — whether alone or combined with IMI — evidenced less than one half the relapse rate of patients who received only medication acutely without continuation medication. The relapse rate for those receiving CT acutely did not differ from that of patients who received medication in *both* acute and continuation phases. Medication continuation (32% relapse) was superior to medication in acute phase only (50% relapse). For acute CT alone, the relapse rate was 21%; it was 15% for COMB. Relapse rates for patients receiving CT (either alone or in combination with medication) was 18%. Most relapses with CT occurred later (mean survival times $= 17.4 \pm 1.2$ months) than those following medication discontinuation (3.3 ± 0.4 months). However, only 44 of the 64 patients completing treatment were followed-up, which demands caution in interpreting results. Relapse predictors included greater neuroticism, more hopelessness, more previous therapists, and more residual depression at end of acute treatment. No predictors differentiated the four treatment conditions.

Shapiro *et al* [67] followed 103 of the 117 completer patients for 1 year. Recovery was declared if a patient had at least 4 months of no symptoms (i.e. BDI score ≤ 9). Relapse was declared if the BDI score was ≥ 15 during a period of remission (before recovery), while recurrence was declared if the BDI score was ≥ 15 after recovery. Of 103 patients, 52% were treatment responders; 57% maintained their gains, 32% partially maintained gains, and 22% suffered a relapse or recurrence. Thus, 29% of patients who entered the trial were asymptomatic throughout the 1-year follow-up — a figure comparable to Shea *et al* [74]. No differences in outcomes or maintenance of gains were found between CT and IPT. No relations between baseline symptom severity and short- or long-term outcome were found, except that patients who were more depressed at baseline tended not to maintain their gains regardless of the treatment type or number of sessions. Those patients who received 8 sessions of IPT were doing less well at 1 year on all measures. There was a nonsignificant trend toward better maintenance of gains with 16 sessions of CT compared to the three other treatment cells (i.e. 8 or 16 weeks of IPT or 8 sessions of CT). A more prolonged exposure to CT, while equivalent to 8 sessions in terms of symptom reduction, seemingly has a better longer-term outcome, a finding consistent with Jarrett *et al* [5].

In one report, acute phase CT responders continued to receive continuation CT either alone or combined with pharmacotherapy [147]. After 6 months of continuation CT, fewer patients who had received CT, whether alone or in combination, had relapsed compared to the medication only group (but medication was uncontrolled after the acute phase). Relapse rates were 6% and 0% vs. 30%, respectively. Over the 2-year naturalistic follow-up, the cumulative proportion of recurrences for patients treated acutely with CT alone was 23%, 21% for CT plus medication, and 78% for medication.

Blackburn and Moore [221] reported relapse/recurrence rates after 24 months of maintenance CT which was preceded by CT or medication in the acute phase. Groups were defined based on treatments during acute and follow-up phases, and medication choice was left to clinician discretion. Group 1 ($n = 26$) received medication in acute *and* follow-up. Group 2 ($n = 22$) received medication in acute followed by CT in follow-up. Group 3 ($n = 27$) received CT in acute followed by CT in follow-up. Acute phase medication consisted of an equivalent of 100 mg/day of AMI (for tricyclics), 45 mg/day of phenelzine (for monoamine-oxidase inhibitors), and 20 mg/day of fluoxetine (for selective serotonin reuptake inhibitors).

Medication management was conducted by consultants, registrars, or GPs seeing patients every 3 weeks for about 30 minutes. The study required at least 50 mg/day of AMI (or equivalent), 30 mg of phenelzine (or equivalent), or 20 mg of fluoxetine (or equivalent) during maintenance. Note that medication doses in either acute or follow-up may have been inadequate.

All three groups benefited equally throughout acute treatment (HAM-D totals decreased from 20 to 10–13). During the 2-year follow-up (treatment provided throughout), all three groups continued to gain slightly in overall symptom reduction. The relapse/recurrence rates were 31% for those maintained on medication (4 of 13), 36% for those switched from medication to CT during follow-up (5 of 14), and 24% for those treated with CT acutely and in follow-up (4 of 17).

Jarrett et al [5] further addressed whether continuing CT provided greater benefit than discontinuing it following acute response to CT treatment in two pilot studies in outpatients with MDD. In study 1, responders to acute CT were followed monthly. Study 2 provided 10 sessions of continuation CT to acute CT responders over 8 months. Follow-up treatments were fully controlled in both studies.

Relapse/recurrence rates for those without continuation CT were 40.4% (6 months), 50.3% (12 months), 66.9% (18 months), and 73.5% (24 months), as compared to those who received continuation CT at 20.0% for 6 months, 27.3% for 12 months, and 36.4% at 18 months and at 24 months (survival analysis).

In a naturalistic, 1-year follow-up ($n = 48$ with MDD) of responders to 16 weeks of CT, 32% had relapsed/recurred [219]. Correlates of relapse included prior depressive episodes, more depressive symptoms, and higher dysfunctional attitudes at baseline, slower acute treatment response, and being unmarried. Patients who fully recovered at end of acute CT (HAM-D score <6) were significantly less likely to relapse (9%) than the partially recovered (52%). These findings and others indicate that full symptom remission should be the aim of treatment because, when not attained, patients are at greater risk for relapse [222].

A recent pilot study suggests the potential value of continuation CT in depressed adolescents [223]. Continuation CT was provided to 17 patients who remitted from MDD for 6 months and then compared to historical controls ($n = 12$) with only acute treatment to remission. Continuation CT had a lower relapse rate (20%) than controls (50%).

Wilson et al [110] examined the effects of CT as an adjunct to acute and maintenance treatment with lithium in reducing depression in a 1-year follow-up of elderly patients with MDD. During acute and continuation phases, 17 of 31 patients received CT along with medication. During 1-year medication maintenance, subjects entered a double-blind, placebo-controlled study of low-dose lithium. Those who had received CT had significantly reduced HAM-D scores during maintenance phase.

In a small study, 48 patients with MDD were randomized to brief CT plus UC or UC only [224]. More subjects ($n = 15$) recovered with CT plus UC than with UC ($n = 8$). When neuroticism scores were controlled, reductions in BDI and HAM-D scores favored CT throughout the 12-month follow-up. Trends favoring CT at follow-up weeks 7, 19, 32, and 58 attained significance at weeks 7 and 58 when controlling for premorbid neuroticism. While treatment was uncontrolled during follow-up, these findings are comparable to Evans *et al* [98] (i.e. acute CT is associated with a better follow-up course than no acute CT).

Indications

Few people have searched for ways to identify individuals who benefit over the longer term from CT, IPT, or other therapies. Frank *et al* [225] searched for predictors of benefit for maintenance IPT in their trial. They found the quality of IPT was clinically and statistically significantly related to the average length of the well interval. Higher quality IPT was associated with longer survival times. Those rated above the median quality ratings survived almost 2 years, while those below it survived <5 months. This important finding indicates that the quality/nature of the therapy itself relates to outcome. It is possible, however, that individuals with more complex depressions, or "neurotic" styles, lead therapists to deviate from recommended IPT, thereby reducing IPT "quality," yet these patients may have a worse prognosis anyway. Thus, whether the relationship between the quality of IPT and outcome is causal remains uncertain. Yet, the benefits associated with IPT are not attributable to the nonspecific effects since therapist time was equivalent in higher and lower quality IPT.

Hayes *et al* [226] conducted a retrospective data analysis on 30 depressed outpatients treated in Hollon *et al* [86]. While all therapists maintained primarily cognitive focus, those that addressed interpersonal and developmental domains were associated with improvement, and the developmental focus predicted a better longer-term recovery and better functioning over the 24-month naturalistic follow-up.

PREVENTING THE ONSET OF DEPRESSION

Logically, it should be possible to identify people at risk for depression and intervene psychologically to reduce their vulnerability toward precipitation of depressive episodes by stressful life events [194]. On the other hand, little research has focused on this potentially very important area (for recent reviews, see [124, 227]).

Lewinsohn *et al* [181, 228] were the first to identify, implement, and evaluate an intervention program aimed at preventing the onset of depression in depressed adolescents. These studies focused on depressed adolescents who had already developed some evidence of the condition based on an elevated depression symptom severity rating score (see previous discussions of BT above).

Most recently, Beardslee and colleagues [229, 230] have designed an intervention to decrease the impact of risk factors on developing depression in not yet symptomatic children and adolescents, by promoting resilience-related behaviors and attitudes — enhancing parental and family functioning — in hopes of preventing the onset of depressions [231–234]. The intervention, consistent with a developmental perspective aimed at ages 8–15 years, is family-centered because of the effects of depression on cognitive [235], interpersonal [236] and marital/family function [237], and used by diverse practitioners.

An extensive review [230] notes that pilot studies of this intervention reveal it to be safe and feasible, with promising results based on assessment of parents in small samples [233]. The effects in parents appear to persist over time [238]. Greater benefits are associated with clinician-facilitated intervention rather than a lecture didactic format [234].

The 18-month follow-up on 37 families revealed sustained effects of the intervention, favouring the clinician-facilitated intervention (more positive self-report and assessor-rated changes in parents) [229]. A large prospective study to determine whether this intervention prevents or delays depression in at-risk offspring is ongoing.

DOES PSYCHOTHERAPY ADD TO THE BENEFITS OBTAINED WITH ANTIDEPRESSANT MEDICATION?

While the combination of medication and psychotherapy is often recommended on clinical grounds for MDD [239], RCT evidence is not yet convincing [12, 46, 239–241]. An extensive review [89] found no advantage of the combination contrasted with either psychotherapy alone or medication alone, as did the Depression Guideline Panel [46], Wexler and Cicchetti [242] and Manning *et al* [243]. Thase [240] conducted a meta-analysis that included 595 depressed outpatients treated with either CBT or IPT alone, or IPT in combination with antidepressants. Among the less severe, single episode patients, the combination strategy had only a modest advantage (~10%) over the psychotherapies alone. By contrast, among the patients with more severe, recurrent depression, combined treatment produced a large and clinically meaningful advantage (~30%). Major studies included Blackburn *et al* [84], Hersen *et al* [209], Murphy *et al* [85] and Beck *et al* [244]. Psychological treatments combined with medication have included CT, BT, BPD, and IPT. One study found that the combination of IPT and medication resulted in better social adjustment 1 year after acute treatment as compared to medication alone [64].

All studies of this issue can be criticized, because they were not conducted in populations defined a priori to be especially likely to benefit from the combination. For example, the Depression Guideline Panel [46] suggested that patients most likely to benefit from combination were those with chronic or complex depressions (i.e. those with comorbid Axis I, Axis II, or GMC), but no RCT specific to this population is available. Secondly, all combination studies to date have used depression-targeted brief psychotherapies (IPT, BT, or CT), not less focused personality-targeted approaches, for which the combination may be especially useful. Finally, most studies have focused on the short-term symptomatic effects of the combination, yet combination treatment may add to medication effects in terms of improved function and delayed relapse in the longer run [241].

A large, multi-site RCT comparing CBT vs. nefazodone alone vs. the combination in acute, continuation and maintenance phase treatment is currently ongoing (Keller and colleagues, personal communication). This will be the first study to target the proper population to gauge the acute or longer-term effects of combined treatment.

Another clinically logical role for therapy is with patients who have responded but not remitted with medication only [46]. Fava and associates have recently conducted such studies [245–248]. In the initial studies [245, 246], 40 patients with MDD who had responded to medication, but who still had residual symptoms, were randomly assigned to receive either CT or CM. Antidepressants were tapered to discontinue in both groups. Those receiving CT had a lower relapse rate (15%) over 2-year follow-up than those in CM (35%), and lower relapse rates (35 vs. 70%) at 4-year and 6-year (50 vs. 75%) follow-up [248]. Whether the findings can be attributed causally to CT per se or to removal of residual symptoms associated with CT is not clear. Other evidence indicates that patients with residual symptoms fare more poorly in the long run (increased relapse/recurrence) than those without such symptoms [98, 222, 249, 250].

Recently, the same group [247, 248] engaged patients with recurrent MDD comparable to the Frank *et al* [6] population. CT for residual symptoms was supplemented with relapse prevention strategies. In the trial 40 MDD patients, once successfully treated with antidepressant medications, were randomly assigned to either this CT or CM. During the 20-week experimental period, antidepressants were tapered to discontinue. Residual symptoms were preferentially benefited by the CT versus CM during the 2-year follow-up, during which treatment was fully controlled. Relapse/recurrence rates were lower with CT (10%) than CM (80%). Since this study replicates and extends prior work, it establishes an important role for therapy, specifically CT, in the attainment of symptom remission in medication responders with residual symptoms.

SUMMARY

The efficacy of depression-targeted, time-limited psychotherapies as acute phase treatments for mild-to-moderately depressed outpatients with MDD is clear. It is often equal to medication, and may be preferred in milder, uncomplicated, nonchronic cases. PST or BBT also appear efficacious in this population. Maintenance treatments appear beneficial but are exceeded by medication. However, converting medication responders into remitters with psychotherapy seems an effective approach.

CT is effective in depressed adolescents. The depressed elderly do as well with IPT, CT, or BT as other adults. What is missing is an ability to match patients to a particular treatment to decide who is benefited by the combination of medication and psychotherapy, and if benefits are obtained acutely, how long should the therapy be continued and for whom. Another major practical question is whether or not these therapies can be used in routine clinical care with equivalently good outcomes to those obtained in research settings.

Consistent Evidence

Clinical management/psychoeducation clearly increases medication adherence in MDD. Cognitive therapy, interpersonal psychotherapy, and behavior therapy have equal acute phase efficacy in adult outpatients with nonpsychotic MDD. Cognitive therapy, interpersonal psychotherapy, and behavior therapy at least equal and may exceed the acute phase efficacy of brief psychodynamic therapy. Cognitive therapy, behavior therapy, or interpersonal psychotherapy equal (but far less often exceed) the acute phase efficacy of medications in outpatients with MDD. The combination of an acute phase symptom-targeted therapy combined with antidepressant medication does not exceed the effects of either treatment alone.

Several predictors of poorer acute phase outcomes are not specific to a particular therapy, but are predictive of poorer outcomes across nearly all therapies including medication. They include, most persuasively, comorbid personality disorders, longer duration of the index episode, and sometimes being unmarried or responding later as opposed to earlier in acute treatment.

Maintenance phase interpersonal psychotherapy (for those treated with interpersonal psychotherapy plus medication in acute and continuation phases) exceeds placebo in two trials, but medication provided greater maintenance prophylaxis than interpersonal psychotherapy alone. Other maintenance phase trials suggest efficacy for cognitive therapy.

Depressed patients who respond but do not remit with medication benefit both symptomatically and prognostically from cognitive therapy to remove residual symptoms compared to others given only clinical management.

Both cognitive therapy and behavior therapy have acute phase efficacy in depressed adolescents. Elderly adults appear to respond as well to maintenance phase interpersonal psychotherapy, acute phase cognitive therapy, and acute phase behavior therapy as nonelderly adults with MDD.

The rationale to treat depressions associated with (but not physiologically caused by) general medical conditions is strong. Problem-solving therapy in depressed primary care or less severely ill outpatients has efficacy against waiting list and is comparable to other active treatments.

Behavioral-marital therapy is an effective acute phase treatment, and effectively improves marital relations in the maritally distressed.

Incomplete Evidence

Acute phase interpersonal psychotherapy may improve longer-term social adjustment. Cognitive therapy and behavior therapy may exceed the acute phase effects of brief psychodynamic therapy.

Indicators as to which depressed patients benefit more or less from each psychotherapy appear insufficiently powerful to be recommended in routine clinical care.

Acute phase cognitive therapy, once discontinued, delays relapses/recurrences as compared to acute phase medication, if it is discontinued, but several trials are flawed.

Moderately strong evidence suggests that providing 6–8 months of continuation phase cognitive therapy (behavior therapy, brief psychodynamic therapy, and interpersonal psychotherapy have not been systematically studied) to acute phase cognitive therapy responders may be associated with delayed or reduced relapse rates as compared to providing only acute phase cognitive therapy.

Depressed patients who fail to respond to a depression-targeted psychotherapy may respond to antidepressant medication.

Areas Still Open to Research

The following questions remain to be answered: Do patients with more chronic/complex depressions preferentially benefit from the combination of medication and psychotherapy? What is the longer-term efficacy (continuation/maintenance phases) for cognitive therapy? What is the efficacy of interpersonal psychotherapy in depressed adolescents? Do patients who fail (or cannot tolerate) an antidepressant medication respond to psychotherapy? Does psychotherapy aimed at depression associated with general medical conditions reduce morbidity or mortality? How effective is it compared to medication? Does psychotherapy to prevent depressions in at-risk individuals (those who have never been ill) or to prevent/delay the evolution from D-NOS to MDD have efficacy? What is the efficacy of cognitive therapy, interpersonal psychotherapy, behavior therapy or brief psychodynamic therapy in dysthymic disorder or D-NOS? Is brief psychodynamic therapy less effective than cognitive therapy or behavior therapy in the acute phase for MDD? Where does psychotherapy fit into an overall depression management program (e.g. is psychotherapy effective if medications fail or cannot be tolerated)? Is computer-assisted (or telephone-assisted) therapy effective? What is the efficacy of psychotherapies for depressed children? What is the efficacy of continuation or maintenance phase therapy for depressed adolescents? Can we develop, implement, and evaluate a widely disseminated "depression inoculation" program using a public health approach? What is the comparative cost-effectiveness of psychotherapy, medication, or the combination in routine primary care and psychiatric clinic settings? Do the therapies used in routine clinical care produce equivalent outcomes to those found in research settings?

ACKNOWLEDGEMENTS

The authors appreciate the secretarial assistance of Fastword, Inc. of Dallas, the technical and secretarial assistance of David Savage, and the administrative support of Kenneth Z. Altshuler, MD, Stanton Sharp Distinguished Chair, Professor and Chairman, Department of Psychiatry, UT Southwestern Medical Center, Dallas, TX.

REFERENCES

1. Rush A.J. (1986) Pharmacotherapy and psychotherapy. In *Clinical Psychopharmacology* (Ed. L.R. Derogatis), pp. 46–67, Addison-Wesley, Menlo Park, CA.
2. Wilkes T.C.R., Belsher G., Rush A.J., Frank E., and Associates (1994) *Cognitive Therapy for Depressed Adolescents*, Guilford Press, New York.
3. Basco M.R., Rush A.J. (1996) *Cognitive-behavioural Therapy for Bipolar Disorder*, Guilford Press, New York.
4. Beck A.T., Rush A.J., Shaw B.F., Emery G. (1979) *Cognitive Therapy of Depression*, Guilford Press, New York.
5. Jarrett R.B., Basco M.R., Riser R., Ramanan J., Marwill M., Rush A.J. (1998) Is there a role for continuation phase cognitive therapy for depressed outpatients? *J. Consult. Clin. Psychol.*, **66**: 1036–1040.

6. Frank E., Kupfer D.J., Perel J.M., Cornes C., Jarrett D.B., Mallinger A.G., Thase M.E., McEachran A.B., Grochocinski V.J. (1990) Three-year outcomes for maintenance therapies in recurrent depression. *Arch. Gen. Psychiatry*, **47**: 1093–1099.

7. American Psychiatric Association (1994) *Diagnostic and Statistical Manual of Mental Disorders, 4th edn (DSM-IV)*. American Psychiatric Association, Washington, DC.

8. World Health Organization (1992) *The ICD-10 Classification of Mental and Behavioural Disorders. Clinical Descriptions and Diagnostic Guidelines*, World Health Organization, Geneva.

9. Judd L.L., Akiskal H.S., Paulus M.P. (1997) The role and clinical significance of subsyndromal depressive symptoms (SSD) in unipolar major depressive disorder. *J. Affect. Disord.*, **45**: 5–17.

10. Depression Guideline Panel (1993) *Clinical Practice Guideline, Number 5: Depression in Primary Care*, vol. 1: *Detection and Diagnosis*, US Department of Health and Human Services, Public Health Service, Agency for Health Care Policy and Research. AHCPR Publication No. 93-0550, Rockville, MD.

11. Kraemer H.C. (1992) *Evaluating Medical Tests: Objective and Quantitative Guidelines*, Sage Publications, Newbury Park, CA.

12. Roth A., Fonagy P., Parry G., Target M., Woods R. (1996) *What Works for Whom? A Critical Review of Psychotherapy Research*, Guilford Press, New York.

13. Basco M.R., Rush A.J. (1995) Compliance with pharmacotherapy in mood disorders. *Psychiatr. Ann.*, **25**: 269–279.

14. Aagaard J., Vestergaard P. (1990) Predictors of outcome in prophylactic lithium treatment: a 2-year prospective study. *J. Affect. Disord.*, **18**: 259–266.

15. Bech P., Vendsberg P.B., Rafaelsen O.J. (1976) Lithium maintenance treatment of manic-melancholic patients: its role in the daily routine. *Acta Psychiatr. Scand.*, **53**: 70–81.

16. Cochran S.D., Gitlin M.J. (1988) Attitudinal correlates of lithium compliance in bipolar affective disorder. *J. Nerv. Ment. Dis.*, **176**: 457–464.

17. Connelly C.E., Davenport Y.B., Nurnberger J.I. (1982) Adherence to treatment regimen in a lithium carbonate clinic. *Arch. Gen. Psychiatry*, **39**: 585–588.

18. Connelly C.E. (1984) Compliance with outpatient lithium therapy. *Perspect. Psychiatr. Care*, **22**: 44–50.

19. Danion J.M., Neureuther C., Krieger-Finance F., Imbs J.L., Singer L. (1987) Compliance with long-term lithium treatment in major affective disorders. *Pharmacopsychiatry*, **20**: 230–231.

20. Fawcett J., Kravitz H.M. (1985) The long-term management of bipolar disorders with lithium, carbamazepine, and antidepressants. *J. Clin. Psychiatry*, **46**: 58–60.

21. Jamison K.R., Gerner R.H., Goodwin F.K. (1979) Patient and physician attitudes toward lithium. *Arch. Gen. Psychiatry*, **36**: 866–869.

22. Kucera-Bozarth K., Beck N.C., Lyss L. (1982) Compliance with lithium regimen. *J. Psychosoc. Nurs. Ment. Health Serv.*, **20**: 11–15.

23. Schwarcz G., Silbergeld S. (1983) Serum lithium spot checks to evaluate medication compliance. *J. Clin. Psychopharmacol.*, **3**: 356–358.

24. Youssel F.A. (1983) Compliance with therapeutic regimens: a follow-up study for patients with affective disorders. *J. Adv. Nurs.*, **8**: 513–517.

25. Altamura A.C., Mauri M. (1985) Plasma concentration, information and therapy adherence during long-term treatment with antidepressants. *Br. J. Clin. Pharmacol.*, **20**: 714–716.

26. Myers E.D., Calvert E.J. (1984) Information, compliance and side effects: a study of patients on antidepressant medication. *Br. J. Clin. Pharmacol.*, **17**: 21–25.

27. Cohen D. (1983) The effectiveness of videotape in patient education on depression. *J. Biocommun.*, **10**: 19–23.
28. Peet M., Harvey N.S. (1991) Lithium maintenance: 1. A standard education program for patients. *Br. J. Psychiatry*, **158**: 197–200.
29. Seltzer A., Roncari I., Grafinkel P. (1980) Effect of patient education on medication compliance. *Can. J. Psychiatry*, **25**: 638–645.
30. Jamison C., Scogin F. (1995) The outcome of cognitive bibliotherapy with depressed adults. *J. Consult. Clin. Psychol.*, **63**: 644–650.
31. Burns D.D. (1980) *Feeling Good. The New Mood Therapy*, William Morrow, New York.
32. Hamilton M. (1960) A rating scale for depression. *J. Neurol. Neurosurg. Psychiatry*, **12**: 56–62.
33. Hamilton M. (1967) Development of a rating scale for primary depressive illness. *Br. J. Soc. Clin. Psychol.*, **6**: 278–296.
34. Scogin F., Jamison C., Gochneaur K. (1989) Comparative efficacy of cognitive and behavioural bibliotherapy for mildly and moderately depressed older adults. *J. Consult. Clin. Psychol.*, **57**: 403–407.
35. Scogin F., Hamblin D., Beutler L. (1987) Bibliotherapy for depressed older adults: a self-help alternative. *Gerontologist*, **27**: 383–387.
36. Catalan J., Gath D.H., Anastasiades P., Bond S.A., Day A., Hall L. (1991) Evaluation of a brief psychological treatment for emotional disorders in primary care. *Psychol. Med.*, **21**: 1013–1018.
37. Mynors-Wallis L.M., Gath D.H., Lloyd-Thomas A.R., Tomlinson D. (1995) Randomised controlled trial comparing problem solving treatment with amitriptyline and placebo for major depression in primary care. *Br. Med. J.*, **310**: 441–445.
38. Arean P.A., Perri M.G., Nezu A.M., Schein R.L., Christopher F., Joseph T.X. (1993) Comparative effectiveness of social problem-solving therapy and reminiscence therapy as treatments for depression in older adults. *J. Consult. Clin. Psychol.*, **61**: 1003–1010.
39. Nezu A.M., Nezu C.M., Perri M.G. (1989) *Problem-solving Therapy for Depression: Theory, Research, and Clinical Guidelines*, Wiley, New York.
40. Nezu A.M., Perri M.G. (1989) Social problem-solving therapy for unipolar depression: an initial dismantling investigation. *J. Consult. Clin. Psychol.*, **57**: 408–413.
41. Hussian R.A., Lawrence P.S. (1981) Social reinforcement of activity in social problem solving training in the treatment of depressed institutionalized elderly. *Cogn. Ther. Res.*, **5**: 57–69.
42. Nezu A.M. (1986) Efficacy of a social problem-solving therapy approach for unipolar depression. *J. Consult. Clin. Psychol.*, **54**: 196–202.
43. McEwen B.S., Stellar E. (1993) Stress and the individual. Mechanisms leading to disease. *Arch. Intern. Med.*, **153**: 2093–2101.
44. Armenian H.K., Pratt L.A., Gallo J., Eaton W.W. (1998) Psychopathology as a predictor of disability: a population-based follow-up study in Baltimore, Maryland. *Am. J. Epidemiol.*, **148**: 269–275.
45. Katon W., Sullivan M.D. (1990) Depression and chronic medical illness. *J. Clin. Psychiatry*, **51** (Suppl.): 3–11.
46. Depression Guideline Panel (1993) *Clinical Practice Guideline, Number 5. Depression in Primary Care*: vol. 2. *Treatment of Major Depression*, US Department of Health and Human Services, Public Health Service, Agency for Health Care Policy and Research. AHCPR Publication No. 93-0551, Rockville, MD.

47. Keitner G.I., Ryan C.E., Miller I.W., Norman W.H. (1992) Recovery and major depression: factors associated with twelve-month outcome. *Am. J. Psychiatry*, **149**: 93–99.

48. Keitner G.I., Ryan C.E., Miller I.W., Kohn R., Epstein N.B. (1991) 12-month outcome of patients with major depression and comorbid psychiatric or medical illness (compound depression). *Am. J. Psychiatry*, **148**: 345–350.

49. Lyness J.M., Caine E.D., Conwell Y., King D.A., Cox C. (1993) Depressive symptoms, medical illness, and functional status in depressed psychiatric inpatients. *Am. J. Psychiatry*, **150**: 910–915.

50. Musselman D.L., Evans D.L., Nemeroff C.B. (1998) The relationship of depression to cardiovascular disease: epidemiology, biology, and treatment. *Arch. Gen. Psychiatry*, **55**: 580–592.

51. Friedman M., Thoresen C.E., Gill J.J., Ulmer D., Powell L.H., Price V.A., Brown B., Thompson L., Rabin D.D., Breall W.S. *et al* (1986) Alteration of type A behaviour and its effects on cardiac recurrences in post myocardial infarction patients: summary of results of the Recurrent Coronary Prevention Project. *Am. Heart J.*, **112**: 653–665.

52. Blumenthal J.A., Jiang W., Babyak M.A., Krantz D.S., Frid D.J., Coleman R.E., Waugh R., Hanson M., Appelbaum M., O'Connor C. *et al* (1997) Stress management and exercise training in cardiac patients with myocardial ischemia. Effects on prognosis and evaluation of mechanisms. *Arch. Intern. Med.*, **157**: 2213–2223.

53. Frasure-Smith N., Lespérance F., Talajic M. (1993) Depression following myocardial infarction. Impact on 6-month survival. *JAMA*, **270**: 1819–1825.

54. Frasure-Smith N., Prince R. (1985) The ischemic heart disease life stress monitoring program: impact on mortality. *Psychosom. Med.*, **47**: 431–445.

55. Frasure-Smith N. (1991) In-hospital symptoms of psychological stress as predictors of long-term outcome after acute myocardial infarction in men. *Am. J. Cardiol.*, **67**: 121–127.

56. Goldberg D.P. (1972) *The Detection of Psychiatric Illness by Questionnaire: A Technique for the Identification of Non-Psychotic Psychiatric Illness*, Oxford University Press, London.

57. Jones D.A., West R.R. (1996) Psychological rehabilitation after myocardial infarction: multicentre randomized controlled trial. *Br. Med. J.*, **313**: 1517–1521.

58. Taylor C.B., Miller N.H., Smith P.M., DeBusk R.F. (1997) The effect of a home-based, case-managed, multifactorial risk-reduction program on reducing psychological distress in patients with cardiovascular disease. *J. Cardiopulm. Rehabil.*, **17**: 157–162.

59. Frasure-Smith N., Lespérance F., Prince R.H., Verrier P., Garber R.A., Juneau M., Wolfson C., Bourassa M.G. (1997) Randomized trial of home-based psychosocial nursing intervention for patients recovering from myocardial infarction. *Lancet*, **350**: 473–479.

60. Klerman G.L., Weissman M.M., Rounsaville B.J., Chevron E.S. (1984) *Interpersonal Psychotherapy of Depression*, Basic Books, New York.

61. Mufson L., Moreau D., Weissman M.M., Wickramaratne P., Martin J., Samoilov A. (1994) Modification of interpersonal psychotherapy with depressed adolescents (IPT-A): phase I and II studies. *J. Am. Acad. Child Adolesc. Psychiatry*, **33**: 695–705.

62. Markowitz J.C., Klerman G.L., Clougherty K.F., Spielman L.A., Jacobsberg L.B., Fishman B., Frances A.J., Kocsis J.H., Perry S.W. III (1995) Individual psychotherapies for depressed HIV-positive patients. *Am. J. Psychiatry*, **152**: 1504–1509.

63. Weissman M.M., Klerman G.L., Paykel E.S., Prusoff B., Hanson B. (1974) Treatment effects on the social adjustment of depressed patients. *Arch. Gen. Psychiatry*, **30**: 771–778.

64. Weissman M.M., Prusoff B.A., Dimascio A., Neu C., Goklaney M., Klerman G.L. (1979) The efficacy of drugs and psychotherapy in the treatment of acute depressive episodes. *Am. J. Psychiatry*, **136**: 555–558.

65. Elkin I., Shea M.T., Watkins J.T., Imber S.D., Sotsky S.M., Collins J.F., Glass D.R., Pilkonis P.A., Leber W.R. *et al* (1989) National Institute of Mental Health Treatment of Depression Collaborative Research Program. General effectiveness of treatments. *Arch. Gen. Psychiatry*, **46**: 971–982.

66. Shapiro D.A., Barkham M., Rees A., Hardy G.E., Reynolds S., Startup M. (1994) Effects of treatment duration and severity of depression on the effectiveness of cognitive-behavioural and psychodynamic-interpersonal psychotherapy. *J. Consult. Clin. Psychol.*, **62**: 522–534.

67. Shapiro D.A., Rees A., Barkham M., Hardy G., Reynolds S., Startup M. (1995) Effects of treatment duration and severity of depression on the maintenance of gains after cognitive-behavioural and psychodynamic-interpersonal psychotherapy. *J. Consult. Clin. Psychol.*, **63**: 378–387.

68. Schulberg H.C., Block M.R., Madonia M.J., Scott C.P., Rodriguez E., Imber S.D., Perel J., Lave J., Houck P.R., Coulehan J.L. (1996) Treating major depression in primary care practice. Eight-month clinical outcomes. *Arch. Gen. Psychiatry*, **53**: 913–919.

69. Klerman G.L., Weissman M.M. (1987) Interpersonal psychotherapy (IPT) and drugs in the treatment of depression. *Pharmacopsychiatry*, **20**: 3–7.

70. Jarrett R.B., Rush A.J. (1994) Short-term psychotherapy of depressive disorders: current status and future directions. *Psychiatry*, **57**: 115–132.

71. Brown C., Schulberg H.C. (1995) The efficacy of psychosocial treatments in primary care. A review of randomized controlled trials. *Gen. Hosp. Psychiatry*, **17**: 414–424.

72. Crits-Christoph P. (1992) The efficacy of brief dynamic psychotherapy: a meta-analysis. *Am. J. Psychiatry*, **149**: 151–158.

73. Anderson E.M., Lambert M.J. (1995) Short-term dynamically oriented psychotherapy: a review and meta-analysis. *Clin. Psychol. Rev.*, **15**: 503–514.

74. Shea M.T., Elkin I., Imber S.D., Sotsky S.M., Watkins J.T., Collins J.F., Pilkonis P.A., Beckham E., Glass D.R., Dolan R.T. *et al* (1992) Course of depressive symptoms over follow-up. Findings from the National Institute of Mental Health Treatment of Depression Collaborative Research Program. *Arch. Gen. Psychiatry*, **49**: 782–787.

75. Elkin I., Gibbons R.D., Shea M.T., Sotsky S.M., Watkins J.T., Pilkonis P.A., Hedeker D. (1995) Initial severity and differential treatment outcome in the National Institute of Mental Health Treatment of Depression Collaborative Research Program. *J. Consult. Clin. Psychol.*, **63**: 841–847.

76. Endicott J., Spitzer R.L., Fleiss J.L., Cohen J. (1976) The global assessment scale. A procedure for measuring overall severity of psychiatric disturbance. *Arch. Gen. Psychiatry*, **33**: 766–771.

77. Barkham M., Rees A., Shapiro D.A., Stiles W.B., Agnew R.M., Halstead J., Culverwell A., Harrington V.M. (1996) Outcomes of time-limited psychotherapy in applied settings: replicating the Second Sheffield Psychotherapy Project. *J. Consult. Clin. Psychol.*, **64**: 1079–1085.

78. Mason B.J., Markowitz J.C., Klerman G.L. (1993) Interpersonal psychotherapy for dysthymic disorders. In *New Applications of Interpersonal Psychotherapy* (Eds G.L. Klerman, M.M. Weissman), pp. 225–264, American Psychiatric Press, Washington, DC.

79. Markowitz J.C. (1998) *Interpersonal Psychotherapy*. Review of Psychiatry Series, American Psychiatric Press, Washington, DC.

80. Markowitz J.C., Kocsis J.H., Fishman B., Spielman L.A., Jacobsberg L.B., Frances A.J., Klerman G.L., Perry S.W. (1998) Treatment of depressive symptoms in human immunodeficiency virus-positive patients. *Arch. Gen. Psychiatry*, **55**: 452–457.

81. Hardy G.E., Barkham M., Shapiro D.A., Reynolds S., Rees A., Stiles W.B. (1995) Credibility and outcome of cognitive-behavioural and psychodynamic-interpersonal psychotherapy. *Br. J. Clin. Psychol.*, **34**: 555–569.

82. Sotsky S.M., Glass D.R., Shea M.T., Pilkonis P.A., Collins J.F., Elkin I., Watkins J.T., Imber S.D., Leber W.R., Moyer J. *et al* (1991) Patient predictors of response to psychotherapy and pharmacotherapy: findings in the NIMH Treatment of Depression Collaborative Research Program. *Am. J. Psychiatry*, **148**: 997–1008.

83. Shea M.T., Pilkonis P.A., Beckham E., Collins J.F., Elkin I., Sotsky S.M., Docherty J.P. (1990) Personality disorders and treatment outcome in the NIMH Treatment of Depression Collaborative Research Program. *Am. J. Psychiatry*, **147**: 711–718.

84. Blackburn I.M., Bishop S., Glen A.I., Whalley L.J., Christie J.E. (1981) The efficacy of cognitive therapy in depression: a treatment trial using cognitive therapy and pharmacotherapy, each alone and in combination. *Br. J. Psychiatry*, **139**: 181–189.

85. Murphy G.E., Simons A.D., Wetzel R.D., Lustman P.J. (1984) Cognitive therapy and pharmacotherapy: singly and together in the treatment of depression. *Arch. Gen. Psychiatry*, **41**: 33–41.

86. Hollon S.D., DeRubeis R.J., Evans M.D., Wiemer M.J., Garvey M.J., Grove W.M., Tuason V.B. (1992) Cognitive therapy and pharmacotherapy for depression. Singly and in combination. *Arch. Gen. Psychiatry*, **49**: 774–781.

87. Dobson K.S. (1989) A meta-analysis of the efficacy of cognitive therapy for depression. *J. Consult. Clin. Psychol.*, **57**: 414–419.

88. Nietzel M.T., Russell R.L., Hemmings K.A., Gretter M.L. (1987) Clinical significance of psychotherapy for unipolar depression: a meta-analytic approach to social comparison. *J. Consult. Clin. Psychol.*, **55**: 156–161.

89. Robinson L.A., Berman J.S., Neimeyer R.A. (1990) Psychotherapy for the treatment of depression: a comprehensive review of controlled outcome research. *Psychol. Bull.*, **108**: 30–49.

90. Steinbrueck S.M., Maxwell S.E., Howard G.S. (1983) A meta-analysis of psychotherapy and drug therapy in the treatment of unipolar depression with adults. *J. Consult. Clin. Psychol.*, **51**: 856–863.

91. Conte H.R., Plutchik R., Wild K.V., Karasu T.B. (1986) Combined psychotherapy and pharmacotherapy for depression. A systematic analysis of the evidence. *Arch. Gen. Psychiatry*, **43**: 471–479.

92. Gaffan E.A., Tsaousis I., Kemp-Wheeler S.M. (1995) Researcher allegiance and meta-analysis: the case of cognitive therapy for depression. *J. Consult. Clin. Psychol.*, **63**: 966–980.

93. Gelder M.G. (1994) Cognitive therapy for depression. In *Research in Mood Disorders: An Update*. Psychiatry in Progress Series (Eds H. Hippius, C.N. Stefanis, F. Müller-Spahn), pp. 115–124, Hogrefe & Huber, Gottingen.

94. Rush A.J., Beck A.T., Kovacs M., Hollon S.D. (1977) Comparative efficacy of cognitive therapy and pharmacotherapy in the treatment of depressed outpatients. *Cogn. Ther. Res.*, **1**: 17–37.

95. Teasdale J.D., Fennell M.J., Hibbert G.A., Amies P.L. (1984) Cognitive therapy for major depressive disorder in primary care. *Br. J. Psychiatry*, **144**: 400–406.

96. Khan A., Dager S.R., Cohen S., Avery D.H., Scherzo B., Dunner D.L. (1991) Chronicity of depressive episode in relation to antidepressant-placebo response. *Neuropsychopharmacol.*, **4**: 125–130.

97. Jacobson N.S., Hollon S.D. (1996) Cognitive-behaviour therapy versus pharmacotherapy: now that the jury's returned its verdict, it's time to present the rest of the evidence. *J. Consult. Clin. Psychol.*, **64**: 74–80.

98. Evans M.D., Hollon S.D., DeRubeis R.J., Piasecki J.M., Grove W.M., Garvey M.J., Tuason V.B. (1992) Differential relapse following cognitive therapy and pharmacotherapy for depression. *Arch. Gen. Psychiatry*, **49**: 802–808.

99. Hautzinger M., De Jong-Meyer R. (1996) Cognitive-behavioural therapy versus pharmacotherapy in depression. In *Interpersonal Factors in the Origin and Course of Affective Disorders* (Eds C. Mundt, M.J. Goldstein, K. Hahlweg, P. Fiedler), pp. 329–340, Gaskell/Royal College of Psychiatrists, London.

100. de Jong-Meyer R., Hautzinger M. (1996) Results of two multicenter treatment studies among patients with endogenous and nonendogenous depression: conclusions and prospects [German]. *Zeitschrift für Klinische Psychologie. Forschung und Praxis*, **25**: 155–160.

101. Hautzinger M., de Jong-Meyer R., Treiber R., Rudolf G.A. (1996) The efficacy of cognitive behaviour therapy and pharmacotherapy, alone or in combination, in nonendogenous unipolar depression [German]. *Zeitschrift für Klinische Psychologie. Forschung und Praxis*, **25**: 130–145.

102. Hautzinger M., Stark R., Treiber R. (1989) *Kognitive Verhaltenstherapie bei Depressionen*. Psychologie Verlag Union, Weinheim.

103. de Jong-Meyer R., Hautzinger M., Rudolf G.A., Strauss W. (1996) The effectiveness of antidepressants and cognitive behaviour therapy in patients with endogenous depression: results of analyses of variance on main and secondary outcome measures. *Zeitschrift für Klinische Psychologie. Forschung und Praxis*, **25**: 93–109.

104. Murphy G.E., Carney R.M., Knesevich M.A., Wetzel R.D., Whitworth P. (1995) Cognitive behaviour therapy, relaxation training, and tricyclic antidepressant medication in the treatment of depression. *Psychol. Rep.*, **77**: 403–420.

105. Zettle R.D., Rains J.C. (1989) Group cognitive and contextual therapies in treatment of depression. *J. Clin. Psychol.*, **45**: 436–445.

106. Free M.L., Oei T.P., Sanders M.R. (1991) Treatment outcome of a group cognitive therapy program for depression. *Int J. Group Psychother.*, **41**: 533–547.

107. Steuer J.L., Mintz J., Hammen C.L., Hill M.A., Jarvik L.F., McCarley T., Motoike P., Rosen R. (1984) Cognitive-behavioural and psychodynamic group psychotherapy in treatment of geriatric depression. *J. Consult. Clin. Psychol.*, **52**: 180–189.

108. Riskind J.H., Beck A.T., Steer R.A. (1985) Cognitive-behavioural therapy in geriatric depression: comment on Steuer *et al. J. Consult. Clin. Psychol.*, **53**: 944–945.

109. Beutler L.E., Scogin F., Kirkish P., Schretlen D., Corbishley A., Hamblin D., Meredith K., Potter R., Bamford C.R., Levenson A.I. (1987) Group cognitive

therapy and alprazolam in the treatment of depression in older adults. *J. Consult. Clin. Psychol.*, **55**: 550–556.

110. Wilson K.C., Scott M., Abou-Saleh M., Burns R., Copeland J.R. (1995) Long-term effects of cognitive-behavioural therapy and lithium therapy on depression in the elderly. *Br. J. Psychiatry*, **167**: 653–658.

111. Stuart S., Bowers W.A. (1995) Cognitive therapy with inpatients: review and meta-analysis. *J. Cognit. Psychother.*, **9**: 85–92.

112. Stuart S., Wright J.H., Thase M.E., Beck A.T. (1997) Cognitive therapy with inpatients. *Gen. Hosp. Psychiatry*, **19**: 42–50.

113. Thase M.E., Bowler K., Harden T. (1991) Cognitive behaviour therapy of endogenous depression. Part 2: Preliminary findings in 16 unmedicated inpatients. *Behav. Ther.*, **22**: 469–477.

114. Simons A.D., Thase M.E. (1992) Biological markers, treatment outcome, and 1-year follow-up in endogenous depression: electroencephalographic sleep studies and response to cognitive therapy. *J. Consult. Clin. Psychol.*, **60**: 392–401.

115. Nofzinger E.A., Thase M.E., Reynolds C.F. III, Frank E., Jennings J.R., Garamoni G.L., Fasiczka A.L., Kupfer D.J. (1993) Sexual function in depressed men. Assessment by self-report, behavioural, and nocturnal penile tumescence measures before and after treatment with cognitive behaviour therapy. *Arch. Gen. Psychiatry*, **50**: 24–30.

116. Thase M.E., Simons A.D., Reynolds C.F. III (1993) Psychobiological correlates of poor response to cognitive behaviour therapy: potential indications for antidepressant pharmacotherapy. *Psychopharmacol. Bull.*, **29**: 293–301.

117. Bowers W.A. (1990) Treatment of depressed inpatients. Cognitive therapy plus medication, relaxation plus medication, and medication alone. *Br. J. Psychiatry*, **156**: 73–78.

118. Miller I.W., Norman W.H., Keitner G.I., Bishop S., Dow M.G. (1989) Cognitive-behavioural treatment of depressed inpatients. *Behav. Ther.*, **20**: 25–47.

119. Ross M., Scott M. (1985) An evaluation of the effectiveness of individual and group cognitive therapy in the treatment of depressed patients in an inner city health centre. *J. Royal Coll. Gen. Pract.*, **35**: 239–242.

120. Scott A.I., Freeman C.P. (1992) Edinburgh primary care depression study: treatment outcome, patient satisfaction, and cost after 16 weeks. *Br. Med. J.*, **304**: 883–887.

121. Vostanis P., Harrington R. (1994) Cognitive-behavioural treatment of depressive disorder in child psychiatric patients: rationale and description of a treatment package. *Eur. Child Adolesc. Psychiatry*, **3**: 111–123.

122. Brent D.A., Holder D., Kolko D., Birmaher B., Baugher M., Roth C., Iyengar S., Johnson B.A. (1997) A clinical psychotherapy trial for adolescent depression comparing cognitive, family, and supportive therapy. *Arch. Gen. Psychiatry*, **54**: 877–885.

123. Lewinsohn P.M., Clarke G.N., Rohde P. (1994) Psychological approaches to the treatment of depression in adolescents. In *Handbook of Depression in Children and Adolescents* (Eds W.M. Reynolds, H.G. Johnston), pp. 309–344, Plenum Press, New York.

124. Harrington R., Whittaker J., Shoebridge P., Campbell F. (1998) Systematic review of efficacy of cognitive behaviour therapies in childhood and adolescent depressive disorder. *Br. Med. J.*, **315**: 1559–1563.

125. Lewinsohn P.M., Clarke G.N., Hops H., Andrews J.A. (1990) Cognitive behavioural treatment for depressed adolescents. *Behav. Ther.*, **21**: 385–401.

126. Reed M.K. (1994) Social skills training to reduce depression in adolescents. *Adolescence*, **29**: 293–302.
127. Vostanis P., Feehan C., Grattan E., Bickerton W.L. (1996) A randomised controlled outpatient trial of cognitive-behavioural treatment for children and adolescents with depression: 9-month follow-up. *J. Affect. Disord.*, **40**: 105–116.
128. Wood A., Harrington R., Moore A. (1996) Controlled trial of a brief cognitive-behavioural intervention in adolescent patients with depressive disorders. *J. Child Psychol. Psychiatry Allied Discip.*, **37**: 737–746.
129. Lewinsohn P.M., Clarke G.N., Rohde P., Hops H., Seeley J. (1997) A course in coping: a cognitive-behavioural approach to treatment of adolescent depression. In *Psychosocial Treatments for Child and Adolescent Disorders* (Eds E.D. Hibbs, P.S. Jensen), pp. 109–135, American Psychiatric Press, Washington, DC.
130. Kahn J.S., Kehle T.J., Jenson W.R., Clark E. (1990) Comparison of cognitive-behavioural, relaxation, and self-modeling interventions for depression among middle-school students. *School Psychol. Rev*, **19**: 196–211.
131. Reynolds W.M., Coats K.I. (1986) A comparison of cognitive-behavioural therapy and relaxation training for the treatment of depression in adolescents. *J. Consult. Clin. Psychol.*, **54**: 653–660.
132. Butler L., Mietzitis S., Friedman R., Cole E. (1980) The effect of two school-based intervention programs on depressive symptoms in preadolescents. *Am. Educ. Res. J.*, **17**: 111–119.
133. Markowitz J.C. (1994) Psychotherapy of dysthymia. *Am. J. Psychiatry*, **151**: 1114–1121.
134. Fennel M.J., Teasdale J.D. (1982) Cognitive therapy with chronic drug refractory depressed outpatients. A note of caution. *Cogn. Ther. Res.*, **6**: 455–460.
135. Harpin R.E., Liberman R.P., Marks I., Stern R., Bohannon W.E. (1982) Cognitive-behaviour therapy for chronically depressed patients. A controlled pilot study. *J. Nerv. Ment. Dis.*, **170**: 295–301.
136. Stravynski A., Sahar A., Verreault R. (1991) A pilot study of the cognitive treatment of dysthymic disorder. *Behav. Psychother.*, **4**: 369–372.
137. McCullough J.P. (1991) Psychotherapy for dysthymia. A naturalistic study of ten patients. *J. Nerv. Ment. Dis.*, **179**: 734–740.
138. Mercier M.A., Stewart J.W., Quitkin F.M. (1992) A pilot sequential study of cognitive therapy and pharmacotherapy of atypical depression. *J. Clin. Psychiatry*, **53**: 166–170.
139. Gonzales L.R., Lewinsohn P.M., Clarke G.N. (1985) Longitudinal follow-up of unipolar depressives: an investigation of predictors of relapse. *J. Consult. Clin. Psychol.*, **53**: 461–469.
140. De Jong R., Treiber R., Henrich G. (1986) Effectiveness of two psychological treatments for inpatients with severe and chronic depressions. *Cogn. Ther. Res.*, **10**: 645–663.
141. Emmelkamp P.M., van Oppen P. (1993) Cognitive interventions in behavioural medicine. *Psychother. Psychosom.*, **59**: 116–130.
142. Fava G.A., Sonino N. (1996) Depression associated with medical illness: Treatment considerations. *CNS Drugs*, **5**: 175–189.
143. Larcombe N.A., Wilson P.H. (1984) An evaluation of cognitive-behaviour therapy for depression in patients with multiple sclerosis. *Br. J. Psychiatry*, **145**: 366–371.
144. Kelly J.A., Murphy D.A., Bahr G.R., Kalichman S.C., Morgan M.G., Stevenson L.Y., Koob J.J., Brasfield T.L., Bernstein B.M. (1993) Outcome of cognitive-behavioural and support group brief therapies for depressed, HIV-infected persons. *Am. J. Psychiatry*, **150**: 1679–1686.

145. Miranda J., Muñoz R. (1994) Intervention for minor depression in primary care patients. *Psychosom. Med.*, **56**: 136–141.
146. Beutler L.E., Engle D., Mohr D., Daldrup R.J., Bergan J., Meredith K., Merry W. (1991) Predictors of differential response to cognitive, experiential, and self-directed psychotherapeutic procedures. *J. Consult. Clin. Psychol.*, **59**: 333–340.
147. Blackburn I.M., Eunson K.M., Bishop S. (1986) A two-year naturalistic follow-up of depressed patients treated with cognitive therapy, pharmacotherapy and a combination of both. *J. Affect. Disord.*, **10**: 67–75.
148. Schulberg H.C., Katon W., Simon G.E., Rush A.J. (1998) Treating major depression in primary care practice: an update of the AHCPR practice guidlines. *Arch. Gen. Psychiatry*, **55**: 1121–1127.
149. Craighead W.E., Craighead L.W., Ilardi S.S. (1998) Psychosocial treatments for major depressive disorder. In *A Guide to Treatments that Work* (Eds P.E. Nathan, J.M. Gorman), pp. 226–239, Oxford University Press, New York.
150. Blatt S.J., Quinlan D.M., Pilkonis P.A., Shea M.T. (1995) Impact of perfectionism and need for approval on the brief treatment of depression: the National Institute of Mental Health Treatment of Depression Collaborative Research Program revisited. *J. Consult. Clin. Psychol.*, **63**: 125–132.
151. Weissman A.N. (1979) The Dysfunctional Attitudes Scale: A validation study. *Dissertation Abstracts International*, **40** (B): 1389–1390.
152. Jacobson N.S., Dobson K.S., Truax P.A., Addis M.E., Koerner K., Gollan J.K., Gortner E., Prince S.E. (1996) A component analysis of cognitive-behavioural treatment for depression. *J. Consult. Clin. Psychol.*, **64**: 295–304.
153. Zettle R.D., Herring E.L. (1995) Treatment utility of the sociotropy/autonomy distinction: implications for cognitive therapy. *J. Clin. Psychol.*, **51**: 280–289.
154. Blatt S.J., Quinlan D.M., Zuroff D.C., Pilkonis P.A. (1996) Interpersonal factors in brief treatment of depression: further analyses of the National Institute of Mental Health Treatment of Depression Collaborative Research Program. *J. Consult. Clin. Psychol.*, **64**: 162–171.
155. Jones E.E., Pulos S.M. (1993) Comparing the process in psychodynamic and cognitive-behavioural therapies. *J. Consult. Clin. Psychol.*, **61**: 306–316.
156. Burns D.D., Nolen-Hoeksema S. (1992) Therapeutic empathy and recovery from depression in cognitive-behavioural therapy: a structural equation model. *J. Consult. Clin. Psychol.*, **60**: 441–449.
157. Krupnick J.L., Sotsky S.M., Simmens S., Moyer J., Elkin I., Watkins J., Pilkonis P.A. (1996) The role of the therapeutic alliance in psychotherapy and pharmacotherapy outcome: findings in the National Institute of Mental Health Treatment of Depression Collaborative Research Program. *J. Consult. Clin. Psychol.*, **64**: 532–539.
158. Patience D.A., McGuire R.J., Scott A.I., Freeman C.P. (1995) The Edinburgh Primary Care Depression Study: personality disorder and outcome. *Br. J. Psychiatry*, **167**: 324–330.
159. Simons A.D., Thase M.E. (1990) Mood disorders. In *Handbook of Outpatient Treatment of Adults: Nonpsychotic Mental Disorders* (Eds M.E. Thase, B.A. Edelstein, M. Hersen), pp. 91–138, Plenum Press, New York.
160. Stewart J.W., Mercier M.A., Agosti V., Guardino M., Quitkin F.M. (1993) Imipramine is effective after unsuccessful cognitive therapy: sequential use of cognitive therapy and imipramine in depressed outpatients. *J. Clin. Psychopharmacol.*, **13**: 114–119.
161. Barker W.A., Scott J., Eccleston D. (1987) The Newcastle chronic depression study: results of a treatment regime. *Int. Clin. Psychopharmacol.*, **2**: 261–272.

162. Scott J. (1992) Can cognitive therapy succeed when other treatments fail? *Behav. Psychother.*, **20**: 25–36.

163. Ferster C.B. (1973) A functional analysis of depression. *Am. Psychol.*, **10**: 857–870.

164. Bandura A. (1977) *Social Learning Theory*, Prentice-Hall, Englewood Cliffs, NJ.

165. Lewinsohn P.M., Antonuccio D.O., Breckenridge J.S., Teri L. (1984) *The Coping With Depression Course*, Castalia Publishing, Eugene, OR.

166. Rehm L.P., Fuchs C.Z., Roth D.M., Kornblith S.J., Romano J.M. (1979) A comparison of self-control and assertive skills treatments of depression. *Behav. Ther.*, **10**: 429–442.

167. Bellack A.S., Hersen M., Himmelhoch J.M. (1983) A comparison of social-skills training, pharmacotherapy and psychotherapy for depression. *Behav. Res. Ther.*, **21**: 101–107.

168. Jacobson N.S., Margolin G. (1979) *Marital Therapy: Strategies Based on Social Learning and Behaviour Exchange Principles*, Brunner/Mazel, New York.

169. Beach S.R., O'Leary K.D. (1992) Treating depression in the context of marital discord: outcome and predictors of response of marital therapy versus cognitive therapy. *Behav. Ther.*, **23**: 507–528.

170. Brown R.A., Lewinsohn P.M. (1984) A psychoeducational approach to the treatment of depression: comparison of group, individual, and minimal contact procedures. *J. Consult. Clin. Psychol.*, **52**: 774–783.

171. Rehm L.P., Kornblith S.J., O'Hara M.W., Lamparski D.M., Romano J.M., Elkin J.I. (1981) An evaluation of major components in a self-control behaviour therapy program for depression. *Behav. Mod.*, **5**: 459–489.

172. Rude S.S. (1986) Relative benefits of assertion or cognitive self-control treatment for depression as a function of proficiency in each domain. *J. Consult. Clin. Psychol.*, **3**: 390–394.

173. Thompson L.W., Gallagher D., Breckenridge J.S. (1987) Comparative effectiveness of psychotherapies for depressed elders. *J. Consult. Clin. Psychol.*, **55**: 385–390.

174. Usaf S.O., Kavanaugh D.J. (1990) Mechanisms of improvement in treatment for depression: test of a self-efficacy and performance model. *J. Cognit. Psychother.*, **4**: 51–70.

175. McLean P.D., Hakstian A.R. (1979) Clinical depression: comparative efficacy of outpatient treatments. *J. Consult. Clin. Psychol.*, **47**: 818–836.

176. Gallagher D.E., Thompson L.W. (1982) Treatment of major depressive disorder in older adult outpatients with brief psychotherapies. *Psychother. Theory Res. Pract.*, **19**: 482–490.

177. Jacobson N.S., Dobson K., Fruzzetti A.E., Schmaling K.B., Salusky S. (1991) Marital therapy as a treatment for depression. *J. Consult. Clin. Psychol.*, **59**: 547–557.

178. Rabin A.S., Koslow N.J., Rehm L.P. (1984) Changes in symptoms of depression during the course of therapy. *Cogn. Ther. Res.*, **8**: 479–488.

179. Kornblith S.J., Rehm L.P., O'Hara M.W., Lamparski D.M. (1983) The contribution of self-reinforcement training and behavioral assignments to the efficacy of self-control therapy. *Cogn. Ther. Res.*, **7**: 499–528.

180. van den Hout J.H., Arntz A., Kunkels F.H. (1995) Efficacy of a self-control therapy program in a psychiatric day-treatment center. *Acta Psychiatr. Scand.*, **92**: 25–29.

181. Clarke G.N., Hawkins W., Murphy M., Sheeber L.B., Lewinsohn P.M., Seeley J.R. (1995) Targeted prevention of unipolar depressive disorder in an at-risk

sample of high school adolescents: a randomized trial of a group cognitive intervention. *J. Am. Acad. Child Adolesc. Psychiatry*, **34**: 312–321.

182. Fine S., Forth A., Gilbert M., Haley G. (1991) Group therapy for adolescent depressive disorder: a comparison of social skills and therapeutic support. *J. Am. Acad. Child Adolesc. Psychiatry*, **30**: 79–85.

183. Stark K.D., Reynolds W.M., Kaslow N.J. (1987) A comparison of the relative efficacy of self-control therapy and a behavioural problem-solving therapy for depression in children. *J. Abnorm. Child Psychol.*, **15**: 91–113.

184. Rohde P., Lewinsohn P.M., Seeley J.R. (1994) Response of depressed adolescents to cognitive-behavioural treatment: do differences in initial severity clarify the comparison of treatments? *J. Consult. Clin. Psychol.*, **62**: 851–854.

185. McLean P., Taylor S. (1992) Severity of unipolar depression and choice of treatment. *Behav. Res. Ther.*, **30**: 443–451.

186. Thase M.E., Simons A.D., Cahalane J., McGeary J., Harden T. (1991) Severity of depression and response to cognitive behaviour therapy. *Am. J. Psychiatry*, **148**: 784–789.

187. Kendall P.C., Morris R.J. (1991) Child therapy: issues and recommendations. *J. Consult. Clin. Psychol.*, **59**: 777–784.

188. Taylor S., McLean P. (1993) Outcome profiles in the treatment of unipolar depression. *Behav. Res. Ther.*, **31**: 325–330.

189. Jacobson N.S., Holtzworth-Munroe A., Schmaling K.B. (1989) Marital therapy and spouse involvement in the treatment of depression, agoraphobia, and alcoholism. *J. Consult. Clin. Psychol.*, **57**: 5–10.

190. Coleman R.E., Miller A.G. (1975) The relationship between depression and marital maladjustment in a clinic population: a multitrait-multimethods study. *J. Consult. Clin. Psychol.*, **43**: 647–651.

191. Paykel E.S., Myers J.K., Dienelt M.N., Klerman G.L., Lindenthal J.J., Pepper M.P. (1969) Life events and depression: a controlled study. *Arch. Gen. Psychiatry*, **21**: 753–760.

192. Hooley J.M., Teasdale J.D. (1989) Predictors of relapse in unipolar depressives: expressed emotion, marital distress, and perceived criticism. *J. Abnorm. Psychol.*, **98**: 229–235.

193. Rounsaville B.J., Weissman M.M., Prusoff B.A., Herceg-Baron R.L. (1979) Marital disputes and treatment outcome in depressed women. *Compr. Psychiatry*, **20**: 483–490.

194. Brown G.W., Harris T.O. (1978) *The Social Origins of Depression*, Tavistock, London.

195. Jacobson N.S., Holtzworth-Munroe A. (1986) Marital therapy: a social learning/cognitive perspective. In *Clinical Handbook of Marital Therapy* (Eds N.S. Jacobson, A.S. Gurman), pp. 29–70, Guilford Press, New York.

196. Hahlweg K., Markman H.J. (1988) Effectiveness of behavioural marital therapy: empirical status of behavioural techniques in preventing and alleviating marital distress. *J. Consult. Clin. Psychol.*, **56**: 440–447.

197. Jacobson N.S., Martin B. (1976) Behavioural marriage therapy: current status. *Psychol. Bull.*, **83**: 540–556.

198. Jacobson N.S., Fruzzetti A.E., Dobson K., Whisman M., Hops H. (1993) Couple therapy as a treatment for depression: II. The effects of relationship quality and therapy on depressive relapse. *J. Consult. Clin. Psychol.*, **61**: 516–519.

199. O'Leary K.D., Beach S.R. (1990) Marital therapy: a viable treatment for depression and marital discord. *Am. J. Psychiatry*, **147**: 183–186.

200. Malan D. (1976) *The Frontiers of Brief Psychotherapy*, Plenum Press, New York.

201. Malan D.H. (1979) *Individual Psychotherapy and the Science of Psychodynamics*, Butterworths, London.
202. Mann J. (1973) *Time-Limited Psychotherapy*, Harvard University Press, Cambridge, MA.
203. Wolberg L.R. (1967) *Short-term Psychotherapy*, Grune & Stratton, New York.
204. Luborsky L. (1984) *Principles of Psychoanalytic Psychotherapy: A Manual for Supportive-Expressive Treatment*, Basic Books, New York.
205. Strupp H.H., Binder J.L. (1984) *Psychotherapy in a New Key*, Basic Books, New York.
206. Covi L., Lipman R.S. (1987) Cognitive behavioural group psychotherapy combined with imipramine in major depression. *Psychopharmacol. Bull.*, **23**: 173–176.
207. Svartberg M., Stiles T.C. (1991) Comparative effects of short-term psychodynamic psychotherapy: a meta-analysis. *J. Consult. Clin. Psychol.*, **59**: 704–714.
208. DiMascio A., Weissman M.M., Prusoff B.A., Neu C., Zwilling M., Klerman G.L. (1979) Differential symptom reduction by drugs and psychotherapy in acute depression. *Arch. Gen. Psychiatry*, **36**: 1450–1456.
209. Hersen M., Bellack A.S., Himmelhoch J.M., Thase M.E. (1984) Effects of social skills training, amitriptyline and psychotherapy in unipolar depressed women. *Behav. Ther.*, **15**: 21–40.
210. Diguer L., Barber J.P., Luborsky L. (1993) Three concomitants: personality disorders, psychiatric severity, and outcome of dynamic psychotherapy of major depression. *Am. J. Psychiatry*, **150**: 1246–1248.
211. Pfohl B., Coryell W., Zimmerman M., Stangl D. (1987) Prognostic validity of self-report and interview measures of personality disorder in depressed in-patients. *J. Clin. Psychiatry*, **48**: 468–472.
212. Weissman M.M., Prusoff B.A., Klerman G.L. (1978) Personality and the prediction of long-term outcome of depression. *Am. J. Psychiatry*, **135**: 797–800.
213. Shea M.T., Widiger T.A., Klein M.H. (1992) Comorbidity of personality disorders and depression: implications for treatment. *J. Consult. Clin. Psychol.*, **60**: 857–868.
214. Reynolds C.F. III, Frank E., Perel M., Imber S.D., Cornes C., Miller M.D., Mazumdar S., Houck P.R., Dew M.A., Stack J.A. *et al* (1999) Nortriptyline and interpersonal psychotherapy as maintenance therapies for recurrent major depressions: a randomized controlled trial in patients older than 59 years. *JAMA*, **281**: 39–45.
215. Gallagher D.E., Thompson L.W. (1983) Effectiveness of psychotherapy for both endogenous and nonendogenous depression in older adult outpatients. *J. Gerontol.*, **38**: 707–712.
216. Gallagher-Thompson D., Hanley-Peterson P., Thompson L.W. (1990) Maintenance of gains versus relapse following brief psychotherapy for depression. *J. Consult. Clin. Psychol.*, **58**: 371–374.
217. Kovacs M., Rush A.J., Beck A.T., Hollon S.D. (1981) Depressed outpatients treated with cognitive therapy or pharmacotherapy. A one-year follow-up. *Arch. Gen. Psychiatry*, **38**: 33–39.
218. Simons A.D., Murphy G.E., Levine J.L., Wetzel R.D. (1986) Cognitive therapy and pharmacotherapy for depression. Sustained improvement over one year. *Arch. Gen. Psychiatry*, **43**: 43–48.
219. Thase M.E., Simons A.D., McGeary J., Cahalane J.F., Hughes C., Harden T., Friedman E. (1992) Relapse after cognitive behaviour therapy of depression: potential implications for longer courses of treatment. *Am. J. Psychiatry*, **149**: 1046–1052.

220. Thase M.E., Simons A.D., Reynolds C.F. III (1996) Abnormal electroencephalographic sleep profiles in major depression: association with response to cognitive behaviour therapy. *Arch. Gen. Psychiatry*, **53**: 99–108.
221. Blackburn I.M., Moore R.G. (1997) Controlled acute and follow-up trial of cognitive therapy and pharmacotherapy in outpatients with recurrent depression. *Br. J. Psychiatry*, **171**: 328–334.
222. Rush A.J., Trivedi M.H. (1995) Treating depression to remission. *Psychiatr. Ann.*, **25**: 704–709.
223. Kroll L., Harrington R., Jayson D., Fraser J., Gowers S. (1996) Pilot study of continuation cognitive-behavioural therapy for major depression in adolescent psychiatric patients. *J. Am. Acad. Child Adolesc. Psychiatry*, **35**: 1156–1161.
224. Scott C., Tacchi M.J., Jones R., Scott J. (1997) Acute and one-year outcome of a randomized controlled trial of brief cognitive therapy for major depressive disorder in primary care. *Br. J. Psychiatry*, **171**: 131–134.
225. Frank E., Kupfer D.J., Wagner E.F., McEachran A.B., Cornes C. (1991) Efficacy of interpersonal psychotherapy as a maintenance treatment of recurrent depression. Contributing factors. *Arch. Gen. Psychiatry*, **48**: 1053–1059.
226. Hayes A.M., Castonguay L.G., Goldfried M.R. (1996) Effectiveness of targeting the vulnerability factors of depression in cognitive therapy. *J. Consult. Clin. Psychol.*, **64**: 623–627.
227. Stark K.D., Rouse L.W., Kurowski C. (1994) Psychological treatment approaches for depression in children. In *Handbook of Depression in Children and Adolescents* (Eds W.M. Reynolds, H.F. Johnston), pp. 275–307, Plenum Press, New York.
228. Lewinsohn P.M. (1987) The Coping with Depression Course. In *Depression Prevention: Research Directions*. The Series in Clinical and Community Psychology (Ed. R.F. Muñoz), pp. 159–170, Hemisphere Publishing, Washington, DC.
229. Beardslee W.R., Salt P., Versage E.M., Gladstone T.R., Wright E.J., Rothberg P.C. (1997) Sustained change in parents receiving preventive interventions for families with depression. *Am. J. Psychiatry*, **154**: 510–515.
230. Beardslee W.R., Versage E.M., Wright E.J., Salt P., Rothberg P.C., Drezner K., Gladstone T.R. (1997) Examination of preventive interventions for families with depression: evidence of change. *Develop. Psychopathol.*, **9**: 109–130.
231. Beardslee W.R., Shwoeri L. (1993) Preventive intervention with children of depressed parents. In *Depression in Children and in Families: Assessments and Interventions* (Ed. G.P. Shoolevar), Guilford Press, New York.
232. Beardslee W.R., Podorefsky D. (1988) Resilient adolescents whose parents have serious affective and other psychiatric disorders: importance of self-understanding and relationships. *Am. J. Psychiatry*, **145**: 63–69.
233. Beardslee W.R., Hoke L., Wheelock I., Rothberg P.C., van de Velde P., Swatling S. (1992) Initial findings on preventive intervention for families with parental affective disorders. *Am. J. Psychiatry*, **149**: 1335–1340.
234. Beardslee W.R., Salt P., Porterfield K., Rothberg P.C., van de Velde P., Swatling S., Hoke L., Moilanen D.L., Wheelock I. (1993) Comparison of preventive interventions for families with parental affective disorder. *J. Am. Acad. Child Adolesc. Psychiatry*, **32**: 254–263.
235. Beck A.T. (1987) *Depression: Causes and Treatment*, University of Pennsylvania Press, Philadelphia.
236. Weissman M.M. (1989) Psychotherapy in the treatment of depression. New technologies and efficacy. In *Treatments of Psychiatric Disorders*, vol. 3 (Ed. American Psychiatric Association), pp. 1814–1823, American Psychiatric Association, Washington, DC.

237. Keitner G.I., Miller I.W. (1990) Family functioning and major depression: an overview. *Am. J. Psychiatry*, **147**: 1128–1137.
238. Beardslee W.R., Wright E., Rothberg P.C., Salt P., Versage E. (1996) Response of families to two preventive intervention strategies: long-term differences in behaviour and attitude change. *J. Am. Acad. Child Adolesc. Psychiatry*, **35**: 774–782.
239. American Psychiatric Association (1993) Practice guideline for major depressive disorder in adults. *Am. J. Psychiatry*, **150** (Suppl.): 1–26.
240. Thase M.E. (1997) Integrating psychotherapy and pharmacotherapy for treatment of major depressive disorder: current status and future considerations. *J. Psychother. Pract. Res.*, **6**: 300–306.
241. Hollon S.D., Fawcett J. (1996) Combined medication and psychotherapy. In *Synopsis of Treatments of Psychiatric Disorders* (Eds G.O. Gabbard, S.D. Atkinson), pp. 523–529, American Psychiatric Press, Washington, DC.
242. Wexler B.E., Cicchetti D.V. (1992) The outpatient treatment of depression. Implications of outcome research for clinical practice. *J. Nerv. Ment. Dis.*, **180**: 277–286.
243. Manning D.W., Markowitz J.C., Frances A.J. (1992) A review of combined psychotherapy and pharmacotherapy in the treatment of depression. *J. Psychother. Pract. Res.*, **1**: 103–116.
244. Beck A.T., Hollon S.D., Young J.E., Bedrosian R.C., Budenz D. (1985) Treatment of depression with cognitive therapy and amitriptyline. *Arch. Gen. Psychiatry*, **42**: 142–148.
245. Fava G.A., Grandi S., Zielezny M., Canestrari R., Morphy M.A. (1994) Cognitive behavioural treatment of residual symptoms in primary major depressive disorder. *Am. J. Psychiatry*, **151**: 1295–1299.
246. Fava G.A., Grandi S., Zielezny M., Rafanelli C., Canestrari R. (1996) Four-year outcome for cognitive behavioural treatment of residual symptoms in major depression. *Am. J. Psychiatry*, **153**: 945–947.
247. Fava G.A., Rafanelli C., Grandi S., Conti S., Belluardo P. (1998) Prevention of recurrent depression with cognitive behavioural therapy: preliminary findings. *Arch. Gen. Psychiatry*, **55**: 816–820.
248. Fava G.A., Rafanelli C., Grandi S., Canestrari R., Morphy M.A. (1998) Six-year outcome for cognitive behavioural treatment of residual symptoms in major depression. *Am. J. Psychiatry*, **155**: 1443–1445.
249. Judd L.L., Akiskal H.S., Maser J.D., Zeller P.J., Endicott J., Coryell W., Paulus M.P., Kunovac J.L., Leon A.C., Mueller T.I., Rice J.A., Keller M.B. (1998) A prospective 12-year study of subsyndromal and syndromal depressive symptoms in unipolar major depressive disorders. *Arch. Gen. Psychiatry*, **55**: 694–700.
250. Keller M.B., Gelenberg A.J., Hirschfeld R.M.A., Rush A.J., Thase M., Kocsis J.H., Markiwotz J.C., Fawcett J.A., Koran L.M., Klein D.N., *et al* (1998) The treatment of depression, Part 2: a double-blind, randomized trial of sertraline or imipramine in chronic depression. *J. Clin. Psychiatry*, **59**: 598–608.

Commentaries

Latest Developments in Psychotherapy for Depression
Myrna M. Weissman[1]

This volume sponsored by the World Psychiatric Association, including the excellent review by Rush and Thase, is timely. Epidemiologic studies, conducted across diverse cultures, show clearly the variation in rates for major depression, but consistency of age of onset, symptom patterns, risk factors and comorbidity worldwide, suggesting that standardized treatments with established efficacy also have worldwide applicability [1]. Psychotherapy, while of increasing interest globally, is declining as a treatment in the United States. A recent study of visits to psychiatrists over the last decade (1985–1995), showed a significant decrease in psychotherapy and an increase in psychotropic medication [2]. The mean duration of visits has gone down and the number of visits which were 10 minutes or less has increased. Shortening of visits was most evident in the patients previously identified as users of psychotherapy.

The decline in psychotherapy in the United States is primarily motivated by economics. The vast majority of Americans receive mental health care under insurance plans that closely monitor the course of treatment, set limits on length and require authorization for further visits. Under the pressure of managed care, which considers pharmacotherapy a less expensive option, fewer patients are being treated with talking therapies. Yet surveys show that 70% of adults with depression say that they want psychotherapy. Many depressed patients need alternatives and adjuncts to pharmacotherapy, because they are unable or unwilling to take medication. The population at greatest risk for depression worldwide, women of childbearing years, are often reluctant to take medication during pregnancy and lactations. Most depressed patients have social and interpersonal problems closely associated with their symptoms. Thus, there is a tension between what the public seems to want and what is being provided in the United States. By contrast, outside

[1]Division of Clinical & Genetic Epidemiology, College of Physicians and Surgeons of Columbia University and New York State Psychiatric Institute, 1051 Riverside Drive, New York, NY 10032, USA

the United States there is a growing interest in psychotherapy. For example in Canada, general practitioners are learning psychotherapy and a few have psychotherapy subspecialties. Requests for training psychotherapists in the newer brief psychotherapies come from all over the world.

The psychotherapy pendulum has swung and will likely rebound. As managed care itself changes, and as access to psychotherapy is choked, there is likely to be a resurgence of psychotherapy in the United States. Those psychotherapies that survive and grow are likely to be those with empirical support. There is already a shaking out of psychotherapy candidates. Evidence-based approaches will increasingly separate therapies of tested efficacy from those reliant solely on belief.

Rush and Thase's review comes at a good time. John Markowitz, in New York, and I have just completed a revision of the methods and evidence for interpersonal psychotherapy (IPT), a treatment developed for depression by my late husband Gerald L. Klerman, and appropriately described in their review [3]. As part of our IPT update we gathered all the adaptations and efficacy data on IPT, much of it still in press. I will mention a few of the developments below.

Because of our strong belief that patients should be informed about the treatment they receive and should be able to make informed choices about options, a patient book has been developed for IPT, which describes the process of therapy and provides guides to facilitating the process. Two independently conducted clinical trials of IPT have been completed with depressed adolescents, a 12-week comparison of IPT to clinical management ($n = 48$) and a 12-week comparison of IPT, CBT and wait list control in Puerto Rico ($n = 71$). Both studies showed the efficacy of IPT in reducing symptoms of depression.

As the next step, a school-based effectiveness study of IPT for depressed adolescents has just been initiated by Mufson in New York. Controlled clinical trial studies of depressed pregnant adolescents are ongoing by Gillies in Toronto; of depressed pregnant women by Spinelli in New York; of postpartum depression by Stuart in Iowa. A controlled clinical trial of IPT and social rhythm therapy as adjunct treatment to medication for bipolar disorder is underway by Frank in Pittsburgh; a clinical trial of IPT compared to an SSRI for dysthymia is being conducted by Markowitz in New York. Our group is testing the efficacy of IPT for depressed mothers bringing their children for treatment of depression. In a separate trial we are testing the efficacy of IPT delivered over the telephone for depressed mothers unwilling or unable to come for treatment in person. Finally, Browne and Steiner in Hamilton, Canada, are studying 700 primary care patients with depressive symptoms treated with sertraline, IPT or the combination for up to 3 months. The preliminary follow-up results show the superiority of sertraline either alone or in combination with IPT in symptom reduction. However, patients who received IPT either alone or in combination with sertraline had economically important containment of, or reduction in, expenditures in use of health and social services and lower expenditures for those on social assistance. This study demonstrates the complexity of determining cost-effectiveness of treatment.

This brief review of recent studies of IPT most likely can be surpassed in number by ongoing studies of cognitive therapy which is more widely known. Despite the practice trends in the United States, studies to determine the efficacy and effectiveness of psychotherapy for depression are continuing. Rush and Thase's scholarly review of evidence-based psychotherapy for depression will be an important guide and stimulus to similar investigations worldwide.

REFERENCES

1. Weissman M.M., Bland R.C., Canino G.J., Faravelli C., Greenwald S., Hwu H.G., Joyce P.R., Karam E.G., Lee C.K., Lellouch J. *et al* (1996) Cross-national epidemiology of major depression and bipolar disorder. *JAMA*, **276**: 293–299.
2. Olfson M., Marcus S., Pincus H. (1999) Trends in office based psychiatric practice. *Am. J. Psychiatry*, **156**: 451–457.
3. Weissman M.M., Markowitz J., Klerman G.L. (1999) *Comprehensive Guide to Interpersonal Psychotherapy*. Basic Books, New York.

3.2
Indications and Planning of Psychotherapies: "Much Ado about Nothing"?

Bruce E. Wampold[1]

Rush and Thase have presented a thorough review of the literature related to the psychotherapeutic treatment of depression. Several conclusions, based on what Rush and Thase referred to as "consistent evidence," or "incomplete evidence," were presented. The goal underlying these conclusions is to be able to specify a particular psychotherapy for a particular disorder, a laudable goal but one which does not seem to be scientifically justified.

The medical model assumes that mental disorders can be diagnosed reliably and that the underlying mechanisms responsible for the constellation of symptoms can be identified. Moreover, the model assumes that one or a

[1]*Department of Counseling Psychology, University of Wisconsin–Madison, 1000 Bascom Mall, Madison, WI 53706, USA*

few treatments of a disorder will be effective because the specific ingredients in those treatments directly affect the underlying mechanism and thus are palliative. However, whether or not a medical model is the optimal way to conceptualize psychotherapeutic treatments is an empirical question for which much evidence has been collected.

An alternative model that explains the effectiveness of psychotherapy is a meaning model, such as the one proposed by Frank and Frank [1]. According to them, all psychotherapeutic treatments intended to be therapeutic, based on sound principles, will be effective because they share common components, including (1) an emotionally charged, confiding relationship with a helping person (i.e. the therapist); (2) a healing setting, in which the patient presents to a professional, who the patient believes can provide help and who is entrusted to work on his or her behalf; (3) a rationale or conceptual scheme that provides a plausible explanation for the patient's symptoms and prescribes a procedure for resolving them; and (4) the active participation of both patient and therapist.

Although the medical model has the trappings of a scientific endeavor, the research evidence appears to support a meaning model. This empirical evidence will be briefly summarized here, particularly as it is related to the treatment of depression.

The assumption that psychotherapeutic treatments are effective because the specific ingredients in the treatments alter the underlying mechanism of a disorder results in several predictions, none of which has much empirical support. The first prediction is that some psychotherapies would be more effective (i.e. the ones with more potent specific ingredients) than would others. However, meta-analyses have confirmed that all psychotherapies intended to be therapeutic are equally effective [2]. This result appears to be generalizable to the treatment of depression, as indicated by meta-analyses [3], the most comprehensive psychotherapy clinical trial [4], and the conclusions of Rush and Thase, who note the general equivalence of the cognitive, interpersonal, and behavioral classes of psychotherapy treatments.

A second prediction of the medical model is that evidence should exist that the specific ingredients of a treatment are necessary to produce effects. However, when the components of cognitive-behavioral treatment for depression (the most widely tested and accepted treatment for depression) are systematically eliminated, the treatment remains effective [5].

A third prediction of the medical model is that adherence to protocols of treatments proven to be effective would be related to outcomes, whereas allegiance to the treatment would be irrelevant. The empirical evidence is the opposite. Adherence to protocols does not seem to be related to outcome [6], whereas allegiance to the treatment, as predicted by the meaning model, is related to outcome [3].

A fourth prediction of the medical model is that treatment differences should be larger than therapist differences. That is, the variance in outcomes should be determined by the differences in the treatments provided to patients rather than by the therapists who deliver the treatments. However, in all studies that examine therapist effects, these effects are an order of magnitude greater than treatment effects [6]. Clearly, the skill of the therapist delivering the treatment is more important than adherence to the protocol or the particular treatment offered.

A fifth prediction of the medical model is that common factors, such as the working alliance, would be marginally related to outcome. However, the working alliance and outcome are strongly related across various therapies [7], a pattern seen in treatments of depression as well [8].

It appears that the empirical evidence supports a meaning model of psychotherapy and thus the treatment specificity implicit in Rush and Thase's review is unjustified. My research [2, 6] and clinical experience indicate that it is important that depressed patients have access to psychotherapy and that they have the freedom to choose, from a set of legitimate therapies, the one that they believe will be effective, and that attention be given to the competence of the therapist, regardless of the type of therapy delivered.

REFERENCES

1. Frank J.D., Frank J.B. (1991) *Persuasion and Healing: A Comparative Study of Psychotherapy* (3rd edn), Johns Hopkins, Baltimore.
2. Wampold B.E., Mondin G.W., Moody M., Stich F., Benson K., Ahn H. (1997) A meta-analysis of outcome studies comparing bona fide psychotherapies: empirically, "All must have prizes". *Psychol. Bull.*, **122**: 203–215.
3. Robinson L.A., Berman J.S., Neimeyer R.A. (1990) Psychotherapy for the treatment of depression: a comprehensive review of controlled outcome research. *Psychol. Bull.*, **108**: 30–49.
4. Elkin I., Shea T., Watkins J.T., Imber S.D., Sotsky S.M., Collins J.F., Glass D.R., Pilkonis P.A., Leber W.R., Docherty J.P. *et al* (1989) National Institute of Mental Health Treatment of Depression Collaborative Research Program: general effectiveness of treatments. *Arch. Gen. Psychiatry*, **46**: 971–982.
5. Jacobson N.S., Dobson K.S., Truax P.A., Addis M.E., Koerner K., Gollan J.K., Gortner E., Price S.E. (1996) A component analysis of cognitive-behavioral treatment for depression. *J. Consult. Clin. Psychol.*, **64**: 295–304.
6. Wampold B.E. (1997) Methodological problems in identifying efficacious psychotherapies. *Psychother. Res.*, **7**: 21–43.
7. Horvath A.O., Symonds B.D. (1991) Relation between working alliance and outcome in psychotherapy: a meta-analysis. *J. Coun. Psychol.*, **38**: 139–149.
8. Krupnick J.L., Simmens S., Moyer J., Elkin I., Watkins J.T., Pilkonis P.A. (1996) The role of the therapeutic alliance in psychotherapy and pharmacotherapy outcome: findings in the National Institute of Mental Health Treatment of Depression Collaborative Research Program. *J. Consult. Clin. Psychol.*, **64**: 532–539.

3.3
The State of Antidepressant Psychotherapy: Growing Strengths, Still Unanswered Questions
John C. Markowitz[1]

Rush and Thase make key clinical points in reviewing the psychotherapy and combined treatment of unipolar depression.

Several treatments have demonstrated efficacy for mood disorders. Although pharmacotherapy is best tested, there is now strong evidence for interpersonal psychotherapy (IPT) and cognitive and behavioral therapies as acute treatments from adolescence to old age, and some data for lengthier treatment. Neither patients nor therapists should yield to depressive despair, as there are good grounds for therapeutic optimism.

A disparity exists between research on psychotherapy of depression and its general clinical practice. The best researched and empirically supported therapies are not necessarily those most prescribed. IPT until recently was available *only* in research settings, although the number of trained clinicians is growing. Conversely, psychodynamic psychotherapy, still the most widely practiced psychotherapy in the United States, has unfortunately little validation as an antidepressant treatment. Research on psychodynamic psychotherapy is desperately needed to validate the treatment many practitioners are providing.

Differential therapeutics [1] — the crucial question of which treatment works best for which patients — remains in its infancy. Rush and Thase mention, with appropriate caveats, potentially important predictive variables, but much remains unknown. Nonetheless, the day has passed when a therapist could indiscriminately prescribe one treatment for all patients. Contemporary clinicians should know what works, and when to prescribe a particular treatment for a particular patient.

We know most about acute therapy, far less about long-term treatment. Continuation and maintenance psychotherapy studies are scarce. Rush and Thase indicate that we know little about optimal dosing of psychotherapy (ideal number of sessions and duration) for acute and ongoing treatment, and about duration of effects of treatments. Medication often stops working when the prescription ends. Psychotherapy may have greater enduring benefits, even if it is not the "cure" for depression some theorists had hoped. Research is needed to ascertain how long psychotherapeutic effects endure, and for which patients.

Even simple psychoeducational talking or reading can aid depressed patients in conjunction with pharmacotherapy. This is not what we ordinarily think of as psychotherapy, and it is interesting that Rush and Thase make

[1]*Cornell University Medical College, 445 East 68th Street, Suite 3N, New York, NY 10021, USA*

this their initial definition of psychotherapy. But the point is valuable: at minimum, even when not doing a formal psychotherapy, pharmacologists can augment the effect of medication by listening to, talking to, informing and reassuring their patients.

A few additional interpersonal references to Rush and Thase's hefty bibliography. A controlled, not yet published trial showed that IPT [2] reduced symptoms of depressed adolescents more than a "clinical monitoring" control ($n = 24$ per group) [3]. Conjoint IPT might be listed among marital therapies [4]. The section on continuation psychotherapy might have mentioned the original IPT study [5]. Steiner *et al* [6] recently concluded a large ($n > 700$) community study in Canada, comparing IPT, sertraline, and combined treatment of dysthymic disorder, finding high response rates across treatments: 51% of IPT subjects improved, albeit significantly less than the 63% for sertraline and 62% for combined treatment. On follow-up, IPT was associated with significant economic savings in direct use of health care and social services, making combined treatment as efficacious as, but less costly than, sertraline. At Cornell, an efficacy study is comparing IPT, sertraline, supportive therapy, and combined treatment for dysthymic disorder [7].

Two aspects of the Frank *et al* [8] maintenance study for recurrent depression mentioned by Rush and Thase deserve emphasis. Although it is tempting to read it as a medication versus psychotherapy competition, all patients initially received combined treatment during the acute and continuation phases. In the 3-year maintenance phase, maintenance IPT—the only tested antidepressant maintenance psychotherapy to date—was delivered, as in Reynolds *et al*'s geriatric study [9], at low, once-monthly doses. By contrast, imipramine was given at its highest ever maintenance dosage.

Combined pharmaco-psychotherapy for depression has never fared worse than monotherapy. Many psychiatrists combine antidepressant treatments, particularly for more complex patients. In my experience, combined treatment is often optimal for chronic and severe depressions. Medication and psychotherapy may use different mechanisms: the former may best prevent symptom recurrence, while the latter can help patients manage their lives and address obstacles that might precipitate future episodes. I agree with Rush and Thase on the need for further study of targeted use of combined treatment, more studies of medically ill depressed patients, and most of their other recommendations.

ACKNOWLEDGEMENTS

Supported in part by grant MH-49635 from the National Institute of Mental Health, and by a fund established in The New York Community Trust by DeWitt–Wallace.

REFERENCES

1. Frances A., Clarkin J.F., Perry S. (1984) *Differential Therapeutics in Psychiatry: The Art and Science of Treatment Selection*, New York: Brunner/Mazel.
2. Mufson L., Moreau D., Weissman M.M., Klerman G.L. (1993) *Interpersonal Therapy for Depressed Adolescents*, Guilford Press, New York.
3. Mufson L., Moreau D., Weissman M.M., Jaffee W. (1997) Preliminary data on the efficacy of interpersonal psychotherapy for depressed adolescents. Poster presentation at the meeting of the American Academy of Child and Adolescent Psychiatry, Toronto, 14–19 October.
4. Foley S.H., Rounsaville B.J., Weissman M.M., Sholomskas D., Chevron E. (1990) Individual versus conjoint interpersonal psychotherapy for depressed patients with marital disputes. *Int. J. Family Psychiatry*, **10**: 29–42.
5. Klerman G.L., DiMascio A., Weissman M.M., Prusoff B.A., Paykel E.S. (1974) Treatment of depression by drugs and psychotherapy. *Am. J. Psychiatry*, **131**: 186–191.
6. Steiner M., Browne G., Roberts J., Gafni A., Byrne C., Bell B., Dunn E. (1998) Sertraline and IPT in dysthymia: one-year follow-up. Poster presented at the 38th Annual Meeting of the NIMH New Clinical Drug Evaluation Unit (NCDEU), Boca Raton, Florida, 10–13 June.
7. Markowitz J.C. (1998) *Interpersonal Psychotherapy for Dysthymic Disorder*, American Psychiatric Press, Washington DC.
8. Frank E., Kupfer D.J., Wagner E.F., McEachran A.B., Cornes C. (1991) Efficacy of interpersonal psychotherapy as a maintenance treatment of recurrent depression. Contributing factors. *Arch. Gen. Psychiatry*, **48**: 1053–1059.
9. Reynolds C.F. III, Frank E., Perel M., Imber S.D., Cornes C., Miller M.D., Mazumdar S., Houck P.R., Dew M.A., Stack J.A. *et al* (1999) Nortriptyline and interpersonal psychotherapy as maintenance therapies for recurrent major depression: a randomized controlled trial in patients older than 59 years. *JAMA*, **281**: 39–45.

3.4

Research on Hot-house Psychotherapy

T. Byram Karasu[1]

Rush and Thase have done a scholarly work on gathering data on efficacy and effectiveness studies of psychotherapies in the treatment of depression. They acknowledge that the lack of evidence of effectiveness of some therapies (i.e. psychoanalytical) should not be interpreted as their lack of effectiveness. Ironically, the term "psychotherapy" originally was applied to this "unstudied" modality, which still is the largest practice form in the Western world. Now, over 100 practices call themselves psychotherapy. The authors' review includes only the evidence-based approaches. They found

[1]*Department of Psychiatry and Behavioral Sciences, Albert Einstein College of Medicine, 1300 Morris Park Avenue, Bronx, NY 10461, USA*

that time-limited therapies are effective in the acute phase of mild to moderate depressed outpatients. One of their own major questions is whether these therapies can be used in routine clinical care with equivalent good outcomes to those obtained in a research setting.

My not-so-humble answer is No. It has been tried for decades. Parloff's [1] longstanding concerns about bridging the gap between clinicians and researchers are expressed in his overall view that "psychotherapy appears to have everything going for it, except . . . credibility." Psychotherapy is a field that does not lend itself to scientific methodology. Einstein [2] exalted the theoretical route to truth expressed in mathematical equations, which subsequently could be tested by actual experiences in the field. In psychotherapy, the study of intersubjective experience, direct inferences could better come from the reality of genuine encounters. In this paradigm, an $n = 1$ design is the only one that matters, and is unreplicable. As Laing [3] says, science means knowledge adequate to its subject. The virtuosity of the researchers trying to fit psychotherapy to scientific research only clouds their methodological lenses.

What Parloff [4] said in 1975 still holds, that psychotherapy research can never deliver unequivocal conclusions. This is because, regardless of how it is homogenized, psychotherapy is not a simple stimulus that produces a simple response; it is a highly complex set of interactions between two people. The communication between patient and therapist is never linear, but omnidirectional. It is cumulatively spiral, mediated by both directions and compounded with a multiplicity of silent influences. It is normless, unless the patient is also given a manual — a script — to follow (as is the therapist).

One of the most vexing dilemmas of the field still remains: to what extent psychotherapy can be considered a precise science, defined by such criteria as measurability, replicability, and empirical validation. And if so grounded, would that practice still be called psychotherapy? Psychotherapy's inclusion into medical practice as a treatment modality has contaminated its very nature and set up the psychotherapists for potential duplicities. Psychotherapy is a sediment of artful education on subjective matters. It is an interpretive discipline, not a natural science. It has no fixed presumed endpoints. The relations between therapist and patient are formless and improvisational. It is not even interpersonal, but transpersonal. Attempts at articulation of such transubjective experience, says Fierman [5], is like trying "to decipher a melody from the grooves" of two records.

Even the time-limited therapies have found out that psychotherapy is timeless. They increased their sessions from 8–12, to 15–40. It has been said that if they try harder, they may discover psychoanalysis. There is now a cognitive maintenance therapy. So, are we one day going to see a paper entitled, "Cognitive therapy, terminable or interminable?" Shortening the gestation periods changes the delivery. What constitutes practice under the umbrella of psychotherapy is its abortive variations, which are not fully alive. There is no microwave equivalent to full gestation. Clinical issues are issues for the lifespan, not phases of life, says Stern [6].

All these therapies should stop calling themselves *psycho*therapy. They do not deal with the "psych." They are part of the appropriate, legitimate clinical care of patients. They are therapies. The involvement of the spouse in the care of a patient, and providing cognitive and emotional guidance, should be part of the clinical routine for depressed as well as for all other disorders. Researchers colluding with funding agencies, and clinicians with insurance companies are ultimately misleading, demoralizing and frustrating for everyone involved. It is a waste of money, energy and intellectual resources, perpetuating the perennial question of whether psychotherapy is effective or not — which has become a burden for some, a business for others. Psychotherapy is not researchable any more than the relationship between friends, lovers, parents and children is researchable. This is even more so, because psychotherapy has elements of all these relationships and also none of them. Therefore, as Jaspers [7] concluded, a terra firma is never established and "the thing," itself, always escapes.

REFERENCES

1. Parloff M. (1981) Psychotherapy evidence and reimbursement decisions: Bambi meets Godzilla. Paper presented at the meeting of the Society for Psychotherapy Research, Aspen, Colorado, 18 June.
2. Einstein A. (1969) Autobiographical notes. In *Albert Einstein: Philosopher-Scientist*, (Ed. P.A. Schilpp), pp. 1–96, Cambridge University Press, London.
3. Laing R.D. (1967) *The Politics of Experience*, Pantheon Books, New York.
4. Parloff M. (1975) Twenty-five years of research in psychotherapy, Albert Einstein College of Medicine, Department of Psychiatry, New York, 17 October.
5. Fierman L. (1965) *Effective Psychotherapy*, Free Press, New York.
6. Stern D. (1985) *The Interpersonal World of the Infant*, Basic Books, New York.
7. Jaspers K. (1963) *General Psychopathology*, University of Chicago Press, Chicago.

3.5
Psychotherapy for Depression: Are Additional Controlled Trials Still Warranted?
Carlo Perris[1]

Rush and Thase provide a definitive review of the efficacy of psychotherapy in patients with a depressive disorder, which greatly expands an earlier

[1]*Svenska Institutet för Kognitiv Psykoterapi, Dalag 9A, 1tr, Sabbatsbergs sjukhus, Box 6041, 113 82 Stockholm, Sweden*

one compiled by the present author for the World Health Organization, and later published in a condensed form [1]. Comparing the present one with earlier reviews, there is reason to be impressed by the amount of research that has accumulated in a short span of time. Rush has been among the first in reporting a controlled trial of cognitive therapy (CT) and pharmacotherapy in depressed outpatients [2]. As the present review clearly shows, the conclusions reached more than two decades ago, concerning the efficacy of CT for depression, have been repeatedly confirmed.

Even though Rush and Thase have mostly focused on reports published in English, there is no reason to expect that a perusal of articles in other languages would evidence contradictory results able to influence their conclusions in a substantial way.

At least three additional randomized controlled trials (RCTs), however, are worth mentioning, all concerning a comparison of CT with fluoxetine [3–5]. Most earlier trials of psychotherapy versus pharmacotherapy have comprized the more traditional antidepressants, hence, it is worth emphasising that equivalence of efficacy of CT and drugs also applies to the new selective serotonin reuptake inhibitors (SSRIs).

Rush and Thase's review is as thorough as possible, covering whatever might be relevant in terms of efficacy. Consequently, I will focus my commentary on future research needs.

Almost all the trials reported so far have utilized the same measures — Beck Depression Inventory (BDI) and Hamilton Rating Scale for Depression (HAM-D) — for assessing efficacy, hence focusing on reduction/elimination of symptoms. Those trials have undoubtedly succeeded in documenting the efficacy of especially CT and interpersonal therapy (IPT) in terms of symptom reduction/elimination in patients of various ages, with various types of depression, and in different settings.

It is well known that all listed antidepressant drugs can claim, on the basis of published controlled trials, an efficacy in about 60–70% patients recruited with almost one third of them showing no superior response to drugs than to placebo. When it comes to psychotherapy, however, there seems to be an overzealous ambition to not be satisfied with less than 100% success.

In a Zeitgeist of economical constraints, there is a fertile ground for the continued conviction that drugs represent the treatment of choice for depression unless there is any severe contraindication to their use. Accordingly, psychotherapy research has been directed toward exploring equivalence of effect. This despite the fact that the use of antidepressants, especially in less stringently defined depression and in young children, is highly controversial, and, probably, untenable from an ethical point of view. On the other hand, there is evidence that CT is both clinically effective and, compared with the new SSRIs, competitively cost-effective. A trial of CT versus fluoxetine [5], in fact, showed that fluoxetine alone may result in 33% higher expected costs compared with CT, whereas combination treatment had 23% higher costs than CT alone.

Approximately half of depressed individuals who are in treatment receive care in the general medical setting. The practice guidelines of the US Department of Health and Human Services, repeatedly quoted by Rush and Thase, assume that treatment in primary care (PC) will largely rely on pharmacotherapy. This is understandable if no innovative models of PC provision are emphasized as a necessary development. An RCT of brief CT for major depression in PC [6], however, has shown that the addition of brief CT to "treatment as usual" resulted at the end of the acute phase in significantly more subjects meeting recovery criteria compared with the control group, and that gains were maintained throughout the 12 months of follow-up. Strategies for a further development and implementation of similar approaches should have the highest priority.

Further RCTs of a traditional type which tend to stereotypy, to add to the plenitude of evidence already at hand concerning the efficacy of psychotherapy in depression, are hardly longer warranted, however sophisticated they might be. Ultimately, the more sophisticated these trials become, the more limited value they have for the treatment of the individual case in real life.

Funds allocated to trials of a traditional type should, instead, be more profitably allotted to search for answers to other types of questions than the efficacy of psychotherapy. The time is now ripe, in fact, for a move to research on effectiveness. Such a move, however, must necessarily imply the planning of more complex research designs in which quality of life, social role performance, costs, use of health services, and both patient and provider satisfaction are assessed besides the elimination of symptoms. A further important field of research should concern carefully planned investigations of to what extent early interventions, similar to those which have been developed for psychotic patients, might be both feasible and effective for patients with vulnerability for depressive conditions.

REFERENCES

1. Perris C., Herlofson J. (1993) Cognitive therapy. In *Treatment of Mental Disorders* (Eds N. Sartorius, G. de Girolamo, G. Andrews, G.A. German, L. Eisenberg), pp. 149–199, American Psychiatric Press, Washington, DC.
2. Rush A.J., Beck A.T., Kovacs M., Hollon S. (1977) Comparative efficacy of cognitive therapy and imipramine in the treatment of depressed outpatients. *Cogn. Ther. Res.*, **1**: 17–37.
3. Appleby L., Warner R., Whitton A., Faragher B. (1997) A controlled study of fluoxetine and cognitive-behavioural counselling in the treatment of postnatal depression. *Br. Med. J.*, **314**: 932–936.

4. Dunner D.L., Schmaling K.B., Hendrikson H., Becker J., Lehman A., Bea C. (1996) Cognitive therapy versus fluoxetine in the treatment of dysthymic disorder. *Depression*, **4**: 34–41.
5. Antonuccio D.O., Thomas M., Danton W.G. (1997) A cost-effectiveness analysis of cognitive behavior therapy and fluoxetine (Prozac) in the treatment of depression. *Behav. Ther.*, **28**: 187–210.
6. Scott C., Tacchi M.J., Jones R., Scott J. (1997) Acute and one-year outcome of a randomized controlled trial of brief cognitive therapy for major depressive disorder in primary care. *Br. J. Psychiatry*, **171**: 131–134.

3.6
Depression: The Evidence for What Works and What Doesn't

John S. McIntyre[1]

John Rush and Michael Thase, two of the world's leading experts on affective disorders, have produced a comprehensive and scholarly review of the research evidence related to the psychotherapeutic treatment of depression. Results of research trials, "especially randomized controlled trials (RCTs)," are presented in a clear and systematic manner.

The review is not in itself a guideline for treatment. As the authors point out, "several features distinguish research studies and routine care application." One of the major distinguishing and confounding realities is the issue of comorbidities. Consistent with Kessler's survey [1], a report from the American Psychiatric Association's Practice Research Network (PRN) noted that 57% of the patients studied had at least two Axis I diagnoses and 39% had an Axis II diagnosis [2]. In many of the RCTs, patients with comorbidities are excluded or not considered. There is clear evidence that these comorbidities influence the efficacy results. For example, as noted by Rush and Thase, Shea *et al* [3] and Hardy *et al* [4] reported that personality pathology was associated with poorer responses of depressed patients to some therapies but not to others. Hence, the generalizability of the results of the RCTs to the patient population at large must be done cautiously.

At the same time, as Rush and Thase stress, "we must not disregard the value of evidence to inform practice." Their work will be very useful in the development of practice guidelines, which also require evidence based on clinical wisdom and consensus and, in addition, must include strategies for the integration and staging of the interventions. Complementing these randomized clinical trials are data obtained from practice-based research networks, which provide a mechanism to study patients, treatments, and

[1] *Department of Psychiatry & Behavioral Health, Unity Health System, 81 Lake Avenue, Rochester, NY 14608, USA*

outcomes in typical clinical settings [5]. The American Psychiatric Association's PRN is a national research initiative that currently consists of 750
psychiatrists and within 2 years will engage 1000 practicing psychiatrists in
collaborative clinical and services research. In these frontline practices, there
are crucial clinical questions that are not answered by generalizations from
clinical trials but may be addressed by data from the PRN.

The therapies reviewed by Rush and Thase include clinical man-
agement/psychoeducation, interpersonal psychotherapy (ITP), cognitive
therapy (CT), behavior therapy (BT), marital therapy (MT), brief
psychodynamic therapy (BPT) and continuation/maintenance therapies.

The section on clinical management includes medication adherence
strategies, bibliotherapy, problem-solving therapy and stress management,
especially for patients with general medical conditions. This is an area which
is crucial for clinicians, because it provides a substrate upon which other
specific psychotherapies and somatic therapies are added. In each of the
American Psychiatric Association's Practice Guidelines these approaches
are integrated in a section entitled "Psychiatric Management" [6]. Central
to these interventions is the establishment of a good therapeutic alliance.
Luborsky et al [7] and Safran [8] have "demonstrated" the importance of the
therapeutic alliance in achieving good outcomes, but these are not controlled
trials. Of course, designing RCTs to address this issue is extremely difficult.

The evidence seems clear that ITP, CT, BT, and BPT have demonstrated
efficacy for the treatment of the acute phase of mild to moderate major
depressive disorder, and the results for all these depression-targeted, short-
term psychotherapies appear equal to results for medication. However,
these beneficial results are not lasting. Klerman and Weissman note that the
percentage of patients who "remained well over the 18-month follow-up
was disappointingly low, ranging from 19% to 30%" [9]. For maintenance
treatment, medication seems more effective.

Although psychodynamic psychotherapy has been extensively studied,
there are few RCTs [10]. A recent excellent text by Cameron et al reviews
guidelines for the psychotherapies and includes the empirical basis for these
treatments [11].

As Rush and Thase point out, it is not clear which patients may respond
better to which therapies and how long the treatment should continue in
order to minimize the possibility of a recurrence. There are very few data
concerning the efficacy of psychotherapies for children who are depressed,
and for adolescents relatively few data for the continuation or maintenance
phase.

Clearly, as documented by Rush and Thase, we have learned much about
what works and what doesn't in the treatment of depression, but much more
needs to be done.

REFERENCES

1. Kessler R.C., McGonagle K.A., Zhao S., Nelson C.B., Hughes M., Eshleman S., Wittchen H.-U., Kendler K.S. (1994) Lifetime and 12-month prevalence of DSM-III-R psychiatric disorders in the United States; results from the National Comorbidity Survey. *Arch. Gen. Psychiatry*, **51**: 8–19.
2. West J.C., Zarin D.A., Pincus H.A., McIntyre J.S. (1996) Characteristics of psychiatric patients. *Psychiatr. Serv.*, **47**: 577.
3. Shea M.T., Pilkonis P.A., Beckham E., Collins J.F., Elkin I., Sotsky S.M., Docherty J.P. (1990) Personality disorders and treatment outcome in the NIMH Treatment of Depression Collaborative Research Program. *Am. J. Psychiatry*, **147**: 711–718.
4. Hardy G.E., Barkham M., Shapiro D.A., Reynolds S., Rees A., Stiles W.B. (1995) Credibility and outcome of cognitive-behavioural and psychodynamic-interpersonal psychotherapy. *Br. J. Clin. Psychol.*, **34**: 555–569.
5. Zarin D.A., Pincus H.A., West J.C., McIntyre J.S. (1997) Practice-based research in psychiatry. *Am. J. Psychiatry*, **154**: 1199–1208.
6. American Psychiatric Association (1994) Practice Guideline for the Treatment of Patients with Bipolar Disorder. *Am. J. Psychiatry*, **151** (Dec. Suppl.).
7. Luborsky L., McLennan A.T., Woody G.E., O'Brien C.P., Ambelbach A. (1985) Therapist success and its determinants. *Arch. Gen. Psychiatry*, **42**: 602–611.
8. Safran J.D. (1993) Breaches in the therapeutic alliance: an arena for negotiating authentic relatedness. *Psychotherapy*, **30**: 11–24.
9. Klerman G., Weissman M. (1992) The course, morbidity and costs of depression. *Arch. Gen. Psychiatry*, **49**: 831–834.
10. Sledge W. (1997) Resource document on medical psychotherapy. *J. Psychother. Pract. Res.*, **6**: 123–129.
11. Cameron P., Ennis J., Deadman J. (1998) *Standards and Guidelines for the Psychotherapies*, University of Toronto Press, Toronto.

3.7
Psychotherapy of Depression: Research and Practice
Robert Michels[1]

Rush and Thase conclude that in research settings some psychotherapies are effective in reducing symptoms in the acute phase treatment of mild to moderate major depression disorder.

The evidence does not allow them to conclude that other psychotherapies are less effective or to evaluate the relative efficacy of medication compared to psychotherapy (although for acute symptom-targeted therapy, they find no value in combining medication and psychotherapy, currently probably the most common regimen in American psychiatry).

They alert us that the evidence is less clear if we consider other depressive disorders, broader measures, longer term outcomes, prophylaxis, or factors

[1]*Department of Psychiatry, New York Hospital — Cornell Medical Center, 418 E. 71 Street, New York, NY 10021, USA*

which might predict which patient will benefit from which treatment. They also point out that efficacy in a research setting is different from effectiveness in routine clinical care.

Most depressed patients never receive appropriate treatment. They are not recognized, if recognized not correctly diagnosed, and if diagnosed not appropriately treated. They often have comorbid problems — medical conditions, personality disorders, or substance abuse — and the treatment of depression, particularly mild, subsyndromal or dysthymic depression, is only one component of the treatment of the patient. The clinician's question is not "Is psychotherapy A an effective treatment for disorder B?" but rather "What is the best way to treat this patient who is depressed along with a number of other problems? Does the research literature help?"

The answer is mixed. Virtually every patient with a major depressive disorder, and probably most other depressive conditions, has a good chance of benefiting from treatment. Both medication and psychotherapy can be helpful. However, we know little about predictors regarding which treatment is most effective in which domain of outcome or for which patient. Although combined treatments fail to show an advantage for short-term symptom improvement, broader measures of outcome, longer follow-up, considerations of comorbidity, and the absence of any indication of a negative interaction have all made combined treatment popular, at least for those not preoccupied with cost control.

Specific psychotherapies based upon a theoretical model of depression have received more research attention than the more prevalent, more vaguely defined therapies. This research generally demonstrates efficacy for the psychotherapy being studied, but little evidence to suggest that this efficacy has any relationship to the specific characteristics of the particular therapy. No one could fault a clinician who uses one of the tested therapies, but the data might fail to convince clinicians who prefer alternative therapies. Furthermore, unlike medication, "pure" psychotherapy is uncommon in the "real world," and mixtures and combinations are the rule rather than the exception. The optimal role of outcome research on psychotherapy may be different from that of the outcome research on drugs. One expects that the drug studied by the investigator is the same as the drug used in the clinic and that the clinician should follow the investigator's protocol. In contrast, clinicians generally borrow principles and strategies from several psychotherapies and modify and integrate them as they use them with patients.

We might conclude that it is probably good if the psychotherapist of a depressed patient recognizes that the patient is depressed, includes discussion of symptoms, problems, behavior patterns, beliefs and attitudes that are part of the depressive syndrome, and tries not to aggravate the depression by psychotherapeutic strategies that lead to self-disapproval and guilt. These principles are embodied in the several specific therapies that have been demonstrated to be efficacious in the treatment of depression, but are not universals in all psychotherapy.

We might further conclude that it would be valuable to study common therapeutic principles used by clinicians in order to see how they influence outcome, and for which groups of patients they are most valuable. For example, good clinicians are uncertain about the value of directly confronting early resistances as opposed to accepting and accommodating to them, exploring the premorbid precursors of depressive patterns, as opposed to emphasizing the precipitant of the episode, and so on. Clinicians would translate research on such general strategies into clinical use far more readily than they would learn entirely new treatments.

One important lesson not emphasized by Rush and Thase is that treatments are not effective if patients do not "adhere" to them. Thus, the several classes of antidepressant drugs differ primarily not in their relative efficacy, but in their relative tendency to encourage adherence, and therefore effectiveness. The same may be true of psychotherapies and drug–psychotherapy combinations. The primary differential therapeutic issue in the psychotherapy of depression may not be which treatment is most efficacious, but rather which is most likely to encourage adherence.

In one passage Rush and Thase discuss the classic problem of specific vs. nonspecific effects of psychotherapy. They note that patients with "higher quality" interpersonal psychotherapy (IPT) do better than those with "lower quality," and that since therapist time was equivalent in high and low quality, the benefits could not be attributed to nonspecific effects. However, this does not follow. Difficult patients may deskill therapists from following what may be an irrelevant manual while at the same time they fail to respond to the nonspecific aspects of therapy, or they may deskill therapists in the unmeasured nonspecific as well as the measured specific aspects of the treatment. The question of specific vs. nonspecific effect remains.

Rush and Thase have done an immense service by reviewing our current state of knowledge, clarifying what is not known and what future directions would be helpful.

3.8

Nosology vs. Personality Directed Psychotherapy and the Gap Between Research and Practice
Christoph Mundt[1]

Randomized trials with different modes of psychotherapy which are compared to each other, to waiting or to placebo conditions follow the model

---

[1] Psychiatric Department, University of Heidelberg, Vosstrasse 4, 69115 Heidelberg, Germany

of methodologically high-standard drug trials which are used as entrance tickets to the market for a new substance. In the future the same criteria will be applied to those forms of psychotherapy which the national health insurances are asked to pay for. Thus, the entrance to the market needs the evidence for efficacy proven by rigorous standards. However, the higher the standards of a trial, the better the acceptance of the results, but the more artificial the therapeutic procedures, the wider the gap to real practice. Manualized therapeutic interventions with an adherence measurement make major changes of the setting impossible. This may be necessary though, for example, to correct initial misconstructions of pathogenetic foci or to incorporate new views on a problem which emerges from the running psychotherapy. The methodologically rigorous randomized trials, although able to ascertain the efficacy of a therapy on a basic level, may be inadequate to evaluate the more complex procedures in naturalistic clinical settings which make use of a variety of salutogenetic mechanisms at any one time. Hence more clear-cut, simple, and short-term psychotherapeutic procedures will have advantages in randomized trials over more complex therapies.

Furthermore, help-seeking behaviour and prejudices concerning drug vs. psychotherapy [1] cause sampling artifacts in randomized trials, because those patients who contact health care agencies with clear preferences for one or the other therapeutic pathway must be excluded. Those patients, however, often go through a help-seeking procedure in natural settings until they find a therapist who meets their demands. The mutual positive motivation and the emerging agreement on a joint focus for psychotherapy, in turn, is a positive predictor for the outcome. The more or less equity of cognitive (CT), behavioural (BT) and brief psychodynamic (BDP) psychotherapies and the ceiling effect of the combination of psychotherapies with medication may open some space for personal choice between patient and therapist.

Nevertheless, there are some minor differential effects of psychotherapies, for example, better outcome for social dysfunction with interpersonal psychotherapy (IPT) [2]. Such differential efficiency raises the question whether the nosological categorization of patients for the purpose of psychotherapy-indication should be replaced or at least complemented by a categorization which isolates pathogenetic mechanisms which can be specifically matched to psychotherapeutic tools. Also the fact that evidence is poor concerning the efficacy of psychotherapies for very severely retarded depression, psychotic depression, or depression with very deeply altered affect raises the question how to specify the target of psychotherapy within the overall psychopathology.

This can be attempted with regard to the quantity and quality of psychopathological elements. Such attempts have been made, for example, by specifying the targets as social adaptation, personality attitudes, hopelessness, and intrapunitiveness. Such a procedure would pose the question whether, for example, retardation is a more suitable target for psychotherapy or for medication or whether automatic negative cognitions with internal locus of control are more accessible through cognitive psychotherapy or through self-directed psychotherapies. Obviously the answer to this question needs both taking into account the extent of the psychopathological particulars and their being embedded in the whole of mentation. Retardation, for example, may be accessible through activation therapy up to a certain degree, but not at the extent of a depressive stupor, whereas this extreme end of retardation usually responds well to electroconvulsive therapy. Activating medication which is clearly efficacious in severely retarded patients, on the other hand, can cause agitation in some cases without improving mood and cognitions. Besides the dimensional quantitative aspect of psychopathological elements, the interaction between different psychopathological realms of dysfunction should be looked at in order to better understand both improvement and adverse effects of psychotherapy. Using one lever — be it activation, cognition, reward experience, re-establishing anaclitic dependency — can pull the whole system up to improvement but can also lead to adverse effects. In such a case, activation, cognitive restructuring, and the elevation of mood do not proceed at the same pace. We observed such adverse effects in cognitively rigid and deeply depressed patients, who presented increased feelings of insufficiency under activation therapy with emerging delusions of guilt.

Psychotherapy needs a focus and hence these elements of psychopathology need teasing apart. What is needed in addition to the nosological categorization is a dimensional quantification of those psychopathological elements which respond to specific psychotherapeutic tools. Of special interest are the degree of insight and accessibility to such a psychopathological area of dysfunction by patients' will and motivation and the degree and direction of the mutual influence of such elements.

As a consequence, this approach would imply the make-up of the premorbid personality, which in many studies is looked at merely in terms of personality disorder comorbidity. A more functional view which also analyses personalities which cannot be categorized as personality disorder could deliver a perspective of how to choose the right psychotherapeutic tool for the right psychopathological target at the most adequate stage of the illness, that is to compose a succession of specific therapeutic steps. The personality feature of perfectionism may serve as an example to illustrate this line of argument. Perfectionism has been shown to have specific impact on the course of depression, probably implying specific interactions with the severity of depression and the social environment [3]. Empirically based functional personality concepts, such as the typus melancholicus personality, suggest therapeutic change of attitudes which are linked to depressogenic dysfunctions if a mismatch between those personality features and the social environment occurs.

One possible way of pursuing this track is the process-analysis of psychotherapy, by which interactions between personality attitudes, psycho-pathological elements of dysfunctions, and response to therapy modules at a defined stage of the therapy can be examined.

REFERENCES

1. Jorm A.F., Korten A.E., Rodgers B., Pollitt P., Jacomb P.A., Christensen H., Jiao Z. (1997) Belief systems of the general public concerning appropriate treatments for mental disorders. *Soc. Psychiatry Psychiatr. Epidemiol.*, **32**: 468–473.
2. Shea M.T., Elkin J., Imber S.D., Sotsky S.M., Watkins J.T., Collins J.F., Pilkonis P.A., Beckham E., Glass D.R., Dolan R.T. *et al* (1992) Course of depressive symptoms over follow-up: findings from the National Institute of Mental Health Treatment of Depression Collaborative Research Programme. *Arch. Gen. Psychiatry*, **49**: 782–787.
3. Mundt C., Goldstein M., Hahlweg K., Fiedler P. (Eds) (1996) *Interpersonal Factors in the Origin and Course of Affective Disorders*, Gaskell, London.

3.9

The Sequential Use of Pharmacotherapy and Psychotherapy in Depressive Disorders

Giovanni A. Fava[1]

Rush and Thase have discussed the very limited evidence suggesting a beneficial effect of the combination of medication and psychotherapy in depression. This is probably due to the fact that the two types of treatment are generally provided at the same time. Administration of treatment in sequential order has been mainly limited to instances of treatment resistance. Cognitive-behavioral strategies have been successful in the management of drug-resistant major depressive disorders [1], to the same extent that imipramine was found to be effective after unsuccessful cognitive therapy of depression [2]. This literature suggests that a trial of a different modality of treatment should be performed before labeling an episode of major depression as "refractory" or "treatment-resistant." Only when both psychotherapeutic and pharmacological approaches have been used in a sequential order, is it justified to define depression as refractory.

The arbitrary nature of the clinical and research decisions along a response continuum that may range from refractory depression to full remission via partial remission is not frequently acknowledged [3, 4]. Treatment of

[1] *Affective Disorders Program, Department of Psychology, University of Bologna, Viale Berti Pichat 5, 40127 Bologna, Italy*

depression by pharmacological means is likely to leave a substantial amount of residual symptomatology in most of the patients [3, 4]. The treatment patients tend to receive appears to be inadequate, or simply partial, even in specialized settings [3]. Using an observer-rated scale — Paykel's Clinical Interview for Depression [5] — that was found to be a suitable and sensitive instrument for detecting subclinical symptomatology [3], only about 10% of patients with major depression successfully treated with antidepressant drugs and judged to be fully remitted had no residual symptoms [6]. These findings were replicated recently [7]. The presence of residual symptoms after completion of drug or psychotherapeutic treatment has been correlated with poor long-term outcome [3, 4]. Further, some residual symptoms of major depression may progress to become prodromal symptoms of relapse [8]. This led to the development of a sequential strategy based on the use of pharmacotherapy in the acute phase of depression and of cognitive-behavioral therapy in its residual phase [6]. The preliminary results of this strategy, both in primary major depressive disorder [9, 10] and in recurrent depression [11] appear to be promising in terms of differential relapse rate. This challenges the assumption that therapeutic strategies that are effective in the short term are the most suitable for long-term treatment and requires a conceptual shift from current maintenance or continuation strategies [12]. There is limited awareness that current techniques of treating depression are geared to acute situations more than to residual phases of illness. Ryff and Singer [13] suggested that the absence of well-being creates conditions of vulnerability to possible future adversities and that the route of recovery lies not exclusively in alleviating the negative, but in engendering the positive. A specific, well-being-enhancing psychotherapeutic strategy (well-being therapy) has been developed [14] and two preliminary studies appear to be promising [11, 15].

REFERENCES

1. Fava G.A., Savron G., Grandi S., Rafanelli C. (1997) Cognitive-behavioral management of drug resistant major depressive disorder. *J. Clin. Psychiatry*, **58**: 278–282.
2. Stewart J.W., Mercier M.A., Agosti V., Guardino M., Quitkin F.M. (1993) Imipramine is effective after unsuccessful cognitive therapy. *J. Clin. Psychopharmacol.*, **13**: 114–119.
3. Fava G.A. (1996) The concept of recovery in affective disorders. *Psychother. Psychosom.*, **65**: 2–13.
4. Fava G.A. (1999) Subclinical symptoms in mood disorders. Pathophysiological and therapeutic implications. *Psychol. Med.*, **29**: 47–61.
5. Paykel E.S. (1985) The Clinical Interview for Depression. *J. Affect Disord.*, **9**: 85–96.
6. Fava G.A., Grandi S., Zielezny M., Canestrari R., Morphy M.A. (1994) Cognitive behavioral treatment of residual symptoms in primary major depressive disorder. *Am. J. Psychiatry*, **151**: 1295–1299.

7. Nierenberg A.A., Keefe B.R., Leslie V.C., Alpert J.E., Pava J.A., Worthington J.J., Rosenbaum J.F., Fava M. (1999) Residual symptoms in depressed patients who respond acutely to fluoxetine. *J. Clin. Psychiatry*, **60**: 221–225.
8. Fava G.A., Kellner R. (1991) Prodromal symptoms in affective disorders. *Am. J. Psychiatry*, **148**: 823–830.
9. Fava G.A., Grandi S., Zielezny M., Rafanelli C., Canestrari R. (1996) Four year outcome for cognitive behavioral treatment of residual symptoms in major depression. *Am. J. Psychiatry*, **153**: 945–947.
10. Fava G.A., Rafanelli C., Grandi S., Canestrari R., Morphy M.A. (1998) Six-year outcome for cognitive behavioral treatment of residual symptoms in major depression. *Am. J. Psychiatry*, **155**: 1443–1445.
11. Fava G.A., Rafanelli C., Grandi S., Conti S., Belluardo P. (1998) Prevention of recurrent depression with cognitive behavioral therapy. *Arch. Gen. Psychiatry*, **55**: 816–820.
12. Fava G.A. (1997) Conceptual obstacles to research progress in affective disorders. *Psychother. Psychosom.*, **66**: 283–285.
13. Ryff C.D., Singer B. (1996) Psychological well-being. *Psychother. Psychosom.*, **65**: 14–23.
14. Fava G.A. (1999) Well-being therapy. Conceptual and technical issues. *Psychother. Psychosom.*, **68**: 171–179.
15. Fava G.A., Rafanelli C., Cazzaro M., Conti S., Grandi S. (1998) Well-being therapy. *Psychol. Med.*, **28**: 475–480.

3.10
Integrating Psychotherapies in Clinical Practice
Raymundo Macías[1]

Three basic points constitute the standpoint for my commentary. Firstly, the idea that human beings are the basis for all our professional efforts. They are an integrative bio-psycho-social unit and we treat sick people, not illnesses. Nevertheless, we have to move permanently from the principle of uniqueness or singularity to the principle of universality, to see what one shares with others, and to use our knowledge of many particular cases to try to generalize for the benefit of all.

Secondly, we have developed our own general concept of psychotherapy, after some 40 years of clinical practice. It is the use of different psychological techniques, by a professional, to heal or help in the process of healing, relieving or soothing emotional pain, anxiety and/or depression, to reduce, alleviate and solve symptoms and problems and, if possible, to restore functioning, thus facilitating the growth and development of patients or persons in need of help, or at least to be able to console or comfort them in their suffering.

[1] *Instituto de la Familia, Jalisco # 8, Tizapán, México, D.F. 01080*

Thus, psychotherapy is a human encounter. We might paraphrase Franz Alexander's "emotional corrective experience" and, integrating other approaches, say it is "a human reparative, reconstructive, growth and healing experience", in which both sides — patients and therapists — benefit.

Thirdly, a basic belief that theories, methods and techniques should be in the service of the patients, not the patients in the service of any of the former, being used to demonstrate that a particular approach is better than another, at any rate not if doing so deprives patients of the benefits they might obtain from more comprehensive treatment. In this light we will add our voice to those who question the use of only "placebo" or "no treatment" at all in control groups that could have benefited from some kind of treatment, just to have more "rigorous" data and prove significant evidence for one particular approach in comparison to another.

We consider, from our clinician and teacher standpoint, rather than from that of a researcher, that a good treatment plan, including all necessary resources for the benefit of the patient, should be tailored to each particular case.

On the other hand, we totally agree with Rush and Thase's comment, in their extremely well-documented and exhaustive review, that though we should be cautious in generalizing from research data to common clinical practice, the value of evidence for informing practice must not be overlooked, and therefore, those responsible for policymaking and administrating health systems, while they should not rely exclusively on research evidence, should certainly not ignore it. We should also consider other forms of therapy, such as Gestalt, systemic, experiential or process groups, which are used frequently and claim good results, yet have no formal control studies to evaluate their efficacy. Yet, generally speaking, clinical populations are usually best served by first using treatment methods with proven efficacy/safety.

Sorrow and depressive mood have been regarded as the characteristics of depression in the traditional approach, for almost 30 years; the cognitive process of the depressive patient, previously considered as a consequence of the affective disturbance, is now seen as the main element. Furthermore, Beck's cognitive model of depressive vulnerability offers an explanation of why some patients develop a major depressive episode after a significant loss or setback, while other people do not. Individual differences in personality determine the types of latent depressive beliefs which are present and as a consequence the types of stressing events that are prone to trigger a depressive episode. Through the development of this theory and approach, numerous questionnaires and evaluation scales have been designed, so taken together this model and these instruments designed more specifically to deal with depressive disorders constitute a standing option for treatment.

Different studies report that cognitive therapy reduces depressive symptoms during the acute phase in the less severe cases as much as antidepressants, yet both combined offer better results. In our experience it is within the field of psychiatry that this can be done, whereas at the primary care level, a great number of depressive problems could be dealt with by general practitioners and family physicians using antidepressants, supportive therapy and a psychoeducational approach to the patient and the family. The importance of a family approach has to be stressed, particularly in dealing with elderly patients, because considering the recursive processes that occur in the family, quite frequently the loss of status of the elder adds to other significant psychological losses the patient might have already experienced, and dealing with a deeply depressed member of the family might become an important stressor to the whole system, sometimes generating intense negative feelings of rejection or aggression that reinforce the whole situation. The same dynamics might not apply only to the depressed elders.

There are some points that Rush and Thase present in their summary as consistent evidence that coincide entirely with our extensive clinical experience, particularly within the institutional mental health program of the social security system in Mexico. The main points are: that good clinical management by the family physician as well as by the specialist using a psychoeducational approach increases medication adherence in the depressed patients and also reduces or delays relapses; that different psychotherapies (cognitive, interpersonal, behavioral) have equal acute phase efficacy in adult nonpsychotic depressed outpatients; that some predictors of poor outcome are not specific to a particular model but are relevant to almost all therapies including medication; that elderly adults appear to respond as well to maintenance and acute phase psychotherapies as nonelderly adults with major depression; and that treating depressions associated with general medical conditions is extremely important.

3.11
Building on the Foundations: Where Next in Therapeutic Outcome Research?

John C. Nemiah[1]

In their review of the recent literature concerning the treatment of depressive disorders, Rush and Thase have accomplished a monumental task. From their survey of the reports of randomized controlled trials of a variety of biological and psychological treatment modalities in patients with major depressive disorders, they provide strong evidence for the effectiveness of

[1] Department of Psychiatry, Dartmouth–Hitchcock Medical Center, One Medical Center Drive, Lebanon, New Hampshire 03756, USA

such therapeutic interventions. The treatment of depression works — a fact that, as Rush and Thase demonstrate, is amply documented by scientific data.

Although a variety of treatment modalities have been examined in experimental investigations, three forms of psychological therapy — interpersonal psychotherapy (IPT), cognitive therapy (CT), and behavioral therapy (BT) — have been the particular focus of extensive study. Indeed, as Rush and Thase point out, there has been a sufficiently extensive investigation of these three forms of treatment to provide conclusive evidence not only that they are consistently effective in their own right, but that they achieve therapeutic results that are on a par with those produced by antidepressant medications. That finding is of major clinical significance and underscores the importance of including psychotherapeutic modalities as a major component of the clinical management of patients with depressive disorders.

It should further be recognized that the same body of evidence pointing to the therapeutic effectiveness of IPT, CT, and BT also indicates that all three of those modalities have "equal efficacy" in the treatment of the acute phase of non-psychotic major depressive disorders. Here, again, research provides us with an encouragingly positive conclusion about the clinical value of the psychotherapies in treating depression. At the same time, however, it reveals a curious finding that warrants the following further considerations.

To begin with, we should note that each of these three forms of psychological treatment is based on distinctly different conceptions of the mechanism of production of depressive symptoms, and each arrives at distinctly different therapeutic goals and procedures based on those different conceptual formulations. For example, interpersonal psychotherapy is concerned primarily with exploring and resolving patients' conflicts in their interpersonal relationships, whereas cognitive therapy focuses on detecting and changing pathogenic beliefs. Behavioral therapy, on the other hand, shifts the focus of attention away from patients' subjective experiences to the delineation and eradication of pathological patterns of learned behavior.

Each of these conceptual models makes sense. Each provides the clinician with a useful and logical explanation of the pathogenesis of patients' symptoms. And each supplies a rationale for a therapeutic approach that has been demonstrated to be highly effective. However, a logical problem is posed by the fact that those same outcome studies also demonstrate that all three treatment modalities are equally effective. No matter which conceptual model of pathogenesis is held or which form of treatment based on it is applied to the clinical management of depressed patients, they recover in equal numbers. It makes no difference, apparently, how we conceive of our patients' illnesses or what techniques we use to treat them. Our patients get well with equal facility.

Here is indeed a curious conclusion that not only leaves us with a superfluity of hypotheses but finds us lacking sufficient data to enable us to judge their relative validity as explanatory models or guides to treatment. Occam's razor is clearly called for to simplify our hypotheses. For example, we might postulate that, despite their apparent differences, the three forms of treatment share a common set of features that explains their therapeutic effectiveness. Perhaps, regardless of individual differences in technical details, all three are therapeutically successful because they offer patients fundamentally the same kind of treatment. All of them provide an organized, intensive treatment program that involves the exposure of patients to a team of actively attentive and enthusiastic therapists. All provide a richly supportive human environment with strongly positive suggestions for recovery. All of them, in other words, surround the patient with a set of conditions inherently conducive to the removal of symptoms and to the restoration of normal functioning. Is it possible, we may ask, that factors of this nature have been at work in some or all of the studies reviewed in this survey?

The questions thus raised are not meant as a criticism or a refutation of the findings of the remarkably extensive and careful investigations of the treatment of depression that Rush and Thase have reviewed for us. On the contrary, they follow logically from those findings and point to future areas of research that have as yet to be examined. Rush and Thase, for example, have pointed to the paucity of investigations and information about the clinical indications for the various forms of therapy, and, by implication, to how little is known about the psychological processes involved in the treatment of and recovery from depression. As this review of recent research has clearly demonstrated, we now know that psychotherapeutic measures are indeed effective in treating depressive disorders. Armed with that knowledge, we are now in a position to move forward to a second generation of investigations designed both to explore in much more detail exactly how those psychotherapeutic measures work and to determine the indications for their use based on an understanding of the psychopathological processes underlying the disorders they are designed to treat. With their admirable summary and synthesis of the initial phases of the investigation of the psychotherapies, Rush and Thase have made the move to the next phase of study that much the easier for us all.

4

Depressive Disorders in Children and Adolescents: A Review

Richard Harrington

Royal Manchester Children's Hospital, Manchester, UK

INTRODUCTION

Until recently it was widely believed that depressive disorders were rare in young people. Young children were thought to be incapable of experiencing many of the phenomena that are characteristic of depressive disorders in adults. Affective disturbance in adolescents was often dismissed as adolescent "turmoil". Over the past 20 years, however, there has been a substantial change in the ways in which mood disturbance among the young has been conceptualized. The use of structured personal interviews has shown that depressive syndromes resembling adult depressive disorders can and do occur among both prepubertal children and adolescents [1]. Indeed, clinical research in the United Kingdom has suggested that as many as one in four referrals to child psychiatrists suffer from a depressive disorder [2]. Depression may be becoming more prevalent among young people [3].

In this chapter, a discussion of the clinical picture and differential diagnosis of depressive disorders in young people precedes a review of their natural history. The most promising psychological and pharmacological treatments for the disorders are then described. The chapter concludes with a discussion of future directions for research.

CLINICAL PICTURE AND DIFFERENTIAL DIAGNOSIS

Diagnosis of Depressive Disorder

Defining the boundaries between extremes of normal behaviour and psychopathology is a dilemma that pervades all of psychiatry. It is especially

Depressive Disorders, Second Edition. Edited by Mario Maj and Norman Sartorius.

problematic to establish the limits of depressive disorder in young people, because of the cognitive and physical changes that take place during this time. Adolescents tend to feel things particularly deeply, and marked mood swings are common during the teens [4]. It can be difficult to distinguish these intense emotional reactions from depressive disorders. By contrast, young children do not find it easy to describe how they are feeling, and often confuse emotions such as anger and sadness [5]. They have particular difficulty in describing certain of the key cognitive symptoms of depression, such as hopelessness and self-denigration. Indeed, there are developmental changes in many of the cognitive abilities that may underlie these depressive cognitions. Thus, for instance, during middle childhood (ages 7–9) the self is conceived in outward, physical terms. If asked to describe themselves, children of this age will tend to frame their descriptions in terms of external characteristics, or what they do. It is only by adolescence that young people will regularly describe themselves in terms of psychological characteristics.

Assessment of young people who present with symptoms of depression must therefore begin with the basic question of diagnosis. This will mean interviewing the child or adolescent alone. It is not enough to rely on accounts obtained from the parents since they may not notice depression in their children, and may not even be aware of suicidal attempts. Indeed, it is now common practice to obtain information from several sources. Children usually give a better account of symptoms related to internal experience, whereas parents are likely to be better informants on overt behavioural difficulties. Accounts from children and parents are usually supplemented by information from other sources, particularly teachers and direct observations.

Although the interviewing of multiple informants may yield much useful information, the diagnosis of depressive disorder in young people can still be very difficult. Standardized diagnostic systems such as DSM-IV [6] and structured psychiatric interviews can help in deciding whether the patient has serious depressive symptomatology that requires treatment. Unfortunately, such diagnostic systems tend to be overinclusive in this age group and many dysphoric children and adolescents who meet criteria for major depression remit within a few weeks [7]. It is important, then, that careful inquiry is made about the impact the young person's symptoms have had on everyday functioning and about the presence of symptoms of unequivocal psychopathological significance, such as suicidal planning or marked weight loss.

Probably the best single indicator of whether or not a young person has a serious depressive disorder is the duration of the problem. Polysymptomatic depressive states that persist for more than 6 weeks usually require intervention.

Efforts to improve the reliability and validity of diagnosis have been focused on two areas: the development of standardized assessment instruments, and biological tests.

A number of factors need to be considered in selecting an instrument to assess depression among the young [8]. In choosing between the questionnaires that are available, it is especially important that the user has a clear idea of what the scale is going to be used for. For example, questionnaires that are good discriminators between depressed and non-depressed children may be ineffective as measures of change during treatment. In clinical settings, self-report questionnaires provide a convenient way of screening for symptoms that are not part of the presenting complaint, and may be useful for measuring treatment response. They are especially helpful in monitoring subjective feelings. In research settings, questionnaires have been used both as a primary source of data and as a screening instrument to select subjects for further in-depth interviews. Unfortunately, many depression questionnaires have low specificity for depressive disorder. This means that if they are used as screens, then many young people who have high scores on the screening questionnaire will turn out not to have a depressive disorder at interview. Many clinicians are unaware of this problem, and tend to assume that a high score on a depression questionnaire means that the adolescent has a high probability of having a depressive disorder [9].

Several standardized interviews have been devised for use with children and many of them will generate depressive diagnoses. These instruments have led to important advances in the assessment of juvenile depression and as a result structured psychiatric interviews are being used more and more as diagnostic tools in clinical settings. Nevertheless, there are several unresolved difficulties [10]. Firstly, although interrater reliability has been reasonable, test–retest reliability has been less good, and affective symptoms are particularly unstable in the younger age groups. Secondly, there is often low agreement between parent and child on depressive features, and it is still not clear how information from different sources should be combined. It is quite common in clinical practice to find that young people report severe feelings of depression that go unrecognized both by parents and by other informants such as teachers.

These problems in making the clinical diagnosis of depression have led to much interest in the use of psychobiological measures as markers of depressive disorder. Probably the best known of these is the dexamethasone suppression test (DST). Unfortunately, the DST is not sufficiently specific to be of much value in making the diagnosis [11]. For example, its results are influenced by many other factors such as weight loss [12]. As a result, few clinicians place great reliance on its findings.

Assessment and Differential Diagnosis of Other Difficulties

Although the accurate diagnosis of depressive disorder is an important part of clinical management, assessment only starts with the diagnosis, it does not stop with it. Depressed children usually have multiple problems, such as educational failure, impaired psychosocial functioning, and comorbid psychiatric disorders. Indeed, it seems that most children who meet research criteria for depressive disorder are given some other primary diagnosis by the clinicians involved in their care [13]. This overlap of depression and other psychiatric diagnoses has been one of the most consistent findings from research in referred clinical populations, where an association has been found with conditions as diverse as conduct disorder, anxiety states, learning problems, hyperactivity, anorexia nervosa and school refusal [14, 15]. Moreover, depressed adolescents tend to come from families with high rates of psychopathology and may have experienced adverse life events [16]. All these problems need to be identified and the causes of each assessed.

The final part of the assessment involves the evaluation of the young person's personal and social resources. There is evidence that being successful at school or in other areas of life can protect young people from the effects of adverse life experiences [17]. The best guide to the child's ability to solve future problems is his or her record in dealing with difficulties in the past. The ability of the family to support the patient should also be evaluated.

AETIOLOGY

The aetiology of child and adolescent depressive disorders is likely to be multifactorial, including both genetic and environmental factors. Genetic factors account for a substantial amount of the variance in liability to bipolar illness in adults, but probably play a less substantial, though still significant, part in unipolar depressive conditions [18]. Interest in the genetics of depressive disorders arising in young people has been stimulated by data from several sources. First, it seems that, among adult samples, earlier age of onset is associated with an increased familial loading for depression [19]. Second, the children of depressed parents have greater than expected rates of depression [20]. Third, there are high rates of affective disorders among the first-degree relatives of depressed child probands [21]. Moreover, there is some specificity in this linkage, to the extent that the risk applies mainly to affective disturbances as opposed to non-affective disorders [22].

It will be appreciated that just because a disorder runs in families, it does not necessarily follow that the linkages are mediated genetically. It is likely that family environmental factors are also important. For instance, discordant intrafamilial relationships seem to be strong predictors of the course of depressive disorders among the young. Children with depression admitted to hospital who return to families showing high levels of criticism and discord have a much worse outcome than children returning to more harmonious environments [23]. Stresses and acute life events outside the family, such as friendship difficulties and bullying, are also likely to be relevant in this age group [24].

Current models of depression in young people also emphasize the importance of bidirectional influences. Depression and its associated symptoms, such as irritability, can be a cause of family and peer difficulties, as well as a consequence. It is possible that negative cycles of interaction are started, in which depression causes family environmental problems, which in turn lead to worsening of the depression [25].

The psychological and biological mechanisms that link these risk factors to depression remain poorly understood. The most influential of the psychological models (which have had important implications for treatment — see below) have been the cognitive theories, which were first developed with cases of adult depression. The main idea behind these theories is that depressed people develop a distorted perception of the world (such as the expectation that things will always go wrong), which is caused by earlier adversity. When the child experiences current adversity, these negative cognitions become manifest, which then leads to depression. The occurrence of distorted negative cognitions has been documented in numerous studies of depressed young people [26].

Biological theories have mainly consisted of straightforward downward extensions of models first developed with adult cases. The best known theory is the amine hypothesis, which proposes that depression is caused by underactivity in cerebral amine systems. This hypothesis arose from studies of adults which found that drugs that alter cerebral amine concentrations, such as imipramine, are also associated with mood changes. Several studies of young people with depressive disorders have reported abnormalities of the biological markers that are thought to reflect the activity of these systems [27]. However, it is still not clear if these abnormalities cause depression.

COURSE AND OUTCOME

By comparison with non-depressed subjects, young people diagnosed as depressed are more likely to have subsequent episodes of depression. Thus studies of children meeting DSM-III criteria for depression have shown that depression in childhood often recurs. For example, Kovacs et al [28] found that about 70% of child patients with a major depressive disorder had another episode within 5 years. This increased risk of recurrence extends into adulthood. Harrington et al [13] followed-up 63 depressed children and adolescents on average 18 years after their initial contact. The depressed group was four times more likely to have an episode of depression after the age of 17 years than a control group who had been matched on a large number of variables, including non-depressive symptoms. This increased risk was maintained well into adulthood and was associated with significantly increased rates of attending psychiatric services and of using medication, as compared to the controls. A preliminary report from a large follow-up study in the United States has found increased suicide rates in depressed adolescent patients [29].

A variety of different factors appear to predict continuity. The characteristics of the index episode are important to the extent that children with "double depression" (major depression and dysthymic disorder) have a worse short-term outcome than children with major depression alone [28]. Older children have a worse prognosis than younger ones, and continuity to adulthood is best predicted by a severe adult-like depressive presentation [13]. Although it is often assumed that continuity of depression is mainly due to the direct persistence of the initial disorder or of premorbid psychological and/or biological vulnerabilities to depression, it should be borne in mind that environmental mechanisms may also be involved [23]. Relapse may also be linked to parental depression [20]. Hammen *et al* [30] found a close temporal relationship between maternal depression and a recurrence of depression in the child, supporting the idea of an environmentally mediated mechanism.

Recovery from the Index Episode

Although the risk of recurrence of juvenile depression is high, it is important to know that the prognosis for the index episode is quite good. The available data suggest that the majority of children with major depression will recover within 2 years. For example, Kovacs *et al* [31] reported that the cumulative probability of recovery from major depression by 1 year after onset was 74% and by 2 years was 92%. This study was based on subjects who in most cases had a previous history of treatment for emotional-behavioural problems. However, Keller *et al* [32] reported very similar findings in a retrospective study of time to recovery from first episode of major depression in young people who had mostly not received treatment. The probability of recovery for adolescent inpatients with major depression also appears to be about 90% by 2 years [33], though those with long-standing depressions recover less quickly than those whose presentation is acute.

It seems, then, that most young people with major depression will recover to a significant extent, but that a substantial proportion of those who recover will relapse.

PRINCIPLES OF TREATMENT

Many of the general principles of treatment follow from the description of the depressed young person's difficulties outlined above. Comorbidity is frequent, there are many complications and there is a high risk of relapse. Other types of adversity are part of the cause and may need intervention in their own right. The course is determined by more than just the presence and severity of depression. Therefore, attention must be paid to biological, familial, educational and peer contributions. As with other child psychiatric disorders, it is important not only to treat the presenting problems but also to foster normal development. A treatment programme therefore has multiple aims: to reduce depression, to treat comorbid disorders, to promote social and emotional adjustment, to improve self-esteem, to relieve family distress and to prevent relapse.

Initial Management

The initial management of depressed young people depends greatly on the nature of the problems identified during the assessment procedure. The assessment may indicate that the reaction of the child is appropriate for the situation. In such a case, and if the depression is mild, a sensible approach can consist of regular meetings, sympathetic discussions with the child and the parents, and encouraging support. These simple interventions, especially if combined with measures to alleviate stress, are often followed by an improvement in mood. In other cases, particularly those with severe depression or suicidal thinking, a more focused form of treatment is indicated.

It is important that the clinician considers a number of key questions early on in the management of depressed young people. The first question is whether the depression is severe enough to warrant admission to hospital. Indications for admission of depressed children are similar to those applicable to their adult counterparts, and include severe suicidality, psychotic symptoms or refusal to eat or drink. A related question is whether the child should remain at school. When the disorder is mild, school can be a valuable distraction from depressive thinking. When the disorder is more severe, symptoms such as poor concentration and motor retardation may add to feelings of hopelessness. It is quite common in such cases that ensuring that the child obtains tuition in the home, or perhaps in a sheltered school, improves mood considerably.

The second question is whether the depression is complicated by other disorders such as behavioural problems. If it is, then as a general rule it is best to sort out these complications before embarking on treatment for the depression. For example, if a child has a major behavioural disorder, then it will be necessary to ensure that appropriate psychosocial measures are being taken to deal with this. Similarly, the depression-like states that are common in adolescents with anorexia nervosa usually respond much better to weight gain than they do to antidepressants.

The third question concerns the management of the stresses that are found in many cases of major depression. It is sometimes possible to alleviate some of these stresses, such as bullying. However, in the majority of cases, acute stressors are just one of a number of causes of the depression. Moreover, such stressors commonly arise out of chronic difficulties such as family discord, and may therefore be very hard to remedy. Symptomatic treatments for depression can therefore be helpful even when it is obvious that the depressive symptoms occur in the context of chronic family or social adversity that one can do little to change.

INDIVIDUAL AND GROUP PSYCHOLOGICAL THERAPIES

Many different individual or group psychosocial interventions have been used with depressed children, including cognitive therapy, psychotherapy, art therapy, and drama therapy (see [34] for a review). Depression is a problem with such pervasive features that one can find abnormalities in almost any domain (e.g. cognitive, interpersonal, psychodynamic) to justify virtually any intervention. This review therefore uses several inclusion criteria [35] to select from the huge array of interventions. The first is whether there is a theory about the mechanisms of disorder and about how treatment reduces dysfunction. The second is whether there has been basic research on these mechanisms independent of treatment outcome studies. The third criterion is whether the treatment has been, or is being, evaluated in randomized controlled trials.

Two individual or group psychological treatments are relatively well developed in respect of these criteria: cognitive-behaviour therapy and interpersonal psychotherapy.

Individual and Group Cognitive-behavioural Therapies

According to cognitive theory, depression is not simply triggered by adversity but rather by the perception and processing of adverse events. Research has shown that depressed children often have low self-esteem and a variety of cognitive distortions such as selectively attending to negative features of an event [25, 36, 37]. In addition, depressed children are more likely than the non-depressed to develop negative attributions [38]. For example, Curry and Craighead [39] found that adolescents with greater depression attributed the cause of positive events to unstable external causes. Depressed children also have low perceived academic and social competence [40].

Although many studies have documented the association between childhood depression and various cognitive distortions, there are many unresolved questions. In particular, it is unclear whether these negative cognitions are a cause or a consequence of depression [26]. Moreover, it is not known whether some cognitive processes are more important than others. Nevertheless, research on cognitive processes in depressed children has provided a useful theoretical basis for planning treatment strategies.

Cognitive-behavioural treatment (CBT) programmes were developed to address the cognitive distortions and deficits identified in depressed children. Many varieties of CBT exist for childhood depression, but they all have the following common characteristics. First, the child is the focus of treatment (although most CBT programmes involve parents). Second, therapists play an active role in treatment; the child and therapist collaborate to solve problems. Third, the therapist teaches the child to monitor and keep a record of thoughts and behaviour; there is much emphasis on diary-keeping and on homework assignments. Fourth, treatment usually combines several different procedures, including behavioural techniques (such as activity scheduling) and cognitive strategies (such as cognitive restructuring).

There have been trials of cognitive-behaviour therapy in samples of children with (a) depressive symptoms, recruited from schools, and (b) depressive disorder.

Treatment in the school setting allows easy access. This is important because epidemiological studies suggest that only a minority of depressed young people come to mental health services for treatment [41]. It is also easier to integrate psychological treatment with work carried out by other professionals, such as teachers. A potential disadvantage is that it may be difficult to maintain privacy. Moreover, school-based group interventions may not be suitable for young people with severe problems, such as children who repeatedly harm themselves.

There have been at least nine controlled studies of CBT in samples of children with depressive symptoms recruited through schools [42–50]. The design has usually been to screen all children with a depression question-naire and then to invite those with a high score to participate in a group intervention. For example, in one of the first randomized controlled trials to suggest that CBT is effective in childhood depression, Reynolds and Coats [42] involved an entire school in a multiple stage screening procedure. They invited those who were screen positive (a high score on a depression question-naire on two occasions) to take part in the study. Cognitive-behaviour therapy consisted of 10 group sessions that emphasized the training of self-control skills such as self-monitoring, problem-solving and self-reinforcement.

Table 4.1 presents results of the six randomized trials that provided quantitative data on outcomes. Tabled information includes the conditions contrasted, duration of therapy, uptake of treatment after screening (i.e. the percentage of children who were screen positive who went on to have treatment) and indices of outcome. As the table indicates, in three of the trials CBT was significantly superior to no treatment. Of the controlled trials not shown in Table 4.1, a non-randomized trial reported that CBT was significantly superior to no treatment [44], as did a randomized trial that did not present quantitative outcome data [46]. One trial has not so far reported whether CBT was more effective than the control intervention [49].

Although these results are promising, they may not necessarily apply to cases with depressive disorder. Table 4.2 summarizes the results of six randomized trials of CBT for children diagnosed with depressive disorder, expressed as the numbers remitted after therapy [51–56]. The table shows studies carried out in community and outpatient samples. The comparison conditions have usually been inactive interventions such as remaining on a waiting list or attention placebo. All studies have shown that CBT was superior to its comparison condition and in four of them this difference was statistically significant [52–54, 56]. A meta-analysis of the studies found a pooled odds ratio in an intent-to-treat analysis of 2.2 (95% confidence interval 1.4–3.5), suggesting significant improvement in the CBT group over the comparison interventions [57].

Table 4.2 omits two additional studies. One non-randomized study reported that therapeutic support was superior to social skills training [58]. The other, a preliminary report from an ongoing study, reported an emerging trend for CBT to be superior to remaining on a waiting list [59].

There are few data regarding the factors that influence treatment outcome. The most consistent finding thus far has been that children with severe depressive disorders respond less well to CBT than children with mild or moderately severe conditions [60–62]. For example, Jayson et al [61] found that only 25% of young people who were unable to function in at least one social domain (e.g. unable to go to school) responded to CBT.

Research has also examined the role that changes in negative cognitions might have in predicting outcome. CBT is not differentially more effective in cases with high cognitive distortion [60, 62]. Lewinsohn et al [53] found that changes in depressogenic cognitions did not account for the superiority of CBT over remaining on a waiting list.

Proponents of cognitive-behavioural therapy have long suggested that it might protect against relapse once treatment has finished. But does CBT really provide such protection? The available data do not yet provide an answer to this question. Two studies have not yet published follow-ups [51, 52] and one provided no follow-up data because the control group was given active treatment immediately after the first phase [53]. In many trials the duration of follow-up was too short (less than 3 months) to determine whether the intervention had any real protective effect [42, 43, 45, 47, 48, 54]. Only four randomized trials have published data on outcomes after a follow-up interval of 6 months or more [7, 50, 56, 63]. Only one of them found a significant long-term effect of treatment. One found that around 50% of patients who remitted with CBT had a further episode within the next 6 months [56]. In

TABLE 4.1 Randomized comparative studies of the cognitive-behavioural therapies in non-diagnosed school samples with depressive symptoms

Study	Age (years)	Cell	Type of CBT NT	Sessions (no.)	Uptake (%)	Subjects randomized (no.)	Subjects evaluated (no.)	Outcome measure	Mean pre	Mean post	Results
Reynolds and Coats, 1986 [42]	Mean = 15.6	CBT RT NT	SC	10 10 0	48	9 11 10	6 8 10	BDI	21.1 17.1 16.9	6.4 5.6 18.3	CBT = RT > NT
Stark et al, 1987 [43]	9–12	CBT BPS NT	SC	12 12 0	64	9 10 9	9 10 9	CDI	21.6 22.4 20.1	8.0 9.0 18.6	SC = BPS > NT
Kahn et al, 1990 [47]	10–14	CBT RT SM NT	CWDC	12 12 14 0	79	17 17 17 17	17 17 17 17	RADS	85.4 83.8 84.3 86.9	53.4 61.8 62.1 80.1	CBT = RT = SM >NT
Liddle and Spence, 1990 [45]	7–11	CBT APC NT	SCT	8 8 0	94	11 10 10	11 10 10	CDI	21.0 22.3 20.7	14.4 19.3 16.9	SCT = APC = NT

continues overleaf

TABLE 4.1 (*continued*)

Study	Age (years)	Cell	Type of CBT	Sessions (no.)	Uptake (%)	Subjects rando-mized (no.)	Subjects evaluated (no.)	Outcome measure	Mean pre	Mean post	Results
Marcotte and Baron, 1993 [48]	14–17	CBT NT	Rational emotive	12 0	58	15 13	12 13	BDI	24.0 21.4	14.2 14.8	CBT = NT
Weisz, et al, 1997 [50]	Mean = 9.6	CBT NT	PASCET	8 0	Not known	16 32	Not known	CDI	18.6 17.8	7.1 11.8	CBT > NT

APC = attention placebo control; BPS = behavioural problem-solving; BDI = Beck Depression Inventory; CBT = cognitive-behaviour therapy; CDI = Children's Depression Inventory; CWDC = Coping With Depression Course; NT = no treatment; PASCET = Primary and Secondary Control Enhancement Training; RADS = Reynolds Adolescent Depression Scale; RT = relaxation training; SC = self-control; SCT = social compe-tence training; SM = self-modelling.

TABLE 4.2 Randomized comparative studies of cognitive-behavioural interventions in samples diagnosed with depressive disorder

Study	Age (years)	Sample	Cell	Type of CBT	Sessions (no.)	Subjects randomized (no.)	Outcome measure	Subjects remitted (no.)	Results
Lewinsohn et al, 1990 [53]	14–18	Adverts & clinics	CBT / NT	CWDC	14 / 0	24 / 24	K-SADS	9/21 / 1/19	CBT > NT
Reed 1994 [54]	14–19	Community	CBT / AP	Structured learning	6 / 6	12 / 6	CR	6/11 / 0/6	CBT > AP
Vostanis et al, 1996 [55]	8–17	Outpatient clinic	CBT / AP	DTP	9 / 9	29 / 28	K-SADS	25/29 / 21/28	CBT = AP
Wood et al, 1996 [56]	9–17	Outpatient clinic	CBT / AP	DTP	8 / 8	25 / 27	K-SADS	13/24 / 5/24	CBT > AP
Brent et al, 1997 [52]	13–18	Outpatient & adverts	CBT / NST	From Beck	14 / 14	37 / 35	K-SADS	21/35 / 12/33	SBFT > NST
Lewinsohn et al, 1996 [78]	13–19	Community	CBT / NT	CWDC	14 / 8	Not known	K-SADS	24/37 / 13/27	CBT = NT

AP = attention placebo; CBT = cognitive-behaviour therapy; CR = clinician rating based on an interview and several depression questionnaires; CWDC = Coping With Depression Course; DTP = Depression Treatment Programme; K-SADS = Kiddie Schedule for Affective Disorders and Schizophrenia; NT = no treatment; NST = non-directive supportive treatment; SBFT = systemic behavioural family therapy.

a separate non-randomized study, the same research group found that the relapse rate was much lower when subjects continued in cognitive therapy for 6 months after remission [64].

In conclusion, there have been more randomized trials of CBT in childhood depression than any other psychological treatment. The outcome evidence makes CBT one of the most promising treatments for both community and outpatient samples. Another advantage is the availability of training manuals for professional therapists [46, 65], which should make it easier to learn the approach. However, formal training in CBT with children is not available in many centres.

Extant research on CBT also has several limitations. First, it is based on samples with mild or moderately severe depression. CBT may not be effective in severely depressed children. Second, much of the published research has compared CBT with inactive conditions such as remaining on a waiting list or psychological placebo. The high rate of spontaneous remission in childhood depression [32] means that it is important to demonstrate that CBT is better than no treatment. Third, we also need to know how CBT compares with other recognized forms of intervention, such as medication. Fourth, it is unclear whether cognitive or behavioural processes correlate with a better outcome. The therapeutic basis for change is therefore uncertain. Finally, it is not known whether CBT has lasting benefits for depressed children. The available evidence suggests that to avoid relapse it may be necessary for some cases to have ongoing treatment or booster sessions. Such sessions are now part of many treatment programmes. Even so, CBT is a highly promising treatment whose efficacy has been demonstrated in several independent studies.

Interpersonal Psychotherapy

Interpersonal psychotherapy (IPT) is based on the premise that depression occurs in the context of interpersonal relationships. It derives from a number of theoretical and empirical sources [66], the most prominent theoretical source being the work of Adolf Meyer [67], whose psychobiological approach to understanding psychiatric disorders emphasized the importance of the environment. The empirical basis for treating childhood depression with IPT comes from research showing a strong association between depression and problems with relationships [68]. Whilst IPT develops from an interpersonal view of depression, it does not assume that interpersonal problems cause depression. The interpersonal context can contribute to the alleviation of the child's depressive symptoms, regardless of the personality organization or biological vulnerability of the individual [69].

IPT is a brief time-limited therapy. The two main goals are to identify and treat, first, the depressive symptoms and second, the problems associated with the onset of depression.

Several trials have evaluated IPT in depressed adults [66]. Moreau, Mufson *et al* [69, 70] modified the therapy for use with depressed adolescents. IPT for adolescents works on five main problem areas. Four of these come from the use of IPT with depressed adults — grief, interpersonal role disputes, role transitions and interpersonal deficits. The fifth area, single-parent families, was added because of its frequent occurrence and the difficulties it creates for the adolescent. The emphasis in therapy is on dealing with current difficulties rather than on problems in the past. Treatment techniques include identifying targets, clarifying roles, and modifying patterns of communication.

There are as yet no published randomized controlled trials of IPT for depressed children, though two are currently underway [59, 71]. However, there is evidence that IPT is effective in the acute phase of depression in adults [72]. Moreover, preliminary data suggest that IPT is both feasible and associated with improvement in adolescents with major depression [73].

Interpersonal psychotherapy is a promising but as yet untested treatment for depression in young people. Its promise stems both from the evidence that it is an effective treatment for depression in adults and from its underlying rationale.

FAMILY THERAPY

There has been a large amount of research on the families of depressed children. There is now strong evidence of an association between depression in children and problems of family members, including mental illness and dysfunctional family relationships [22, 25, 74]. This association is likely to reflect environmental mechanisms as well as genetic processes [21]. Family factors associated with the onset and course of juvenile depressive disorder include high parental criticism [75], family discord [76] and poor communication between parents and child [25].

There are widely differing definitions of the activity of family therapy, but most therapies have the following features in common [77]. First, they typically involve face-to-face work with more than one family member. Second, therapeutic work focuses on altering the interactions among family members. Third, practitioners think of improvement at two levels — that of the presenting problem and that of the relationship patterns associated with the problem.

Two kinds of work have been undertaken with the families of depressed children. The first, exemplified by the research of Lewinsohn, Clarke *et al* [51, 53], consists of parental attendance at a course run in parallel with the child's treatment [78]. The aim of this course is to help parents promote the adolescent's learning of new skills. Parents also learn problem-solving and communication skills. Adolescents and parents practise these skills in joint sessions.

The second approach involves conjoint family work. In this approach the primary focus is usually within the treatment sessions, which aim directly to change family communication patterns and methods of solving problems. The therapist may also help the family to see depression from the relational function it may have within the family.

There have been at least four randomized controlled trials of family therapy in childhood depression. Two included cases with major depression [7, 52] and involved a family intervention only. Two examined the value of parental sessions given in parallel with CBT to children diagnosed with either major depression or dysthymic disorder [51, 53].

Table 4.3 presents the findings, expressed as remission from depressive disorder, and shows that the results have so far been negative. Neither of the studies of a parallel parental course have found that this significantly augments individual therapy.

On present evidence it would be premature, however, to conclude that family therapy is ineffective in childhood depression. With only four trials completed as yet, it could be that significant benefits will emerge in future studies. The association between childhood depression and family dysfunction is so strong that further studies of family interventions are certainly indicated. However, until there is a firmer empirical basis for family therapy, other interventions will be the treatment of choice.

PSYCHOSOCIAL PREVENTION OF CHILDHOOD DEPRESSION

There is a strong theoretical case for preventing depression in childhood. Although the evidence reviewed earlier suggests that some effective psychological treatments are available, many children fail to respond (Table 4.2). Moreover, only a minority of depressed children ever come for help [41].

It is customary to distinguish between two types of primary preventive strategy: universal and targeted programmes. Universal programmes involve all individuals in a population regardless of their level of risk. Typically, such programmes involve either attempts to change levels of depression directly [79] or efforts to develop strengths that might protect against depression [80]. These programmes have usually consisted of educational sessions and cognitive-behavioural techniques, particularly techniques to develop social skills.

Targeted programmes aim to prevent depression in a population known to be at risk. The best established risk factors for depressive disorder in childhood are depressive symptoms and a family history of depression [81]. Interventions for children with depressive symptoms are similar to those described earlier. Family interventions typically involve an educational

TABLE 4.3 Randomized comparative studies of family interventions in samples diagnosed with depressive disorder

Study	Age (years)	Sample	Cell	Family intervention	Sessions (no.)	Subjects randomized (no.)	Outcome measure	Subjects remitted (no.)	Results
Lewinsohn et al, 1990 [53]	14–18	Adverts & clinics	CBT CBT-P	Parental course in parallel with CBT	14 14 + 14	24 21	K-SADS	9/21 9/19	CBT-P = CBT
Brent et al, 1997 [52]	13–18	Outpatient & adverts	SBFT NST	Functional therapy and problem-solving	14 14	35 35	K-SADS	9/31 12/33	SBFT = NST
Clarke et al, 1997 [51]	13–19	Community	CBT CBT-P	Parental course in parallel with CBT	14 14 + 14	Not known	K-SADS	24/37 22/32	CBT-P = CBT
Harrington et al, 1998 [7]	11–16	Clinical, DSP[a]	FPS RC		5 3	56 53	K-SADS	28/51 36/51	FPS = RC

[a]The numbers shown here are based on the subsample with major depression.
CBT = cognitive-behaviour therapy; CBT-P = cognitive-behaviour therapy with parental sessions; DSP = deliberate self-poisoning; FPS = family problem-solving; K-SADS = Kiddie Schedule for Affective Disorders and Schizophrenia; NST = non-directive supportive treatment; RC = routine care; SBFT = systemic behavioural family therapy.

programme about depression plus elements that target some of the problems that are common in families with a depressed parent, such as poor intrafamilial communication [82].

Clarke et al [79] have conducted two randomized trials of universal interventions designed to reduce depressive symptoms in the general population of children. Neither has shown significant benefits. However, the three published trials of interventions in high-risk groups have produced promising findings. King and Kirschenbaum [80] studied primary school children with a high score on a screening questionnaire. They found that a programme of social skills training and consultation with parents and teachers was significantly better than consultation alone in reducing depressive symptoms. In a study of bereaved families, Sandler et al [83] found that a programme of help for the whole family reduced depressive symptoms in the child.

Research has also examined the efficacy of CBT in preventing depressive disorder. Clarke et al [84] randomly allocated schoolchildren with a high score on a depression questionnaire to CBT or to no treatment. The CBT group had a significantly reduced risk of depressive disorder during the next year.

Two studies not included in Table 4.4 also require some comment. Jaycox et al [85] conducted a non-randomized study that compared CBT with no treatment in children identified as at high risk because of depressive symptoms and their reports of parental conflict. CBT was associated with a significant reduction in depressive symptoms and with improved behaviour in the classroom. Beardslee et al [82, 86] conducted a randomized trial with families in which at least one parent had an affective disorder. They compared a clinician-facilitated educational preventive programme with a lecture group. No data are yet available on rates of depressive disorders in the offspring, but early findings indicate that there are useful changes in the family's knowledge about depression and in intrafamilial communication.

Research on the prevention of depression in children is necessarily at an early stage. The preliminary evidence suggests that universal programmes that aim to reduce depression across the whole population may not be effective. Universal programmes have a number of advantages over targeted interventions [87] but it may be better for such programmes to concentrate on increasing factors that could protect against depression rather than trying to reduce depression itself [79].

Several studies have suggested that interventions targeted at high-risk groups may be effective in reducing the risk of depression. A strength of these studies is that preventive programmes have huge potential to reduce the burden of suffering arising from depression. A challenge for targeted approaches is to increase the proportion of individuals who are willing to take part. The uptake of psychological treatments offered to individuals

TABLE 4.4 Randomized studies of interventions to prevent depression in children

Study	Age (years)	Sample	Cell	Uptake (%)	Follow-up	Subjects randomized (no.)	Subjects evaluated (no.)	Outcome	Results
Clarke et al, 1993 [79]	14–15	School: all students	EI AP	"All students"	12 weeks	567 (both groups)	279 234	CES-D	EI = AP
Clarke et al, 1993 [79]	14–15	School: all students	BST AP	"All students"	12 weeks	190 190	151 149	CES-D	BST = AP
King and Kirschenbaum, 1990 [80]	8	School: high score on AML	FS PS	73%	Unclear	36 42	21 25	CDRS-R	FS > PS
Sandler et al, 1992 [83]	7–17	Bereaved families	FBP NT	52%	None	35 37	24 31	CAS	FBP > NT
Clarke et al, 1995 [84]	Mean = 15	School: high score on CES-D	CBT NT	36%	1 year	76 74	55 71	K-SADS	CBT > NT

AP = attention placebo; AML = Activity Mood screening questionnaire; BST = behavioural skills training; CAS = Child Assessment Schedule; CBT = cognitive-behaviour therapy; CES-D = Centre for Epidemiological Studies Depression Scale; EI = educational intervention; FBP = family bereavement programme; FS = full service — social skills groups & consultation; K-SADS = Kiddie Schedule for Affective Disorders and Schizophrenia; NT = no treatment; PS = partial service — consultation only.

identified as at risk because of a high score on a screening questionnaire has often been low (Tables 4.1 and 4.4). Future studies must also pay greater attention to the possible harmful effects that might result from targeting at-risk children for treatment [88].

PHARMACOLOGICAL TREATMENTS

Theoretical Basis

Three types of investigations have provided information on possible neuro-biological abnormalities in depressed young people. The first is the study of cortisol secretion, measured by investigations such as the DST. Several studies have shown that, in comparison with non-depressed patients, depressed young people are less likely to show suppression of cortisol secretion when the exogenous corticosteroid dexamethasone is administered [11]. The specificity of the DST for depressive disorder is, however, less for young people than it is for adults [89]. The second investigation is the study of sleep. Polysomnographic (PSG) studies of depressed adults have found that they tend to show abnormalities of sleep, including shortened rapid eye movement (REM) latency (time from the start of sleep to the first period of REM sleep) and reduced slow wave sleep [90]. Many PSG studies with depressed adolescents have shown sleep abnormalities, mainly of REM sleep [91–96]. These generally positive results contrast with the mainly negative results with children, in whom, with one or two exceptions [e.g. 93] studies comparing depressed cases with controls have shown few differences [97–99].

The third type of biologically informative investigation has been the study of growth hormone (GH) secretion. A variety of pharmacological challenge agents that stimulate release of GH have been studied in depressed adults. The idea has been to investigate the activity of certain neuronal pathways, particularly the monoamine pathways, as these are thought to be implicated in the aetiology of depression. Studies of adults with major depression have tended to show blunted GH response to provocative stimuli [100], which has also been demonstrated in prepubertal children both during major depression [101–103] and after recovery [104]. Interestingly, however, the results with adolescents have been negative. Though some studies have reported high levels of GH in adolescents with major depression [105], GH provocation studies with depressed adolescents [101, 105–107] have not found the blunting of GH response that has been reported in prepubertal children.

In interpreting these findings it should be noted that many of these biological investigations may be influenced by factors other than depression. For example, weight loss can lead to a positive DST [108]. Antidepressants can cause blunting of GH response in provocation tests, even if they are stopped months before the test [12]. Moreover, much biological research in this age group has relied on normal control groups rather than groups with non-depressive psychiatric disorder, so it is unclear whether the results are specific to depression or would also be found in other child psychiatric disorders. All in all, however, the results of biological investigations suggest that adolescents with depressive conditions resemble depressed adults in their sleep patterns and in their response to the DST. But the results with depressed prepubertal children have been less consistent.

Tricyclic Antidepressants

Most of the research on pharmacotherapy has been with the tricyclic antidepressants (TCAs), especially imipramine and nortriptyline. The results from early open trials were encouraging, with several studies reporting that TCAs were associated with high response rates [109, 110]. However, as indicates, with one exception [111], none of the controlled double-blind trials have found any significant differences between oral TCAs and placebo [112–121].

There are several possible reasons for the apparent failure of the oral TCA studies [122]. First, it is difficult to do randomized drug trials in this age group. Consent must in practice be obtained from two people, and many parents are reluctant to allow their children into a study in which one of the treatments is medication. This may be especially difficult in studies involving TCAs, where regular monitoring of cardiac function is required. Second, some TCA studies have been based on very severe cases of depression in inpatient samples. Indeed, the pooled response rate across the TCA trials in both children and adolescents is only around one third [123], much less than in studies with adults. Third, it is likely that juvenile depressive disorders are heterogeneous. Drug effects may only be apparent in certain subgroups and TCA trials have generally been too small to permit meaningful subgroup analysis. It could be that there is a small effect of medication that would have been detected in larger trials. Fourth, there may be developmental variations in the metabolism of TCAs, such as their rate of elimination from the body [124], which make it hard to get the dosage right. Fifth, it has been suggested that young people differ from adults both in the relative balance of the cerebral neurotransmitters on which TCAs are thought to act [125] and in the hormonal milieu of the brain [126]. Finally, some of the studies have had methodological problems [123]. The sample size in many of them has been small and interim analyses were conducted in some.

In summary, the evidence thus far does not support the efficacy of the TCAs in child or adolescent depression. This finding, together with the evidence about their potential toxicity [127], makes them second line treatments.

TABLE 4.5 Randomized, double-blind, placebo-controlled studies of tricyclic antidepressants for child and adolescent depression

Study	Age (years)	Treatment	TCA dose	TCA treatment duration (weeks)	Subjects randomized (no.)	Subjects evaluated (no.)	Outcome measure	Results
Kramer and Feiguine, 1981 [112]	13–17	Amitriptyline Placebo	Maximum 200mg/day	6	10 10	10 10	DACL	TCA = placebo
Petti and Law, 1982 [113]	6–12	Imipramine Placebo	5mg/kg/day	6	3 3	3 3	BID	TCA = placebo
Kashani et al, 1984 [114]	Mean = 10.8	Amitriptyline Placebo	1.5mg/kg/day	4 each	9; crossover design	9; crossover design	BID	TCA = placebo
Preskorn et al, 1987 [111]	6–12	Imipramine Placebo	Maximum 5mg/kg/day	6	10 12	Not known	CDRS	TCA > placebo
Puig-Antich et al, 1987 [115]	Mean = 9	Imipramine Placebo	Maximum 5mg/kg/day	5	16 22	16 22	K-SADS	TCA = placebo
Geller et al, 1989 [116]	6–12	Nortriptyline Placebo	"Fixed" plasma levels	8	60 (both groups)	26 24	K-SADS	TCA = placebo
Hughes et al, 1990 [117]	6–12	Imipramine Placebo	ND	6	31 (both groups)	13 14	DICA	TCA = placebo
Geller et al, 1990 [118]	12–17	Nortriptyline Placebo	"Fixed" plasma levels	8	35 (both groups)	12 19	K-SADS	TCA = placebo
Kutcher et al, 1994 [119]	15–19	Desipramine Placebo	200mg/day	6	30 30	18 dropped out	HAM-D	TCA = placebo
Kye et al, 1996 [120]	12–17	Amitriptyline Placebo	5mg/kg/day	8	18 13	12 10	K-SADS	TCA = placebo
Birmaher et al, 1998 [121]	12–18	Amitriptyline Placebo	5mg/kg/day	10	13 14	13 14	HAM-D	TCA = placebo

BID = Bellevue Index of Depression; CDRS = Children's Depression Rating Scale; DACL = Depression Adjective Checklist; DICA = Diagnostic Interview Schedule for Adolescents; HAM-D = Hamilton Depression Rating Scale; K-SADS = Kiddie Schedule for Affective Disorders and Schizophrenia, ND = No data; TCA = Tricyclic antidepressant

Other Antidepressants

A recent report suggests that the selective serotonin reuptake inhibitor (SSRI) fluoxetine may be of benefit to children and adolescents with major depression [93]. It is too early to say whether this finding is robust — a small previous trial with fluoxetine produced a negative result [128]. Nevertheless, it clearly raises the possibility that young people may be more responsive to antidepressants than previously thought. The study by Emslie *et al* [93] did not find that children responded differently from adolescents. Negative results have been reported in a trial with venlafaxine [129].

DEVELOPING A TREATMENT STRATEGY

Table 4.6 shows the steps in the management of moderately severe depressive disorder in adolescents which are discussed below. Adolescents with severe depression, which we define as a Global Assessment Scale [130] score of 30 or less (which means that the adolescent is unable to function in most activities of daily life) seldom respond to CBT alone [61].

Step 1. In clinical samples, mild and moderately severe depressive disorders in adolescents remit rapidly in around a third of cases [81, 131].
Step 2. This suggests that a sensible initial approach should consist of a thorough assessment, sympathetic discussions with the adolescent and the family, and encouraging support. These simple interventions, especially if combined with measures to alleviate stress, are often followed by improvement in mood.
Step 3. However, about two thirds of depressed adolescents will not remit within a month, and these cases should be offered further treatment.
Step 4. The best treatment for major depression in adolescence is not yet clearly established. Fluoxetine is probably cheaper than CBT and appears to

TABLE 4.6   Steps in the management of moderately severe depression in adolescents

Step 1.	Assessment: how severe is the depression?
Step 2.	Mild or moderate depression may respond to support and simple measures to reduce stress.
Step 3.	Reassess after 2–3 weeks.
Step 4.	If no response, start CBT.
Step 5.	Reassess after 6–8 weeks.
Step 6.	Those who are doing well with CBT should continue. Those who are partially responding may benefit from augmentation with another treatment such as fluoxetine. Failure to respond should trigger a review of reasons for treatment resistance.
Step 7.	Subjects who still fail to respond may benefit from other treatments.

CBT = cognitive-behavioural therapy.

have fewer side effects than TCAs [132]. However, its benefits have not yet been established in multiple trials. This suggests that, if it is available, CBT is probably the first choice treatment.

Step 5. A meta-analysis [57] of CBT studies found that around a third of clinically depressed adolescents had not improved by the end of the CBT course. Therefore, patients should be reassessed after about 6–8 weeks to determine whether there has been a response or not.

Step 6. By this stage, there are likely to be two groups who still need help: those who have failed to respond or are getting worse, and those who have partially improved but are still symptomatic. If an adolescent is resistant to the effects of CBT, then the reasons for this should be reviewed. It may be that other problems besides depression are present. Common causes of treatment resistance include undiagnosed psychosocial stressors such as abuse, chronic family difficulties, and emerging personality problems. Less common but important causes are undiagnosed physical disorders, such as endocrine disturbances and drug abuse. Review may also indicate some specific reasons for the failure of CBT. For example, CBT is less effective when given by an inexperienced therapist who tells the adolescent what to do rather than giving the patient the opportunity to work it out on his or her own.

Step 7. If the review does not show a simple way of improving the adolescent's mental state, then a different line of treatment should be pursued. In some instances, this means starting an antidepressant, such as an SSRI. In other cases it may be necessary to provide treatments such as family therapy.

SUMMARY

Consistent Evidence

There is now consistent evidence that depressive disorders in young people are associated with significant impairment, such as poor peer relationships and impaired academic performance. Moreover, there is a high risk of relapse, which may extend into adult life. Depression in young people is not, then, "normal" or something that children will naturally grow out of. It can be a serious disorder that requires psychiatric treatment.

There are a large number of potential treatments for childhood depression. Unfortunately, little outcome evidence exists for most of them. This review highlighted the five that have been most researched: CBT, family therapy, IPT, TCAs and SSRIs. All of these treatments are based on theories about the mechanisms of childhood depression that have led to testable hypotheses.

CBT has been evaluated in several trials, and there is now consistent evidence that it is an effective treatment both for depressive symptoms and for mild depressive disorders.

There is also consistent evidence that TCAs are not effective. Of course, many of the TCA trials conducted thus far have been too small. Nevertheless, given the side effects of these drugs, there is no justification for considering TCAs as a first line treatment.

Incomplete Evidence

The results of a systematic and relatively large trial of fluoxetine [133] have produced evidence that it may be effective in reducing depression. However, given the failure of the TCA trials, replication is needed. Interpersonal psychotherapy is a promising but also relatively untested treatment. It is unclear whether any intervention, psychological or pharmacological, reduces the relapse risk.

Areas Still Open to Research

Future research must address many unresolved issues. Perhaps the most pressing need is for more trials of the main psychological treatment alternatives to CBT, such as IPT and family therapy. CBT also requires further evaluation in clinical samples. A key question for future research is how CBT compares with other treatments, such as antidepressant medication. These studies will need to measure costs as well as effectiveness. More trials of antidepressant medications such as fluoxetine and paroxetine are required.

Future studies also need to tackle some of the problems of the published trials. Randomization was poorly described in both pharmacological and psychological studies. The methods used to allocate subjects were unclear and very few studies described who conducted the randomization. Few trials stated how the final sample size was reached or what the rules were for stopping the study and analysing the data. This last point is important because it is quite common in this literature to find reports of interim analyses from ongoing trials. For instance, a recent summary of psychosocial treatment research on children, funded by the National Institute of Mental Health [134], contained three such reports. Frequent analysis of data can lead to both false positive and false negative results [135]. Few studies provided evidence for successful blinding of outcome assessors.

Another limitation is that in the majority of the studies conducted so far depression has been the main focus of outcome assessment. There has been neglect of other domains, such as comorbid disorders, academic performance and social impairment, despite the evidence of a strong association between childhood depression and problems in all of these areas [34]. Moreover, follow-up intervals have seldom exceeded a year. Yet we know that childhood depression, like depression in adult life, is a recurrent problem. Treatments that do not seem to work in the short term may be effective in the long term [136].

In conclusion, significant issues need to be addressed to advance research in this field. We cannot yet say that any intervention alters the long-term prognosis of childhood depression. However, some promising treatments exist for management of the acute episode.

ACKNOWLEDGEMENTS

The MacArthur Foundation Research Network on Psychopathology and Development and the North West Regional Health Authority supported this work. Portions of this article are based on a review in the *British Journal of Psychiatry* and the author is grateful for permission to reproduce them here.

REFERENCES

1. Angold A., Costello E.J., Worthman C.M. (1998) Puberty and depression: the roles of age, pubertal status and pubertal timing. *Psychol. Med.*, **28**: 51–61.
2. Kolvin I., Barrett M.L., Bhate S.R., Berney T.P., Famuyiwa O.O., Fundudis T., Tyrer S. (1991) The Newcastle Child Depression Project: diagnosis and classification of depression. *Br. J. Psychiatry*, **159** (Suppl. 11): 9–21.
3. Fombonne E. (1995) Depressive disorders: time trends and putative explanatory mechanisms. In *Psychosocial Disorders in Young People: Time Trends and Their Origins* (Eds M. Rutter, D. Smith), pp. 544–615, Wiley, Chichester.
4. Rutter M., Graham P., Chadwick O.F., Yule W. (1976) Adolescent turmoil: fact or fiction? *J. Child Psychol. Psychiatry*, **17**: 35–56.
5. Kovacs M. (1986) A developmental perspective on methods and measures in the assessment of depressive disorders: the clinical interview. In *Depression in Young People: Developmental and Clinical Perspectives* (Eds M. Rutter, C.E. Izard, R.B. Read), pp. 435–465, Guilford, New York.
6. American Psychiatric Association (1994) *Diagnostic and Statistical Manual of Mental Disorders*, 4th edn, American Psychiatric Association, Washington, DC.
7. Harrington R.C., Kerfoot M., Dyer E., McNiven F., Gill J., Harrington V., Woodham A., Byford S. (1998) Randomized trial of a home based family intervention for children who have deliberately poisoned themselves. *J. Am. Acad. Child Adolesc. Psychiatry*, **37**: 512–518.
8. Harrington R.C., Shariff A. (1992) Choosing an instrument to assess depression in young people. *Newsletter Assoc. Child Psychol. Psychiatry*, **14**: 279–282.
9. Clark A., Harrington R. (1999) On diagnosing rare disorders rarely: appropriate use of screening instruments. *J. Child Psychol. Psychiatry*, **40**: 287–290.
10. Harrington R.C. (1994) Affective disorders. In *Child and Adolescent Psychiatry: Modern Approaches*, 3rd edn (Eds M. Rutter, E. Taylor, L. Hersov), pp. 330–350, Blackwell Scientific, Oxford.
11. Casat C.D., Powell K. (1988) The dexamethasone suppression test in children and adolescents with major depressive disorder: a review. *J. Clin. Psychiatry*, **49**: 390–393.

12. Cowen P.J., Wood A.J. (1991) Biological markers of depression. *Psychol. Med.*, **21**: 831–836.
13. Harrington R.C., Fudge H., Rutter M., Pickles A., Hill J. (1990) Adult outcomes of childhood and adolescent depression: I. Psychiatric status. *Arch. Gen. Psychiatry*, **47**: 465–473.
14. Harrington R.C., Fudge H., Rutter M., Pickles A., Hill J. (1991) Adult outcomes of childhood and adolescent depression: II. Risk for antisocial disorders. *J. Am. Acad. Child Adolesc. Psychiatry*, **30**: 434–439.
15. Brady E.U., Kendall P.C. (1992) Comorbidity of anxiety and depression in children and adolescents. *Psychol. Bull.*, **111**: 244–255.
16. Goodyer I.M., Altham P.M.E. (1991) Lifetime exit events and recent social and family adversities in anxious and depressed school-age children and adolescents — I. *J. Affect. Disord.*, **21**: 219–228.
17. Garmezy N., Masten A.S. (1994) Chronic adversities. In *Child and Adolescent Psychiatry: Modern Approaches*, 3rd edn (Eds M. Rutter, E. Taylor, L. Hersov), pp. 191–208, Blackwell Scientific, Oxford.
18. Kendler K.S., Kessler R.C., Walters E.E., MacLean C., Neale M.C., Heath A.C., Eaves L.J. (1995) Stressful life events, genetic liability, and onset of an episode of major depression in women. *Am. J. Psychiatry*, **152**: 833–842.
19. Strober M. (1992) Relevance of early age-of-onset in genetic studies of bipolar affective disorder. *J. Am. Acad. Child Adolesc. Psychiatry*, **31**: 606–610.
20. Radke-Yarrow M., Nottelmann E., Martinez P., Fox M.B., Belmont B. (1992) Young children of affectively ill parents: a longitudinal study of psychosocial development. *J. Am. Acad. Child Adolesc. Psychiatry*, **31**: 68–77.
21. Harrington R.C. (1996) Family-genetic findings in child and adolescent depressive disorders. *Int. Rev. Psychiatry*, **8**: 355–368.
22. Harrington R.C., Fudge H., Rutter M., Bredenkamp D., Groothues C., Pridham J. (1993) Child and adult depression: a test of continuities with data from a family study. *Br. J. Psychiatry*, **162**: 627–633.
23. Asarnow J.R., Goldstein M.J., Carlson G.A., Perdue S., Bates S., Keller J. (1988) Childhood-onset depressive disorders. A follow-up study of rates of rehospitalization and out-of-home placement among child psychiatric inpatients. *J. Affect. Disord.*, **15**: 245–253.
24. Goodyer I.M., Wright C., Altham P.M.E. (1989) Recent friendships in anxious and depressed school-age children. *Psychol. Med.*, **19**: 165–174.
25. Hammen C. (1991) *Depression Runs in Families. The Social Context of Risk and Resilience in Children of Depressed Mothers*, Springer-Verlag, New York.
26. Harrington R.C., Wood A., Verduyn C. (1998) Clinically depressed adolescents. In *Cognitive Behaviour Therapy for Children and Families* (Ed. P. Graham), pp. 156–193, Cambridge University Press, Cambridge.
27. Yaylayan S., Weller E.B., Weller R.A. (1992) Neurobiology of depression. In *Clinical Guide to Depression in Children and Adolescents* (Eds M. Shafii, S.L. Shafii), pp. 65–88, American Psychiatric Press, Washington, DC.
28. Kovacs M., Feinberg T.L., Crouse-Novak M., Paulauskas S.L., Pollock M., Finkelstein R. (1984) Depressive disorders in childhood. II. A longitudinal study of the risk for a subsequent major depression. *Arch. Gen. Psychiatry*, **41**: 643–649.
29. Rao U., Weissman M.M., Martin J.A., Hammond R.W. (1993) Childhood depression and risk of suicide: preliminary report of a longitudinal study. *J. Am. Acad. Child Adolesc. Psychiatry*, **32**: 21–27.

30. Hammen C., Burge D., Adrian C. (1991) Timing of mother and child depression in a longitudinal study of children at risk. *J. Consult. Clin. Psychol.*, **59**: 341–345.
31. Kovacs M., Feinberg T.L., Crouse-Novak M.A., Paulauskas S.L., Finkelstein R. (1984) Depressive disorders in childhood. I. A longitudinal prospective study of characteristics and recovery. *Arch. Gen. Psychiatry*, **41**: 229–237.
32. Keller M.B., Beardslee W., Lavori P.W., Wunder J., Dors D.L., Samuelson H. (1988) Course of major depression in non-referred adolescents: a retrospective study. *J. Affect. Disord.*, **15**: 235–243.
33. Strober M., Lampert C., Schmidt S., Morrell W. (1993) The course of major depressive disorder in adolescents: I. Recovery and risk of manic switching in a 24-month prospective, naturalistic follow-up of psychotic and nonpsychotic subtypes. *J. Am. Acad. Child Adolesc. Psychiatry*, **32**: 34–42.
34. Harrington R.C. (1993) *Depressive Disorder in Childhood and Adolescence*, Wiley, Chichester.
35. Kazdin A.E. (1997) Practitioner review: psychosocial treatments for conduct disorder in children. *J. Child Psychol. Psychiatry*, **38**: 161–178.
36. Kendall P.C., Stark K.D., Adam T. (1990) Cognitive deficit or cognitive distortion in childhood depression. *J. Abnorm. Child Psychol.*, **18**: 255–270.
37. McCauley E., Mitchell J.R., Burke P., Moss S. (1988) Cognitive attributes of depression in children and adolescents. *J. Consult. Clin. Psychol.*, **56**: 903–908.
38. Kaslow N.J., Rehm L.P., Pollack S.L., Siegel A.W. (1988) Attributional style and self-control behavior in depressed and nondepressed children and their parents. *J. Abnorm. Child Psychol.*, **16**: 163–175.
39. Curry J.F., Craighead W.E. (1990) Attributional style in clinically depressed and conduct disordered adolescents. *J. Consult. Clin. Psychol.*, **58**: 109–116.
40. Cole D.A. (1990) Relation of social and academic competence to depressive symptoms in childhood. *J. Abnorm. Psychol.*, **99**: 422–429.
41. Cooper P.J., Goodyer I. (1993) A community study of depression in adolescent girls: I—Estimates of symptom and syndrome prevalence. *Br. J. Psychiatry*, **163**: 369–374.
42. Reynolds W.M., Coats K.I. (1986) A comparison of cognitive-behavioural therapy and relaxation training for the treatment of depression in adolescents. *J. Consult. Clin. Psychol.*, **54**: 653–660.
43. Stark K.D., Reynolds W.M., Kaslow N. (1987) A comparison of the relative efficacy of self-control therapy and a behavioral problem-solving therapy for depression in children. *J. Abnorm. Child Psychol.*, **15**: 91–113.
44. Butler L., Meizitis S., Friedman R., Cole E. (1980) The effect of two school-based intervention programs on depressive symptoms in pre-adolescents. *Am. Educ. Res. J.*, **17**: 111–119.
45. Liddle B., Spence S.H. (1990) Cognitive-behaviour therapy with depressed primary school children: a cautionary note. *Behav. Psychotherapy*, **18**: 85–102.
46. Stark K.D. (1990) *Childhood Depression: School-based Intervention*, Guilford, New York.
47. Kahn J.S., Kehle T.J., Jenson W.R., Clark E. (1990) Comparison of cognitive-behavioral, relaxation, and self-modeling interventions for depression among middle-school students. *School Psychol. Rev.*, **2**: 196–211.
48. Marcotte D., Baron P. (1993) L'efficacité d'une stratégie d'intervention emotivo-rationnelle auprès d'adolescents dépressifs du milieu scolaire. *Can. J. Counselling*, **27**: 77–92.
49. Rehm L.P., Sharp R.N. (1996) Strategies for childhood depression. In *Cognitive Therapy with Children and Adolescents: A Casebook for Clinical Practice* (Eds

M.A. Reineke, F.M. Dattilio, A. Freeman), pp. 103–123, Guilford Press, New York.

50. Weisz J.R., Thurber C.A., Sweeney L., Proffitt V.D., LeGagnoux G.L. (1997) Brief treatment of mild-to-moderate child depression using primary and secondary control enhancement training. *J. Consult. Clin. Psychol.*, **65**: 703–707.

51. Clarke G.N., Lewinsohn P., Seeley J. (1997) The second Oregon cognitive-behaviour therapy study with depressive disorder in adolescents. Personal communication.

52. Brent D., Holder D., Kolko D., Birmaher B., Baugher M., Roth C., Iyengar S., Johnson B. (1997) A clinical psychotherapy trial for adolescent depression comparing cognitive, family, and supportive treatments. *Arch. Gen. Psychiatry*, **54**: 877–885.

53. Lewinsohn P.M., Clarke G.N., Hops H., Andrews J. (1990) Cognitive-behavioural treatment for depressed adolescents. *Behav. Ther.*, **21**: 385–401.

54. Reed M.K. (1994) Social skills training to reduce depression in adolescents. *Adolescence*, **29**: 293–302.

55. Vostanis P., Feehan C., Grattan E., Bickerton W. (1996) Treatment for children and adolescents with depression: lessons from a controlled trial. *Clin. Child Psychol. Psychiatry*, **1**: 199–212.

56. Wood A.J., Harrington R.C., Moore A. (1996) Controlled trial of a brief cognitive-behavioural intervention in adolescent patients with depressive disorders. *J. Child Psychol. Psychiatry*, **37**: 737–746.

57. Harrington R.C., Whittaker J., Shoebridge P., Campbell F. (1998) Systematic review of efficacy of cognitive behaviour therapies in child and adolescent depressive disorder. *Br. Med. J.*, **316**: 1559–1563.

58. Fine S., Forth A., Gilbert M., Haley G. (1991) Group therapy for adolescent depressive disorder: a comparison of social skills and therapeutic support. *J. Am. Acad. Child Adolesc. Psychiatry*, **30**: 79–75.

59. Rossello J., Bernal G. (1996) Adapting cognitive-behavioural and interpersonal treatments for depressed Puerto Rican adolescents. In *Psychosocial Treatments for Child and Adolescent Disorders: Empirically Based Strategies for Clinical Practice* (Eds E.D. Hibbs, P.S. Jensen), pp. 157–185, American Psychological Association, Washington, DC.

60. Brent D.A., Kolko D.J., Birmaher B., Baugher M., Bridge J. (1999) A clinical trial for adolescent depression: predictors of additional treatment in the acute and follow-up phases of the trial. *J. Am. Acad. Child Adolesc. Psychiatry*, **38**: 263–270.

61. Jayson D., Wood A.J., Kroll L., Fraser J., Harrington R.C. (1998) Which depressed patients respond to cognitive-behavioral treatment? *J. Am. Acad. Child Adolesc. Psychiatry*, **37**: 35–39.

62. Clarke G.N., Hops H., Lewinsohn P.M., Andrews J.A., Seeley J.R., Williams J.A. (1992) Cognitive-behavioral group treatment of adolescent depression: prediction of outcome. *Behav. Ther.*, **23**: 341–354.

63. Vostanis P., Feehan C., Grattan E., Bickerton W. (1996) A randomized controlled out-patient trial of cognitive-behavioural treatment for children and adolescents with depression: 9-month follow-up. *J. Affect. Disord.*, **40**: 105–116.

64. Kroll L., Harrington R.C., Gowers S., Frazer J., Jayson D. (1996) Continuation of cognitive-behavioural treatment in adolescent patients who have remitted from major depression. Feasibility and comparison with historical controls. *J. Am. Acad. Child Adolesc. Psychiatry*, **35**: 1156–1161.

65. Wilkes T.C.R., Belsher G., Rush A.J., Frank E. (1994), *Cognitive Therapy for Depressed Adolescents*, Guilford, New York.

66. Klerman G.L., Weissman M.M. (1992) Interpersonal psychotherapy. In *Handbook of Affective Disorders*, 2nd edn (Ed. E.S. Paykel), pp. 501–510, Churchill Livingstone, Edinburgh.

67. Meyer A. (1957) *Psychobiology: a Science of Man*, Thomas, Springfield, IL.

68. Goodyer I.M., Herbert J., Tamplin A., Secher S.M., Pearson J. (1997) Short-term outcome of major depression: II. Life events, family dysfunction, and friendship difficulties as predictors of persistent disorder. *J. Am. Acad. Child Adolesc. Psychiatry*, **36**: 474–480.

69. Moreau D., Mufson L., Weissman M.M., Klerman G.L. (1991) Interpersonal psychotherapy for adolescent depression: description of modification and preliminary application. *J. Am. Acad. Child Adolesc. Psychiatry*, **30**: 642–651.

70. Mufson L., Moreau D., Weissman M.M., Klerman G.L. (1993) *Interpersonal Psychotherapy for Depressed Adolescents*, Guilford, New York.

71. Mufson L., Moreau D., Weissman M.M. (1996) Focus on relationships: interpersonal psychotherapy for adolescent depression. In *Psychosocial Treatments for Child and Adolescent Disorders: Empirically Based Strategies for Clinical Practice* (Eds E.D. Hibbs, P.S. Jensen), pp. 137–155, American Psychological Association, Washington, DC.

72. Elkin I., Shea T., Watkins J.T., Imber S.D., Sotsky S.M., Collins J.F., Glass D.R., Pilkonis P.A., Leber W.R., Docherty J.P. *et al* (1989) National Institute of Mental Health Treatment of Depression Collaborative Research Program. General effectiveness of treatments. *Arch. Gen. Psychiatry*, **46**: 971–982.

73. Mufson L., Fairbanks J. (1996) Interpersonal psychotherapy for depressed adolescents: a one-year naturalistic follow-up study. *J. Am. Acad. Child Adolesc. Psychiatry*, **35**: 1145–1155.

74. Goodyer I.M., Cooper P.J., Vize C., Ashby L. (1993) Depression in 11 to 16 year old girls: the role of past parental psychopathology and exposure to recent life events. *J. Child Psychol. Psychiatry*, **34**: 1103–1115.

75. Asarnow J.R., Goldstein M.J., Tompson M., Guthrie D. (1993) One-year outcomes of depressive disorders in child psychiatric inpatients: evaluation of the prognostic power of a brief measure of expressed emotion. *J. Child Psychol. Psychiatry*, **34**: 129–137.

76. Harrington R.C., Rutter M., Weissman M., Fudge H., Groothues C., Bredenkamp D., Rende R., Pickles A., Wickramaratne P. (1997) Psychiatric disorders in the relatives of depressed probands. I. Comparison of prepubertal, adolescent and early adult onset forms. *J. Affect. Disord.* **42**: 9–22.

77. Gorell Barnes G. (1994) Family therapy. In *Child and Adolescent Psychiatry: Modern Approaches*, 3rd edn (Eds M. Rutter, E. Taylor, L. Hersov), pp. 946–965, Blackwell Scientific, Oxford.

78. Lewinsohn P.M., Clarke G.N., Rohde P., Hops H., Seeley J.R. (1996) A course in coping: a cognitive-behavioral approach to the treatment of adolescent depression. In *Psychosocial Treatments for Child and Adolescent Disorders. Empirically Based Strategies for Clinical Practice* (Eds E. Hibbs, P.S. Jensen), pp. 109–135, American Psychological Association, Washington, DC.

79. Clarke G.N., Hawkins W., Murphy M., Sheeber L. (1993) School-based primary prevention of depressive symptomatology in adolescents. Findings from two studies. *J. Adolesc. Res.*, **8**: 183–204.

80. King C.A., Kirschenbaum D.S. (1990) An experimental evaluation of a school-based program for children at risk: Wisconsin early intervention. *J. Comm. Psychol.*, **18**: 167–177.

81. Harrington R.C., Vostanis P. (1995) Longitudinal perspectives and affective disorder in children and adolescents. In *The Depressed Child and Adolescent. Developmental and Clinical Perspectives* (Ed. I.M. Goodyer), pp. 311–341, Cambridge University Press, Cambridge.

82. Beardslee W.R., Salt P., Porterfield K., Rothberg P.C., Velde P.v.D., Swatling S., Hoke L., Moilanen D.L., Wheelock I. (1993) Comparison of preventive interventions for families with parental affective disorder. *J. Am. Acad. Child Adolesc. Psychiatry*, **32**: 254–263.

83. Sandler I.N., West S.G., Baca L., Pillow D.R., Gersten J.C., Rogosch F., Virdin L., Beals J., Reynolds K.D., Kallgren C., *et al* (1992) Linking empirically based theory and evaluation: the family bereavement program. *Am. J. Comm. Psychol.*, **20**: 491–521.

84. Clarke G.N., Hawkins W., Murphy M., Sheeber L.B., Lewinsohn P.M., Seeley J.R. (1995) Targeted prevention of unipolar depressive disorder in an at-risk sample of high school adolescents: a randomized trial of a group cognitive intervention. *J. Am. Acad. Child Adolesc. Psychiatry*, **34**: 312–321.

85. Jaycox L.H., Reivich K.J., Gillham J., Seligman M.E.P. (1994) Prevention of depressive symptoms in school children. *Behav. Res. Ther.*, **32**: 801–816.

86. Beardslee W.R., Wright E., Rothberg P.C., Salt P., Versage E. (1996) Response of families to two preventive intervention strategies: long-term differences in behavior and attitude change. *J. Am. Acad. Child Adolesc. Psychiatry*, **35**: 774–782.

87. Graham P. (1994) Prevention. In *Child and Adolescent Psychiatry: Modern Approaches*, 3rd edn (Eds M. Rutter, E. Taylor, L. Hersov), pp. 815–828, Blackwell Scientific, Oxford.

88. Harrington R.C., Clark A. (1998) Prevention and early intervention for depression in adolescence and early adult life. *Eur. Arch. Psychiatry Clin. Neurosci.*, **248**: 32–45.

89. Ferguson H.B., Bawden H.N. (1988) Psychobiological measures. In *Assessment and Diagnosis in Child Psychopathology* (Eds M. Rutter, A.H. Tuma, I.S. Lann), pp. 232–263, Guilford, New York.

90. Benca R.M., Obermeyer W.H., Thisted R.A., Gillin J.C. (1992) Sleep and psychiatric disorders. A meta-analysis. *Arch. Gen. Psychiatry*, **49**: 651–668.

91. Appelboom-Fondu J., Kerkhofs M., Mendlewicz J. (1988) Depression in adolescents and young adults—polysomnographic and neuroendocrine aspects. *J. Affect. Disord.*, **14**: 35–40.

92. Cashman M.A., Coble P., McCann B.S., Taska L., Reynolds C.F., Kupfer D.J. (1986) Sleep markers for major depressive disorder in adolescent patients. *Sleep Res.*, **15**: 91.

93. Emslie G.J., Roffwarg H.P., Rush A.J., Weinberg W.A., Parkin-Feigenbaum L. (1987) Sleep EEG findings in depressed children and adolescents. *Am. J. Psychiatry*, **144**: 668–670.

94. Kutcher S., Williamson P., Marton P., Szalai J. (1992) REM latency in endogenously depressed adolescents. *Br. J. Psychiatry*, **161**: 399–402.

95. Lahmeyer H.W., Poznanski E.O., Bellur S.N. (1983) EEG sleep in depressed adolescents. *Am. J. Psychiatry*, **140**: 1150–1153.

96. Riemann D., Schmidt M.H. (1993) REM sleep distribution in adolescents with major depression and schizophrenia. *Sleep Res.*, **22**: 554.

97. Dahl R.E., Ryan N.D., Birmaher B., Al-Shabbout M., Williamson D.E., Neidig M., Nelson B., Puig-Antich J. (1991) Electroencephalographic sleep measures in prepubertal depression. *Psychiatry Res.*, **38**: 201–214.

98. Puig-Antich J., Goetz R., Hanlon C., Davies M., Thompson J., Chambers W.J., Tabrizi M.A., Weitzman E.D. (1982) Sleep architecture and REM sleep measures in prepubertal children with major depression during an episode. A controlled study. *Arch. Gen. Psychiatry*, **39**: 932–939.

99. Young W., Knowles J.B., MacLean A.W., Boag L., McConville B.J. (1982) The sleep of childhood depressives: comparison with age-matched controls. *Biol. Psychiatry*, **17**: 1163–1168.

100. Checkley S. (1992) Neuroendocrinology. In *Handbook of Affective Disorders*, 2nd edn (Ed. E.S. Paykel), pp. 255–266, Churchill Livingstone, Edinburgh.

101. Jensen J.B., Garfinkel B.D. (1990) Growth hormone dysregulation in children with major depressive disorder. *J. Am. Acad. Child Adolesc. Psychiatry*, **29**: 295–301.

102. Puig-Antich J., Goetz R., Davies M., Fein M., Hanlon C., Chambers W.J., Tabrizi M.A., Sachar E.J., Weitzman E.D. (1984) Growth hormone secretion in prepubertal major depressive children. II. Sleep related plasma concentration during a depressive episode. *Arch. Gen. Psychiatry*, **41**: 463–466.

103. Ryan N.D., Dahl R.E., Birmaher B., Williamson D.E., Iyengar S., Nelson B., Puig-Antich J., Perel J.M. (1994) Stimulatory tests of growth hormone secretion in prepubertal major depression: depressed versus normal children. *J. Am. Acad. Child Adolesc. Psychiatry*, **33**: 824–833.

104. Puig-Antich J., Novacenko H., Tabrizi M.A., Ambrosini P., Goetz R., Bianca J., Sachar E.J. (1984) Growth hormone secretion in prepubertal major depressive children. III. Response to insulin induced hypoglycemia in a drug-free, fully recovered clinical state. *Arch. Gen. Psychiatry*, **41**: 471–475.

105. Kutcher S., Malkin D., Silverberg J., Marton P., Williamson P., Malkin A., Szalai J., Katic M. (1991) Nocturnal cortisol, thyroid stimulating hormone, and growth hormone secretory profiles in depressed adolescents. *J. Am. Acad. Child Adolesc. Psychiatry*, **30**: 407–414.

106. Dahl R.E., Ryan N.D., Williamson D.E., Ambrosini P.J., Rabinovich H., Novacenko H., Nelson B., Puig-Antich J. (1992) Regulation of sleep and growth hormone in adolescent depression. *J. Am. Acad. Child Adolesc. Psychiatry*, **31**: 615–621.

107. Waterman G.S., Ryan N.D., Puig-Antich J., Meyer V., Ambosini P.J., Rabinovich H., Stull S., Novacenko H., Williamson D.E., Nelson B. (1991) Hormonal responses to dextroamphetamine in depressed and normal adolescents. *J. Am. Acad. Child Adolesc. Psychiatry*, **30**: 415–422.

108. Mullen P.E., Linsell C.R., Parker D. (1986) Influence of sleep disruption and calorie restriction on biological markers for depression. *Lancet*, **ii**: 1051–1055.

109. Weinberg W.A., Rutman J., Sullivan L., Penick E.C., Dietz S.G. (1973) Depression in children referred to an educational diagnostic centre: diagnosis and treatment. *J. Paediatrics*, **83**: 1065–1072.

110. Geller B., Cooper T., Chestnut E., Anker J.A., Schuchter M.D. (1986) Preliminary data on the relationship between nortriptyline plasma level and response in depressed children. *Am. J. Psychiatry*, **143**: 1283–1286.

111. Preskorn S.H., Weller E.B., Hughes C.W., Weller R.A., Bolte K. (1987) Depression in prepubertal children: dexamethasone nonsuppression predicts differential response to imipramine vs. placebo. *Psychopharmacol. Bull.*, **23**: 128–133.

112. Kramer A.D., Feiguine R.J. (1981) Clinical effects of amitriptyline in adolescent depression. *J. Am. Acad. Child Adolesc. Psychiatry*, **20**: 636–644.

113. Petti T.A., Law W. (1982) Imipramine treatment of depressed children: a double-blind pilot study. *J. Clin. Psychopharmacol.*, **2**: 107–110.

114. Kashani J.H., Shekim W.O., Reid J.C. (1984) Amitriptyline in children with major depressive disorder: a double-blind crossover pilot study. *J. Am. Acad. Child Adolesc. Psychiatry*, **23**: 348–351.

115. Puig-Antich J., Perel J.M., Lupatkin W., Chambers W.J., Tabrizi M.A., King J., Goetz R., Davies M., Stiller R. (1987) Imipramine in prepubertal major depressive disorders. *Arch. Gen. Psychiatry*, **44**: 81–89.

116. Geller B., Cooper T., McCombs H., Graham D., Wells J. (1989) Double-blind placebo-controlled study of nortriptyline in depressed children using a "fixed plasma level" design. *Psychopharmacol. Bull.*, **25**: 101–108.

117. Hughes C.W., Preskorn S.H., Weller E., Weller R., Hassanein R., Tucker S. (1990) The effect of concomitant disorders in childhood depression on predicting clinical response. *Psychopharmacol. Bull.*, **26**: 235–238.

118. Geller B., Cooper T.B., Graham D.L., Marsteller F.A., Bryant D.M. (1990) Double-blind placebo-controlled study of nortriptyline in depressed adolescents using a "fixed plasma level" design. *Psychopharmacol. Bull.*, **26**: 85–90.

119. Kutcher S., Boulos C., Ward B., Marton P., Simeon J., Ferguson H.B., Szalai J., Katic M., Roberts N., Dubois C., *et al* (1994) Response to desipramine treatment in adolescent depression: a fixed-dose, placebo-controlled trial. *J. Am. Acad. Child Adolesc. Psychiatry*, **33**: 686–694.

120. Kye C.H., Waterman G.S., Ryan N.D., Birmaher B., Williamson D.E., Iyengar S., Dachille S. (1996) A randomized, controlled trial of amitriptyline in the acute treatment of adolescent major depression. *J. Am. Acad. Child Adolesc. Psychiatry*, **35**: 1139–1144.

121. Birmaher B., Waterman G.S., Ryan N.D., Perel J., McNabb J., Balach L., Beaudry M.B., Nasr F.N., Karambelkar J., Elterich G. *et al* (1998) Randomized, controlled trial of amitriptyline versus placebo for adolescents with "treatment resistant" major depression. *J. Am. Acad. Child Adolesc. Psychiatry*, **37**: 527–535.

122. Ryan N.D. (1990) Pharmacotherapy of adolescent major depression. Beyond TCAs. *Psychopharmacol. Bull.*, **26**: 75–79.

123. Hazell P., O'Connell D., Heathcote D., Robertson J., Henry D. (1995) Efficacy of tricyclic drugs in treating child and adolescent depression: a meta-analysis. *Br. Med. J.*, **310**: 897–901.

124. Geller B. (1991) Psychopharmacology of children and adolescents: pharmacokinetics and relationships of plasma/serum levels to response. *Psychopharmacol. Bull.*, **27**: 401–409.

125. Strober M., Freeman R., Rigali J. (1990) The pharmacotherapy of depressive illness in adolescence: I. An open label trial of imipramine. *Psychopharmacol. Bull.*, **26**: 80–84.

126. Ryan N.D., Puig-Antich J., Cooper T., Rabinovich H., Ambrosini P., Davies M., King J., Torres D., Fried J. (1986) Imipramine in adolescent major depression: plasma level and clinical response. *Acta Psychiatr. Scand.*, **73**: 275–288.

127. Henry J.A. (1992) Toxicity of antidepressants: comparisons with fluoxetine. *Int. Clin. Psychopharmacol.*, **6** (Suppl. 6): 22–27.

128. Simeon J.G., Dinicola V.F., Ferguson H.B., Copping W. (1990) Adolescent depression: a placebo-controlled fluoxetine treatment study and follow-up. *Progr. Neuro-Psychopharmacol. Biol. Psychiatry*, **14**: 791–795.

129. Mandoki M.W., Tapia M.R., Sumner G.S., Parker J.L. (1997) Venlafaxine in the treatment of children and adolescents with major depression. *Psychopharmacol. Bull.*, **33**: 149–154.
130. Shaffer D., Gould M.S., Brasic J., Ambrosini P., Fisher P., Bird H., Aluwahlia S. (1983) A children's Global Assessment Scale (C-GAS). *Arch. Gen. Psychiatry*, **40**: 1228–1231.
131. Kerfoot M., Dyer E., Harrington V., Woodham A., Harrington R.C. (1996) Correlates and short-term course of self-poisoning in adolescents. *Br. J. Psychiatry*, **168**: 38–42.
132. Ambrosini P.J., Bianchi M.D., Rabinovich H., Elia J. (1993) Antidepressant treatments in children and adolescents I. Affective disorders. *J. Am. Acad. Child Adolesc. Psychiatry*, **32**: 1–6.
133. Emslie G., Rush A., Weinberg W., Kowatch R., Hughes C., Carmody T., Rintelmann J. (1997) A double-blind, randomized placebo-controlled trial of fluoxetine in depressed children and adolescents. *Arch. Gen. Psychiatry*, **54**: 1031–1037.
134. Hibbs E.D., Jensen P.S. (Eds) (1996) *Psychosocial Treatments for Child and Adolescent Disorders. Empirically Based Strategies for Clinical Practice.* American Psychological Association, Washington, DC.
135. Pocock S.J. (1983) *Clinical Trials: A Practical Approach*, Wiley, Chichester.
136. Kolvin I., Garside R.F., Nicol A.R., Macmillan A., Wolstenholme F., Leitch I.M. (1981) *Help Starts Here*, Tavistock, London.

Commentaries

4.1
Towards an Understanding of Early Onset Depression

James F. Leckman[1]

Reports in the scientific literature concerning childhood depression have increased three-fold over the past two decades. In 1999, with nearly a hundred reports appearing per annum, Prof. Harrington's timely paper provides a useful overview of this potentially lethal disorder and a guide to some of the most promising treatment strategies presently available. This commentary touches on a range of topics, from phenomenology to genetics and the role of epigenetic factors, before considering the prospects for newly emerging treatments. It closes with a brief comment on the merits of dynamical and evolutionary perspectives on this form of developmental psychopathology.

Recent studies of adult depression and the criteria used to guide diagnostic decisions have found little empirical support for most of the thresholds used in the DSM-IV criteria for major depression [1]. Most of the relevant characteristics appeared to be continuous traits, suggesting that major depression — as specified by DSM-IV — may best be seen as a diagnostic convention imposed on a continuum of depressive symptoms of varying severity and duration. While comparable studies have not been completed in child and adolescent populations, there would appear to be little doubt that similar results would pertain. One could also credibly argue that clinically relevant dimensions would extend, in most cases, beyond depressed mood and would include other troubling affects, particularly anxiety. Indeed, twin studies have suggested that both an individual's vulnerability to develop anxiety and his depression are governed in part by the same set of genes [2].

Longitudinal studies have begun to document complex interactions between adverse life events (including adverse perinatal events), somatic illnesses, maternal depression, diagnoses of depression and anxiety, treatment response, and risks of recurrence and subsequent physical

[1]Child Study Center, Sterling Hall of Medicine, Yale University School of Medicine, PO Box 207900, New Haven, CT 06520-7900, USA

illnesses. In one example, investigators at the Oregon Research Institute found that major depressive disorder (MDD) in adolescence was associated with maternal emotional problems during gestation and with not being breastfed [3]. In another study, Pat Cohen and her colleagues at Columbia found that physical illness at all ages increased the risk of new-onset major depressive disorder (MDD), and that MDD also predicted subsequent illhealth [4]. Finally, David Brent and his colleagues at the University of Pittsburgh have reported that for depressed adolescents comorbid anxiety is a predictor of poor response to psychosocial treatments in general [5]. Although cognitive-behavioral therapy (CBT) outcomes were less affected by comorbid anxiety, the efficacy of CBT plummeted in the presence of maternal depressive symptoms. As proposed by Kendler, it appears likely that genetic factors can interact with environmental factors to influence the vulnerability to MDD in subtle ways. In the absence of heritable risk factors, children appear to be less vulnerable to psychosocial adversity [6]. In contrast, the presence of heritable risk factors has been associated with an increased risk of exposure to high-risk environments. Ongoing longitudinal studies of twins have the promise of clarifying these associations. Beyond statistical analyses, it is also increasingly likely that some of the specific vulnerability genes will be identified. Although in most cases their individual effects are likely to be modest and highly dependent on the individual's genetic background, it is possible that genes of moderate effect will also be detected. Such discoveries may guide future pathophysiological and therapeutic research.

As reviewed in Harrington's chapter, CBT is gaining greater acceptance in the treatment of childhood depression. Additional work is needed to refine these methods and to implement them throughout the mental health profession. However, just as advances are being made in this arena, we appear to be on the cusp of a new era in psychopharmacology, with the advent of substance P and corticotropin-releasing factor analogues. These agents are just beginning to be used in Phase II and III clinical trials and the initial results are quite promising [7]. Whether they will be suitable for use in children is unclear at the moment, but their side-effect profile appears remarkably benign.

The developing brain is a self-organizing system that has evolved from a rudimentary design first established in our remote chordate ancestors more than 450 million years ago. Although dynamical and evolutionary perspectives on affective syndromes may be heuristically useful in providing a theoretical framework to integrate interdisciplinary research [8], application of these approaches to unipolar depression has lagged behind and has failed to yield a coherent model. Why do depressive states emerge and dominate the cognitive-behavioral repertoire of affected individuals? Is it a plea to other members of the social group, or a mode of conservation and self-protective withdrawal during times of stress and cognitive reorganization, or is it simply a consequence of psychosocial adversity, and if untreated a prelude to the apoptosis of the individual (suicide)?

REFERENCES

1. Kendler K.S., Gardner C.O. Jr. (1998) Boundaries of major depression: an evalua-tion of DSM-IV criteria. *Am. J. Psychiatry*, **155**: 172–177.
2. Kendler K.S. (1996) Major depression and generalized anxiety disorder. Same genes, (partly) different environments — revisited. *Br. J. Psychiatry*, **30** (Suppl.): 68–75.
3. Allen N.B., Lewinsohn P.M., Seeley J.R. (1998) Prenatal and perinatal influences on risk for psychopathology in childhood and adolescence. *Develop. Psychopathol.*, **10**: 513–529.
4. Cohen P., Pine D.S., Must A., Kasen S., Brook J. (1998) Prospective associations between somatic illness and mental illness from childhood to adulthood. *Am. J. Epidemiol.*, **147**: 232–239.
5. Brent D.A., Kolko D.J., Birmaher B., Baugher M., Bridge J., Roth C., Holder D. (1998) Predictors of treatment efficacy in a clinical trial of three psychosocial treatments for adolescent depression. *J. Am. Acad. Child Adolesc. Psychiatry*, **37**: 906–914.
6. Kendler K.S. (1998) Anna-Monika-Prize paper. Major depression and the envi-ronment: a psychiatric genetic perspective. *Pharmacopsychiatry*, **31**: 5–9.
7. Kramer M.S., Cutler N., Feighner J., Shrivastava R., Carman J., Sramek J.J., Reines S.A., Liu G., Snavely D., Wyatt-Knowles E. *et al* (1998) Distinct mechanism for antidepressant activity by blockade of central substance P receptors. *Science*, **281**: 1640–1645.
8. Leckman J.F., Mayes L.C. (1998) Understanding developmental psychopathology: how useful are evolutionary accounts? *J. Am. Acad. Child Adolesc. Psychiatry*, **37**: 1011–1021.

4.2

Depression In Youth: Trends in Diagnosis

Stephen V. Faraone[1]

Two decades ago, few argued with the idea that diagnosing depression in children "would appear to be premature and treatment unwarranted" [1]. But, having raised the diagnosis of youth depression to well-reasoned, textbook respectability, Prof. Harrington shows that the opposite is true. Far from being rare, youth depression is a common affliction having clinical implications.

To what can we attribute the evolution of thinking about youth depression? Assuredly, the data reviewed by Harrington show that youth depression,

[1]*Pediatric Psychopharmacology Unit of the Child Psychiatry Service, Massachusetts General Hospital, Harvard Medical School, 15 Parkman Street, Boston, MA 02114, USA*

having had its day in the court of scientific inquiry, has won the day. But this required two paradigmatic shifts in diagnostic thinking: the shift from hierarchical to non-hierarchical diagnoses and the shift from diagnoses that downplayed developmental differences to those that were sensitive to the variations of psychopathology through the life cycle.

Childhood depression's struggle for respectability was due, in part, to its pervasive comorbidity with other disorders. Comorbidity had obscured youth depression due to the hierarchical diagnosis paradigm, which assumes psychiatric disorders are discrete entities that co-occur infrequently. Consider the third edition of the American Psychiatric Association's *Diagnostic and Statistical Manual* (DSM), which told clinicians that if two disorders co-occurred, then the disorder higher in the hierarchy should be diagnosed. A more pervasive disorder high on the hierarchy could exhibit the symptoms of a less pervasive disorder lower on the hierarchy.

The revised edition of DSM-III moved away from hierarchical diagnosis, a trend that continued with the publication of DSM-IV. Nevertheless, DSM-IV retains hierarchical guidelines for the differential diagnosis of depression in youth. For instance, it posits that dysphoria and mood lability are associated features of attention deficit hyperactivity disorder (ADHD) and warns clinicians not to overdiagnose depression in ADHD children whose mood disturbance is characterized by irritability rather than by sadness or loss of interest. Given that chronic irritability is usually the primary mood disturbance in depressed youth, this guideline impels clinicians to diagnose ADHD but not depression when faced with a child who seems to have both disorders.

The DSM's comments about ADHD and depression are vague enough to allow for much variability in their implementation. A clinician who adopts a strict hierarchical view will see fewer cases of depression than one who adopts a more lax interpretation. These clinicians agree on the signs and symptoms expressed by apparently depressed youth but disagree as to whether the diagnosis of depression is warranted. Ultimately, research studies will determine when it is and is not valid to diagnose depression in the presence of another disorder. For example, a meta-analysis of family studies showed a familial link between depression and ADHD, suggesting the validity of diagnosing both disorders in youth [2].

Because ignoring comorbidity will limit treatment options, the conservative clinician will take an empirical approach to diagnosis. This method simply applies diagnostic criteria and diagnoses all disorders that are evident. Eventually, research will lead to firm guidelines about how to treat youth who have depression in the context of another disorder. Until then, we must use clinical judgement to select treatment options based on the range of disorders observed.

Children stand on the shifting sands of physical, emotional, social and neuropsychological development. Although recognized for decades, developmental change has only recently had tangible consequences for youth depression. DSM-IV explicitly accommodates developmental changes in two ways: it allows the depressed mood to be irritable and lists failure to make expected weight gains as a sign of the disorder.

Yet this may not be enough. As Richard Harrington has shown, developmental change creates diagnostic questions: Is the sad and sullen adolescent depressed? Is the angry 7 year old capable of discriminating anger from sadness? How does the ennui of adolescence differ from the loss of energy of depression? How does a 6 year old express worthlessness?

Although most of these questions remain to be answered, systematic research shows that the expression of depression in youth differs from the typical adult picture. Depressed youth are frequently irritable, their course is frequently chronic, their onset is often insidious and comorbid disorders are common. More work is needed to determine how these, and other developmental differences should be incorporated into diagnostic criteria.

Due to the growing acceptance of comorbidity and the use of developmentally sensitive diagnoses, youth depression is no longer the pariah that it was two decades ago. Nevertheless, depressed children are still underidentified.

Both researchers and clinicians need to work within a theoretical framework that accommodates comorbidity and developmental sensitivity. Perhaps a diagnostic nomenclature of the future will incorporate age- or stage-specific, norm-referenced criteria, using psychometric methods to adapt diagnoses to developmental transitions. Such an approach has worked effectively for the assessment of adaptive functioning and intellectual performance. Perhaps it should be considered for the diagnosis of depression.

REFERENCES

1. Lefkowitz M.M., Burton N. (1978) Childhood depression: A critique of the concept. *Psychol. Bull.*, **85**: 716–726.
2. Faraone S., Biederman J. (1997) Do attention deficit hyperactivity disorder and major depression share familial risk factors? *J. Nerv. Ment. Dis.*, **185**: 533–541.

4.3
Depressive Disorders in Childhood and Adolescence: State of the Art
Peter M. Lewinsohn[1]

The empirical study of childhood/adolescent depression is of relatively recent origin. Initially, depression in children/adolescents was thought

[1] *Oregon Research Institute, Eugene 97403-1983, USA*

not to exist or to manifest itself by non-depressive symptoms such as somatic complaints, behavioral difficulties, or academic failure [1, 2]. Subsequent work [3–9] revealed that depressive disorders can and do occur during childhood/adolescence. The results of recent studies indicate that depression is more prevalent during childhood/adolescence than had previously been thought [10–12], and the lifetime prevalence during adolescence has been estimated as high as 20% [13].

Prof. Harrington presents an integration of this rapidly growing area of empirical and clinically important research. His work has been in the forefront of this area. He points to specific issues about which we need more information. I would like to add two more.

The first is the gender issue. Beginning at age 12–13 depression is already twice as prevalent in girls. Girls not only report significantly more depressive symptomatology, they also report less satisfaction with their appearance on various measures of body image, and significantly lower self-esteem. There may be important gender differences that need to be taken into consideration in treatment. Modifications of existing treatment protocols to reflect gender-related psychosocial problems may be needed.

Another topic that deserves more attention is the linkage between depression and physical morbidity and functional impairment due to physical morbidity. First identified as a risk factor by Reinherz and her colleagues in 1989 [14], recent studies [15] also suggest that depression is a risk factor for health-related problems and vice versa. Assessment of physical health status should be part of the diagnostic evaluation of depressed young people.

As Harrington suggests, an important thrust for the future likely will be efforts to modify existing treatments to make them more sensitive to the fact that close to 50% of depressed young people have another mental disorder, the most common being conduct, substance use, anxiety, and attention deficit disorders [16].

REFERENCES

1. Sperling M. (1959) Equivalents of depression in children. *J. Hillside Hospital*, **8**: 138–148.
2. Toolan J.M. (1969) Depression in children and adolescents. In *Adolescence: Psychosocial Perspective* (Eds G. Caplan, S. Lebovici), pp. 264–270, Basic Books, New York.
3. Carlson G.A., Strober M. (1978) Affective disorder in adolescence: issues in misdiagnosis. *J. Clin. Psychiatry*, **39**: 63–66.
4. Cytryn L., McKnew D.H. Jr. (1972) Proposed classification of childhood depression. *Am. J. Psychiatry*, **129**: 149–155.
5. Kovacs M., Beck A.T. (1977) An empirical-clinical approach toward a definition of childhood depression. In *Depression in Childhood: Diagnosis, Treatment, and Conceptual Models* (Eds J.G. Schulterbrandt, A. Raskin), pp. 1–25, Raven Press, New York.

6. Poznanski E.O., Zrull J.P. (1970) Childhood depression: clinical characteristics of overtly depressed children. *Arch. Gen. Psychiatry*, **23**: 8–15.
7. Puig-Antich J., Weston B. (1983) The diagnosis and treatment of major depressive disorder in childhood. *Ann. Rev. Med.*, **34**: 231–245.
8. Rutter M., Tizard J., Yule W., Graham P., Whitmore K. (1976) Research report: Isle of Wight Studies 1964–1974. *Psychol. Med.*, **6**: 313–332.
9. Weinberg W.A., Rutman J., Sullivan L., Penick E.C., Dietz S.G. (1973) Depression in children referred to an educational diagnostic center: diagnosis and treatment. *J. Pediatrics*, **83**: 1065–1072.
10. Angold A. (1988) Childhood and adolescent depression: I. Epidemiological and aetiological aspects. *Br. J. Psychiatry*, **152**: 601–617.
11. Fleming J.E., Offord D.R. (1990) Epidemiology of childhood depressive disorders: a critical review. *J. Am. Acad. Child Adolesc. Psychiatry*, **29**: 571–580.
12. Rutter M. (1988) *Studies of Psychosocial Risk*, Cambridge University Press, Cambridge.
13. Lewinsohn P.M., Hops H., Roberts R.E., Seeley J.R., Andrews J.A. (1993) Adolescent psychopathology: I. Prevalence and incidence of depression and other DSM-III-R disorders in high school students. *J. Abnorm. Psychol.*, **102**: 133–144.
14. Reinherz H.Z., Stewart-Berghauer G., Pakiz B., Frost A.K., Moeykens B.A., Holmes W.M. (1989) The relationship of early risk and current mediators to depressive symptomatology in adolescence. *J. Am. Acad. Child Adolesc. Psychiatry*, **28**: 942–947.
15. Lewinsohn P.M., Seeley J.R., Hibbard J., Rohde P., Sack W.H. (1996) Cross-sectional and prospective relationships between physical morbidity and depression in older adolescents. *J. Am. Acad. Child Adolesc. Psychiatry*, **35**: 1120–1129.
16. Lewinsohn P.M., Rohde P., Seeley J.R. (1998) Major depressive disorder in older adolescents: prevalence, risk factors, and clinical implications. *Clin. Psychol. Rev.*, **18**: 765–794.

4.4
"At least in the form seen in adults." A Commentary on Major Depressive Disorder in Youth

Gabrielle A. Carlson[1]

The point at which I began doing research on mood disorders in young people [1], in adults, unipolar/bipolar distinctions had replaced previous dichotomies, bipolar disorder was responding to lithium, and unipolar depression was responding to tricyclic antidepressants. "Depressive reactions" were "apparently rare in children, at least in the form seen in adults" [2]. The research thrust was to demonstrate that major mood disorders occurred in youths, that they were phenomenologically

[1]*Department of Child and Adolescent Psychiatry, State University of New York at Stony Brook, Stony Brook, New York 1794-8790, USA*

similar to those in adults and would thus respond to the same treatments.

In the past 20+ years, we have learned that depression is far from rare in young people. In community samples, depending on the age group and criteria being used, prevalence ranges from 2 to 20% [3]. In clinical samples, rates of 60% in children and adolescents were found at UCLA Neuropsychiatric Institute in 1977–78 [4]. In 1991, a similar survey of outpatient and inpatient mental health facilities in Suffolk County, New York, revealed depression as a primary concern occurred in 63% of 532 adolescent inpatients and outpatients, and 39% of 616 child inpatients and outpatients. In other words, it has remained a prominent concern in mental health facilities.

Unlike adult depression, where the subject him/herself usually describes the problem, young people are brought in by caretakers who describe what they see, not necessarily what the child experiences. One has to dig for child/adolescent major depression. When it is diagnosed, it is almost invariably nested within other psychopathology. Young people spontaneously presenting for care with uncomplicated major depression or bipolar disorder are indeed rare.

As noted in Prof. Harrington's review, the depressive disorder usually begins after the onset of another psychiatric disorder. Cantwell and I [5] pointed this out using the primary/secondary distinction. Definitions change, however. DSM-IV rediagnosis of the 14 youths who had met criteria for primary major depression using criteria available in 1978 revealed that 3 had prior social phobia, 2 had attention deficit hyperactivity disorder, primarily inattentive type (one including severe learning disabilities), 2 probably had Asperger's disorder. Four young people (all over age 12) had bipolar disorder (1 with bipolar depression, 3 with bipolar II disorder). Only three were really primary.

Community studies also demonstrate higher rates of comorbidity in youth than in adults. The following odds ratios reveal considerably more comorbidity in youth [3, 6]: anxiety 4.2 in adults, mean 6.5 (range 4.4–10.4) in children/adolescents; conduct disorder 1.3 in adults, mean 5.5 (range 2.2–16) in children/adolescents, substance abuse 1.8 in adults, mean 5.6 (range 3.1–8.6) in children/adolescents.

The implications of high rates of comorbidity for treatment are considerable. The fact that young people have not shown significant improvement on tricyclic antidepressants (TCAs) has been attributed to their age, different neurotransmitter systems, and so on. In fact, adults with comorbid anxiety disorders, bipolar disorder and substance abuse (the upward extension of externalizing disorders) also respond poorly to TCAs [7].

The other phenomenological differences between youths and adults with depression are the relatively higher rates of bipolar disorder and higher rates of depression switching to mania. The switch rate from psychotic depression in adults was 3% [8]; it was 28% in adolescents [9]. However, as with major depression, bipolar disorder in children is highly comorbid, less so in adolescents [10]. Treatment implications are similar. Data would suggest that lithium responsivity is poorer in people of any age with comorbidity [11].

In conclusion, then, it appears that depression, as it exists in adults, is rare in children if one looks only for uncomplicated, non-comorbid depression. On the other hand, comorbidity complicates childhood disorders as it does adult disorders, and secondary depression in both age groups may be remarkably similar in terms of treatment response and prognosis.

REFERENCES

1. Carlson G.A., Davenport Y., Jamison K. (1977) A comparison of outcome in adolescent and late onset bipolar manic-depressive illness. *Am. J. Psychiatry*, **134**: 919–922.
2. Slater E., Roth M. (1967) *Child Psychiatry in Clinical Psychiatry*, Williams and Wilkins, London.
3. Costello E.J., Angold A., Sweeney M.E. (1998) Comorbidity with depression in children and adolescents. In *Comorbidity in Affective Disorders* (Ed. M. Tohen), pp. 179–196, Dekker, New York.
4. Carlson G.A., Cantwell D.P. (1980) A survey of depressive symptoms, syndrome and disorder in a child psychiatry population. *J. Child Psychol. Psychiatry*, **21**: 19–25.
5. Carlson G.A., Cantwell D.P. (1980) Unmasking masked depression in children and adolescents. *Am. J. Psychiatry*, **137**: 445–449.
6. Kessler R. (1998) Comorbidity of unipolar and bipolar depression with other psychiatric disorders in a general population survey. In *Comorbidity in Affective Disorders* (Ed. M. Tohen), pp. 1–25, Dekker, New York.
7. Aliopoulous J., Zisook S. (1996) Tricyclic antidepressant medications. In *Predictors of Treatment Response in Mood Disorders* (Ed. P. Goodnick), pp. 1–36, American Psychiatric Press, Washington, DC.
8. Johnson J., Horwath E., Weissman M.M. (1991) The validity of major depression with psychotic features based on a community study. *Arch. Gen. Psychiatry*, **48**: 1075–1081.
9. Strober M., Lampert C., Schmidt S., Morrell W. (1993) The course of major depressive disorder in adolescents: recovery and risk of manic switching in a 24-month prospective, naturalistic follow-up of psychotic and non-psychotic subtypes. *J. Amer. Acad. Child Adolesc. Psychiatry*, **32**: 34–42.
10. Carlson G.A. (1999) Mania and ADHD-comorbidity and confusion. *J. Affect. Disord.* (in press).
11. Abou-Saleh M.T. (1993) Who responds to prophylactic lithium therapy? *Br. J. Psychiatry*, **163** (Suppl. 21): 20–26.

4.5
The "Atypicality" of Depression in Youth

Joseph Biederman[1] and Thomas Spencer[1]

In contrast to the enormous advances over the last two decades on the psychobiological and therapeutic foundation of adult depression [1], childhood depression continues to be supported by a weak scientific basis with its attendant impact in diagnosis, identification and therapeutics. Although the reasons for this state of affairs remain unclear, several lines of evidence suggest that depression in youth may have unique features compared to adult depression that compound its identification. These include dysphoria and irritability as the predominant mood disturbance rather than sadness and melancholia [2], "mood reactivity" as seen in atypical forms of adult depression [3], insidious onset and a chronic course rather than acuteness and episodicity [2, 4], male preponderance or equal gender representation [5] rather than female preponderance, an increased personal and familial risk for bipolar disorder [6] and a much larger spectrum of comorbidity than seen in adult depression [2, 5]. Consistent with this atypical profile by adult standards, is the pharmacological evidence documenting selective efficacy for serotonergic drugs [7] and absence of responsivity to tricyclic antidepressants [3].

While some investigators suggest that juvenile depression follows a largely remitting course [8], others stress its chronicity [2, 4]. These contradictory findings may be accounted for by different definitions of remission. Although most reports examining rates of remission in depressed youth limit themselves to syndromatic remission, using this definition, a youth who loses a single symptom of depression can be considered "remitted" even though he or she remains quite ill and dysfunctional. A stricter definition of remission would be that of "symptomatic" remission in which the youth no longer has symptoms of depression, and an even stricter definition of remission would be that of functional remission in which the depressed youth no longer has symptoms of depression or dysfunction. Considering the critical importance of interpersonal functioning, careful consideration should be given to regaining functional status and not merely symptom decline in assessing recovery from depression in youth.

Fortunately, emerging data from controlled clinical trials documented that cognitive-behavioral therapy (CBT) shows promise in controlling symptoms of depression in the young [9]. Equally promising are results from two recent large randomized placebo-controlled clinical trials documenting significant separation from placebo for the serotonergic specific reuptake inhibitors

[1] *Pediatric Psychopharmacology Unit, Massachusetts General Hospital, WACC 725, 15 Parkman Street, Boston, MA 02114, USA*

(SSRIs) fluoxetine [7] and paroxetine [10] in depressed youth. Considering the safety profile of SSRIs, these findings are most welcomed.

While familiality suggests that genes may play a role in the etiology of depression in youth, it also suggests that youth may become depressed as a consequence of a poor environment generated by a depressed parent. Irrespective of its biological or psychosocial underpinnings, the development of a depressive syndrome in a child is a serious matter, since it is commonly associated with a high degree of morbidity and dysfunction. However, the atypical clinical picture, its fluctuating course, the high levels of irritability, aggression, oppositionalism, anxiety, school and behavioral difficulties [2] greatly complicate its identification in youth. Considering that depression is a major risk factor for suicide and that suicide is a leading cause of mortality in the young [11, 12], failing to identify depression in youth can have dire consequences.

While the choice of treatment can vary within different settings, it is important to emphasize that the major hurdle facing depressed youth today continues to be underidentification. We hope that this worrisome state of affairs will soon be alleviated by scientific advances and aggressive educational efforts focused on juvenile mood disorders.

REFERENCES

1. Musselman D., DeBattista C., Nathan K., Kilts C., Schatzberg A., Nemeroff C. (1998) Biology of mood disorders. In *Textbook of Psychopharmacology* (Ed. D. Kupfer), pp. 549–588, American Psychiatric Press, Washington, DC.
2. Biederman J., Faraone S.V., Mick E., Lelon E. (1995) Psychiatric comorbidity among referred juveniles with major depression: fact or artifact? *J. Am. Acad. Child Adolesc. Psychiatry*, **34**: 579–590.
3. Nierenberg A.A., Alpert J.E., Pava J., Rosenbaum J.F., Fava M. (1998) Course and treatment of atypical depression. *J. Clin. Psychiatry*, **59**: 5–9.
4. Kovacs M., Feinberg T.L., Crouse-Novak M., Paulauskas S.L., Finkelstein R. (1984) Depressive disorders in childhood: I. A longitudinal prospective study of characteristics and recovery. *Arch. Gen. Psychiatry*, **41**: 229–237.
5. Angold A., Costello E.J. (1993) Depressive comorbidity in children and adolescents: empirical, theoretical and methodological issues. *Am. J. Psychiatry*, **150**: 1779–1791.
6. Geller B., Fox L., Clark K. (1994) Rate and predictors of prepubertal bipolarity during follow-up of 6- to 12-year-old depressed children. *J. Am. Acad. Child Adolesc. Psychiatry*, **33**: 461–468.
7. Emslie G., Rush J., Weinberg W., Kowatch R., Hughes C., Carmody T., Rintelmann J. (1997) A double-blind, randomized, placebo-controlled trial of fluoxetine in children and adolescents with depression. *Arch. Gen. Psychiatry*, **54**: 1031–1037.
8. Harrington R., Fudge H., Rutter M., Pickles A., Hill J. (1990) Adult outcomes of childhood and adolescent depression. I: Psychiatric status. *Arch. Gen. Psychiatry*, **47**: 465–473.

9. Brent D.A., Holder D., Kolko D. (1997) A clinical psychotherapy trial for adolescent depression comparing cognitive, family and supportive therapy. *Arch. Gen. Psychiatry*, **54**: 877–882.

10. Wagner K., Birmaher B., Carlson G., Clarke G., Emslie G., Geller B., Keller M., Klein R., Kutcher S., Papatheodorou G. *et al* (1998) Safety of paroxetine and imipramine in the treatment of adolescent depression. Presented at the NCDEU Meeting, Boca Raton, 10–13 June.

11. Ryan N.D., Puig-Antich J., Ambrosini P., Rabinovich H., Robinson D., Nelson B., Iyengar S., Twomey J. (1987) The clinical picture of major depression in children and adolescents. *Arch. Gen. Psychiatry*, **44**: 854–861.

12. Brent D.A., Kolko D.J., Allan M.J., Brown R.V. (1990) Suicidality in affectively disordered adolescent inpatients. *J. Am. Acad. Child Adolesc. Psychiatry*, **29**: 586–593.

4.6
How the Study of Early Onset Depression Challenges Us to Produce a New Paradigm for Understanding Mood Disorders

Stanley P. Kutcher[1]

Early onset depressive disorder is an area of increasing investigation across a variety of domains. Yet its current, and by extension, future elucidation is hampered by a conceptual paradigm that may be confusing at best and distracting at worse. Indeed, much of our activity directed towards understanding early onset depressive disorder can be likened to the response of the person who, when asked why he was searching for his hat in front of a shop window instead of in an adjacent park where it had blown away, replied "because the light is much better here".

As studies of diagnosis and treatment of depression in children and teens have shown us, our concept of depression has, it can be argued, become so broad that its utility as a medical diagnosis is now suspect. Indeed, the very word "depression" is used by professions and the public alike to denote everything from personal experiences arising from "the slings and arrows of outrageous fortune" to profound and even life-threatening states of psychophysical inertia.

Perhaps fueled by the now popular perspective of health as a utopian state (as defined by the World Health Organization), the construct of and subsequent identification of "depression" now encompasses everything from socially induced distress to expected (but not tolerated) dysphoria arising from adversity to an intense psychophysiological state in which an individual's usual cognitive, behavioural and affective heterogeneity is replaced

[1] *Department of Psychiatry, Dalhousie University, QE II Health Sciences Centre, Abbie J. Lane Building, 5909 Jubilee Road, Suite 4082, Halifax, Nova Scotia, B3H 2E2, Canada*

by a homogeneous pattern of constricted variability. For example, low-grade but persistent unhappiness can now be "diagnosed" as dysthymia, and even brief dysphoric experiences of low intensity can be somehow construed as minor depression. Thus, clinical depression (as a medical term) may be conceptually and actively confused with distress and unhappiness. The wish to sanitize the human condition, even if it arises primarily from altruistic foundations, seems to underlie our ever increasing diagnosis of "depression". In support of this perspective, recent studies have now demonstrated that antidepressant medications used by "normal" individuals will not only enhance their quality of life, but will also make them easier to live with as described by their significant relations.

This "diagnostic extension" of the concept of depression is further complicated by the confusion of comorbidity, as recent debates on the diagnosis of bipolar disorder in young people have demonstrated. It is a leap of something akin to faith to believe that 60, 70 or 80% of "depressed" youngsters have an additional and unique psychiatric disorder! Perhaps in our syndromatically based diagnostic developments we have debased the mathematical foundations of set theory and have happily developed what we feel are unique categories using shared elements. For example, a set of golf clubs cannot be confused with a set of hockey sticks, because the elements, although superficially similar, are essentially different, yet concentration and sleep problems (for example) can be used to define both depression and anxiety. Additionally, in many cases, we have assumed, and not confirmed, that diagnostic elements are part of the implied pathoetiology of a "disorder" (e.g. early morning awakening in depression) instead of an example of a homeostatic mechanism arising from within the organism which may serve to redirect a variety of cognitive, behavioural or affective disturbances.

Our conceptual model(s) of "depression" have been elevated to the status of organizing principles without sufficient critical examination. What is the validity of our definitions? What is the predictive attribution of what we call depression? Where is the independent experimental evidence that will allow us to either confirm or reject, with some degree of certainty, the model, which we apply? Have we become so broad in our conceptual framework that, in our desire to be of help, we have lost sight of the boundaries between "disease", "disorder" and usual experience? Perhaps there are no such boundaries?

The available literature on the treatment of "depression" in young people substantiates this concern. Arguably, the "best " evidence for psychological treatment — cognitive-behaviour therapy (CBT) — is less than impressive in its superiority over true placebo therapy. Although CBT is theory-based and has been informed by years of research, it still cannot be demonstrated to be associated with cognitive theories of pathoetiology. Critical studies of depressed teens, for example, have shown that substantial numbers do not exhibit the expected cognitive set, that the presence of the expected cognitive set is not predictive of response to CBT, and that successful pharmacotherapy in the absence of CBT provides remission of negative cognition and that there is no evidence that negative cognitions are a cause rather than a consequence of depression. Thus, the construct is neither necessary nor sufficient for either diagnosis or treatment. Such critical assessment should raise concern either with the model of the disorder (depression), or the mode of initiation/intervention (CBT), or both.

What the study of early onset depression provides for us, is the opportunity to review and challenge our conceptual paradigm of mood disorders. As Kuhn has demonstrably argued, conventional perspectives in scientific thought continue until the anomalies are such that they demand a critical re-evaluation of the conceptual framework itself. Perhaps this is what the studies of early onset depression are leading to.

Some consideration must be given to a perspective that understands disorders of mood not as depression or mania (and stops in between) but as neurologically mediated disturbances in the amplitude, frequency and synchronicity of a variety of mood states. For example, depressed individuals could be understood not as having a "depressed mood", but as exhibiting a mood state in which the various components that make up mood (i.e. joy, happiness, sadness, irritability, enthusiasm, grief, etc.) have lost their independent trajectories and have become "glued" together in an extremely stable and undifferentiated state of variable duration and severity. Alternatively, manic individuals could be understood not as having a "manic mood", but as exhibiting a mood state in which the various components have become super-desynchronized — so much so that the expected heterogeneity of individual states is overexpressed and that the subsequent effect is one of extreme affective instability of variable duration and severity. "Normal" mood states would be somewhere in between and could exhibit a degree of responsive and yet biologically determined desynchronization that would allow for environmental impact as an external modifier of behaviour, while at the same time allowing for the intergenerational transmission of genetically determined properties for excessive synchronization or desynchronization. Each individual's ontogenetic development could then be expected to recapitulate phylogenetic patterns. Thus, the childhood years would be associated with a critical period in which external impactors on neural development might be expected to modify the genetically based central nervous system propensity for mood synchronization. The adolescent years would be associated with the expression and "fine tuning" of the organism's ability to synchronize mood — as the "normal" development of mood in teenagers shows. Subsequent life cycle development would then fit on this neural background, and the effects of both external (e.g. stressors) and internal (e.g. CNS degeneration) factors would be expected to express these synchronies/desynchronies. Treatments for disrupted mood states would not be focused on antidepressant or antimanic amelioration, rather they would be developed toward setting mood states into a relative state of chaotic desynchronization.

Richard Harrington's chapter on depression in children and adolescents has clearly outlined the anomalies in our paradigm as it pertains to understanding disorders of mood. Will further research be directed towards identifying further anomalies or will it take a new direction?

4.7
Adult and Childhood Depressions May in Fact be Different Illnesses
Alvin A. Rosenfeld[1]

For centuries, social reformers have pointed out that children could be self-denigrating and hopelessly despondent. More than 150 years ago Charles Dickens crafted poignant portraits of miserably unhappy children on society's margins. To him, these children's emotions were reactions to terribly depriving external circumstances. Others have traditionally contended that some part of the way these children feel and act emerges from inner, inherited deficiencies. The new twist the 1980s introduced was the growing consensus that, contrary to psychoanalytic theorizing, children actually could be diagnosed as being clinically, psychiatrically depressed more or less *in the same way as adults were*. This paradigm was widely accepted; it seemed likely to make treating depressed children more successful. To date, that promise has not been fulfilled. In some ways the new paradigm diverted child psychiatric attention away from a major contributor to extreme childhood misery, the truly terrible circumstances some children live in.

Classifying a child's misery correctly becomes a semantic exercise unless that categorization contributes to a superior understanding and/or better potential or actual interventions. Like many hypotheses in child psychiatry, the current childhood depression paradigm derived in large part from an advance in general psychiatry: adults with unipolar depressions were being treated very successfully with tricyclic antidepressants. For them, tricyclic medications have been shown to be highly effective [1]. Might these medications also relieve children's suffering? After all, in contemporary practice, clinicians certainly see some children from organized, supportive families — perhaps with a genetic loading for depression — who suffer from major depressions that look remarkably like the adult condition. Today,

[1] 4 East 89th Street, New York, NY 10128, USA

some of these children improve with medication. But theirs are responses in the uncontrolled, single case study world that constitutes office practice.

While the hypothesis that childhood depression is like adult depression and therefore highly treatable with antidepressants was worth testing, as Prof. Harrington writes, "with the exception of Preskorn *et al* all of the controlled double-blind trials have found no significant differences between oral tricyclics and placebo." The findings with selective serotonin reuptake inhibitors (SSRIs) are similar. Although clinicians use these medications because they seem to help some children, as yet, careful scientific study has delineated no specific group of children who respond to antidepressants the same way as adults do. Perhaps, in a year or two, available scientific facts with SSRIs will be different. But today they are not. In fact, considerable evidence indicates that placebos are as highly effective in treating childhood depressions. Were we reacting fully scientifically, we would be funding far more research investigating why this remarkably safe intervention works far better for children than for adults.

Yet many child psychiatrists continue to accept the "children can be depressed in something like the adult fashion" paradigm as if it were on the verge of being proven. Unfortunately, as this new paradigm became accepted, the field simultaneously did not really discard, but did de-emphasize one that considered children's depression as a reaction to miserable living conditions, emotionally and/or materially. It is hard to keep your spirits up if you doubt you will eat today. But particularly during Ronald Reagan's presidency, getting social research funded became difficult in America. Some of the most severely depressed, hopeless children who clinicians see are the abused and neglected ones in the foster care system. In one California study, foster children use about ten times the mental health services that other similarly indigent children do [2]. These children's real life experiences likely would have persuaded all but the most invulnerable child that life is miserable and that they are helpless, hopeless, and useless. These children usually have been living in chaotic homes with grossly disturbed, often substance-abusing, sometimes criminal, parents. Studies of foster care populations are seriously methodologically flawed. Yet in aggregate they suggest that a very high percentage of these children have emotional difficulties, including many with major depressions [2].

Some foster care research data parallel findings that Harrington's paper reports: depressed children live in families with adverse environments, high parental criticism, family discord, and poor communication between parent and child. It might be more parsimonious to conclude that to date, data about childhood depression's etiology points to "an environmentally mediated mechanism" with familial discord as a primary associated factor.

A conservative reading of available data suggests that childhood depression is a final common pathway with numerous possible etiologies. One may be a biological depression or genetic vulnerability. But more children become clinically depressed because of real external circumstances in everyday life. Cases of these two types ought not to be comingled in research samples. When the environmental paradigm fits, the child's depression may be an appropriate reaction to stressful real life situations. Those children need adequate social and familial interventions which assure that they live in decent, emotionally supportive circumstances. Child psychiatrists who want to ameliorate depressions in more children while sticking to the data, might better focus on changing the family environment, assuring that more children have living situations that approximate the "average expectable." Maybe Charles Dickens was right after all!

Note: Since adolescents were considered social adults as recently as 75 years ago, this commentary focuses on pre-pubertal children.

REFERENCES

1. Reynolds C.F.III, Frank E., Perel, J.M., Imber S.D., Cornes C., Miller M.D., Mazumdar S., Houck P.R., Dew M.A., Stack J.A. *et al* (1999) Nortriptyline and interpersonal psychotherapy as maintenance therapies for recurrent major depression: a randomized controlled trial in patients older than 59 years, *JAMA*, **281**: 39–45.
2. Rosenfeld A.A., Pilowsky D.J., Fine P., Thorpe M., Fein E., Simms M.D., Halfon N., Irwin M., Alfaro J., Saletsky R. *et al* (1997) Foster care: an update, *J. Am. Acad. Child Adolesc. Psychiatry*, **36**: 448–457.

4.8

Taking Stock and Moving on: Current Issues and Challenges Concerning Child and Adolescent Depressive Disorders

Cheryl A. King[1]

The last 20 years have witnessed a tremendous surge in research on prepubertal and adolescent depression. The cumulative result is an empirically based description or picture of a condition whose existence was disputed just one generation ago. Scientific studies indicate — and both the mental health delivery system and popular culture now acknowledge — the relatively high prevalence of depressive disorders among youth. As is clear from Prof. Harrington's comprehensive review, findings from multiple studies converge on the clinical presentation, course and outcome, and psychosocial correlates of depressive disorders.

[1]*Department of Child and Adolescent Psychiatry, University of Michigan Medical Center, 1500 East Medical Center Drive, Ann Arbor, MI 48109, USA*

It is also clear from Harrington's review, however, that there are few known efficacious treatments for prepubertal and adolescent depression. Treatments that have garnered some empirical support, such as cognitive-behavioral therapy and fluoxetine, have not emerged as "cures" or "across the board" treatments of choice. Cognitive-behavioral therapy has the most evidence supporting its effectiveness, but may have little or no impact on the more severe depressive disorders and the suicidal thoughts and behaviors that are common among depressed youth. Fluoxetine needs further study to ascertain the extent of its effectiveness and to determine whether or not initial positive findings replicate. Thus, there are promising leads, but at this juncture, treatment protocols for depressed youth are suggestive rather than definitive.

It is within this context that Harrington puts forward his suggested treatment guidelines. Rather than proclaim, he makes suggestions based on a strong mix of empirical findings, clinical experience, and common sense. I would like to extend his discussion and comment on several issues that have substantial implications for clinical practice and further research. These are: (1) the problem of diagnostic threshold; (2) developmental considerations; (3) the subcategorization of depressive disorders; and (4) suicidality.

Clinical experience suggests that many young people exist — at least for hours or days at a time — at, near, or just over the diagnostic threshold for a depressive disorder. And, despite high reliability and concurrent validity for total counts of depressive symptoms, research on structured diagnostic interviews shows relatively poor reliability in determining whether or not symptoms meet the diagnostic threshold [1]. If an adolescent near the diagnostic threshold presents for an evaluation, will the youth be diagnosed with a depressive disorder? Is a simple count of five symptoms plus "significant" psychosocial impairment adequate for a diagnosis of major depressive disorder? Is the count ever "simple" for near threshold cases? That is, when is a symptom a symptom? How many have counted three definite and three likely, or four definite and two possible, as close enough to five symptoms? What is significant fatigue? What is low self-esteem in a young teenage girl? How do we count irritability in a teenager with severe school performance problems and severely punishing parents?

Even when combined with a developmental interview, a cross-sectional evaluation of a possibly depressed child or adolescent may be inadequate. Harrington's conservative approach, evident in the suggestion to begin with "a thorough assessment, sympathetic discussion with the adolescent and family, and encouraging support" is sensible for youth at or near the diagnostic threshold — especially when combined with efforts to alleviate stress. The empirical data indicating that a significant minority of depressive disorders remit rapidly should not be ignored [2, 3]. For the subset of youth who are improved at follow-up, diagnostic labeling will have been avoided.

In addition, the tendency of providers to assume that all improvements are due to their prescribed treatment — resulting in the continuation of possibly unneeded treatment — will have been circumvented. This strategy would benefit treatment efficacy research as well, resulting in inclusion of only those youth with clear depressive disorders.

A developmental perspective enables us to view prepubertal children and adolescents as individuals on a life course or developmental trajectory. Their family/social contexts and relationships, psychological characteristics, life experiences, and psychiatric conditions influence each other across time. In this transactional model of influence, the notion of impact is extremely important. The clinician might ask, "How can I best move this child onto a healthier developmental trajectory?" For a 10 year old, a school intervention to promote friendship development or reduce the risk of school failure may be most critical. For a 14 year old, treatment of emerging alcohol abuse may be most critical. This is not to argue that treatment of the depressive symptoms should not occur. Rather, we must avoid the temptation to see such treatment as sufficient and to view all psychosocial problems as emerging or resulting from the depressive symptoms. In a transactional model of mutual influence, successful symptomatic relief will have a positive ripple effect. But other interventions may have as much or more impact, and deserve careful consideration.

Depressive disorders characterize a highly heterogeneous group of prepubertal children and adolescents. As presented by Harrington, these youth have a broad range of psychosocial strengths and weaknesses and, more often than not, comorbid psychiatric conditions. Given our rich understanding of the phenomenology and course of these comorbid conditions, it behooves us to focus more efforts on understanding the course that prepubertal and adolescent depression takes when it occurs with different comorbid conditions. The 13-year-old depressed girl with social phobia and a history of separation anxiety will undoubtedly have a different course and benefit from a different treatment "package" than a 16-year-old depressed boy with conduct disorder and severe alcohol abuse. Although this may seem like common sense in clinical practice, as researchers we still need to develop, describe and package, and evaluate treatments accordingly.

Approximately 70% of youth with major depressive disorders report significant suicidal thoughts at some time during the course of their depression. The empirical evidence is clear that youth with depressive disorders are at increased risk for suicide attempts and completed suicide, and that this risk may be increased further in the presence of comorbid mental disorders or substance abuse [4]. Follow-up studies suggest that the risk period may not be outgrown [5]. Although depressive disorders are highly prevalent during childhood and adolescence, and the tragedy of suicide is a relatively rare event, suicide risk must be carefully assessed in each depressed child. Involvement of parents and guardians is essential if there are any concerns about possible suicide risk. An open channel of communication with provision of psychoeducation concerning signals of increased risk and the availability of emergency services is recommended.

REFERENCES

1. King C.A., Katz S.H., Ghaziuddin N., Brand E., Hill E., McGovern L. (1997) Diagnosis and assessment of depression and suicidality using the NIMH Diagnostic Interview Schedule for Children (DISC-2.3). *J. Abnorm. Child Psychol.*, **25**: 173–181.
2. Shain B.N., King C.A., Naylor M., Alessi N. (1991) Chronic depression and hospital course in adolescents. *J. Am. Acad. Child Adolesc. Psychiatry*, **30**: 428–433.
3. Harrington R.C., Vostanis P. (1995) Longitudinal perspectives and affective disorder in children and adolescents. In *The Depressed Child and Adolescent: Developmental and Clinical Perspectives* (Ed. I.M. Goodyer), pp. 311–341, Cambridge University Press, Cambridge.
4. King C.A. (1997) Suicidal behavior in adolescence. In *Review of Suicidology* (Eds R.W. Maris, M.M. Silverman, S.S. Canetto), pp. 61–95, Guilford Press, New York.
5. Rao U., Weissman M.M., Martin J.A., Hammond R.W. (1993) Childhood depression and risk of suicide: a preliminary report of a longitudinal study. *J. Am. Acad. Child Adolesc. Psychiatry*, **32**: 21–33.

4.9

Increasing Awareness of Depressive Disorders in Childhood: Implications for World Child and Adolescent Mental Health

John A. Corbett[1]

The increasing awareness that depressive disorders in childhood can be recognized more frequently than was previously thought has important implications both for prevention and for the provision of services. This explosion of interest parallels attempts to destigmatize depression in adults.

In the United Kingdom, the "Defeat Depression Campaign" organized by the Royal College of Psychiatrists and carried out between 1991 and 1996 was aimed at education of the public about depression in adults, its treatment and encouragement of earlier treatment seeking. The findings of research into the efficacy of this initiative have recently been reported by Paykel and his colleagues on behalf of the College [1]. Surveys of public attitudes were conducted, involving over 2000 households sampled to be representative of the population of the UK prior to the campaign, which

[1] *Department of Psychiatry, University of Birmingham, North Warwickshire NHS Trust, Lea Castle, Nr Kidderminster, DY10 3PP, UK*

involved newspaper and magazine articles, radio and television programmes and other media activities. The survey was repeated in March 1995 and June 1997 and showed significant positive changes regarding attitudes to depression, reported experience of it, attitudes to antidepressants and, less consistently, to help from general practitioners. Changes were of the order of 5–10% and throughout attitudes to depression and to treatment by counselling were very favourable, whereas antidepressants were regarded as addictive and less effective.

Prof. Harrington has shown that research findings concerning adult depression cannot easily be extrapolated onto work with children and adolescents. However, education and awareness of the subject might be approached in the same way. Anna Freud [2] pointed out that children do not tend to complain about their feelings or symptoms, and it is usually other people, particularly parents and teachers, who tend to complain about them. There is, however, in all areas of work with young people an increasing awareness of the need to listen to them and develop skills in eliciting information about feelings and emotionally laden topics such as experience of abuse and other significant life events. This is a core skill for child psychiatrists and it is particularly relevant, in parts of the world where there are few psychiatrists, to the training of all mental health workers. There are of course opportunities during general education to include teaching on mental health issues which will not only improve awareness of young people but assist in the recruitment and training of health professionals and volunteers.

Much of the research on depression in young people has been reported from academic centres in Europe and America, and now that methods have been established for carrying out such studies these need to be extended to other parts of the world. One outstanding issue concerns the changing pattern in diagnosis of depressive disorders with age and the different ways in which depressive affect in young people is experienced by the youngsters themselves and by adults responsible for them.

An important recent study from Puura and colleagues [3], reporting their findings from the Finnish national study, adds significantly to our knowledge about how international studies might be carried out.

In order to find out whether parents and teachers report depressive symptoms in children with self-reported depression, over 5000 Finnish 8–9 year olds were assessed using the Childhood Depression Inventory (CDI) as part of a wider study of child health — 381 had a cut-off score above 17. Teachers reported those with high CDI scores as having poor school performance, restlessness, somatic complaints, unresponsiveness, being bullied and being absent from school, while parents reported depressed mood, unpopularity, social withdrawal, disobedience, inattentiveness and stealing.

In clinical practice, parents and teachers do not always respond empathetically to suggestions that children behaving negatively may be depressed, but an increased awareness and more positive view about treatment of depression by adults is clearly one key to this important issue.

One particular way in which transcultural studies of depression in young people may be examined is to look at markers such as suicide and parasuicide and drug taking in young people and relate these to the diagnosis of depressive disorders in the community.

Here the evidence is somewhat conflicting, for while suicide is relatively uncommon in young children there are clearly wide variations in suicide and attempted suicide in adolescents and young adults. If there is conti-nuity between depression in young children and adolescents, as there seems to be between symptoms of the sort reported from Finland and adolescent turmoil and depression, it is likely that adolescent suicide (at least in a proportion of cases) is an end stage of repeated social failure, low self-esteem and despair. The finding of an increased rate of affective disorders in adoles-cents with pervasive and other severe developmental disorders, although not often presenting as suicide, but frequently with other forms of self-harm, would tend to support this [4].

On the other hand, international studies of the wide variation in youth suicide rates suggest that the picture is more complicated than this. Kelleher [5], reviewing youth suicide trends in the Republic of Ireland, points out that in a country with a population of 3.5 million, 94% of whom are Roman Catholic, traditionally the suicide rate has been very low but has risen over the past 20 years. Although this rise can be partly explained by improvement in the method of collecting statistics, this cannot account for more than 40% of the ten-fold rise in the ratio in males of suicide to undetermined death since the late 1980s. There has been a slight rise in the suicide rate in young adult females, but overall this rate has been stable for the past 20 years.

For 15–24 year olds, the ratio of male to female suicide in Ireland is 7.1:1 for the years 1988–92, and this represented the highest ratio of all countries that returned suicide statistics to the World Health Organization (WHO) over this 5-year period. Of the ten countries with the highest male: female suicide ratios in this time period, seven were English-speaking and were at one time part of the British Empire. Kelleher concludes that if the differences are not artefactual, this would suggest that some shared cultural heritage is influencing suicide behaviour in young people. Although the increase is consistent with an increased prevalence of mood disorder, this seems unlikely to be more than a partial explanation and it is likely that depressed young men today more readily act upon thoughts of suicide than in previous generations, and this in itself may be related to social and cultural change in societies where such changes in rates have been reported.

Such changes will include the increased academic pressures on adolescents, the loosening of religious and family ties, and the availability of illegal drugs to young people. The latter does not appear so important in the Irish studies, but the fact that young people resort to illicit drugs and substances such as solvents to either elevate mood or block out negative affective experiences, may be contrasted with the negative views of adults concerning antidepressants and the relative inefficacy of tricyclic antidepressants in children and adolescents.

It may be that the newer generation of selective serotonin reuptake inhibitors (SSRI) type antidepressants will be found to be more effective in severe depressive disorders in young people, but the recent emphasis on psychological treatments for depression in children and adolescents recently reported by Harrington et al [6] is more encouraging.

Hopefully, the clinical experience of such approaches to treatment will lead to a clarification of strategies for prevention aimed at earlier identification and effective counselling, together with measures which can be employed on a community-wide basis to help vulnerable children to cope with the increasing pressures of a postmodern world.

REFERENCES

1. Paykel E.S., Hart D., Priest R.G. (1998) Changes in public attitudes to depression during the Defeat Depression Campaign. *Br. J. Psychiatry*, **173**: 519–523.
2. Freud A. (1946) *The Psychoanalytical Treatment of Children*. Image, London.
3. Puura K., Almqvist F., Tamminen Piha J., Kumpulainen K., Räsänen E., Moilanen I., Koivisto A.-M. (1998) Children with symptoms of depression. What do the adults see? *J. Child Psychol. Psychiatry*, **39**: 577–585.
4. Corbett J. (1999) Describing developmental disability (in preparation).
5. Kelleher M.J. (1998) Youth suicide trends in the Republic of Ireland. *Br. J. Psychiatry*, **173**: 196–197.
6. Harrington R., Whittaker J., Shoebridge P. (1998) Psychological treatment of depression in children and adolescents. A review of treatment research. *Br. J. Psychiatry*, **173**: 291–298.

4.10

Some Unsolved Problems in Childhood Depression: A Clinician's View

Helmut Remschmidt[1]

Richard Harrington's article starts with the statement that, until recently, it was widely believed that depressive disorders were rare in young people. This statement has to be changed by recent studies that have demonstrated not only the occurrence of depressive states in children and adolescents,

[1] *Department of Child and Adolescent Psychiatry, Philipps-University, D-35033 Marburg, Germany*

but also increasing rates with age. A review of the literature of psychiatric and behavioural disorders in children and adolescents reveals very clearly that depression and suicidal behaviour belong to those disorders that have increased since the end of the Second World War [1]. Among these increasing disorders are further alcohol and drug abuse, delinquency and obesity.

However, this view was quite different in earlier days of child and adolescent psychiatry. According to Carlson and Garber [2] five major schools of thought with regard to depressive disorder in childhood and adolescence can be distinguished. The *first* school, mainly represented by psychoanalytic theorists, stated that there is no depression before puberty, with the consequence that childhood depression was more or less ignored. The *second* perspective assumed that depression in childhood is a "masked depression", which meant that children would express their depressive behaviour by other symptoms which were called "depression equivalents", such as somatic complaints, conduct problems or delinquency [3]. The *third* perspective assumed that the core symptomatology of depressive children is like that of adults, but there are some additional childhood-specific symptoms such as social withdrawal, aggression, negativism, conduct problems and school refusal, though Cantwell [4] pointed out that essential features should be distinguished from associated ones. The *fourth* perspective assumed that childhood depression does not show any difference in comparison to depression in adulthood (isomorphism), which led to the DSM-III classification criteria of depression in childhood [5]. Finally, the *fifth* school of thought, supported by developmental psychologists, suggested that an isomorphism between child depression and depression in adulthood must be unrealistic, leading to the notion that, in spite of similarities between depression in childhood and in adulthood, there are specific manifestations with regard to age and development concerning children's cognitive, linguistic and socio-emotional capacities which influence the expression of depressive symptomatology over time [6].

On the basis of the last view, it can be questioned whether the diagnostic criteria of the current classification systems ICD-10 and DSM-IV are really appropriate. The critique of these classification systems from a developmental perspective can be based on several arguments, including neglecting causal processes, longitudinal course, phases of life, and the judgement of developmental appropriateness of possibly abnormal behaviour [7]. In that view, many child psychiatric disorders can be explained in terms of aberrant or delayed developmental processes which are naturally different from adult development. With regard to these problems, depression in childhood and adolescence can be looked upon at different levels: the symptom level, the syndrome level and the level of disorder, characterized by a certain minimal duration, a clear impairment and a characteristic course and outcome.

The same problems with reference to an *adequate diagnosis* (which are present in spite of some standardized instruments) arise with regard to *aetiology*, which is currently seen in terms of a *multifactorial* approach. However, it remains uncertain to what extent the different factors (genetics, adverse family influences, recent life events, etc.) contribute to the manifestation and the course of the disorder. Harrington gives a well-balanced view of these factors in his review. Finally, also all modern *treatment approaches* are based on this multifactorial perspective. However, in spite of several studies using cognitive-behavioural therapy (CBT), family interventions and tricyclic antidepressants, the results are, on the whole, not very impressive. I agree with Harrington's review that cognitive-behavioural therapy, interpersonal therapy (which was not much studied) and the modern selective serotonin reuptake inhibitors (SSRIs) are promising tools for the treatment of depression. However, if one looks at the most frequently practised therapy, CBT, this method seems to be appropriate only for depressive symptoms and mild depressive disorders. The non-efficacy of tricyclic antidepressants in children and adolescents, based on double-blind placebo-controlled studies, is still a matter of controversy, because several clinicians are convinced of the efficacy of these drugs in cases they have treated. But nevertheless, the results have to be respected and the modern SSRIs should be given priority, especially considering the danger of the cardiotoxic effect of tricyclic antidepressants. In spite of the poor research on SSRIs, this group of antidepressants seems to be promising, not only because of their low rate of adverse effects, but also because of their pharmacological mechanism. The same applies to the modern reversible monoamine oxidase inhibitors, which have been useful in the treatment of hyperkinetic children and children with major depressive disorder. In severe cases, especially in bipolar or monopolar depressive disorders, lithium salts have been demonstrated to be useful. Nevertheless, the whole field of psychopharmacology of depression in children and adolescents is still underdeveloped, and strong efforts are necessary in order to understand the basic mechanisms of drug action and to establish rational and safe therapeutic regimes.

REFERENCES

1. Remschmidt H. (1996) Increase in the rates of psychiatric disorders in children and adolescents: fact or fiction? Presented at the Xth World Congress of Psychiatry, Madrid, 23–28 August.
2. Carlson G.A., Garber J. (1986) Developmental issues in the classification of depression in children. In *Depression in Young People* (Eds M. Rutter, C.E. Izard, P.B. Read), pp. 399–434, Guilford Press, New York.
3. Toolan J.H. (1962) Depression in children and adolescents. *Am. J. Orthopsychiatry*, **32**: 404–414.

4. Cantwell D.P. (1983) Depression in childhood: clinical picture and diagnostic criteria. In *Affective Disorders in Childhood and Adolescence: An Update* (Eds D.P. Cantwell, G.A. Carlson), pp. 3–18, Spectrum, New York.
5. Cytryn L., McKnew H.D. Jr., Benney W.E. Jr. (1980) Diagnosis of depression in children: a reassessment. *Am. J. Psychiatry*, **337**: 22–25.
6. Cicchetti D., Schneider-Rosen K. (1986) An organizational approach to childhood depression. In *Depression in Young People. Developmental and Clinical Perspectives* (Eds M. Rutter, C.E. Izard, P.B. Read), pp. 71–134, Guilford Press, New York.
7. Graham P., Skuse D. (1992) The developmental perspective in classification. In *Developmental Psychopathology* (Eds H. Remschmidt, M.H. Schmidt), pp. 1–6, Hogrefe & Huber, Lewiston, NJ.

4.11
Childhood Depression: Some Unresolved Research Questions

Eric Fombonne[1]

Depression in children and adolescents has received increasing attention over the last 20 years. The number of published research and clinical articles has grown exponentially and nothing indicates that this trend is abating. As pointed out by Richard Harrington, much of this trend reflects changes in psychiatric research in general, with an increased emphasis on direct interviewing of subjects (including children) with standardized procedures, and on the use of symptom-oriented approaches to child psychiatric diagnoses. However, there is also the possibility that the growing focus on affective disorders amongst youth reflected a genuine increase in the incidence of these conditions. Careful reviews of the adult epidemiological literature have concluded that lifetime rates of depressive disorders have increased for birth cohorts born in the post-Second World War era [1]. Furthermore, a decreasing age of onset was simultaneously reported, meaning that depression now appears not only more frequently but also at an earlier age, that is during adolescent years. Although data are more scarce for trends over time in rates of depression amongst child and adolescent samples, the limited evidence points toward the same conclusion [2–5]. However, the magnitude of the increase remains unknown and most probably is lower than sometimes claimed; the specificity of the increase regarding depression is also unclear, since other types of emotional and behavioural disturbances have also increased during the same period [2, 6]. What remains poorly understood is the exact nature of the psychosocial changes which are responsible for this secular increase in depression. The monitoring and elucidation of

[1]*Department of Child and Adolescent Psychiatry, Institute of Psychiatry, De Crespigny Park, Denmark Hill, London SE5 8AF, UK*

fluctuations over time in the incidence of affective disorders amongst youth should therefore appear on the future research agenda of several groups.

Harrington's review provides an admirable summary of the current research findings and challenges in the area of childhood depression. Yet a persisting problem in this field about definition and measurement should be strongly emphasized. Firstly, in spite of studies showing strong similarities of depressive symptomatology between children and adolescents with depression [7], developmental differences exist in the phenomenology of affective disturbances which are not adequately reflected in current measurement procedures, be it in the diagnostic criteria, in the cut-offs used to define caseness on continuous measures, or in the layout of questions in research schedules. Secondly, the use of multiple informants in most research protocols means, in practice, that the "best estimate" procedure described in Harrington's chapter is used to generate diagnoses of depression. This undoubtedly leads to an overinclusive definition which might dilute samples and bias results towards the null hypothesis. Thirdly, the measurement of depression occurring within the context of another psychiatric disorder (as is the rule) provides even more challenges to its adequate assessment. For example, children with conduct disorders often present with depressive *symptoms* which have lasted for some time. In order to meet criteria for major depression, it is necessary to find evidence of impairment arising from the depressive symptomatology. How is that achieved, and how does one differentiate, within a given child, the impairment of functioning due to one disorder from that due to another disorder? Because a conduct-disordered child is impaired in several areas of functioning (by the conduct symptoms), he will de facto fulfil all criteria for major depression, even though the child might just present with a transient depressive syndrome which often is an associated feature of chronic disruptive problems.

Measurement issues are therefore far from being a side issue in depression research. Many randomized clinical trials, particularly those concerned with the efficacy of antidepressant drugs, have failed to properly address them. Thus, significant improvements are often seen using data from one informant only but not with those from the others [8, 9]. Or, results have not taken into account the high rates of comorbid disorders and their confounding effects on drug response; thus, a recent study failing to demonstrate a benefit of high doses of tricyclic medications for treatment-resistant depression was based on a sample including 54% of comorbid depression with conduct disorder [10]. Evidence from other studies shows that comorbid depression with conduct disorder is less likely to respond to antidepressant medication [11] and may confound treatment studies.

Finally, psychological treatment studies have accumulated which show efficacy for short-term interventions. Their results are nevertheless not always consistent with theoretical predictions; for example, gains with cognitive-behavioural therapy (CBT) do not follow parallel changes in cognitive dysfunction. Similarly, family therapy or parental components of interventions do not add any benefit, although disturbances in family background of depressed children represent a well-documented risk factor. The available conceptual models of depression, therefore, need to be considered at best as working hypotheses. Further outlining our current knowledge limits, it is worth also keeping in mind that, thus far, we have little understanding of two major defining features of child and adolescent depression: namely, that its incidence rises enormously during mid-adolescence and that it affects twice as many girls as boys.

Explanatory models which could account for these two features are desperately sought for.

REFERENCES

1. Fombonne E. (1994) Increased rates of depression: update of epidemiological findings and analytical problems. *Acta Psychiatr. Scand.*, **90**: 145–156.
2. Achenbach T.M., Howell C.T. (1993) Are American children's problems getting worse? A 13-year comparison. *J. Am. Acad. Child Adolesc. Psychiatry*, **32**: 1145–1154.
3. Fombonne E. (1999) Time trends in affective disorders. In *Historical and Geographical Influences on Psychopathology* (Eds P. Cohen, C. Slomkowski, L. Robins), pp. 115–139, Lawrence Erlbaum Mahwah, NJ.
4. Ryan N.D., Williamson D.E., Iyengar S., Orvaschel H., Reich T., Dahl R.E., Puig-Antich J. (1992) A secular increase in child and adolescent onset affective disorder. *J. Am. Acad. Child Adolesc. Psychiatry*, **31**: 600–605.
5. Kovacs M., Gatsonis C. (1994) Secular trends in age at onset of major depressive disorder in a clinical sample of children. *J. Psychiatr. Res.*, **28**: 319–329.
6. Fombonne E. (1998) Increased rates of psychosocial disorders in youth. *Eur. Arch. Psychiatry Clin. Neurosci.*, **248**: 14–21.
7. Ryan N., Puig-Antich J., Ambrosini P., Rabinovich H., Robinson D., Nelson B., Iyengar S., Twomey J. (1987) The clinical picture of major depression in children and adolescents. *Arch. Gen. Psychiatry*, **44**: 854–861.
8. Wood A., Harrington R., Moore A. (1996) Controlled trial of a brief cognitive-behavioural intervention in adolescent patients with depressive disorders. *J. Child Psychol. Psychiatry*, **37**: 737–746.
9. Emslie G.J., Rush A.J., Weinberg W.A., Kowatch R.A., Hughes D.W., Carmody T., Rintelmann L. (1997) A double-blind randomized, placebo-controlled trial of fluoxetine in children and adolescents with depression. *Arch. Gen. Psychiatry*, **54**: 1031–1037.
10. Birmaher B., Waterman S., Ryan N., Perel J., McNabb J., Balach L., Beaudry M., Nasr F., Karambelkar J., Elterich G. et al (1998) Randomized, controlled trial of amitriptyline versus placebo for adolescents with "treatment resistant" major depression. *J. Am. Acad. Child Adolesc. Psychiatry*, **37**: 527–535.
11. Hughes C., Sheldon H., Preskorn S., Weller E., Weller R., Hassanein R., Tucker S. (1990) The effect of concomitant disorder in childhood depression on predicting treatment response. *Psychopharmacol. Bull.*, **26**: 235–238.

4.12
Research Trends in Depressive Disorders of Youth
Benedetto Vitiello[1]

After decades of separation between child and adult psychiatry, with respect to nosology and treatment approach, there has been a recent rapprochement between the two fields. Focus has been on the continuity of psychopathology across the age span, with the adoption of the same diagnostic criteria for youth as in adults. This approach is well grounded in the fact that most psychiatric disorders that affect adults have their inception in youth and continue into adulthood [1]. Valid diagnoses can be obtained utilizing similar criteria across age. In both the 10th edition of the *International Classification of Diseases* (ICD-10) [2] and the 4th edition of the *Diagnostic and Statistical Manual of Mental Disorders* (DSM-IV) [3], the criteria for depressive disorders in youth are basically the same as in adults. In DSM-IV, the only differences are that in youth mood can be "irritable" as well as "depressed," and the minimum duration of mood disturbance for a diagnosis of dysthymic disorder is 1 year, rather than 2 years as in adults. The reports that a specific psychotherapy such as cognitive-behavioral therapy is also effective in youth support the theoretical and practical integration across age. This rapprochement, however, should not come at the cost of a decreased sensitivity to developmental differences in illness presentation, course and treatment response. The review by Richard Harrington highlights these differences and their implications for both practitioners and researchers.

In youth, mood is more reactive and the diagnosis of depressive disorders less stable than in adults. Because of this, it is more difficult to demonstrate the efficacy of specific treatments, either pharmacological or psychosocial, versus control conditions, such as placebo or non-specific clinical contact. As pointed out in the review, there is no evidence that oral tricyclic antidepressants are more efficacious than placebo in youth. In fact, the response to placebo has been as high as 70% [4]. This high and unpredictable placebo response makes it difficult to interpret the results of uncontrolled studies, however encouraging they may be. More recently, the attention has shifted to the selective serotonin reuptake inhibitors, as a class of safer and better tolerated antidepressants. Following an 8-week trial of fluoxetine in 96 patients aged 7–17 years with major depression, there was greater improvement on fluoxetine (56%) than on placebo (33%) [5]. Notably, only 31% of the patients treated with fluoxetine had reached complete remission at the end of the study. In another trial, 275 adolescents (aged 12–19 years) were randomized to receive paroxetine, imipramine, or placebo for 8 weeks.

[1]*Child and Adolescent Treatment and Preventive Interventions Research Branch, National Institute of Mental Health, 5600 Fishers Lane, Rockville, MD 20857, USA*

In the preliminary report of this study, paroxetine, but not imipramine, was better than placebo [6].

The treatment approach recommended by Harrington is based on the current state-of-the-art of the field, as also reflected in the guidelines of the American Academy of Child and Adolescent Psychiatry [7]. The efficacy of cognitive-behavioral therapy for youth with depression is fairly well documented [8], and the results of new studies on interpersonal therapy will soon be reported. Further research data are needed before evidence-based treatment guidelines can be fully developed.

Thus, compared with adult depression, depressive disorders in youth present with similarities, but also distinctive features that impact on patient management and call for specific research efforts. While spontaneous remission is more likely than in adults, recurrence is quite common and response to treatment is often unsatisfactory or incomplete, at least in the short term. Clearly, more comprehensively effective treatment and preventive strategies are needed. The current data are limited in terms of number of studies, sample sizes, type of patients enrolled, and duration of treatment. No comparisons between pharmacological and psychosocial modalities have been reported, nor has the efficacy of combined vs. single treatments been studied. Larger clinical trials comparing the effects of different therapeutic modalities, in more representative samples of patients, and for longer duration of treatment are needed.

Note: Throughout the commentary, the term "youth" is used to indicate both "children" and "adolescents." The opinions and assertions contained in this commentary are the private views of the author and are not to be construed as official or as reflecting the views of the Department of Health and Human Services or the National Institute of Mental Health.

REFERENCES

1. Lewinsohn P.M., Rohde P., Klein D.N., Seeley J.R. (1999) Natural course of adolescent major depressive disorder: I. Continuity into young adulthood. *J. Am. Acad. Child Adolesc. Psychiatry*, **38**: 56–63.
2. World Health Organization (1992) *The ICD-10 Classification of Mental and Behavioural Disorders. Clinical Description and Diagnostic Guidelines*, World Health Organization, Geneva.
3. American Psychiatric Association (1994) *Diagnostic and Statistical Manual of Mental Disorders*, 4th edn, American Psychiatric Association, Washington, DC.
4. Birmaher B., Waterman G.S., Ryan N.D., Perel J., McNabb J., Balch L., Beaudry M.B., Nasr F.N., Karambelkar J., Elterich G. *et al* (1998) Randomized controlled trial of amitriptyline versus placebo for adolescents with "treatment resistant" major depression. *J. Am. Acad. Child Adolesc. Psychiatry*, **37**: 527–535.
5. Emslie G.J., Rush A.J., Weiberg W.A., Kowatch R.A., Hughes C.W., Carmody T., Rintelmann J. (1997) A double-blind, randomized, placebo-controlled trial of fluoxetine in children and adolescents with depression. *Arch. Gen. Psychiatry*, **54**: 1031–1037.

6. Keller M.B., Ryan N.D., Birmaher B., Klein R.G., Strober M., Wagner K.D., Weller E.B. (1998) Paroxetine and imipramine in the treatment of adolescent depression. Presented at the 151st Annual Meeting of the American Psychiatric Association, Toronto, 2 June.
7. American Academy of Child and Adolescent Psychiatry (1998) Summary of the practice parameters for the assessment and treatment of children and adolescents with depressive disorders. *J. Am. Acad. Child Adolesc. Psychiatry*, **37**: 1234–1238.
8. Harrington R., Whittaker J., Shoebridge P. (1998) Psychological treatment of depression in children and adolescents. *Br. J. Psychiatry*, **173**: 291–298.

4.13
The Nature of First Episode Major Depression in Childhood and Adolescence

Ian Goodyer[1]

Prof. Harrington's paper provides a clear and comprehensive overview of the current knowledge regarding major depressive disorder in children and adolescents. The review begins by emphasizing the importance of direct examination of the mental state of the child together with parental information which should include the duration of the disorder and the degree of psychosocial impairment, as these crucial aspects of the presenting complaint will help the clinician to determine the correct treatment. The advances in developing standardized assessment procedures for use in research now need to be complemented by pragmatic procedures for use in routine clinical settings. Current methods and procedures for diagnostic assessment are based on adult criteria and the validity of these for children under the age of 6 is not at all clear. Clinicians should bear in mind that, in younger children and perhaps in those who are learning disabled or may have communication difficulties, social withdrawal from usual activities and irritable mood may be indicators of a depressive illness.

The section of the review on causation highlights how we have yet to unravel the multifactorial processes involved in onset. It is worth emphasizing that diagnostic heterogeneity may indicate aetiological heterogeneity. Concurrent non-depressive comorbid conditions are beginning to provide phenotypic clues that there may be different subtypes of depressive disorder [1]. These preliminary findings are potentially of great interest and, if replicated, will aid the targeting of treatments at the appropriate subgroup.

Harrington highlights the striking lack of clear-cut findings regarding aetiology at the psychological and neurobiological level. For example, it has

[1]*Developmental Psychiatry Section, University of Cambridge, Douglas House, 18b Trumpington Road, Cambridge CB2 2AH, UK*

yet to be established if there are enduring biases in negative views about the self, the world or the future in young people that predict the onset of depression. There is, however, increasing clarity regarding the definition and measurement of negative cognitions [2]. One substantial advance is the finding that negative biases about the self may not be apparent to a well person except under conditions of current low mood [3]. Self-reports about negative cognitions in the last few days or weeks may therefore fail to evaluate these more latent processes. Further studies should incorporate child versions of these experimental procedures to assess self-precept under different mood states and help clarify which negative cognitive elements are associated with major depression in young people.

It is notable that the superiority of the cognitive-behavioural approach does not appear to be due to specific changes in depressogenic cognitions present at the time of assessment. This is an unexpected finding that, if replicated, raises questions regarding the mechanisms by which this treatment is efficacious. Interpersonal psychotherapy, by contrast, focuses on the here and now relationships and, whilst it is not entirely clear how, appears to aid the young person in overcoming real life difficulties. It seems possible that these two conversational treatments may have a common set of therapeutic processes, and a comparative trial of the two may be more informative than further studies of one type against a no-treatment group.

Harrington's discussion of the role of cortisol hypersecretion in the pathophysiology of depression in young people is somewhat pessimistic. Loss of diurnal rhythm in selected adrenal steroids occurs in around 50% of depressed young people, and this abnormality appears to exert significant effects on the risk for persistent depression independent of the severity or duration of disorder at presentation [4, 5]. It is not clear if this is more likely in postpubertal adolescents compared to prepubertal children. Cortisol hypersecretion does not appear to correlate with self-reports of depression and may increase the risk for further negative life events [6]. Whilst these findings clearly require replication, they suggest that where hypersecretion is found, treatments that normalize diurnal rhythm may be adjunctive to other treatments. The overall lack of systematic trials of pharmacological agents is particularly worrying. As Harrington notes, the current findings emphasize the need for studies to compare treatments against each other in pragmatic trials including pharmacological versus psychological therapies.

REFERENCES

1. Angold A., Costello E.J., Erkani A. (1999) Comorbidity. *J. Child Psychol. Psychiatry*, 40: 57–88.
2. Ingram R., Miranda J., Segal Z. (1998) *Cognitive Vulnerability to Depression*. Guilford Press, New York.

3. Teasdale J.D., Barnard P.J. (1993) *Affect, Cognition and Change: Remodelling Depressive Thought*, Lawrence Erlbaum, Hillsdale, NJ.
4. Goodyer I.M., Herbert J., Altham P.M.E., Pearson J., Secher S., Shiers S. (1996) Adrenal secretion during major depression in 8 to 16 year olds. I: Altered diurnal rhythms in salivary cortisol and dehydroepiandrosterone (DHEA) at presentation. *Psychol. Med.*, **26**: 245–256.
5. Herbert J., Goodyer I.M., Altham P.M.E., Pearson J., Secher S., Shiers S. (1996) Adrenal secretion and major depression in 8 to 16 year olds. II. Influence of co-morbidity at presentation. *Psychol. Med.*, **26**: 257–263.
6. Goodyer I.M., Herbert J., Altham P.M.E. (1998) Adrenal steroid secretion and major depression in 8 to 16 year olds. III. Influence of the cortisol/DHEA ratio at presentation on subsequent rates of disappointing life events and persistent major depression. *Psychol. Med.*, **28**: 265–275.

4.14

Clinical Update of Child and Adolescent Depression

Sam Tyano[1]

Prof. Harrington's review contributes a lot to our knowledge and is an important addition to the literature in this field. Harrington reviews most of the current literature and puts an emphasis on valid and reliable diagnosis and on future directions for research.

However, we would like to bring to light another perspective of this important issue of depression in the various ages from childhood to adolescence, and put more emphasis on the purely clinical perspective. We believe that in the depressive disorders of childhood and adolescence the clinical perspective is complicated and unique, for a number of reasons.

The variability of the clinical picture is one of the complicating, as well as confusing elements in these disorders [1]. Its occurrence through the different ages is fascinating, as well as significant to the understanding of the disorder.

Depression in children, especially the younger ones, is frequently masked, and may seem like irritability, moodiness, inattention, apathy or agitation, or even may be confused with syndromes such as attention-deficit/hyperactivity disorder (ADHD), conduct disorders and separation anxiety [1, 2]. It may also involve many somatic symptoms that might blur the picture [2].

Another specific characteristic of depression in childhood is its close connection to anxiety. This is the only age group in which the two syndromes are inseparable. Adolescence, in a way, is the fork, the crossroads where these two syndromes are divided. This close connection is described in ICD-10, as the "mixed disorders of conduct and emotions" [3]. This category applies

[1]*Gehah Mental Health Center, POB 102, Petach-Tikva 49100, Israel*

to childhood disorders, which represent both aggressive, unsocialized or oppositional behavior and unconcealed symptoms of depression and anxiety. This connection of depression and anxiety is important to the understanding as well as to the treatment of this age group, which is different from all other age groups.

Depression in adolescents also has some specific characteristics, which are age-exclusive, and form an important trigger in the transformation from the childhood clinical picture to the adult one. Of the many characteristics involved, two will be discussed here. The first is the increasing importance of the biological axis in the breakthrough of puberty. The bodily changes, namely the changed hormonal balance, happen at about the same time as the elevated rate of depression. This is also the age when the depressive characteristics become more similar to those of adults. This overlap of changes indicates considerable likelihood of a connection between the changed body image, the physical–hormonal changes and the initiation of adolescent depression.

The other unique characteristic of adolescent depression is organization and integration towards the fourth organizer [4]. The fourth organizer, which allows the adolescent to choose by himself to have and thus to incorporate his sexual body, has to be differentiated from depression. It must be seen as a normal developmental stage, while the depression is morbid.

Another feature of depressive disorders in childhood and adolescence, which evolves from their clinical characteristics discussed here, is their extensive comorbidity [5]. Some 40–90% of youth with depressive disorders have other psychiatric disorders, and 20–50% have two or more comorbid diagnoses [5]. The list of comorbid disorders includes cognitive and behavioral as well as emotional disorders. It covers the whole psychiatric scale, including psychotic disorders, anxiety disorders, learning disorders, ADHD, post-traumatic stress disorder (PTSD), adjustment disorder (with depressed mood) and bereavement. It also includes general medical conditions such as cancer and hypothyroidism. The differential diagnosis from ADHD is especially complicated, because of the high overlapping rate between the symptoms [6]. It should be noted that in the bipolar disorders there is so much symptom overlapping that a subgroup of "bad ADHD" or a prodrome to bipolar disorder is suggested [7].

The last subject that we would like to mention is the treatment of depressive disorders. This intriguing question arises mainly in children and less in adolescents, whose clinical picture becomes more similar to that of adults as they grow up. The treatment of depression in children consists of psychotherapy as well as psychopharmacological agents [1, 5, 8]. While the psychotherapy most commonly used is cognitive-behavioral therapy (CBT), which is thought to be superior to the other psychotherapies, there are also many reports of successful treatment with other methods [5]. Pharmacological interventions were also found to be successful, but there are two reservations. First, in depressive children there is a high placebo effect, as high as the response rate to most of the antidepressants used [8]. Another reservation, very similar to the first, is that psychotherapies have the same response rate as pharmacological interventions [5].

Overall, the choice of the initial treatment seems to depend on "patient factors" such as severity, chronicity, age, contextual issues, and so on, as well as on "therapist factors", such as clinician availability, motivation and expertise [9]. From the clinical point of view, there is an emerging recognition that the integration of several psychotherapeutic techniques is in the best interests of the patient [5].

The issue of depressive disorders in children and adolescents is an intriguing, complicated and most of all a highly variable one. We have tried to emphasize the diversity of its clinical picture, and the several items evolving from it.

REFERENCES

1. Bidermaher B., Ryan N.D., Williamson D.E., Brent D.A., Kaufman J., Dahl R.E., Perel J., Nelson B. (1996) Childhood and adolescent depression: a review of the past 10 years. Part I. *J. Am. Acad. Child Adolesc. Psychiatry*, **35**: 1427–1439.
2. Ryan N.D., Puig-Antich J., Ambrosini P., Coplan J.D., Weissman M.M. (1987) The clinical picture of major depression in children and adolescents. *Arch. Gen. Psychiatry*, **44**: 854–861.
3. World Health Organization (1992) *The ICD-10 Classification of Mental and Behavioural Disorders: Clinical Descriptions and Diagnostic Guidelines*, World Health Organization, Geneva.
4. Tyano S. (1998) The adolescent and death: the fourth organizer of adolescence. In *The Adolescent in Turmoil* (Ed. A.Z. Schwarzberg), pp. 73–81, Praeger, Westport, CT.
5. American Academy of Child and Adolescent Psychiatry (1998) AACAP official action: Practice Parameters for the Assessment and Treatment of Children and Adolescents with Depressive Disorders. *J. Am. Acad. Child Adolesc. Psychiatry*, **37** (Suppl.): 63S–83S.
6. Barkley R.A. (1990) Differential diagnosis. In *Attention Deficit Hyperactivity Disorder. A Handbook for Diagnosis and Treatment* (Ed. R. A. Barkley), pp. 191–196, Guilford Press, New York.
7. Biederman J. (1998) Resolved: mania is mistaken for ADHD in prepubertal children. *J. Am. Acad. Child Adolesc. Psychiatry*, **37**: 1091–1093.
8. Bidermaher B., Ryan N.D., Williamson D.E., Brent D.A., Kaufman J. (1996) Childhood and adolescent depression: a review of the past 10 years. Part II. *J. Am. Acad. Child Adolesc. Psychiatry*, **35**: 1575–1583.
9. Jacobson N.S., Dobson K.S., Truax P.A., Addis M.E., Koerner K., Gollan J.K., Gortner E., Prince S.E. (1996) A component analysis of cognitive behavioral treatment for depression. *J. Consult. Clin. Psychol.*, **64**: 295–304.

4.15
Treatment Controversies in Childhood Depression

Carrie M. Borchardt[1]

Prof. Harrington provides us with a thoughtful and up-to-date review of childhood depression. I will focus my comments on a couple of the more controversial treatment issues: the relative roles of pharmacotherapy and psychotherapy, and treatment issues regarding comorbid school refusal.

As described in the review, research has shown treatments for depression in this age group to be helpful. This particularly applies to cognitive-behavioral therapy (CBT) and selective serotonin reuptake inhibitors (SSRIs). However, more research is needed on other psychotherapies and other medications, as well as comparative studies which examine various treatment modalities, either singly or in combination. Until we have that, the role of pharmacotherapy relative to psychotherapy will remain controversial.

Some early studies of the use of tricyclic antidepressants to treat children and adolescents with depression suggested they were helpful, and those medications were enthusiastically prescribed for that purpose. However, later studies with improved methodology and sample size failed to definitively demonstrate efficacy. Possibly as a result of that experience, we have become more cautious about the use of antidepressants in children and adolescents. That caution is reflected in the treatment recommendations of the review above, as well as in the Practice Parameters for the Assessment and Treatment of Children and Adolescents with Depressive Disorders [1]. These are part of an effort by the American Academy of Child and Adolescent Psychiatry to develop practice parameters for psychiatric disorders which affect children and adolescents.

The practice parameters suggest that antidepressants may be indicated in more severe depressions, in chronic or recurrent depression, and in those who fail a course of psychotherapy. The SSRIs are the current antidepressants of choice, as there are data to support their benefit and low toxicity in young people. An 8-week, double-blind, placebo-controlled trial of fluoxetine in children and adolescents (ages 7–17 years) with major depression found significantly greater improvement in the active medication group [2]. This study had a reasonable number of subjects, 48 per group. However, complete remission occurred in less than a third of subjects, a result which may be explained in part by the short duration of treatment. Replication of these findings is needed, as well as methodologically sound studies with good sample sizes utilizing other medications.

Once beyond the acute phase of treatment, we find even less research describing maintenance treatment for child and adolescent depression. This

[1] *Division of Child and Adolescent Psychiatry, Box 95 Mayo, 420 Delaware Street SE, Minneapolis, MN 55455, USA*

is true for psychotherapy as well as pharmacotherapy. The substantial rates of recurrence of major depression cited in the review demonstrate the need for effective maintenance or preventive treatment.

As mentioned in the review, difficulties at school can be a complication of depression in childhood and adolescence. Poor concentration and low motivation contribute to difficulties with completing school work, and the student may receive lower grades and/or fall behind in his or her assignments. Students may also struggle with anxiety symptoms. Studies have shown 30–75% of depressed youth have a comorbid anxiety disorder [3]. This can contribute to school refusal. Studies of comorbidity in a school refusal clinic have found that about half of the patients have a depressive disorder [4].

Our group is involved in ongoing investigations regarding school refusal. Most of our subjects have comorbid anxiety and depressive disorders. In our clinic, we frequently recommend modifications in the school program, including special education services to remediate academic delays, smaller classes and/or modified requirements to assist with triggers of panic, close monitoring and mentoring. We do not recommend home-schooling for depressed patients (whether or not they have school refusal), because our experience is that it is often very difficult to return children and adolescents to school after a prolonged absence. Others have found this, also [5]. We are therefore very concerned about contributing to the development of school refusal in depressed children and adolescents. In a recently completed treatment study of school refusal for adolescents with comorbid anxiety disorders and major depression [6], we noted that some subjects are receiving home-schooling at 1-year follow-up. Future study of the data relative to that issue would provide a better basis for decisions regarding home tuition.

REFERENCES

1. American Academy of Child and Adolescent Psychiatry (1998) Practice parameters for the assessment and treatment of children and adolescents with depressive disorders. *J. Am. Acad. Child Adolesc. Psychiatry*, **37** (Suppl.): 63S–83S.
2. Emslie G.J., Rush J., Weinberg W.A., Kowatch R.A., Hughes C.W., Carmody T., Rintelmann J. (1997) A double-blind, randomized, placebo-controlled trial of fluoxetine in children and adolescents with depression. *Arch. Gen. Psychiatry*, **54**: 1031–1037.
3. Kovacs M. (1990) Comorbid anxiety disorders in childhood-onset depressions. In *Comorbidity of Mood and Anxiety Disorders* (Eds J.D. Maser, C.R. Cloninger), pp. 271–281, American Psychiatric Press, Washington, DC.
4. Bernstein G.A. (1991) Comorbidity and severity of anxiety and depressive disorders in a clinic sample. *J. Am. Acad. Child Adolesc. Psychiatry*, **30**: 43–50.
5. Blagg N.R., Yule W. (1984) The behavioural treatment of school refusal—a comparative study. *Behav. Res. Ther.*, **22**: 119–127.

6. Bernstein G.A., Borchardt C.M., Perwien A.R., Crosby R.D., Kushner M.G., Thuras P.D. (1998) Treatment of school refusal with imipramine. Presented at the 45th Annual Meeting of the American Academy of Child and Adolescent Psychiatry, Anaheim, California, 27 October–1 November.

4.16

Psychotherapy for Childhood Depression

Israel Kolvin,[1] Judith Trowell,[1] John Tsiantis,[1] Fredrik Almqvist,[1] and Hartwin Sadowski[1]

Issues discussed in this commentary relate to therapy: the ethics of the random allocation of depressed children to treatment and no-treatment categories; duration of cognitive-behaviour therapy (and interpersonal therapy); arguments in favour of psychodynamic psychotherapy approaches for depressed children.

In Table 4.2 of Prof. Harrington's review there is evidence from those major studies with relatively larger sample sizes and randomization that cognitive-behaviour therapy (CBT) gives rise to higher rates of remission than attention placebo or non-directive supportive treatment, and very much greater effect compared to no treatment, with the percentage remitting being 43% and 5% respectively. With sound evidence of the efficacy of CBT for childhood depression, in the future the use of no-treatment control groups or even placebo control groups should no longer be entertained. Previous designs are both unacceptable ethically and clinically unwelcome to knowledgeable parents. Preferably a comparison design should be used where the alternative therapy groups are equally credible.

The studies listed by Harrington suggest that in CBT efficacy is combined with brief duration and rather few sessions. However, two of the listed studies indicate there was a doubling of sessions from 14 to 28 [1, 2], and Wood et al [3] report that half the patients who had remitted had a further episode within the next 6 months, but, with continuation of CBT for 6 months, the relapse rate was much lower. These are the so-called "booster" sessions, but it can be argued that the concept of a "booster" is a misnomer. What is required for an optimum effect is doubling the number of sessions with a concomitant doubling of the duration of therapy. The eventual number of sessions is unlikely to be substantially less than in brief focused individual psychodynamic psychotherapy.

A recent study of brief CBT for depressive disorder in adolescents [3] showed, at the end of therapy, a clear advantage of CBT over relaxation

[1]*Tavistock and Portman NHS Trust, 120 Belsize Lane, London NW3 2BA, UK*

approaches on some measures; however, this significant advantage did not last and by 6 months post-therapy was no longer present, partly due to the high relapse rate in the CBT group and partly because of the continuing effects of the relaxation therapy. Another study of a heterogeneous group of depressive conditions (only a minority with major depressive disorders) also indicates a rapid response to CBT by the end of treatment, but a rapid decay thereafter [4]. Hence, other psychotherapies need to be identified which have effects that are evident at the end of therapy and which are maintained at follow-up at least 6 months after therapy is terminated.

Gaps remain in the information regarding the utility of psychological treatment of major depression in childhood. More needs to be known about individual psychodynamic psychotherapy, especially as it holds promise of the persistence of effects and thus prevention of relapse; in addition, it can be used in clinics where group therapy is not always practical. Is there evidence from preliminary studies or pilot studies for this?

Previously Wrate et al [5] studied 72 clinical cases attending as outpatients or inpatients a university child psychiatry department, using a quasi-experimental design. Cases were studied in a systematic way approximately 15 and 27 months after intake. Over 8 in 10 of these had had individual psychotherapy, together with social casework for the family. An algorithm combining evidence of neurotic disorder with impairment (category 300 of ICD-9) with high mood scores on a systematic child interview allowed a posthoc diagnosis of depression. On the basis of these joint criteria, approximately 31% of the sample were found to have clinical depression on presentation. Of those diagnosed as depressed at intake, over 50% showed comorbidity with conduct disorder — which is indicative of the complexity of psychopathology in this sample. In those who were depressed, clinical depression reduced by 91% at first follow-up and 95.5% by the second follow-up. These findings offer support of the efficacy of individual psychodynamic psychotherapy combined with multimodal approaches for depressed children.

Tebbutt et al [6] have reported a worrying continuity of depression in sexually abused children over a long time span (5 years) and stated that treatment appeared to have little effect on depression. In an ongoing study of psychotherapy for sexually abused girls [7] the children were interviewed using semi-structured interviews (K-SADS). The extent of psychiatric disturbance in this female cohort was substantial. For these reasons, it was thought unlikely that the disorder would improve spontaneously. Some 59% of the subjects entering therapy were judged to show major depressive disorder at reception but few presented with depression at the end of treatment and the treatment effects were maintained [8]. This amounts to a better outcome than most studies of depressed children, especially those studies which precluded children who had been sexually abused.

While CBT approaches appear promising in the short term, psychodynamic psychotherapy holds the promise of more fundamental and lasting changes in childhood depression by improving the subjects' capacity to resolve internal and external conflicts as they grow up. With the serious nature of childhood/adolescent depression it is crucial that treatments with known efficacy and *more than transitory effects* be provided promptly and skilfully. The above preliminary studies add confidence to the notion of longer term utility of psychodynamic psychotherapy, which is being examined in a multicentre trial (London — I. Kolvin and J. Trowell; Athens — J. Tsiantis; Helsinki — F. Almqvist).

REFERENCES

1. Lewinsohn P.M., Clarke G.N., Hops H., Andrews J. (1990) Cognitive-behavioural treatment for depressed adolescents. *Behav. Ther.*, **21**: 385–401.
2. Clarke G.N., Lewinsohn P., Seeley J. (1997) The second Oregon cognitive-behaviour therapy study with depressive disorder in adolescents. Personal communication to R. Harrington.
3. Wood A.J., Harrington R.C., Moore A. (1996) Controlled trial of a brief cognitive-behavioural intervention in adolescent patients with depressive disorders. *J. Child Psychol. Psychiatry*, **37**: 737–746.
4. Vostanis P., Feehan C., Grattan E. (1998) Two year outcome of children treated for depression. *Eur. Child Adolesc. Psychiatry*, **7**: 12–18.
5. Wrate R., Kolvin I., Garside R., Wolstenholme F., Hulbert C.M., Leitch I. (1995) Helping seriously disturbed children. In *Longitudinal Studies in Child Psychology and Psychiatry* (Ed. A. Nicol), pp. 265–318, Wiley, Chichester.
6. Tebbutt J., Swanston R.K., Oates R., O'Toole B.J. (1997) Five years after child sexual abuse: persisting dysfunction and problems of prediction. *J. Am. Acad. Child Adolesc. Psychiatry*, **36**: 330–339.
7. Trowell J., Kolvin I., Weeramanthri T., Berelowitz M., Leitch I. (1998) Treating girls who have been sexually abused. Report to Department of Health, United States.
8. Trowell J., Kolvin I. (1999) Lessons from a psychotherapy outcome study with sexually abused girls. *Clin. Child Psychol. Psychiatry*, **4**: 79–89.

4.17
Role of Neurobiological and Genetic Factors in Treatment of Childhood Depression

Barbara Geller[1]

In striking contrast to the multitude of positive treatment studies for adults with major depressive disorders (MDD), there are few controlled

[1] *Washington University School of Medicine, 4940 Children's Place, Box 8134, St Louis, MO 63110, USA*

investigations that have demonstrated efficacy for child MDD. As future controlled studies are developed, there will be an escalating need for incorporation of burgeoning neurobiological and familial/molecular genetic findings.

In this regard, several neurobiological and familial-genetic differences between child versus adult populations may account, in part, for the disparate tricyclic antidepressant (TCA) findings to which Prof. Harrington refers in his review. For example, cortisol suppression and rapid eye movement (REM) sleep latency patterns follow developmental trajectories that do not begin to mimic findings in adults until adolescence [1, 2]. Furthermore, in study populations of prepubertal subjects who were either offspring of depressed parents or who were entered as part of pharmacological or neuroendocrine investigations of child MDD, there have been consistent findings of familial loading of mood disorders [3–5]. These findings were not replicated in a clinical case sample [6], perhaps because of differences in study recruitment methods. Regardless of the reason for these disparate results, however, treatment designs that use family history (FH) may be useful. Geller *et al* [7] used this approach after observing that 32% of severe, prepubertal MDD subjects developed bipolar disorders (BP) and that switching was predicted by FH of BP or multigenerational/loaded MDD [8]. Thus, it seemed reasonable to perform a controlled study of lithium for prepubertal MDD with FH predictors of future BP. Although this study had a negative outcome, it is premature to discontinue use of FH in future designs.

Environmental influences on age of onset of MDD include a study of offspring of depressed parents in which familial factors were significant for child and adult onset of MDD, but not for adolescent onset [5]. This is consistent with findings of a significant association between certain life events and the onset of adolescent MDD [9]. Other observations comprised an inverse association of marital disharmony and parental hostility with familial loading in child MDD [6].

Unraveling environmental versus genetic factors and their interaction will be crucial for establishing appropriate length of treatment. More biologically determined MDD may, similar to BP, require indefinite maintenance, while more environmentally related MDD may be responsive to time-limited strategies.

Preventive interventions also need to be considered. In this regard, infant offspring of depressed versus non-depressed mothers were shown to have decreased left frontal electroencephalographic activity [10]. This type of data underscores the need for developing prevention studies that include parental treatment.

With regard to defining subtypes, it has been shown that adolescent twins with MDD had a significantly smaller subgenual prefrontal cortex (SGPFC) [11], a finding that replicated work in unipolar adults [12]. Strong support of these magnetic resonance imaging (MRI) findings in adult MDD came from neuropathological data that showed a significantly lower number of glial cells in the SGPFC [13]. Thus, although not yet at the point of clinical testing, imaging may be diagnostic in the future.

In summary, the field can anticipate treatment paradigms that target specific neurobiological and familial/molecular genetic subtypes.

REFERENCES

1. Puig-Antich J., Goetz D., Hanlon C., Davies M., Thompson J., Chambers W.J., Tabrizi M.A., Weitzman E.D. (1982) Sleep architecture and REM sleep measures in prepubertal children with major depression: a controlled study. *Arch. Gen. Psychiatry*, **39**: 932–939.
2. Puig-Antich J., Dahl R., Ryan N., Novacenko H., Goetz D., Goetz R., Twomey J., Klepper T. (1989) Cortisol secretion in prepubertal children with major depressive disorder. Episode and recovery. *Arch. Gen. Psychiatry*, **46**: 801–809.
3. Puig-Antich J., Goetz D., Davies M., Kaplan T., Davies S., Ostrow L., Asnis L., Twomey J., Iyengar S., Ryan N.D. (1989) A controlled family history study of prepubertal major depressive disorder. *Arch. Gen. Psychiatry*, **46**: 406–418.
4. Neuman R.J., Geller B., Rice J.P., Todd R.D. (1997) Increased prevalence and earlier onset of mood disorders among relatives of prepubertal versus adult probands. *J. Am. Acad. Child Adolesc. Psychiatry*, **36**: 466–473.
5. Wickramaratne P.J., Weissman M.M. (1998) Onset of psychopathology in offspring by developmental phase and parental depression. *J. Am. Acad. Child Adolesc. Psychiatry*, **37**: 933–942.
6. Harrington R., Rutter M., Weissman M., Fudge H., Groothues C., Bredenkamp D., Pickles A., Rende R., Wickramaratne P.J. (1997) Psychiatric disorders in the relatives of depressed probands. I. Comparison of prepubertal, adolescent and early adult onset cases. *J. Affect. Disord.*, **42**: 9–22.
7. Geller B., Cooper T.B., Zimerman B., Frazier J., Williams M., Heath J., Warner K. (1998) Lithium for prepubertal depressed children with family history predictors of future bipolarity: a double-blind, placebo-controlled study. *J. Affect. Disord.*, (in press).
8. Geller B., Clark K., Fox L.W. (1994) Rate and predictors of prepubertal bipolarity during follow-up of 6 to 12 year old depressed children. *J. Am. Acad. Child Adolesc. Psychiatry*, **33**: 461–468.
9. Williamson D.E., Birmaher B., Frank E., Anderson B.P., Matty M.K., Kupfer D.J. (1998) Nature of life events and difficulties in depressed adolescents. *J. Am. Child Adolesc. Psychiatry*, **37**: 1049–1057.
10. Dawson G., Frey K., Panagiotides H., Osterling J., Hessl D. (1997) Infants of depressed mothers exhibit atypical frontal brain activity: a replication and extension of previous findings. *J. Child Psychiat. Psychol.*, **38**: 179–186.
11. Botteron K.N., Raichle M.E., Heath A.C., Price J.L., Sternhell K.E., Singer T.M., Todd R.D. (1999) An epidemiological twin study of prefrontal neuromorphometry in early onset depression. Annual Meeting of Society for Biological Psychiatry (submitted).
12. Drevets W.C., Price J.L., Simpson J.R. Jr, Todd R.D., Reich T., Vannier M., Raichle M.E. (1997) Subgenual prefrontal cortex abnormalities in mood disorders. *Nature*, **386**: 824–827.

13. Ongur D., Drevets W.C., Price J.L. (1998) Glial reduction in the subgenualpre-frontal cortex in mood. *Proc. Natl. Acad. Sci.*, **95**: 13290–13295.

4.18
Depression in the Family
Richard Todd[1]

Prof. Harrington ably reviews studies of the impact of family environment and genetics on the etiology and course of early onset depression. However, recent studies across the lifespan suggest that the heritability of depression has been systematically underestimated and that major determinants of the presence of illness and comorbidity may be genetic in origin.

Heritabilities for major depressive disorder of 40–50% have been reported for population and clinic-based samples of adult twins [1–4]. In part this moderate heritability appears to be due to the poor reliability (temporal stability) of a lifetime diagnosis of mild major depression [1, 4, 5]. Compared to such cross-sectional analyses, analyses of longitudinal data increase heritability estimates for persistent major depression from about 40 to 70% [1], the latter figure comparable to manic-depressive disorder and schizophrenia. In a new birth records-based, twin study of adolescent females, we have found a cross-sectional heritability of 0.55 for major depression ($n = 986$ twin pairs). Interestingly, all of these studies have also found little evidence for shared environmental effects on the transmission of depression.

An unresolved issue is whether depression represents a continuum of differences in sadness or is a discrete state of illness. Recent studies of twins have supported both views. For example, estimated heritability for the *number* of depressive symptoms is about 70% in a general sample of twin children and adolescents, with increasing heritability from childhood to adolescence [6]. In contrast, latent class analysis suggests three genetically discrete syndromes of depression in the general population [7]. Using the same sample of young adult female twins, Kendler and Gardner [8] argued for the presence of a continuum of depressive symptoms and severities with respect to *predicting* recurrence risk for depression in twins. In our population-based study of female adolescent twins, we found higher heritabilities for symptom counts than for categorical diagnoses of depression.

Depression has also been reported to be frequently comorbid with a variety of other disorders such as anxiety and alcoholism. In young adult twins the

[1]*Department of Psychiatry, Box 8134, Washington University School of Medicine, 4940 Children's Place, St Louis, MO 63110, USA*

genetic contributions to depression appear to be completely overlapping with the genetic contributions to generalized anxiety disorder (reviewed in [9]). In adolescent female twins, we find substantial overlap of depression with both anxiety disorders and disruptive behavior disorders. The overlap with anxiety is largely genetic, while the overlap with disruptive behavior disorders is largely environmental. When the extended family members of children with prepubertal onset depression or manic-depressive illness are examined, increased rates of both affective disorders and alcoholism are found [10]. In family studies of adults, the comorbidity of major depressive disorder and alcoholism appears to be largely through environmental mechanisms, with only limited overlap of genetic factors (reviewed in [11]).

In summary, child and adolescent depression are highly familial disorders which appear to have major genetic determinants of risk, but which have complex determinants of course and comorbidity. Whether depression is best viewed as a discrete illness or as the severe end of a continuum of mood disturbance is unclear. Only by understanding these distinctions and mechanisms of interaction are we likely to make significant progress in diagnosis and in understanding who responds to what type of treatment. The power of such investigations will be greatly enhanced by using a family/genetic perspective to look more powerfully at the effects of both genes and environment.

REFERENCES

1. Kendler K.S., Neale M.C., Kessler R.C., Heath A.C., Eaves L.J. (1993) The lifetime history of major depression in women: reliability and heritability. *Arch. Gen. Psychiatry*, **50**: 863–870.
2. Lyons M.J., Eisen S.A., Goldberg J., True W., Lin N., Meyer J.M., Toomey R., Faraone S.V., Merla-Ramos M., Tsuang M.T. (1998) A registry-based twin study of depression in men. *Arch. Gen. Psychiatry*, **55**: 468–472.
3. Torgersen S. (1986) Genetic factors in moderately severe and mild affective disorders. *Arch. Gen. Psychiatry*, **43**: 222–226.
4. McGuffin P., Katz R., Watkins S., Rutherford J. (1996) A hospital-based twin register of the heritability of DSM-IV unipolar depression. *Arch. Gen. Psychiatry*, **53**: 126–136.
5. Rice J.P., Rochberg N., Endicott J., Lavori P.W., Miller C. (1992) Stability of psychiatry diagnoses: an application to the affective disorders. *Arch. Gen. Psychiatry*, **49**: 824–830.
6. Tharpar A., McGuffin P. (1994) A twin study of depressive symptoms in childhood. *Br. J. Psychiatry*, **165**: 259–265.
7. Kendler K.S., Eaves L.J., Walters E.E., Neale M.C., Heath A.C., Kessler R.C. (1996) The identification and validation of distinct depressive syndromes in a population-based sample of female twins. *Arch. Gen. Psychiatry*, **53**: 391–399.
8. Kendler K.S., Gardner C.O. (1998) Boundaries of major depression: an evaluation of DSM-IV. *Am. J. Psychiatry*, **155**: 172–177.

9. Todd R.D., Heath A. (1996) The genetic architecture of depression and anxiety in youth. *Curr. Opin. Psychiatry*, **9**: 257–261.
10. Todd R.D., Geller B., Neuman R., Fox L., Hickok J. (1996) Increased prevalence of alcoholism in relatives of depressed and bipolar children. *J. Am. Acad. Child Adolesc. Psychiatry*, **35**: 716–724.
11. Todd R.D. (1997) The link between parental alcoholism and childhood mood disorders: a familial/genetic perspective. *Medscape Mental Health*, **2** (4).

5

Depressive Disorders in the Elderly: A Review

Edmond Chiu[1], David Ames[1], Brian Draper[2] and John Snowdon[3]

[1]*University of Melbourne, Australia;* [2]*University of New South Wales and Prince of Wales Hospital, Sydney, Australia;* [3]*University of Sydney, Australia*

INTRODUCTION

This paper provides an overview of the literature on depression in the elderly, and draws the attention of the readers to some, but not all, important issues related to this condition, which is still awaiting further exploration in its clinical presentation, epidemiology, treatment and prognosis. Aetiological factors are also briefly considered in the chapter.

The summary of available evidence is not meant to be exhaustive. It serves to highlight issues of some importance as viewed by the authors. Readers may have other equally or more urgent considerations within their own frameworks.

An exciting future for the study of depression in the elderly is anticipated. The developments in neuroimaging, neuropsychopharmacology and molecular biology will herald a very vigorous body of data which will make this review obsolete in the not too distant future, requiring a total revision and reconceptualization of the subject. The authors eagerly look forward to such development.

PRESENTATION AND DIAGNOSIS OF DEPRESSION IN THE ELDERLY

Is Depression in Old Age Different from Depression in Younger Adults?

The currently used diagnostic systems (DSM-IV [1] and ICD-10 [2]) do not identify any clinical features which are different in old age depression

Depressive Disorders, Second Edition. Edited by Mario Maj and Norman Sartorius.
© 2002 John Wiley & Sons Ltd.

compared with depression in younger adults. Studies comparing depression in older vs. younger adults have produced inconsistent results. Brown et al [3] reflected on the essential similarity between younger and older patients and between patients with early or late onset. The similarity in the "core" phenomenological picture is supported by Baldwin [4], Blazer et al [5], Burvill et al [6], Greenwald and Kramer-Ginsberg [7] and Brodaty et al [8]. On the other hand, Georgotas [9] observed that elderly people with depressive disorders complained less of subjective lowering of mood than younger persons. Hypochondriasis (overconcern with the fear of bodily illness) was found more often in older compared with younger patients [10]. De Alarcon [11] and Good et al [12] reported the preponderance of somatic complaints. Gurland [10] reported greater agitation, which was also noted by Winokur et al [13], whereas a more "endogenous" picture was reported by Blazer et al [14]. More recent studies have reported other differences: Blazer et al [5] detected more weight loss and constipation in older patients but fewer suicidal thoughts; Burvill et al [6] found lower Hamilton Rating Scale for Depression (HAM-D) and Mini Mental State Examination (MMSE) scores and more "organic" features on neuroimaging by computed tomography (CT) scans; Baldwin [4] and Gurland et al [15] noted that older age was related to physical disability, health problems and adverse environments.

The more frequent occurrence of delusions reported by Hordern [16] was supported by Meyers et al [17] and Meyers and Greenberg [18], but not confirmed by the work of Nelson and Bowers [19] and Nelson et al [20].

Most of the above studies were conducted in samples of inpatients, leading to the criticism that the subjects may be more severely ill and do not necessarily reflect a general picture of the elderly living in the community. Oxman et al [21], examining symptom patterns in patients fulfilling Research Diagnostic Criteria (RDC [22]) for minor depressive disorder, identified three symptoms — irritability, feeling pushed to get things done, and loss of interest — as age-related. Kivelä and Pahkala [23–25], in their series of studies based on community samples, found that older males have more initial and middle insomnia, loss of interest and depressed mood, whereas older females have more anxiety, somatic symptoms, initial insomnia, loss of interest and depressed mood.

Downes et al [26] employed a scalar analysis to examine the hierarchical organization of depressive symptoms in old age. Highly rated affective symptoms included worrying, crying, feeling life being not worth living, and the future being frightening, while highly rated somatic symptoms were subjective slowing, restlessness and hypochrondriacal preoccupations.

The Epidemiological Catchment Area (ECA) community sample at Piedmont, including 1606 subjects over 60 years, was examined by Fredman et al [27]. They reported rates of 14.8% for sleep disturbance, 10% for thought of death and 5% for depressed mood. Since only 5% of community subjects reported depressed mood, it is understandable that only 1.7% of the sample received the diagnosis of major depression, using the strict categorical diagnostic approach of DSM-III.

Is Depression in the Older Person Necessarily Associated with Cognitive Impairment and Structural Abnormalities?

The concept of depressive "pseudodementia" [28] with rapid onset of loss of interest, mental slowing, poor concentration, impaired memory and orientation, in the presence of severe depression associated with self-deprecation, guilt, loss of appetite and suicidal thoughts, has gained certain status, especially when it has been shown that the cognitive deficits responded well to antidepressant therapy.

Alexopoulos et al [29] followed up 57 depressed patients annually over an average period of 3 years. Their survival analysis revealed an almost five-fold increase in the risk of developing dementia over those 3 years for those presenting originally with what was considered to be "reversible dementia". They were unable to identify clinical predictors of eventual dementia as neuropsychological and imaging data were not systematically recorded at baseline. The study of Reding et al [30], however, identified that the presence of cerebrovascular, extrapyramidal or spinocerebellar disorder, together with development of confusion on low doses of tricyclic drugs, were good baseline predictors of future development of dementia.

Abas et al [31] found that 70% of her depressive subjects had memory deficits and cognitive slowing, the severity of which was comparable to a group of patients with Alzheimer's disease. However, aphasia and apraxia rarely occurred in depressive subjects, whose poor memory was improved by the use of cues, suggesting that the basis of deficits is the unreliable retrieval of memories laid down, whereas deficits in Alzheimer's disease are related to the earliest (registration) stage of memory establishment.

The current evidence seems to suggest that depression in the elderly is often associated with cognitive impairment, which may persist in a small proportion of patients. There is currently no conclusive evidence to characterize the group of patients who will proceed to irreversible dementia.

Subtypes of Depression in the Elderly

The fact that the current diagnostic categories do not adequately describe older individuals with depression [32] raises the necessity for additional diagnostic categories to be examined to adequately classify depressive disorders experienced by the elderly. In particular, the addition has been suggested of minor depression [33, 34] or subsyndromal depression, being a collection of less severe though potentially dysfunctional disorders which cause significant suffering in the elderly. The establishment of diagnostic criteria for subsyndromal depression is an issue awaiting further debate and research. The debate should also include whether a dimensional (spectrum disorder) approach may be more appropriate than the current orthodoxy of a categorical approach.

In non-Western cultural environments, the diagnosis of "major depression" may not apply to some patients who present with "depressive disorder equivalents" [35]. Many Asian patients have somatic, psychomotor and vegetative symptoms without dysphoria or depressed mood and prefer the culturally more acceptable diagnosis of "neurasthenia" [36, 37].

Caine [38] was cogent in his argument that the syndromatically defined diagnoses which have occupied nosology in the last two decades, while enhancing research vigour and reliability, leading the movement of psychiatric research from the anecdotal to the scientific, unfortunately have also created an environment of "intentional suppression of variability" by which the confounding factors (medical illnesses, heterogeneous symptom clusters) have been "defined out" of studies. The "secondary" (symptomatic/organic) psychiatric syndromes have been subjected to an unsatisfactory dichotomous decision-making process, which separates the clinical environment from the heuristical, and has driven research in a direction which is increasingly unrelated to the reality of depressive disorders in the elderly.

Baldwin [39], in his comprehensive review, suggested that a delusional subtype may be justified. Delusions are usually persecutory and hypochrondriacal, are not associated with a different outcome, and constantly recur in subsequent episodes. Meyers and Greenberg [18] found that delusions predominate in female depressed subjects, and Kivelä and Pahkala [40] reported that only 1% of a community sample had depressive delusions. Such limited supportive evidence awaits further replication before delusional depression can be accepted as a distinct entity.

The coexistence or the development of depression in patients with dementia has been observed. A review by Wragg and Jeste [41] noted that depressed mood occurred in 0–80% (mean 41%) of subjects, while depressive disorder (including dysthymia) was reported in 0–86% (mean 19%) of subjects. Greenwald *et al* [42] and Rovner [43] reported a prevalence rate of 17% and 11%, respectively, of major depression in patients with Alzheimer's disease. Further, more severe cognitive impairment was noted to be associated with major depression. Burns *et al* [44] found depressive symptoms in some two thirds of subjects with Alzheimer's disease, while Kumar [45] found that 50% of carers thought that subjects with dementia were depressed, and Reifler *et al* [46] and Merriam *et al* [47] reported a figure of 26% and 86%, respectively.

Vascular depression is a relatively new concept suggested by the studies of Alexopoulos [29] and Krishnan [48] and Krishnan *et al* [49, 50]. The neuroimaging studies of Pearlson *et al* [51], Rabins *et al* [52], Sackheim [53] and Zubenko [54] add to the possibilities that structural substrate abnormality of the brain may play a role in the aetiology of a possible subtype of depression in the elderly. The presence of vascular pathology linked to depression in old age, supported by clinical and neuroimaging evidence, has interesting heuristic, preventive and treatment implications. To establish this as a new subtype of depression will require further research.

In summary, depression in the elderly has similar core features to depression of the younger adult. However, there are some phenomenological differences. The presentation of depression in the elderly may be difficult to detect in special situations such as dementia. The categorical nosological approach to diagnosis excludes a large number of elderly patients whose clinical presentation does not meet strict criteria, but who are nevertheless suffering from a depressive disorder. The subtyping of depression using concepts appropriate to the younger adult is unsatisfactory. Further research is warranted especially on minor (subsyndromal) depression, delusional depression, vascular depression and culturally determined subtypes.

EPIDEMIOLOGY OF DEPRESSION IN OLD AGE

There is conflicting evidence concerning the prevalence of depression in old age. There have been several large surveys of adult populations that purported to show a lower rate of depressive disorders among elderly than among younger adults [55–57]. The latest of these studies found that 1.7% of persons aged 65 years or more manifested affective disorders, in contrast to rates of 5.0% in the 55–64 age group and 6.4% or more in age groups of 18–54 years [57]. One sixth of the affective disorders were labelled as dysthymia while five sixths had "depression".

The two large North American surveys provided data concerning major depressive episode, dysthymia and manic episode: in the Epidemiologic Catchment Area study [ECA] [55], the 1-month prevalence rate of major depressive episode in those aged 65 years or more was 0.7%, while the rate for dysthymia was 1.8%. In the Canadian study [56], the 6-month prevalence rate of major depressive episode was 1.2% and the lifetime prevalence of dysthymia was 3.3%.

In contrast, there have been a number of studies of older adults that have shown high rates of depression. Blazer and Williams [58] found that 14.7% of a community sample aged 65 years or more showed significant dysphoric symptoms: 3.7% had major depression, 6.5% were dysphoric with physical health impairment and 4.5% were "simply dysphoric". Since then, studies in various countries [59–64] have shown that depression, variously described as "pervasive" or "cases", ranged in prevalence from 11.5 to 17.7%. Copeland *et al* [63] estimated that the incidence of cases of depression in old age was at least 2.37% per year. In a recent article for a mainly non-psychiatrist readership, Macdonald [65] wrote that "the prevalence of depression among people aged over 65 is 15% in the general community, 25% in general practice patients".

Not all studies of depression in old age have reported such high rates. Henderson *et al* [66] found that only 0.4% of a sample of Canberra (Australian) residents aged 70 years or more had major depression, and 0.6% had dsythymia. Elsewhere in Australia, Kay *et al* [60] had previously reported that 10.2% of an elderly sample had major depression. Prevalence figures from studies limited to elderly populations have varied to an astonishing extent. Copeland [67] reanalysed data from a London sample (65 years+) to show that 4.6% had major depression and 6.3% dysthymic disorder, but major depression rates of only 1–2% have been reported recently in other European studies (i.e. more similar to the large North American survey results). These studies showed differing rates of dysthymic disorder. In Spain [68], 1% had major depression, 1.3% dysthymic disorder and 2.5% adjustment disorder with depressed mood — a total of 4.8% with "any depression". In Finland [69], 2.2% had major depression, 11.9% dysthymic disorder, 2% atypical depression and 0.5% cyclothymic disorder. In The Netherlands [70], the prevalence of major depression escalated from 1.3% at age 55–59 to 2.7% at age 80–85 years, while the prevalence of minor depression ranged from 9.4% (age 55–59) to 16.7% (80–85 years).

In an ECA "offshoot" study, during which psychiatrists interviewed subjects who had scored positive ($n = 810$) on questions screening for mental morbidity, Romanoski *et al* [71] found that the prevalence of DSM-III depressive disorders increased with age (4.9% at ages 25–44 and 45–64, 5.5% at age 65 years or more), but that proportionally far more of the old age depressions were "depressive disorders other than major depression". The percentage of elderly subjects who were actively depressed, but were not diagnosed as having a DSM-III depressive disorder, was nearly double the rate in those aged 25–44 and 45–64 years.

There have been studies limited to the "very elderly": Girling *et al* [72] estimated the prevalence of DSM-III-R major depressive disorder in a community sample aged 77 years or more to be 2.4%, but this figure did not include a similar percentage of people with dementia who had a "depressive syndrome". Skoog [73] reported that 13% of non-demented people aged 85 years or more, including some in institutions, fulfilled criteria for major depressive syndrome, and a further 6.6% had dysthymia. Roberts *et al* [74] reported the prevalence of major depressive episodes among American samples aged 50–69 years ($n = 1482$) and 70 years or more ($n = 737$) to be, respectively, 7.4% and 12.1%.

Sampling and methodological differences may explain some of the discrepancies between the findings of these and other studies. It is likely that researchers vary somewhat in their understanding or interpretation of DSM descriptions such as "markedly diminished" and "most of the day" [1]. Even if ratings were believed to be reliable, it is likely that differences in selection and screening processes, exclusion criteria and interview techniques result in differing response rates and a differing likelihood of achieving full cooperation during interviews.

Lyness et al [75] provided evidence that some older patients with clinically significant depression underreport their symptoms. Elderly persons with depression may not acknowledge being sad, down or depressed in mood [76, 77]. Knauper and Wittchen [78] found that older and younger subjects reported depressive symptoms equally frequently, but that elderly people more often attributed such symptoms to coexisting physical illness. Disability and impairments (which are more prevalent in old age) may make it difficult to take part in surveys. Unless interview arrangements can be adapted to ensure participation of a truly representative sample of elderly people, bias will affect results.

The ECA study's methodology has been criticized [79]. Henderson et al [66] used a schedule which (in contrast to the ECA's Diagnostic Interview Schedule) did not exclude symptoms of depression that might be attributable to medical illness, medication, drugs or alcohol. In spite of thus avoiding one of the ECA study's sources of bias, their findings led them to conclude that the prevalence of depression in old age in Canberra may be lower than in younger age groups.

Many clinicians, after reviewing the above-mentioned evidence, have concluded that depression becomes less common in old age. Explanations for this low prevalence have been sought, including the suggestion of a cohort effect [32]. A higher mortality rate among depressed people could lead to a reduced prevalence of depression in old age. Exposure to adverse experiences during earlier years might induce increased resistance to depression later in life [76].

The following key questions should be asked:

1. How do we define depression? Reifler [80] states that when geriatric psychiatrists talk about depression in elderly persons, they are usually referring to major depression. Is this correct? Evidence quoted above [e.g. 59, 63] would suggest that some psychiatrists disagree. If it *is* so, is it appropriate?
2. Do we believe that (in spite of conflicting evidence) the prevalence of major depression, and maybe of dysthymia, is lower in old age than among younger age groups? If so, what are the clinical implications? Would this belief affect conclusions about the need for clinical services among elderly people?

3. Do we believe that major depression and dysthymia are more severe conditions and need more attention/services than other forms of clinically significant depression? Does a diagnosis of major depression trigger a "usual" clinical response, different from management approaches to cases of depression that do not fulfil criteria for major depression or dysthymia?

The relevance of the above questions becomes obvious when we consider why researchers seek to obtain epidemiological data. Jenkins *et al* [81] outlined reasons for carrying out large-scale community studies of psychiatric morbidity. Firstly, effective policy needs to be based on epidemiology. Secondly, such studies allow needs to be assessed and thus are useful in planning services.

As well as providing data on health care needs, epidemiological data lead to insights about aetiology, prevention and treatment of disorders [82]. However, meaningful conclusions about factors related to clinically significant depressions will be limited if a majority of cases of depression are excluded from consideration in such studies. And clearly, the validity of conclusions about service needs must be in doubt if, through *strict application of diagnostic criteria* (as in Henderson *et al*'s study), only a small, select proportion of the cases of depression are identified as in need of services. Researchers apply diagnostic criteria in the same way to young and old, even though it is recognized that comorbid physical changes and other factors associated with ageing may lead to "masking" of depressive features. Caine *et al* [38] commented that affective disturbances often are not expressed symptomatically among elderly patients in the same stereotypic fashion as that encountered among younger patients. They added that current use of rigorous diagnostic criteria might prove highly reliable but not especially valid.

Taking Henderson *et al*'s [66] study as an example, 1% of community residents aged over 70 years were labelled as depressed (i.e. they fulfilled criteria for major depressive episode or dysthymia), but it is likely that (based on other reports mentioned above) far more than 1% of elderly people had clinical depressions but did not fulfil criteria for the two affective disorders on which the study focused. Yet there is evidence [e.g. 83] that the clinical and prognostic consequences are just as serious in a large proportion of those other depressions as they are in major depression or dysthymia. The difficulty (for Henderson and others) is that alternative diagnostic categories have not yet been well defined as discrete and meaningful entities. Blazer [32] declared that "there is a need for additional diagnostic categories to describe the complex ways that depression presents in older adults". He stated that although DSM-III-R is not "age biased", it fails to accommodate correlates of age such as comorbid cognitive impairment and comorbid physical illness. He referred to the suggested category of "minor depression" but commented that this is probably a collection of less severe though potentially dysfunctional disorders, rather than a single entity.

Thus, in answer to the first question it is apparent that researchers and clinicians differ in their understanding of the term "depression". There is some (disputed) evidence that the prevalence of major depression and dysthymia as defined by the DSM system is lower in old age than in youth. But the third question is more important. To answer it, we must review evidence about the correlates of old age depressions, including those that do not conform to strict DSM criteria for diagnosing major depression and dysthymia.

CORRELATES OF DEPRESSION IN OLD AGE

Health and Disability

Both cross-sectional and longitudinal studies have provided evidence of a close relationship between physical health and depression [84]. Blazer et al [33] found that chronic illness and disability, analysed as separate variables, were both significantly associated with depression rating scores. In a study of depression in a large community sample of older adults, Kennedy et al [85] reported that poor health and disability explained 35% of the total variance, and outranked demographic, social support and life event characteristics in their association with depressive symptoms. In a longitudinal study, they found that increasing disability and declining health preceded the emergence of depression in many subjects, and changes in health provided "a major if incomplete" explanation of the remission or persistence of depressive symptoms.

Henderson et al [66] reported significant associations between scores of elderly subjects on a continuous measure of depression on the one hand, and self-ratings of health, pain, disability in activities of daily living, and infor- mant ratings of disability, on the other. In a longitudinal study, Henderson et al [86] found that, after controlling for initial depression scores, the only significant predictive psychological and physical health variables were neuroticism, the number of medical conditions and the number of physical symptoms.

Caution is needed, however, when interpreting the evidence. Self-ratings concerning symptoms and health may be influenced by mood. Subjective measures of pain and physical health have a much stronger relation with depression scores than do objective health measures [87].

In an important series of papers, Prince et al [64, 88] suggested that associations between physical health changes and depression scores relate mainly to the degrees of consequent functional impairment and handicap (i.e.

disadvantage in performance of a normal role). They showed that handicap due to disability was the most important predictor of the onset of pervasive depression, but that maintenance of depression was related more to low levels of social support and participation than to disablement. Previously, Gurland et al [59] had suggested that disability is the most important determinant of the rates and outcomes of all types of chronic depression in old age.

It is well recognized that the prevalence of depression is considerably increased among people with serious medical problems, such as cancer, Parkinson's disease and stroke [89]. Valvanne et al [90] reported a strong association between major depression and objective ratings of ill-health and functional incapacity in subjects aged 75, 80 and 85 years. In a study of medical inpatients aged over 60 years, the strongest correlate of major depression was severity of medical illness [91]: 22% and 28%, respectively, of these patients experienced major or minor depression. Minor depression was less strongly correlated with medical illness severity.

Burvill et al [92] reported that the prevalence of major depression 4 months after stroke was 15%, while 8% had minor depression. Morris et al [93], examining patients 8 weeks after acute stroke, reported that major depression following stroke was independent of stroke severity. However, minor depression after a stroke was related to level of disability and was best construed (the authors stated) as a psychological reaction to the functional consequences of stroke. Those with minor depression were physically more disabled, but scored lower on a depression rating than those with major depression.

In a longitudinal community study of 646 subjects aged 55–85 years, Beekman et al [84] found that chronic physical illness and functional limitations were associated with minor but not major depression. Minor depression was defined as "all clinically relevant depressive syndromes not fulfilling rigorous diagnostic criteria for major depression". They cautioned that their measurement of physical health variables had relied on subject reports, but concluded that major depression has its origins in longstanding personal vulnerability, while minor depression is more often a reaction to stresses encountered in later life. It is relevant to note that "minor depression" includes "adjustment disorder with depressed mood". Broadhead et al [34] similarly had reported an association of physical illness with minor more than with major depression.

It has been reported that elderly people with physical illness are given more support by relatives [94]; however, the potential stress-buffering role of social support has been found to be limited to subjects with minor depression [84]. This, too, may have implications concerning use of resources.

The prevalence of various chronic medical conditions is much higher in old age [38]. The importance of physical ill-health and disability in relation to onset and persistence of depression in old age is undoubted. This has implications as regards treatment. The above discussion has focused on the need to consider minor depressions as well as major depression. There is good reason to consider both psychological and biological treatment approaches in cases associated with disability or physical ill-health.

Dementia

The prevalence of depression among persons with dementia is high (12% with major depression, compared to 4% of non-demented persons aged 75 years+), and depression is associated with increased levels of disability in this population [95]. The high prevalence of depression in nursing homes (where most residents have dementia and many have chronic physical illnesses) has been documented [96, 97]. Clarification concerning the multi-factorial aetiology of such cases, the relative importance of physical health factors, and trials of treatments that differ according to the way the depression presents, is awaited.

Social Factors

There is strong evidence of associations between social factors and the onset of late life depression [98]. Social factors may also relate to differential patterns of recovery from major [99] and non-major depressions.

Murphy [100] referred to the role of recent life events in precipitating depression; she had found that depressed elderly patients were at least twice as likely as normal subjects to have experienced a severe event in the previous year. She suggested that the higher prevalence of depression among working-class people compared to middle-class subjects could be explained by their greater liability to suffer from severe adverse events (including physical illnesses). Furthermore, persistent major social difficulties (e.g. housing, finance or family problems) were also associated with depression. Murphy found that having no confidant at all was associated with an increased risk of depression, but only in conjunction with a severe life event.

Emmerson et al [101] reported an increase in severe life events in the 3 months prior to onset of late life depression. Lack of confidant was reported by men (45% compared to 3% of controls) but not women (6% vs. 4%).

Others have reported that living alone is associated with an increased risk of depression in old age [62, 102, 103], and there are higher rates of depression among those who are widowed or divorced [55, 103]. The rate of depression has been found to be higher among women in some studies [66, 68, 104], though whether this might relate to their greater likelihood of living alone and without a spouse has not been clarified. Green et al [105] found that feelings of loneliness were predictive of having depression at 3-year follow-up.

Having perceptions of adequate social support is protective against depression in old age [106]. Henderson *et al* [86] reported that social support from close friends was one of the factors accounting for differences in depression score in a follow-up study of 709 elderly people, some of them being in nursing homes.

Some studies have reported a negative association between depression in old age and educational level [68]; Pahkala *et al* [69] found this applied to men only.

George [99] referred to recent research suggesting that physiological mechanisms such as immune functioning or cardiovascular reactivity might be responsible for precipitation of depression by stressful events, experiences or situations. However, she commented that the effects of social factors on the onset of, and recovery from, depression tend to be weaker in old age than for younger adults. She also pointed out that there had been inadequate investigation of social factors in relation to diagnostic subtypes of depression in old age. In particular, it would seem important to examine the interaction between social factors, personality variables and onset/outcome of different subtypes. George [99] and Murphy [107] have pointed to a need for studies examining interactions between the multiple determinants of late-life depression, using an integrated approach which brings together the biological and psychosocial perspectives.

Kendler *et al* [108], exploring a model for the prediction of major depressive episodes in a sample of women (mean age 30 years), concluded that at least four major and interacting risk factor domains need consideration in order to understand their aetiology: traumatic experiences, genetic factors, temperament and interpersonal relations. In this younger population, the effects of physical health, disability and brain changes were not discussed. Extension of the model is needed to account for some of the associations observed in relation to late-life depression.

Relevant to interaction models, Rozzini *et al* [109] used multiple regression to show that co-occurrence of multiple disadvantage conditions (e.g. disability, poor social support and low income) is independently associated with an increased occurrence of symptomatic depression. Cervilla and Prince [110] found that the presence of cognitive impairment modifies the association between life events and social support deficits and depression.

Biological Factors

There is now an extensive literature concerning brain changes associated with different types of depression. For example, Austin and Mitchell [111] proposed investigation of a hypothesis that the prefrontal cortex and basal ganglia are primary sites of dysfunction in melancholia. Depression occurs with increased frequency in patients with disorders involving basal ganglia pathology. Regional deficits of functional (neural) activity are consistently detected during brain neuroimaging of individuals with ongoing affective symptoms [112].

Neuroimaging studies give support for a view that a neurodegenerative process underlies the development of a proportion of late-onset depressions. Magnetic resonance imaging (MRI) revealed more subcortical white matter hyperintensities in the brains of subjects whose first depressive episode occurred after the age of 50 years. This accords with evidence of a lack of association between late-onset depression and family history of affective illness [8, 113, 114].

It has been suggested that the association of hyperintensities and late-onset depression is a function of cerebrovascular disease [115]. Hickie et al [114] hypothesized that cerebrovascular insufficiency in older persons leads to changes in subcortical structures which then provide a structural basis for development of depression. However, Lyness et al [116] found no difference in cerebrovascular risk factors between older patients with major depression and normal controls. Nor were these factors associated with age of onset of depression. Reasons for the association have not yet been demonstrated.

It is of interest that although rates of psychotic and melancholic depression appear to increase with age, no difference was found between early-onset and late-onset depression in levels of psychomotor disturbance [117]. It might have been expected that age-related changes in the basal ganglia might result in more psychomotor retardation in late-onset cases. Again there is a need for more studies.

In the area of neurochemistry and neuroendocrinology, early studies have given some indication of the possible fertile areas of research. The age-related reduction of cortical serotoninergic binding [118] and of dopaminergic function [119] points towards a possible predisposition of the elderly towards depressive disorders. The reduction of cerebrospinal fluid (CSF), homovanillic acid (HVA), metabolite of dopamine, was found by Brown and Gershon [120] to be associated with increased brain, plasma and CSF monoamine oxidase B (MAO-B) activity. Karlsson [121] reported an increased turnover of noradrenaline and serotonin in normal ageing brain, whereas the principal metabolite of noradrenaline, MHPG (3-methoxy-4-hydroxyphenylglycol) did not show significant alteration with age. These reported changes do not clarify the role of monoamine neurotransmitters in the development of depressive disorders in the elderly.

The influence of neuroendocrine changes in the elderly is equally unclear. Studies with the dexamethasone suppression test (DST), although showing non-suppression to occur more frequently in the elderly depressives than in younger patients, and detecting some correlation between DST normalization and clinical improvement in elderly patients with depression, also showed the positivity of the test in some 30% of patients with Alzheimer's disease, thus demonstrating an unsatisfactory specificity in old age depression [122]. The association between DST and the presence of leukoariosis reported by Krishnan [48], whilst providing some support for the concept of "vascular depression", adds a confounding factor in the understanding of the role of DST as a marker in elderly depression.

Similarly, the blunted thyroid-stimulating hormone (TSH) response to thyrotropin-releasing hormone (TRH) occurs both in depression in the elderly and in a third of Alzheimer's disease subjects [123, 124]. Targum *et al* [125], by demonstrating the variability of TRH test response in depressed and normal elderly subjects, call into further question the specificity of TSH response for elderly depression.

TREATMENT OF DEPRESSION IN OLD AGE

The advent of an evidence-based approach to psychiatry has highlighted limitations in our knowledge about the efficacy and effectiveness of the treatment of depression in old age. Clinicians have long recognized that, due to the biological, psychological and social effects of ageing, older people with depression require adjustments to treatment protocols. These adjustments have primarily relied on accumulated clinical wisdom, due to the lack of data from controlled studies, which often excluded the elderly.

Numerous factors affect the quality of available evidence. There are doubts about whether the data obtained from most existing randomized controlled trials (RCTs) of antidepressants can be generalized, due to the use of samples not typical of routine clinical practice. For example, only 4.2% of depressed elderly patients referred for inclusion in a phase III antidepressant study could be recruited [126]. Application of stringent exclusion criteria regarding concomitant medication, physical and psychiatric comorbidity was the main reason.

The "old", physically ill and institutionalized elderly are underrepresented in RCTs, despite the latter two having the highest rates of depression. Further, the presence of comorbid acute or serious physical illness reduces the chance of recovery [127, 128]. Yet, it is information regarding the safety, acceptability and effectiveness of treatments in such patients that is of the greatest benefit to the clinician. In addition, RCTs of antidepressants focus on acute treatment, rather than treatment resistance or relapse prevention. There have been few prospective studies that have examined these issues and none of them has been controlled [129–131].

Most RCTs of depression treatment in old age involve the use of antide-pressant medication alone. In routine clinical practice, effective management often requires a combination of interventions [132]. There have been few studies that have examined the effectiveness of combining antidepressants with psychotherapy [133], let alone other non-pharmacological interventions such as exercise, music therapy and social groups, despite their frequent use by clinicians. Yet the combination of antidepressants and psychotherapy may have a better outcome for the acute treatment and maintenance of major depression in the elderly than either modality alone [134]. More complex questions of which combination/s of interventions best suit particular subtypes of depression, or depressions complicated by comorbid conditions, remain largely unaddressed.

The effectiveness of treatment also depends on the skills of the clinician. There is evidence that mental health specialists obtain better outcomes for depression in old age compared with other health professionals. For example, an RCT of the treatment of depression in the frail elderly living at home by a psychogeriatric team showed that significantly more of the intervention group (58%), than the general practitioner (GP) managed control group (25%), had recovered after 6 months [135]. It has been suggested that investigation of variations in recovery rates between centres in multicentre drug trials may yield important information on the nuances of treatment, but this is hampered by the small sample size at each centre [132]. This is particularly important in the evaluation of psychosocial treatments [136]. Effectiveness may also depend on the model of service delivery utilized. For example, the use of clinical pathways for old age depression has been shown to improve the processes of inpatient care and reduce length of stay [137]. Better clinical outcomes have been obtained in specialty psychiatric units as compared to general medical wards [138].

The interface between specialists and primary care has been examined with mixed results [139, 140]. While there is evidence that collaborations between psychogeriatric services and general practitioners (GPs) can improve the detection of depression and the treatment strategies employed [140], improved treatment outcomes are more elusive. The style of collaboration is important. Pure consultative models are ineffective [141, 142]. "Shared care", where there is greater educational and supervisory interaction between the specialist service and the GP, may provide better outcomes, with one RCT showing a significant reduction in depressive symptoms over a $9\frac{1}{2}$-month programme [143].

Few elderly depressives seen in primary care have uncomplicated major depressions; most have minor depressions [144]. Yet the treatment of minor depression, dysthymia, depression secondary to a general medical condition and atypical depressions has been infrequently researched [145, 146]. To a certain extent, the lack of RCTs for these conditions is reflected in the relative neglect of psychotherapy research in old age.

Most controlled trials focus on symptom resolution as determined by changes on various depression rating scales as their main outcome measure. It has been recommended by the National Institute of Mental Health

(NIMH)/MacArthur Foundation Workshop that outcome assessment measures be expanded beyond symptomatology, to include function, disability, morbidity, mortality, quality of life and service use. The widespread adoption of standardized outcome measures was also recommended [136]. Self-perceived outcome measures should also be included [147].

In reviewing the efficacy and effectiveness of depression treatments in old age, we shall focus on patients with problems more typical of clinical practice, especially the physically ill, those with comorbid dementia, nursing home residents, non-major depressives and patients with resistant depression.

Pharmacological Treatment

Since 1964, more than 70 RCTs of the use of antidepressants in old age have been published. Most subjects have been physically well, independently living, "young" old outpatients with non-psychotic major depression and without comorbid psychiatric disorders ("uncomplicated major depression").

Reviews and meta-analyses have concluded that antidepressants are efficacious, with around 50–60% of patients improving as compared to about 30% with placebo [133, 148, 149]. Age alone does not appear to significantly affect the general efficacy of antidepressants in the acute treatment of uncomplicated major depression.

On broader outcome measures, there is some evidence that the selective serotonin reuptake inhibitor (SSRI) fluoxetine may significantly improve functional health and well-being, as measured on the 36-item Short-Form Health Status Survey, compared with placebo [150]. Further, a comparison of sertraline and nortriptyline found that quality of life and cognitive measures were significantly better with sertraline, despite lack of significant differences on depression scales [151]. Self-perceived outcome measures suggest that the elderly may have a delayed onset of antidepressant activity compared with younger patients, that is not detected on depression scales [152].

Acute treatment response is influenced by a number of factors. Older patients whose first episode of major depression occurred before the age of 60 have been found to take 5–6 weeks longer to achieve remission than late-onset depressives [153]. Delayed response has also been found to occur in patients with high baseline anxiety and with outpatient treatment [154]. Poor acute response to pharmacotherapy has been reported to occur in patients with MRI scan hyperintensities in the frontal deep white matter, basal ganglia and pontine reticular formation [155]. Several strategies have been reported to improve the acute response to SSRIs, including one night of total sleep deprivation at the start of therapy [156] and augmentation with oestrogen replacement therapy [157].

Whether specific antidepressants have greater efficacy and effectiveness is unclear even within the narrow focus of uncomplicated major depression. Of the older tricyclic agents (TCAs), it is generally agreed that the secondary amine TCAs (nortriptyline, desipramine) have fewer adverse effects in the elderly [149]. Despite this, tertiary amine TCAs (e.g. amitriptyline, imipramine) have been frequently and inappropriately used as comparators for the newer agents, that is SSRIs, reversible inhibitors of monoamine oxidase A (RIMA), selective noradrenaline and serotonin reuptake inhibitors (SNRIs), $5HT_2$ receptor antagonists and adrenoreceptor antagonists. This has limited the interpretation of studies in the elderly [147]. Non-standard ascertainment of adverse effects of all agents under study has also been a problem [147]. Further, with some of the newer agents (e.g. SNRIs, $5HT_2$ receptor antagonists) there is little or no data available in the elderly.

Meta-analyses of RCTs of SSRIs and RIMA in mixed age groups have shown them to have similar efficacy to TCAs but with better tolerability [158, 159]. Similar conclusions have been drawn in the elderly [149], particularly the "old" old [160]. Effectiveness of treatment with SSRIs is probably enhanced by the greater likelihood of maintaining an adequate dose than with other antidepressants [161].

These advantages may only apply in mild to moderate depression, as doubts have been expressed about their efficacy in severe and melancholic depression [162–165]. In addition, the elderly may not tolerate SSRIs as well as younger people, being more prone to extrapyramidal symptoms and weight loss [166]. The choice of the SSRI may depend on the propensity of an individual agent to cause adverse effects, especially due to pharmacokinetic drug interactions caused by an inhibitory effect on the hepatic cytochrome P450 metabolic system. In this regard, sertraline and citalopram have the least inhibitory effect and may be the SSRIs of choice [167].

Depression Associated with Physical Illness

The stability of the physical illness has a major influence on acute treatment outcome. In acute serious physical illnesses, depression outcome may relate more to changes in the course of physical illness and placebo effect rather than any specific medication effect [168]. Further, RCTs have recruitment difficulties in this population. In one study 90% of patients were excluded because of contraindications to the proposed treatment with a TCA [169]. Drop-out rates of 27–49% following recruitment and incidental mortality of subjects have been reported [170–172].

Placebo-controlled studies have not demonstrated a significant effect of antidepressants in depression associated with acute severe physical illnesses, although small sample sizes limit interpretation of results [see Table 5.1]. In

TABLE 5.1 Controlled trials of antidepressant treatment of depression in elderly patients with acute physical illness

Authors	Patients (no.)	Illnesses and setting	Mean age (years)	Drug	Daily dose, duration	Completers	Side effects	Outcome: comments
Schifano et al, 1990 [170]	48	Geriatric medical inpatients	75	Maprotiline (Map) vs. Mianserin (Mia)	112.5–150 mg (Map); 67.5–90 mg (Mia), 4 weeks	65% (Map) 80% (Mia)	Map = Mia	Mia > Map; short trial, ? any better than placebo response
Tan et al, 1994 [171]	63	General medical inpatients	80	Lofepramine (Lof) vs. Placebo (Pla)	70 mg, 4 weeks	72% (Lof) 74% (Pla)	Lof = 38% Pla = 31%	Lof = Pla; low dose, short trial
Andersen et al, 1994 [173]	28	Acute post-stroke and depression	68.2 (Cit) 65.8 (Pla)	Citalopram (Cit) vs. Pla	10–40 mg, 6 weeks	?	+Nausea and vomiting with Cit	Cit = Pla; 50% recovery both groups
Evans et al, 1997 [172]	82	Geriatric medical inpatients	80.4	Fluoxetine (Flu) vs. Pla	20 mg, 8 weeks	53.8% (Flu) 48.8% (Pla)	Flu = Pla +Gastro-intestinal side effects with Flu	Flu = Pla; Flu trend to better outcome

each of these studies, the antidepressants were well tolerated apart from gastrointestinal upsets with fluoxetine and lofepramine, although data on patients withdrawn due to adverse events were not supplied.

In contrast, the efficacy of antidepressant therapy in depressed older patients with stable or chronic physical illness has been more clearly established, although at times the antidepressant effect may be indirect, for example, by pain reduction [168]. Four placebo-controlled studies of nortriptyline have yielded positive results in the reduction of depressive symptoms in chronically ill patients [174, 175], post-stroke depression [176] and chronic obstructive pulmonary disease [177]. Adverse effects were common, with 17–35% patients withdrawing from studies [175–177]. Low dose doxepin was also found to be effective, with fewer adverse effects, in a 3-week placebo-controlled trial of 24 elderly patients with non-major depression in a rehabilitation unit [178].

However, concerns about the side effects of TCAs, particularly anti-cholinergic effects, orthostatic hypotension and cardiac toxicity, limit their usefulness in the physically ill elderly. The more tolerable and less toxic new-generation antidepressants are potentially the drugs of choice, but there have been few RCTs in the physically ill elderly. A recent RCT of paroxetine and nortriptyline in depressed mixed age patients with ischaemic heart disease demonstrated this potential advantage by finding that, while efficacy was similar, nortriptyline induced an increased heart rate, orthostatic hypotension and heart rate variability [179]. Two RCTs of SSRIs have shown efficacy in the elderly with chronic physical illnesses and post-stroke depression after more than 7 weeks treated with fluoxetine [180] and citalopram respectively [173].

Psychostimulants such as methylphenidate have been proposed as an alternative pharmacological strategy in the physically ill, due to rapid onset of action and favourable cardiovascular profile, but sound controlled studies are lacking [133], with existing studies showing only limited effect [181]. There is also doubt about their safety profile in acutely ill patients [182].

Depression Associated with Dementia

The evidence for the efficacy of antidepressants is limited, as noted by the five RCTs listed in Table 5.2.

The placebo-controlled studies recorded a large placebo response. Only one study of moclobemide with a large sample size of 511 demonstrated a significantly higher response rate with the antidepressant [187], although two studies showed significantly fewer depressive symptoms with citalopram [184] and maprotiline [186]. A comparison of trazodone and folic acid found no significant differences between the agents and while there was a

TABLE 5.2 Controlled trials of antidepressant treatment of depression in elderly patients with dementia

Authors	Patients (no.)	Mean age (years)	Diagnosis	Drug	Daily dose, duration	Comple-ters	Side effects	Outcome: comments
Reifler et al, 1989 [183]	33	72	DSM-III dementia and major depression	Imipramine (Imi) vs. Placebo (Pla)	83 mg (mean); 8 weeks	81.2% (Imi) 88.2% (Pla)	Imi = Pla, +Cognitive impairment with Imi	Imi = Pla, Both improved from baseline
Nyth et al, 1992 [184]	29	65+	DSM-III dementia and major depression	Citalopram (Cit) vs. Pla	10–30 mg; 6 weeks	63%	37% Cit 25% Pla	Cit > Pla
Passeri et al, 1993 [185]	96	65+	Dementia and depression (HAM-D > 17)	Folate (Fol) vs. Trazodone (Tra)	50 mg (Fol), 100 mg (Tra); 8 weeks	100%	1 patient on Tra	Fol = Tra Excluded placebo responders at 2 weeks run-in
Fuchs et al, 1993 [186]	127	65+	DSM-III-R dementia with mild depression	Maprotiline (Map) vs. Pla	75 mg; 8 weeks	78%	17.7% Map 8.1% Pla	Map > Pla on Geriatric Depression Scale
Roth et al, 1996 [187]	511	74.6 (median)	DSM-III dementia and depression	Moclobe-mide (Moc) vs. Pla	400 mg; 6 weeks	85.2% (Moc) 81.4% (Pla)	49.2% Moc 41.3% Pla	Moc > Pla High placebo response

reduction in depressive symptoms, the mean HAM-D scores for both groups remained above 18 after 8 weeks treatment [185].

The impact of these agents on cognitive and behavioural measures needs also to be taken into consideration. Moclobemide was found to improve cognitive function [187], while citalopram improved associated behavioural disturbances including agitation, irritability and restlessness [184, 188]. It has also been reported that sertraline may act on food refusal and affective symptoms in severe dementia where traditional diagnostic criteria for depression are not applicable [189]. In contrast, imipramine was found to further impair cognition [183].

Depression in Residential Care

Antidepressant treatment is frequently inadequate in residential care, with low rates of prescription and inadequate dosages [190–192]. Treatment studies have to contend with the confounding effects of poor physical health, dementia and old age. Few have been undertaken.

The only placebo-controlled trial of antidepressant treatment of major depression in elderly nursing home residents found that nortriptyline was effective in significantly improving depressed mood and reducing suicidality. However, 34% of subjects had adverse events that required termination of treatment, demonstrating the vulnerability of these patients and the need for careful monitoring [175]. In an open-label trial of SSRIs in "old" old depressed nursing home residents, good responses were obtained in those with major depressive disorder (93%), but not in depression associated with dementia (7%) [193].

Non-major Depression

The NIMH Treatment of Depression Collaborative Research Project found no advantage for active medication over placebo among less severely depressed outpatients [194]. Since these findings, several studies have demonstrated that antidepressants may have some efficacy in the elderly with prolonged depressive reactions [195], reactive depression [196] and mild depression [197]. While these studies may challenge the NIMH findings, at this stage there is insufficient evidence to revise them.

Conclusions

In summary, age and chronic stable physical illnesses do not appear to influence the efficacy of antidepressants in major depression. Despite limited research, SSRIs are recommended for first line pharmacotherapy in major depression of mild–moderate severity. The higher rates of adverse effects associated with TCAs reduce their effectiveness, but the secondary amine nortriptyline may be the antidepressant of choice in severe major depression. The efficacy of antidepressant treatment of depression in the elderly with acute or serious physical illnesses is unproven. There is only limited evidence supporting the efficacy of antidepressants in depression complicating dementia and in non-major depression, with SSRIs and moclobemide being drugs of choice largely due to tolerability.

Psychosocial Interventions

There have been relatively few outcome studies of psychosocial interventions for depression in old age. Despite the limited evidence, reviews of psychosocial interventions in general [198] and cognitive-behavioural approaches in particular [199–200] have concluded that they are effective treatments.

A meta-analysis of 17 studies of psychosocial interventions in the elderly found an overall effect size of 0.78 vs. no treatment or placebo control [198]. This did not significantly vary with depression severity or between group and individual treatments. No clear superiority was found for any system of psychotherapy (cognitive, behavioural, reminiscence, psychodynamic, interpersonal, supportive or eclectic). This level of efficacy is similar to that found for the psychotherapy of depression across the age range [201].

A quantitative review of cognitive therapy in the elderly identified only seven studies published between 1981 and 1994 that provided outcome data [200]. Only 362 patients were treated — 120 with cognitive therapy, of whom 75% were in group therapy. Most patients were community-dwelling outpatients. The authors commented on the lack of information provided in the studies about the type and severity of depression being treated and concomitant physical illnesses. Cognitive therapy was found to show a 66% improvement over psychodynamic therapy, 60% improvement over behaviour therapy and 89% improvement over waiting list controls.

Depression Associated with Physical Illness

The use of psychosocial interventions in depressed older patients with acute physical illnesses has not been studied, despite the well-recognized importance of psychological support in these patients [172]. There is also little information regarding the effectiveness of psychosocial interventions in the elderly with chronic physical illnesses, although common treatment issues have been identified for applying cognitive-behavioural therapy [202]. Initial research has suggested that brief psychotherapy is feasible, acceptable and effective in providing short-term symptom reduction in medically ill elderly patients [203]. Most RCTs of psychosocial interventions fail to provide data on physical health. An exception compared psychodynamic and cognitive group therapies in 53 depressed older subjects, 90% of whom had concomitant medical conditions [204]. Cognitive therapy was found to be more effective than psychodynamic therapy. Studies are required to examine the effectiveness of psychosocial interventions in older patients with acute and chronic physical illnesses who meet diagnostic criteria for depression.

Depression Associated with Dementia

Psychosocial treatments have been infrequently attempted. A recent RCT of behavioural treatments, involving the use of pleasant events and problem-solving in 72 community-living patient/caregiver dyads, demonstrated a significant improvement in depressive symptoms in both the patient and caregiver: 60% of patients improved as compared to only 20% of controls. Importantly, improvements were maintained for 6 months [205]. In contrast, three different group interventions in a residential care setting were found to be ineffective in reducing depressive symptoms in a controlled trial [206].

Depression in Residential Care

There have been a number of RCTs of psychosocial interventions for depression in nursing homes; all have involved group therapies including cognitive therapy, reminiscence, problem-solving, social reinforcement, music therapy, focused visual imagery, education/discussion and planned social activities. The studies have many methodological weaknesses that include failure to use diagnostic criteria for depression, small sample sizes, lack of physical health measures, non-blind ratings and inadequate reporting of outcomes [206–210]. This limits interpretation of the results.

Four studies reported a significant reduction of depressive symptoms at the end of the programme with groups using cognitive therapy, reminiscence, problem-solving and planned social activities respectively [207–210]. However, it is noteworthy that cognitive therapy and social reinforcement were ineffective in other studies [206, 207]. The only study employing diagnostic criteria reported a response rate of 45% with planned social activities [210], although a second study reported that 25% improved on clinical cut-off scores on the BDI with a problem-solving group [207]. In studies with longer follow-up, treatment effects were not sustained 2–3 months after completion of the groups [207, 210].

Non-major Depression

Psychosocial interventions, which have similar efficacy in non-major depression as compared with major depression [198], are usually preferred as the initial treatment approach. Apart from the various types of psychotherapy previously mentioned, a range of other psychosocial interventions has been investigated in RCTs.

Progressive resistance training was found to significantly reduce depressive symptoms and improve quality of life measures as compared with an attention-control group in a 10-week programme involving 32 elderly subjects with mild to moderate depressions [211]. Intensity of training was a significant independent predictor of decrease in depression scores. In contrast, aerobic exercise in a walking group was not found to have a significantly different effect than a social contact group in the treatment of moderate depression in old age [212].

Music therapy, provided either in an 8-week home-based programme or a self-administered programme, was found to reduce depressive symptoms and distress and to improve self-esteem compared with waiting list controls in 30 older patients with major and minor depression [213]. Improvements were maintained over a 9-month follow-up. Interpersonal counselling for older medically ill patients with depressive symptoms, not meeting criteria for major depression or dysthymia, was only found to have a significant advantage over usual care after 6-months treatment [203].

Conclusions

In summary, psychosocial interventions have been found to be efficacious in major and non-major depressions, being the treatments of choice in the latter. Cognitive therapy may be the modality of choice, but not all agree. The interaction of physical health, old age and cognitive decline upon these treatments has not been taken into sufficient account in existing studies. RCTs of psychosocial treatments in nursing homes suggest that a range of group therapies may have a short-term effect, which is not sustained for more than a few months without an ongoing structured programme. The very promising outcomes obtained with behavioural treatments in dementia require replication.

Electroconvulsive Therapy (ECT)

ECT has an important role in the management of severe depression in late life. Surveys of clinical practice indicate that there are higher rates of prescription of ECT in the elderly [214, 215]. This is probably due to the greater risk of psychosis, suicidality, marked motor change and malnutrition associated with severe late life depression [8, 216]. These features not only require a rapid, effective response, but psychosis in particular has been found to be predictive of ECT outcome in most [217–219], but not all studies [220–222]. Other reasons include the greater likelihood of medication-resistance related to brain white-matter lesions in elderly depressives [114] and better response rates to ECT in the elderly [223].

A meta-analysis of the efficacy of ECT in severe depression has demonstrated its superiority over other treatments [224]. Yet, only one study of real vs. simulated ECT has provided separate analyses to show efficacy in older patients [225]. There have also been few comparisons of ECT with antidepressant medication in the elderly and there are methodological limitations. Yet in each study ECT was found to be superior in antidepressant-resistant depression [226], psychotic depression [222] and major depression [128, 227].

Most studies of the effectiveness of ECT have been limited by retrospective design, but they consistently report that 70–97% of older patients show at least moderate improvement [219, 220, 226, 228–236]. Ratings of good outcomes show greater variability, with a range of 23–97%, but with most studies between 45 and 75%. Of interest, in prospective studies that used treatment protocols, results are better, with 71–88% of subjects having good outcomes [219, 225]. Poor response has been reported to be associated with concomitant development of physical illness [127, 237], medication resistance in some [238, 239] but not all studies [225, 234], and being "old" old in some [236] but not all studies [225, 234].

For many years, the choice of electrode placement in the elderly was largely based on balancing the increased efficacy associated with bilateral administration [240, 241] with the lower rates of cognitive dysfunction associated with unilateral administration [242, 243]. Despite limited data in older patients, it is now generally agreed that, with unilateral ECT, high stimulus dosage (2.5 times seizure threshold) is more efficacious than the traditional low dosage (just above threshold) regimen, with similar outcomes to bilateral ECT [243]. However, there is disagreement about whether there should be a fixed or titrated dosage schedule [243, 244]. According to Abrams [244], studies using a fixed stimulus dosage schedule show a greater response rate than those using titrated schedules, without evidence of the excessive cognitive dysfunction predicted by Sackheim *et al* [243]. In support of this, comparison of a titrated moderate dosage schedule with a fixed high dosage schedule, in 19 elderly patients, found that patients on the fixed dosage schedule responded faster and received fewer treatments [245]. For bilateral ECT, there is no advantage in using a high stimulus dosage regimen [243].

Post-ECT confusion has been reported to occur in 18–52% of elderly patients [232, 234, 236]. Pre-ECT cognitive status and post-ictal disorientation have been found to predict retrograde amnesia in a mixed-age sample [246]. In contrast, cognitive impairment associated with depression in the elderly has been found to improve after ECT [223, 247]. This apparent paradox occurs because cognitive impairment associated with depression relates to the acquisition of information, while the cognitive impairment induced by ECT is amnestic in nature [216].

Relapse rates range around 30–60% over 6 months, but are reduced by two thirds by maintenance antidepressants, mood stabilizers and occasionally ECT [244]. The timing of the introduction of the maintenance agent, choice of agent and dosage are issues that have not been addressed in the elderly.

ECT is generally safe in the elderly. There is evidence that complications, particularly cardio-respiratory problems, falls and confusion, are more likely in patients over 75 and with the concurrent use of medication [234, 236]. This appears to be mainly a function of premorbid health, particularly cardiac [244, 248]. Despite this, ECT may be a safer treatment for the older severely depressed cardiac patient than antidepressants, particularly with cardiac monitoring and pulse oximetry throughout the procedure [248]. Further, in the hospitalized elderly, the adverse effects and mortality associated with ECT have been reported to be less than those associated with the use of antidepressants [227, 249].

There have been no prospective studies of ECT in dementia patients with depression. A controlled retrospective series of 21 elderly dementia patients found that there were no significant differences in ECT response in comparison with patients without dementia, although there were higher rates of post-ECT confusion [250]. An earlier literature review found that depression improved in 73% of patients, cognition improved in 29% and cognition worsened, usually transiently, in 21% [251]. Thus the outcome of ECT in severe depression associated with dementia appears similar to that found in the elderly without dementia.

In summary, although there is a dearth of well-designed studies of ECT in old age, the available evidence suggests that it is the most effective treatment available for severe depression, particularly when a rapid response is required and psychosis is present. Suprathreshold unilateral application is recommended as the initial approach. Maintenance therapy with antidepressants, mood stabilizers or ECT is required following recovery. Randomized trials of types of ECT and comparisons with pharmacotherapy are required in a number of clinical situations, including psychotic depression, medication-resistant depression, the "old" old and the physically ill.

TREATMENT-RESISTANT DEPRESSION

While the prevalence of true non-response to treatment is unknown, it has been estimated that 18–40% of elderly depressives may be treatment-resistant [252]. Apparent treatment resistance in the elderly may occur due to an underlying medical cause of depression, subtherapeutic drug levels, inadequate length of trials, intolerance of side effects and non-compliance [253]. Factors that may contribute to treatment resistance include coexisting physical illness, concomitant drugs (especially benzodiazepines) and underlying cerebral pathology [252].

Although guidelines for treatment approaches have been devised, there have been few studies in the elderly [252]. Subsequent courses of antidepressants may need to be longer, a minimum of 6 weeks [131]. Lithium augmentation may not be as effective in older patients due to intolerance [130]. ECT may be the most effective treatment. A randomized study of 39 subjects with antidepressant-resistant depression demonstrated the superiority of ECT over paroxetine, with 71% of the ECT group fulfilling response criteria and the ECT response being faster [226]. Non-pharmacological treatments should also be considered, but data are lacking [254].

PROGNOSIS OF DEPRESSION IN OLD AGE

The landmark study of Roth [255] overturned a long-standing belief that the outcome of late-life depression was uniformly malign. However, the comforting dictum that depression in the elderly usually has a good outcome was called into question by Murphy [237] 28 years later, and for the last decade and a half a series of studies has added fuel to the fire of controversy about the fate of old people with depressive disorders.

Factors which will affect the outcome of cohorts of elderly depressed patients include the definitions of depression, recovery and relapse employed by researchers, the instruments used and the source of the cohort followed. It is unethical to conduct naturalistic long-term studies on untreated patients who present for clinical assessment and care, but epidemiological studies of community-resident elderly often include many depressed subjects who are not receiving treatment.

Criteria for Study Validity

Cole and Bellavance [256] identify six criteria by which the validity of a prognostic study may be assessed [257]. These are:

1. *Formation of an inception cohort.* Depression should be identified at an early uniform point in its course, so that those patients with multiple relapses or chronicity who have multiple chances of inclusion do not make the prognosis appear worse than it is. Cole and Bellavance argue that only patients with "first" episodes of depression (whether this should be first in lifetime or first in old age is arguable) should be included.
2. *Description of referral pattern.* Bias may occur where experts are referred problem cases (centripedal bias), when they follow "interesting cases" (popularity bias) and when referral filter bias leads to services dealing with cases which are not representative of the general population. All studies based in specialist services are prone to these biases, which may

have a huge effect, as the majority of depressed subjects identified in community surveys never reach specialist services. Even studies based in primary care would be subject to some bias, as not all individuals with depression present to or are recognized by general practitioners. Only community-based studies with random selection of subjects can overcome this form of bias. However, the challenges inherent in undertaking such research with meaningful numbers of subjects are huge. Some surveys of elderly people yield a prevalence of major depressive disorder below 1% [66].

3. *Completion of follow-up.* A few dropouts and lost cases are bound to occur in even the best conducted study, but when 20% or more of the inception cohort is lost the study may arbitrarily be deemed unsatisfactory.

4. *Development of objective outcome criteria.* Outcomes need to be rated in explicit categories which are objective and can be related to normal clinical practice. This is harder than it sounds. While it may not be too difficult to agree on which patients have remained continuously well since recovery from the index episode and which have died, the threshold for dementia may be hard to operationalize and the distinction between continuous illness and depressive invalidism or multiple relapses can be exceptionally hard to standardize, especially if review assessments are conducted at 1-year intervals or greater and there are no hard data to determine the exact nature and severity of symptoms which affected patients in the interim. Even division into "good" and "bad" outcome categories is tricky. Many researchers class all but those who remain well after recovery from an index episode as having "bad" outcomes, but has a patient who suffers a 4-week relapse of major depression in a 6-year follow-up really done badly? A more realistic approach may be to quantify outcomes by counting the number of weeks ill and well since recovery, but this may be hard without very frequent and costly assessments. Another approach is to use continuous variables such as depression scale scores rather than rigid categories of outcome, but should one rely on observer-rated or self-rated scales?

5. *Blind outcome assessment.* Expectations about the course of the disorder, knowledge of presenting features and subsequent events which could affect prognosis may bias clinical raters who should be blind to such data when rating outcome.

6. *Adjustment for extraneous prognostic factors.* Disability, dementia, personality, physical illness, treatments and social factors may affect prognosis. Eliminating or accounting for the influence of such factors represents a significant challenge but would be attempted in a putative ideal study.

In addition to the factors enumerated above, other issues, which should be addressed, include:

1. *Use of operationalized diagnostic criteria.* Studies prior to 1980 tended not to use operationalized diagnostic criteria such as those of DSM-III [258]. The use of such criteria may aid the generalizability and replicability of studies, though it is still possible for researchers trained in different traditions to apply such seemingly objective criteria in diverse ways [259]. Because all such systems contain theoretical biases, it may be useful to diagnose cases by more than one system simultaneously (e.g. DSM-IV and ICD-10) and to report both sets of results [260].

2. *Use of structured assessment interviews.* Trained interviewers using structured assessment tools will elicit key data in a more reliable way than interviewers who are untrained and use ad hoc interview techniques. Most early studies and some quite recent ones used idiosyncratic interview techniques, which do not permit replication.

3. *Prospective design.* Retrospective studies, especially those that utilize case note entries to rate disorder severity and outcome [e.g. 127] are open to considerable criticism, especially as Murphy [237] found case note entries to be at marked variance with the results of a structured interview.

4. *Power.* In order to assess the impact of a mere 20 variables on prognosis it is necessary to have a sample size of 200 subjects or more, otherwise statistical power will be insufficient. Yet, hardly any studies have included this many subjects. Combining subjects in meta-analyses may be one way to get around this problem.

Results of Studies Conducted to Date

Psychiatric Hospital and Outpatient Studies

Cole and Bellavance [256] identified 16 studies published since 1950 in English or French [127, 233, 237, 261–273] languages. Only Murphy's study [237] formed an inception cohort (all subjects were experiencing their first episode of depression since age 60). No study gave an adequate account of referral pattern and potential sample biases. The studies by Magni *et al* [267] and Agbayewa [268] lost 32% and 45% of their cohorts to follow-up, but the other studies followed over 80% of their cohorts. Only three studies [271–273] specified criteria for outcome categories, which ranged from 2 to 8 separate categories between studies. No study had blind outcome assessment and none adjusted for all possible extraneous outcome influences, though several accounted for some. No study related treatments received to prognosis. Three of the studies did not use operationalized diagnostic criteria; most avoided use of structured interviews and at least two had a retrospective design. No study included 200 or more subjects.

When study results were combined, 60% of subjects were free from depression at follow-up, and 14–22% were continuously ill. In studies which went on for less than 2 years, 25–68% of subjects had been continuously well after recovery from the index episode (mean 43.7%, 95% CI 36.0–51.3%), 11–25% had relapsed and then recovered again (mean 15.8%, 13.6–18.0%), 3–69% had been continuously ill (mean 22.2%, 14.1–30.3%), and 8–40% had other outcomes such as death or dementia (mean 22.5%, 15.2–29.7%). Studies which exceeded 2 years in duration found that 18–34% (mean 27.3%, 16.8–37.8%) of subjects were continuously well after initial recovery, 23–52% (mean 32.5%, 28.8–36.1%) were well after having at least one relapse, 7–30% (mean 14.2%, 1.8–26.7%) were continuously ill with depression and 23–39% (mean 30.9%, 20.7–41.2%) had other outcomes. Poor outcome was inconsistently associated with physical illness, cognitive impairment and depressive severity, whereas social factors apart from severe intervening life events were not associated with outcome. In Post's studies [262, 263], length of time ill with depression before presentation was a strong predictor of poor outcome, but of course selecting a proper inception cohort would remove this factor from the equation.

The Old Age Depression Interest Group [274] study compared the efficacy of dothiepin and placebo in 69 elderly patients who had recovered from major depression. Drug treatment reduced the risk of relapse by a factor of 2.5, whereas a prolonged index depressive episode trebled the chance of relapse. Although this study did not use structured interviews, it does report on the long-term impact of a prophylactic treatment for depression in the elderly and thus actually has some applicability in practice.

Stoudemire et al [275] focused on cognitive outcome in 55 elderly patients treated for depression with antidepressants or ECT and followed for 4 years. After 4 years, 83.7% exhibited "clinically meaningful improvements", though 50% experienced a rehospitalization.

A retrospective study conducted in Ireland [276], on 86 elderly patients treated by an old age psychiatry service, found 37% to be dead at 1 year. Of those who survived, 50% were depression free and 7% demented. Those seen on domiciliary visits did best and those with physical illness or cognitive impairment at baseline did worst.

Another case note study of 54 elderly compared with 56 younger subjects [277] found little difference between the two groups. A year after receiving hospital treatment for depression, 44.4% of the elderly had recovered and remained well, 24% had relapsed but recovered again, 13% had some residual symptoms and 5.5% were continuously ill. Both longer duration of illness at presentation and higher number of previous depressions predicted a poorer outcome for the elderly subjects.

Lee and Lawlor [278] for a mean period of 19 months followed, 51 elderly patients presenting to a Dublin old age service with major depression and 49 with other depressive diagnoses. Good outcomes were reported in 57% of those with major depression and 41% of the remainder. No predictor of outcome could be found in the major depression group (in which 18% of subjects died), though being younger, having had more psychiatric admissions and not requiring benzodiazepines were associated with good outcome in the group with other depressive diagnoses.

Flint and Rifat [279] reported that of 19 elderly patients with psychotic major depression remitting after ECT and 68 non-psychotic patients who got better with medication, the psychotic group had earlier and more frequent relapses. Of the 16 psychotic subjects completing the study, 6 did well, 9 became depressed again and 1 died, while in the larger group 50 completed the study, of whom 30 did well, 10 had another depression, 3 died, 1 could not tolerate medication, 2 became manic and 4 became physically ill.

A recent study [280] supported the idea that severe deep white matter lesions (DWMLs) detected on MRI have a bad prognostic impact. No subject with such lesions had a good outcome in a study of 60 Australian subjects with major depression aged 55 and over. Severe DWMLs were the only factor associated with poor outcome in an analysis which also examined the impact of age, sex, length of time ill before treatment, diastolic blood pressure and the presence of cardiovascular risk factors.

Studies of Elderly Medical Inpatients

Cole and Bellavance [281] reviewed eight studies [282–289], all of them methodologically flawed, which found that after 3 months or less 18% of depressed medical inpatients were well, 43% depressed and 22% dead. The figures at 12 months and over were respectively 19, 29 and 53%. More severe depression, depression which preceded admission, and more serious physical illness were associated with adverse outcomes.

Studies in Primary Care

No methodologically acceptable study of elderly depressed patients in primary care followed for over a year could be identified for this review.

Community Studies

Five studies identified by Cole and Bellavance [63, 290–293] had small samples of depressed subjects (23–123, excluding those diagnosed with dysthymia rather than major depression by Kivelä et al [292]), but generally were better designed than the hospital-based studies. No study accounted for or eliminated all extraneous prognostic factors. All used structured or semi-structured interviews and some reported that follow-up was blind to initial diagnosis.

When the five studies were divided according to follow-up period, 22–46% of subjects followed for less than 2 years were well (mean 34.1%, 14–54.3%), and 6–32% (mean 19%, 3.6–34.4%) of those in studies which followed subjects for more than 2 years were well. Continuous illness was reported in 14–44% (mean 27.1%, 5.5–48.7%) of subjects in studies of 2 years or less, and 14–36% (mean 27%, 9.9–44.2%) of participants in longer studies. Other outcomes (usually death but including relapse, dementia and other psychiatric disorders) affected 28–34% of those in studies less than 2 years (mean 30.7%, 12.2–49.2%), and 27–58% (mean 44.3%, 29.6–59%) of individuals followed for over 2 years. In three studies rates of antidepressant prescribing were 4% [63], 9% [290] and 33% [293]. The rate of psychiatric referral was noted by Forsell et al [293] to be 2 in 34. Kivelä et al [292] found physical illness and social factors to be unrelated to outcome, while O'Connor et al [291] and Forsell et al [293] found that patients with dementia were less likely than cognitively intact subjects to be depressed at follow-up. One investigator from the studies reviewed by Cole and Bellavance subsequently reported additional data. Kivelä [294] reported that after 5 years 12% of her original cohort of 42 subjects with major depression remained well, 26% were still depressed, 12% were demented, 45% dead and 5% untraceable. A higher prevalence of physical illness at baseline was related to poor long-term outcome.

Of studies not reviewed by Cole and Bellavance, Livingstone et al [295] followed up 62 subjects diagnosed as depressed after 2.6 years. Recovery had occurred in 34%, 39% were still depressed and 27% were dead, but there was a high dropout rate. More severely depressed subjects at baseline and females tended to do worse. A 1-year study of 238 Dutch subjects by Beekman et al [296] used only a 20-item scale to assess depression, but data were collected on five occasions after study entry. Chronic depression affected 14%, 8% were depressed at baseline but recovered, 16% had an incident depression, 10% had a variable course and 52% were never depressed. Of those depressed at baseline, 43% had chronic depression, 32% recovered without relapse and 25% remitted and then relapsed. Health-related variables predicted both onset and course of depression. In a study using the same 20-item scale, Kennedy et al [297] screened and followed 1577 elderly Americans, of whom 211 were classed as depressed. They found 46% remained depressed for 2 years, while 114 recovered. Again, worsening health was associated with depression persistence, as was advanced age.

Studies of Residential Populations

After a 4-year follow-up period, 6 in 35 surviving residents who had screened positive for depression in 12 British local authority homes for the elderly had recovered and most of the remaining 75 initially classed as depressed were dead [298]. In a second cohort, 28% of 60 depressed residents were no longer depressed after 1 year [299]. In both these cohorts, depression score and an expressed wish to die when screened were associated with mortality [300]. In a nursing home study of 454 new admissions, conducted in the USA by Rovner *et al* [190], major depressive disorder was positively associated with mortality at 1 year.

Suicide

Lindesay [301] reviewed the data on suicide in the elderly, showing that older persons have the highest suicide rate of all age groups, with depressive disorder as the major risk factor. However, they are less likely to engage in acts of deliberate self-harm unless they have suffered from a depressive disorder or other mental disorders. The predictive value of previous attempts and somatic symptoms presenting to primary care physicians was noted, as well as the increased vulnerability on the anniversary of significant personal losses.

Recommendations for Future Research and Clinical Practice

The main conclusion produced after reviewing research in this field is one of disappointment at the inadequacy of our research methodology and our inability to make useful links between alterable prognostic factors and outcomes. Depression is the commonest disorder seen by old age psychiatrists and if it cannot be studied effectively enough to permit modification of adverse prognostic factors, then the whole point of research in our field must be called into question. Large studies are needed with explicit diagnostic criteria, thorough documentation and measurement of possible prognostic factors (including treatments), which follow patients at frequent intervals for more than 2 years. Outcome categories need to be operationalized, and independent measurement must be made of quality of life, general function and physical health. Outcome should be rated blind and every aspect of the study should have demonstrated reliability. Studies are urgently needed in primary care, though given the poor quality of studies in psychiatric settings the psychiatrists might do better to alert the general practitioners to the deficiency and ask them to do the studies themselves, rather than stepping into general practices to conduct such research.

In the meantime, all we can say is that, although specialist service-based studies probably overstate the malignity of the prognosis of late-life depression, most people who have one episode will have another if we wait long enough. The longer they have been depressed and the more physically ill they are, the worse they will do. The risk of death among those elderly people who have had an episode of depression is almost certainly raised. It therefore seems prudent to treat depressed old people energetically, to follow them closely in order to retreat relapses at an early stage [302]. The liberal use of prophylactic antidepressants is to be encouraged, and precise criteria for which drugs to use, for how long and in whom are urgently awaited.

SUMMARY

Consistent Evidence

- Presentation of depression in the elderly is similar to younger adults in the "core" features, but different in having less dysphoric mood and more somatic concern.
- The current categorical diagnostic systems (ICD-10, DSM-IV) do not include a large number of elderly with significant depressive symptoms which do not satisfy syndromic criteria, and who therefore are not included in prevalence and other studies. A "subsyndrome" category may need to be considered in the future revisions of diagnostic systems.
- Antidepressants are effective in treatment of depression in old age. The high rate of adverse affects of the tricyclic group mitigates against its use in the elderly. The lower rate of adverse events in the newer antidepressants (SSRIs) makes them more acceptable. However, nortriptyline has a role in severe depression in the elderly.
- Electroconvulsive therapy (ECT) has demonstrated efficacy in treatment of old age depression with the benefit of rapid response in the severely ill with and without psychotic symptoms.
- The suicide rate in the elderly is high. Presentation with somatic complaints to a physician preceding the suicidal acts is frequent. Deliberate self-harm is usually associated with depressive disorders and other mental disorders.

Incomplete Evidence

- Various subtypes of depression are being considered. Delusional depression and vascular depression appear to have some clinical validity.
- Despite differing methodological approaches in the definition of depression in epidemiological studies, there is some evidence to suggest that the prevalence of major depression in the elderly is lower than that in younger adults.
- Outcome of depression in the elderly is little different to that in younger patients. Poor outcome is associated with physical illness, cognitive impairment and severity of depressive symptoms. Depression in the elderly is associated with excess physical disability and increased mortality.

- Psychosocial interventions are useful in major and non-major depression, but there is some disagreement on the modality of choice.
- Neuroendocrine and neurochemical studies show some data, but with low specificity for depression.

Areas Still Open to Research

- Characterization of "subsyndromal" or "subthreshold" depression is needed to accommodate those elderly suffering with significant depressive symptoms who do not reach "criteria" of existing syndromal diagnosis.
- The relationship between cognitive impairment and depression in the elderly requires exploration. Is depression of late onset a prodrome of cognitive impairment? Is cognitive impairment a necessary consequence of depression of late onset? If so, what are the biological mechanisms underlying this relationship?
- Cardiovascular disease, especially hypertension, is a possible risk factor of both vascular dementia and depression. Further exploration of the relationship between these three conditions will yield possible preventive approaches.
- New epidemiological data using common assessment schedules which will include non-syndromal subtypes and risk factors will help to clarify uncertainties in this area.
- Psychosocial factors in the development of depressive disorders and its management will need more vigorous research.
- Randomized control trials and post-marketing observational studies of new antidepressants in older subjects will yield relevant information to clinicians in the management of elderly depressives in the community.
- Outcome research requires larger samples, consistent methodology and adequate length of follow-up with independent operationalized measurements.
- Treatment-resistant depression needs clear definition with subsequent consistent research approaches.
- Maintenance treatment with antidepressants and ECT requires long-term follow-up studies to demonstrate efficacy in the elderly.
- Management of depressed elderly in residential settings must account for confounding factors of poor physical health, dementia and the patients in the "old" old age group.

ACKNOWLEDGEMENTS

The authors would like to thank Monica Williams for her assistance in literature search and reference sorting and Roz Seath for preparation of the manuscript. The section on correlates of depression in old age had the benefit of a draft paper by Dr O. Forlenza.

REFERENCES

1. American Psychiatric Association (1994) *Diagnostic and Statistical Manual of Mental Disorders*, 4th edn, American Psychiatric Association, Washington, DC.
2. World Health Organization (1992) *The ICD-10 Classification of Mental and Behavioural Disorders: Clinical Descriptions and Diagnostic Guidelines*, World Health Organization, Geneva.
3. Brown R.P., Sweeney J., Loutsch R., Kocsis J., Frances A. (1984) Involutional melancholia revisited. *Am. J. Psychiatry*, **141**: 24–28.
4. Baldwin R.C. (1990) Age of onset of depression in the elderly. *Br. J. Psychiatry*, **156**: 445–446.
5. Blazer D., Bachar J.R., Hughes D.C. (1987) Major depression with melancholia: a comparison of middle-aged and elderly adults. *J. Am. Geriatr. Soc.*, **35**: 927–932.
6. Burvill P.W., Hall W.D., Stampfer H.G., Emmerson J.P. (1989) A comparison of early-onset and late-onset depressive illness in the elderly. *Br. J. Psychiatry*, **155**: 673–679.
7. Greenwald B.S., Kramer-Ginsberg E. (1988) Age at onset in geriatric depression: relationship to clinical variables. *J. Affect. Disord.*, **15**: 61–68.
8. Brodaty H., Peters K., Boyce P., Hickie I., Parker G., Mitchell P., Wilhelm K. (1991) Age and depression. *J. Affect. Disord.*, **23**: 137–149.
9. Georgotas A. (1983) Affective disorders in the elderly: diagnostic and research considerations. *Age Ageing*, **12**: 1–10.
10. Gurland B.J. (1976) The comparative frequency of depression in various adult age groups. *J. Gerontol.*, **31**: 283–292.
11. De Alarcon R.D. (1964) Hypochondriasis and depression in the aged. *Gerontol. Clin.*, **6**: 266–277.
12. Good W.R., Vlachonikolis I., Griffiths P., Griffiths R.A. (1987) The structure of depressive symptoms in the elderly. *Br. J. Psychiatry*, **150**: 463–470.
13. Winokur G., Morrison J., Clancy J., Crowe R. (1973) The Iowa 500: familial and clinical findings favour two kinds of depressive illness. *Compr. Psychiatry*, **14**: 99–107.
14. Blazer D., George L., Landerman R. (1986) The phenomenology of late life depression. In *Psychiatric Disorders in the Elderly* (Eds P.E. Bebbington, R. Jacoby), pp. 143–152, Mental Health Foundation, London.
15. Gurland B.J., Wilder D.E., Berkman C. (1988) Depression and disability in the elderly: reciprocal relations and changes with age. *Int. J. Geriatr. Psychiatry*, **3**: 163–179.
16. Hordern A., Holt N.F., Burt C.G., Gordon W.F. (1963) Amitriptyline in depressive states: phenomenology and prognostic considerations. *Br. J. Psychiatry*, **109**: 815–825.
17. Meyers B.S., Kalayam B., Mei-Tal V. (1984) Late-onset delusional depression: a distinct clinical entity? *J. Clin. Psychiatry*, **45**: 347–349.
18. Meyers B.S., Greenberg R. (1986) Late-life delusional depression. *J. Affect. Disord.*, **11**: 133–137.
19. Nelson J.C., Bowers M.B. (1978) Delusional unipolar depression: description and drug response. *Arch. Gen. Psychiatry*, **35**: 1321–1328.

20. Nelson J.C., Conwell Y., Kim K., Mazure C. (1989) Age at onset in late-life delusional depression. *Am. J. Psychiatry*, **146**: 785–786.
21. Oxman T.E., Barrett J.E., Barrett J., Gerber P. (1990) Symptomatology of late-life minor depression among primary care patients. *Psychosomatics*, **31**: 174–180.
22. Spitzer R.L., Endicott J. (1978) *Research Diagnostic Criteria for a Selected Group of Functional Disorders*, 3rd edn, New York State Psychiatric Institute, New York.
23. Kivelä S.-L., Pahkala K. (1988) Clinician-rated symptoms and signs of depression in aged Finns. *Int. J. Soc. Psychiatry*, **34**: 274–284.
24. Kivelä S.-L., Pahkala K. (1988) Factor structure of the Hamilton Rating Scale for Depression among depressed elderly Finns. *Zeitschrift für Psychologie*, **196**: 389–399.
25. Kivelä S.-L., Pahkala K. (1988) Symptoms of depression among old people in Finland. *Zeitschrift für Gerontologie*, **21**: 257–263.
26. Downes J.J., Davis A.D.M., Copeland J.R.M. (1988) Organisation of depressive symptoms in the elderly population; hierarchal patterns and Guttman scales. *Psychol. Ageing*, **3**: 367–374.
27. Fredman L., Schoenbach V.J., Kaplan B.H., Blazer D.G., James S.A., Kleinbaum D.G., Yankaskas B. (1989) The association between depressive symptoms and mortality among older patients in the Epidemiologic Catchment Area–Piedmont Health Survey. *J. Gerontol.*, **44**: 149–156.
28. Kral V.A., Emery O.B. (1989) Long-term follow-up of depressive pseudo-dementia of the aged. *Can. J. Psychiatry*, **34**: 445–446.
29. Alexopoulos G.S., Young R.C., Shindledecker R.D. (1992) Brain computed tomography findings in geriatric depression and primary degenerative dementia. *Biol. Psychiatry*, **31**: 591–599.
30. Reding M., Haycox J., Blass J. (1985) Depression in patients referred to a dementia clinic. *Arch. Neurol.*, **42**: 894–896.
31. Abas M.A., Sahakian B.J., Levy R. (1990) Neuropsychological deficits and CT scan changes in elderly depressives. *Psychol. Med.*, **20**: 507–520.
32. Blazer D.G. (1994) Epidemiology of late-life depression. In *Diagnosis and Treatment of Depression in Late Life* (Eds L.S. Schneider, C.F. Reynolds, B.D. Lebowitz, A.J. Friedhoff), pp. 9–19, American Psychiatric Press, Washington, DC.
33. Blazer D., Burchett B., Service C., George L.K. (1991). The association of age and depression among the elderly: an epidemiologic exploration. *J. Gerontol.*, **46**: M210–215.
34. Broadhead W.E., Blazer D.G., George L.K., Tse C.K. (1990). Depression, disability days, and days lost from work in a prospective epidemiological survey. *JAMA*, **264**: 2524–2528.
35. Kleinman A.M. (1977) Depression, somatization and the "new cross-cultural psychiatry". *Soc. Sci. Med.*, **11**: 3–10.
36. Lee S. (1998) Estranged bodies, simulated harmony and misplaced cultures: neurasthenia in contemporary Chinese society. *Psychosom. Med.*, **60**: 448–457.
37. Kleinman A. (1986) *Social Origin of Distress and Disease: Depression, Neurasthenia and Pain in Modern China*, Yale University Press, New Haven, CT.
38. Caine E.D., Lyness J.M., King D.A., Connors L. (1994) Clinical and etiological heterogeneity of mood disorders in elderly patients. In *Diagnosis and Treatment of Depression in Late Life* (Eds L.S. Schneider, C.F. Reynolds, B.D. Lebowitz, A.J. Friedhoff), pp. 21–53, American Psychiatric Press, Washington, DC.
39. Baldwin R.C. (1992) The nature, prevalence and frequency of depressive delusions. In *Delusions and Hallucinations in Old Age* (Eds C. Katona, R. Levy), pp. 97–114, Gaskell, London.

40. Kivelä S.-L., Pahkala K. (1989) Delusional depression in the elderly: a community study. *Zeitschrift für Gerontologie*, **22**: 236–241.

41. Wragg R.E., Jeste D.V. (1989) Overview of depression and psychosis in Alzheimer's disease. *Am. J. Psychiatry*, **146**: 577–586.

42. Greenwald B.S., Kramer-Ginsberg E., Marin D.B., Laitman L.B., Hermann C.K., Mohs R.C., Davis K.L. (1989) Dementia with coexisting major depression. *Am. J. Psychiatry*, **146**: 1472–1478.

43. Rovner B.W., Broadhead J., Spencer M., Carson K., Folstein M.F. (1989) Depression and Alzheimer's disease. *Am. J. Psychiatry*, **146**: 350–353.

44. Burns A., Jacoby R., Levy R. (1990) Psychiatric phenomena in Alzheimer's disease. *Br. J. Psychiatry*, **157**: 72–94.

45. Kumar A., Koss E., Metzler D., Moore A., Friedland R.P. (1988) Behavioral symptomatology in dementia of the Alzheimer type. *Alz. Dis. Assoc. Disord.*, **2**: 363–365.

46. Reifler B.V., Larson E., Hanley R. (1982) Coexistence of cognitive impairment and depression in geriatric outpatients. *Am. J. Psychiatry*, **139**: 623–626.

47. Merriam A.E., Aronson M.K., Gatson P., Wey S.L., Katz I. (1988) The psychiatric symptoms of Alzheimer's disease. *J. Am. Geriatr. Soc.*, **36**: 7–12.

48. Krishnan K.R.R. (1991) Organic bases of depression in the elderly. *Ann. Rev. Med.*, **42**: 261–266.

49. Krishnan K.R.R., Goli V., Ellinwood F.H., France R.D., Blazer D.F., Nemeroff C.B. (1988) Leukoencephalopathy in patients diagnosed as major depressive. *Biol. Psychiatry*, **23**: 519–522.

50. Krishnan K.R., McDonald W.M., Doriaiswamy P.M., Tupler L.A., Husain M., Boyko O.B., Figiel G.S., Ellinwood E.H. Jr. (1993) Neuroanatomical substrates of depression in the elderly. *Eur. Arch. Psychiatry Clin. Neurosci.*, **243**: 41–46.

51. Pearlson G.D., Rabins P.V., Kim W.S., Speedie L.J., Moberg P.J., Burns A., Bascom M.J. (1989) Structural brain CT changes and cognitive deficits in elderly depressives with and without reversible dementia ("pseudodementia"). *Psychol. Med.*, **19**: 573–584.

52. Rabins P.V., Pearlson G.D., Aylward E., Kumar A.J., Dowell K. (1991) Cortical magnetic resonance imaging changes in elderly inpatients with major depression. *Am. J. Psychiatry*, **148**: 617–620.

53. Sackheim H.A., Prohovnik I., Moeller J.R., Brown R.P., Apter S., Prudic J., Devanand D.P., Mukherjee S. (1990) Regional cerebral blood flow in mood disorders, I: comparison of major depressive and normal controls at rest. *Arch. Gen. Psychiatry*, **47**: 60–70.

54. Zubenko G.S., Sullivan P., Nelson J.P., Belle S.H., Huff F.J., Wolf G.L. (1990) Brain imaging abnormalities in mental disorders of late life. *Arch. Neurol.*, **47**: 1107–1111.

55. Regier D.A., Farmer M.E., Rae D.S., Myers J.K., Kramer M., Robins L.N., George L.K., Karno M., Locke B.Z. (1993) One-month prevalence of mental disorders in the United States and sociodemographic characteristics: the Epidemiologic Catchment Area study. *Acta Psychiatr. Scand.*, **88**: 35–47.

56. Bland R.C., Newman S.C., Orn H. (1988) Prevalence of psychiatric disorders in the elderly in Edmonton. *Acta Psychiatr. Scand.*, **77** (Suppl. 338): 57–63.

57. Australian Bureau of Statistics (1998) *Mental Health and Wellbeing: Profile of Adults, Australia 1997*, Australian Bureau of Statistics, Canberra.

58. Blazer D., Williams C.D. (1980) Epidemiology of dysphoria and depression in an elderly population. *Am. J. Psychiatry*, **137**: 439–444.

59. Gurland B.J., Copeland J., Kuriansky J., Kelleher M., Sharpe L., Dean L.L. (1983) *The Mind and Mood of Aging*, Croom Helm, London.

60. Kay D.W.K., Henderson A.S., Scott R., Wilson J., Rickwood D., Grayson D.A. (1985) The prevalence of dementia and depression among the elderly living in the Hobart community: the effect of the diagnostic criteria on the prevalence rates. *Psychol. Med.*, **15**: 771–788.

61. Lindsay J., Briggs K., Murphy E. (1989) The Guy's/Age Concern Survey. Prevalence rates of cognitive impairment, depression and anxiety in an urban elderly community. *Br. J. Psychiatry*, **155**: 317–329.

62. Livingston G., Hawkins A., Graham N., Blizard B., Mann A.H. (1990) The Gospel Oak Study: prevalence rates of dementia, depression and activity limitation among elderly residents in inner London. *Psychol. Med.*, **20**: 137–146.

63. Copeland J.R.M., Davidson I.A., Dewey M.E., Gilmore C., Larkin B.A., McWilliam C., Saunders P.A., Scott A., Sharma V., Sullivan C. (1992) Alzheimer's disease, other dementias, depression and pseudodementia: prevalence, incidence and three-year outcome in Liverpool. *Br. J. Psychiatry*, **161**: 230–239.

64. Prince M.J., Harwood R.H., Thomas A., Mann A.H. (1998) A prospective population-based cohort study of the effects of disablement and social milieu on the onset and maintenance of late-life depression. The Gospel Oak Project VII. *Psychol. Med.*, **28**: 337–350.

65. Macdonald A.J.D. (1997) Mental health in old age. *Br. Med. J.*, **315**: 413–417.

66. Henderson A.S., Jorm A.F., Mackinnon A., Christensen H., Scott L.R., Korten A.E., Doyle C. (1993) The prevalence of depressive disorders and the distribution of depressive symptoms in later life: a survey using Draft ICD-10 and DSM-III-R. *Psychol. Med.*, **23**: 719–729.

67. Copeland J.R.M., Gurland B.J., Dewey M.E., Kelleher M.J., Smith A.M.R., Davidson I.A. (1987) Is there more dementia, depression and neurosis in New York? A comparative study of the elderly in New York and London using the computer diagnosis AGECAT. *Br. J. Psychiatry*, **151**: 466–473.

68. Lobo A., Saz P., Marcos G., Dia J.-L., De-la-Camara C. (1995) The prevalence of dementia and depression in the elderly community in a Southern European population. *Arch. Gen. Psychiatry*, **52**: 497–506.

69. Pahkala K., Kesti E., Kongas-Saviaro P., Laippala P., Kivelä S.-L. (1995) Prevalence of depression in an aged population in Finland. *Soc. Psychiatry Psychiatr. Epidemiol.*, **30**: 99–106.

70. Beekman A.T.F., Deeg D.J.H., van Tilburg T., Smit J.H., Hooijer C., van Tilburg W. (1995) Major and minor depression in later life: a study of prevalence and risk factors. *J. Affect. Disord.*, **36**: 65–75.

71. Romanoski A.J., Folstein M.F., Nestadt G., Chahal R., Merchant A., Brown C.H., Gruenberg E.M., McHugh P.R. (1992) The epidemiology of psychiatrist-ascertained depression and DSM-III depressive disorders. *Psychol. Med.*, **22**: 629–655.

72. Girling D.M., Barkley C., Paykel E.S., Gehlhaar E., Brayne C., Gill C., Mathewson D., Huppert F.A. (1995) The prevalence of depression in a cohort of the very elderly. *J. Affect. Disord.*, **34**: 319–329.

73. Skoog I. (1993) The prevalence of psychotic depressive and anxiety syndromes in demented and non-demented 85-year-olds. *Int. J. Geriatr. Psychiatry*, **8**: 247–253.

74. Roberts R.E., Kaplan G.A., Shema S.J., Strawbridge W.J. (1997) Does growing old increase the risk for depression? *Am. J. Psychiatry*, **154**: 1384–1390.

75. Lyness J.M., Cox C., Curry J., Conwell Y., King D.A., Caine E.D. (1995) Older age and the under-reporting of depressive symptoms. *J. Am. Geriatr. Soc.*, **43**: 216–221.

76. Henderson A.S. (1994) Does ageing protect against depression? *Soc. Psychiatry Psychiatr. Epidemiol.*, **29**: 107–109.

77. Gallo J.J., Rabins P.V., Lyketsos C.G., Tien A.Y., Anthony J.C. (1997) Depression without sadness: functional outcomes of nondysphoric depression in later life. *J. Am. Geriatr. Soc.*, **45**: 570–578.

78. Knäuper B., Wittchen H.-U. (1994) Diagnosing major depression in the elderly: evidence for response bias in standardized diagnostic interviews. *J. Psychiatr. Res.*, **28**: 147–164.

79. Snowdon J. (1990) The prevalence of depression in old age. *Int. J. Geriatr. Psychiatry*, **5**: 141–144.

80. Reifler B.V. (1994) Depression: diagnosis and comorbidity. In *Diagnosis and Treatment of Depression in Late Life* (Eds L.S. Schneider, C.F. Reynolds, B.D. Lebowitz, A.J. Friedhoff), pp. 55–59, American Psychiatric Press, Washington, DC.

81. Jenkins R., Bebbington P., Brugha T., Farrell M., Gill B., Lewis G., Meltzer H., Petticrew M. (1997) The National Psychiatric Morbidity Survey of Great Britain — Strategy and methods. *Psychol. Med.*, **27**: 765–774.

82. Swartz M.S., Blazer D.G. (1986) The distribution of affective disorders in old age. In *Affective Disorders in the Elderly* (Ed. E. Murphy), pp. 13–39, Churchill Livingstone, Edinburgh.

83. Wells K.B., Stewart A., Hays R.D. (1989) The functioning and well-being of depressed patients: results from the Medical Outcomes Study. *JAMA*, **262**: 914–919.

84. Beekman A.T.F., Penninx B.W.J.H., Deeg D.J.H., Orwel J., Braam A.W., van Tilburg W. (1997) Depression and physical health in late life: results from the Longitudinal Aging Study Amsterdam (LASA). *J. Affect. Disord.*, **46**: 219–231.

85. Kennedy G.J., Kelman H.R., Thomas C., Wisniewski W., Metz H., Bijur P.E. (1989) Hierarchy of characteristics associated with depressive symptoms in an urban elderly sample. *Am. J. Psychiatry*, **146**: 220–225.

86. Henderson A.S., Korten A.E., Jacomb P.A., Mackinnon A.J., Jorm A.F., Christensen H., Rodgers B. (1997) The course of depression in the elderly: a longitudinal community-based study in Australia. *Psychol. Med.*, **27**: 119–129.

87. Beekman A.T.F., Kriegsman D.M.W., Deeg D.J.H., van Tilburg W. (1995) The association of physical health and depressive symptoms in the older population: age and sex differences. *Soc. Psychiatry Psychiatr. Epidemiol.*, **30**: 32–38.

88. Prince M.J., Harwood R.H., Blizard R.A., Thomas A., Mann A.H. (1997) Impairment, disability and handicap as risk factors for depression in old age. The Gospel Oak Project V. *Psychol. Med.*, **27**: 311–321.

89. Snowdon J. (1994) The epidemiology of affective disorders in old age. In *Functional Psychiatric Disorders of the Elderly* (Eds E. Chiu, D. Ames), pp. 95–110, Cambridge University Press, Cambridge.

90. Valvanne J., Juva K., Erkinjuntti T., Tilvis R. (1996) Major depression in the elderly: a population study in Helsinki. *Int. Psychogeriatr.*, **8**: 437–443.

91. Koenig H.G. (1997) Differences in psychosocial and health correlates of major and minor depression in medically ill older adults. *J. Am. Geriatr. Soc.*, **45**: 1487–1495.

92. Burvill P.W., Johnson G.A., Jamrozik K.D., Anderson C.S., Stewart-Wynne E.G., Chakera T.M.H. (1995) Prevalence of depression after stroke: the Perth community stroke study. *Br. J. Psychiatry*, **166**: 320–327.

93. Morris P.L.P., Shields R.B., Hopwood M.J., Robinson R.G., Raphael B. (1994) Are there two depressive syndromes after stroke? *J. Nerv. Ment. Dis.*, **182**: 230–234.

94. Grant I., Patterson T.L., Yager J. (1988) Social supports in relation to physical health and symptoms of depression in the elderly. *Am. J. Psychiatry*, **145**: 1254–1258.

95. Forsell Y., Winblad B. (1998) Major depression in a population of demented and nondemented older people: prevalence and correlates. *J. Am. Geriatr. Soc.*, **46**: 27–30.

96. Parmelee P.A., Katz I.R., Lawton M.P. (1989) Depression among institutionalized aged: assessment and prevalence estimation. *J. Gerontol.*, **44**: M22–M29.

97. Ames D. (1994) Depression in nursing and residential homes. In *Functional Psychiatric Disorders of the Elderly* (Eds E. Chiu, D. Ames), pp. 142–162, Cambridge University Press, Cambridge.

98. Kivelä S.-L., Kongas-Savario P., Laippala P., Pahkala K., Kesti E. (1996) Social and psychosocial factors predicting depression in old age: a longitudinal study. *Int. Psychogeriatr.*, **8**: 635–644.

99. George L.K. (1994) Social factors and depression in late life. In *Diagnosis and Treatment of Depression in Late Life* (Eds L.S. Schneider, C.F. Reynolds, D. Lebowitz, A.J. Friedhoff), pp. 131–153, American Psychiatric Press, Washington, DC.

100. Murphy E. (1986) Social factors in late life depression. In *Affective Disorders in the Elderly* (Ed. E. Murphy), pp. 78–96, Churchill-Livingstone, Edinburgh.

101. Emmerson J.P., Burvill P.W., Finlay-Jones R., Hall W. (1989) Life events, life difficulties and confiding relationships in the depressed elderly. *Br. J. Psychiatry*, **155**: 787–792.

102. Kennedy G.J., Kelman H.R., Thomas C. (1990) The emergence of depressive symptoms in late life: the importance of declining health and increasing disability. *J. Comm. Health*, **15**: 93–104.

103. Pahkala K., Kivelä S.-L., Laippala P. (1991) Social and environmental factors and major depression in old age. *Zeitschrift für Gerontologie*, **24**: 17–23.

104. Lehtinen V., Joukamaa M. (1994) Epidemiology of depression: prevalence, risk factors and treatment situation. *Acta Psychiatr. Scand.*, **377** (Suppl.): 7–10.

105. Green B.H., Copeland J.R.M., Dewey M.E., Sharma V., Saunders P.A., Davidson I.A., Sullivan C., McWilliam C. (1992) Risk factors for depression in elderly people: a prospective study. *Acta Psychiatr. Scand.*, **86**: 213–217.

106. George L.K., Blazer D.G., Hughes D.C., Fowler N. (1989) Social support and the outcome of major depression. *Br. J. Psychiatry*, **154**: 478–485.

107. Murphy E. (1996) Author's retrospective. Social origins of depression in old age. *Int. J. Geriatr. Psychiatry*, **11**: 500–502.

108. Kendler K.S., Kessler R.C., Neale M.C., Heath A.C., Eaves L.J. (1993) The prediction of major depression in women: toward an integrated etiologic model. *Am. J. Psychiatry*, **150**: 1139–1148.

109. Rozzini R., Frisoni G.B., Ferrucci L., Trabucchi M. (1997) Co-occurrence of disadvantage conditions in elderly subjects with depressive symptoms. *J. Affect. Disord.*, **46**: 247–254.

110. Cervilla J.A., Prince M.J. (1997) Cognitive impairment and social distress pathways to depression in the elderly: a cross-sectional study. *Int. J. Geriatr. Psychiatry*, **12**: 995–1000.

111. Austin M.-P., Mitchell P. (1995) The anatomy of melancholia: does frontal-subcortical pathophysiology underpin its psychomotor and cognitive manifestations? *Psychol. Med.*, **25**: 665–672.

112. Grasby P.M., Bench C. (1997) Neuroimaging of mood disorders. *Curr. Opin. Psychiatry*, **10**: 73–78.

113. Conwell Y., Nelson J.C., Kim K.M., Mazure C.M. (1989) Depression in late life: age of onset as marker of a sub-type. *J. Affect. Disord.*, **17**: 189–195.

114. Hickie I., Scott E., Mitchell P., Wilhelm K., Austin M.-P., Bennett B. (1995) Subcortical hyperintensities on magnetic resonance imaging: clinical correlates and prognostic significance in patients with severe depression. *Biol. Psychiatry*, **37**: 151–160.

115. Greenwald B.S., Kramer-Ginsberg E., Krishnan K.R.R., Ashtari M., Aupperle P.M., Patel M. (1996) MRI signal hyperintensities in geriatric depression. *Am. J. Psychiatry*, **153**: 1212–1215.

116. Lyness J.M., Caine E.D., Cox C., King D.A., Conwell Y., Olivares T. (1998) Cerebrovascular risk factors and later-life major depression. *Am. J. Geriatr. Psychiatry*, **6**: 5–13.

117. Brodaty H., Luscombe G., Parker G., Wilhelm K., Hickie I., Austin M.P., Mitchell P. (1997) Increased rate of psychosis and psychomotor change in depression with age. *Psychol. Med.*, **27**: 1205–1213.

118. Sparks L.D. (1989) Aging and Alzheimer's disease. Altered cortical serotonergic binding. *Arch. Neurol.*, **46**: 138–140.

119. Wong D.F., Wagner H.N. Jr, Dannals R.F., Links J.M., Frost J.J., Ravert H.T., Wilson A.A., Rosenbaum A.E., Gjedde A., Douglas K.H. *et al* (1984) Effects of age on dopamine and serotonin receptors measured by positron tomography in the living human brain. *Science*, **226**: 1393–1396.

120. Brown A.S., Gershon S. (1993) Dopamine and depression. *J. Neural Transm.*, **91**: 75–109.

121. Karlsson I. (1993) Neurotransmitter changes in aging and dementia. *Nordic J. Psychiatry*, **47** (Suppl.): 41–44.

122. Alexopoulos G.S., Young R.C., Haycox J.A., Shamoian C.A., Blass J.P. (1985) Dexamethasone suppression test in depression with reversible dementia. *Psychiatry Res.*, **16**: 277–285.

123. Sunderland T., Tariot P.N., Mueller E.A. (1985) TRH stimulation test in dementia of the Alzheimer type and elderly controls. *Psychiatry Res.*, **16**: 269–275.

124. Molchan S.E., Lawlor B.A., Hill J.L., Mellow A.M., Davis C.L., Martinez R., Sunderland T. (1991) The TRH stimulation test in Alzheimer's disease and major depression. *Biol. Psychiatry*, **30**: 567–576.

125. Targum S.D., Marshall L.E., Fishman P. (1992) Variability of TRH test response in depressed and normal elderly subjects. *Biol. Psychiatry*, **31**: 787–793.

126. Yastrubetskaya O., Chiu E., O'Connell S. (1997) Is good clinical research practice for clinical trials good clinical practice? *Int. J. Geriatr. Psychiatry*, **12**: 227–231.

127. Baldwin R., Jolley D. (1986) The prognosis of depression in old age. *Br. J. Psychiatry*, **149**: 574–583.

128. Zubenko G.S., Mulsant B.H., Rifai A.H., Sweet R.A., Pasternak R.E., Marino L.J. Jr, Tu X.M. (1994) Impact of acute psychiatric inpatient treatment on major depression in late life and prediction of response. *Am. J. Psychiatry*, **151**: 987–994.

129. Reynolds C.F. III, Frank E., Perel J.M., Miller M.D., Cornes C., Rifai A.H., Pollock B.G., Mazumdar S., George C.J., Houck P.R. *et al* (1994) Treatment of consecutive episodes of major depression in the elderly. *Am. J. Psychiatry*, **151**: 1740–1743.

130. Flint A.J., Rifat S.L. (1994) A prospective study of lithium augmentation in antidepressant-resistant geriatric depression. *J. Clin. Psychopharmacol.*, **14**: 353–356.

131. Flint A.J., Rifat S.L. (1996) The effect of sequential antidepressant treatment on geriatric depression. *J. Affect. Disord.*, **36**: 95–105.

132. Banerjee S., Dickinson E. (1997) Evidence based health care in old age psychiatry. *Int. J. Psychiatry Med.*, **27**: 283–292.

133. Schneider L.S., Olin J.T. (1995) Efficacy of acute treatment for geriatric depression. *Int. Psychogeriatr.*, **7** (Suppl.): 7–25.

134. Reynolds C.F. III, Frank E., Perel J.M., Imber S.D., Cornes C., Morycz R.K., Mazumdar S., Miller M.D., Pollock B.G., Rifai A.H. *et al* (1992) Combined pharmacotherapy and psychotherapy in the acute and continuation treatment of elderly patients with recurrent major depression: a preliminary report. *Am. J. Psychiatry*, **149**: 1687–1692.

135. Banerjee S., Shamash K., Macdonald A., Mann A.H. (1996) Randomized controlled trial of effect of intervention by psychogeriatric team on depression in frail elderly people at home. *Br. Med. J.*, **313**: 1058–1061.

136. Lebowitz B.D., Martinez R.A., Niederehe G., Pearson V.L., Reynolds C.F. III, Rudorfer M.V., Schneider L.S., Kupfer D.J. (1995) NIMH/MacArthur Foundation Workshop Report. Treatment of depression in late life. *Psychopharmacol. Bull.*, **31**: 185–202.

137. Bultema J.K., Mailliard L., Getzfrid M.K., Lerner R.D., Colone M. (1996) Geriatric patients with depression. Improving outcomes using a multidisciplinary clinical path model. *JAMA*, **26**: 31–38.

138. Norquist G., Wells K.B., Rogers W.H., Davis L.M., Kahn K., Brook R. (1995) Quality of care for depressed elderly patients hospitalized in the specialty psychiatric units or general medical wards. *Arch. Gen. Psychiatry*, **52**: 695–701.

139. Blanchard M.R., Waterreus A., Mann A.H. (1995) The effect of primary care nurse interventions upon older people screened as depressed. *Int. J. Geriatr. Psychiatry*, **10**: 289–298.

140. Callahan C.M., Hendrie H.C., Dittus R.S., Brater D.C., Hui S.L., Tierney W.M. (1994) Improving treatment of late-life depression in primary care: a randomized clinical trial. *J. Am. Geriatr. Soc.*, **42**: 839–846.

141. Ames D. (1990) Depression among elderly residents of local-authority residential homes: its nature and the efficacy of intervention. *Br. J. Psychiatry*, **156**: 667–675.

142. Seidel G., Smith C., Hafner R.J., Holme G. (1992) A psychogeriatric community outreach service: description and evaluation. *Int. J. Geriatr. Psychiatry*, **7**: 347–350.

143. Llewellyn-Jones R., Baikie K.A., Andrews C., Pond D., Willcock S.M., Castell S., Smithers H.E., Cohen J., Baikie A., Snowdon J.S. *et al* (1997) A controlled trial of shared care for late life depression in residential care. *Aust. N. Zeal. J. Psychiatry*, **31** (Suppl. 1): A7.

144. Callahan C.M., Hendrie H.C., Tierney W.M. (1996) The recognition and treatment of late-life depression: a view from primary care. *Int. J. Psychiatry Med.*, **26**: 155–171.

145. Beck D.A., Koenig H.G. (1996) Minor depression: a review of the literature. *Int. J. Psychiatry Med.*, **26**: 177–209.

146. Draper B., Anstey K. (1996) Psychosocial stressors, physical illness and the spectrum of depression in elderly inpatients. *Aust. N. Zeal. J. Psychiatry*, **30**: 567–572.

147. Rigler S.K., Studenski S., Duncan P.W. (1998) Pharmacologic treatment of geriatric depression: key issues in interpreting the evidence. *J. Am. Geriatr. Soc.*, **46**: 106–110.

148. Gerson S.C., Plotkin D.A., Jarvik L.F. (1988) Antidepressant drug studies, 1964–1988: empirical evidence for aging patients. *J. Clin. Psychopharmacol.*, **8**: 311–322.

149. Anstey K., Brodaty H. (1995) Antidepressants and the elderly: double-blind trials 1987–1992. *Int. J. Geriatr. Psychiatry*, **10**: 265–279.

150. Heiligenstein J.H., Ware J.E. Jr, Beusterien K.M., Roback P.J., Andrejasich C., Tollefson G.D. (1995) Acute effects of fluoxetine versus placebo on functional health and well-being in late-life depression. *Int. Psychogeriatr.*, **7** (Suppl.): 125–137.

151. McEntee W., Ko G., Richter E. (1996) Sertraline and nortriptyline: heart rate, cognitive improvement and quality of life in depressed elderly. Presented at the 20th CINP Congress, Melbourne, 23–27 June.

152. Möller H.J., Muller H., Volz H.P. (1996) How to assess the onset of antidepressant effect: comparison of global ratings and findings based on depression scales. *Pharmacopsychiatry*, **29**: 57–62.

153. Reynolds C.F. III, Dew M.A., Frank E., Begley A.E., Miller M.D., Cornes C., Mazumdar S., Perel J.M., Kupfer D.J. (1998) Effects of age at onset of first lifetime episode of recurrent major depression on treatment response and illness course in elderly patients. *Am. J. Psychiatry*, **155**: 795–799.

154. Flint A.J., Rifat S.L. (1997) Effect of demographic and clinical variables on time to antidepressant response in geriatric depression. *Depress. Anxiety*, **5**: 103–107.

155. Simpson S.W., Jackson A., Baldwin R.C., Burns A. (1997) Subcortical hyperintensities in late-life depression: acute response to treatment and neuropsychological impairment. *Int. Psychogeriatr.*, **9**: 257–275.

156. Bump G.M., Reynolds C.F. III, Smith G., Pollock B.G., Dew M.A., Mazumdar S., Geary M., Houck P.R., Kupfer D.J. (1997) Accelerating response in geriatric depression: a pilot study combining sleep deprivation and paroxetine. *Depress. Anxiety*, **6**: 113–118.

157. Schneider L.S., Small G.W., Hamilton S.H., Bystritsky A., Nemeroff C.B., Meyers B.S. (1997) Estrogen replacement and response to fluoxetine in a multicenter geriatric depression trial. Fluoxetine Collaborative Study Group. *Am. J. Geriatr. Psychiatry*, **5**: 97–106.

158. Montgomery S.A., Kasper S. (1995) Comparison of compliance between serotonin reuptake inhibitors and tricyclic antidepressants: a meta-analysis. *Int. Clin. Psychopharmacol.*, **9** (Suppl. 4): 33–40.

159. Delini-Stula A., Mikkelsen H., Angst J. (1995) Therapeutic efficacy of antidepressants in agitated anxious depression — a meta-analysis of moclobemide studies. *J. Affect. Disord.*, **35**: 21–30.

160. Finkel S.I. (1996) Efficacy and tolerability of antidepressant therapy in the old-old. *J. Clin. Psychiatry*, **57** (Suppl. 5): 23–28.

161. Shasha M., Lyons J.S., O'Mahoney M.T., Rosenberg A., Miller S.I., Howard K.I. (1997) Serotonin reuptake inhibitors and the adequacy of antidepressant treatment. *Int. J. Psychiatry Med.*, **27**: 83–92.

162. Danish University Antidepressant Group (1986) Citalopram: clinical effect profile in comparison with clomipramine: a controlled multicenter study. *Psychopharmacology*, **90**: 131–138.

163. Danish University Antidepressant Group (1990) Paroxetine: a selective serotonin reuptake inhibitor showing better tolerance, but weaker antidepressant effect than clomipramine in a controlled multicenter study. *J. Affect. Disord.*, **18**: 289–299.

164. Roose S.P., Glassman A.H., Attia E., Woodring S. (1994) Comparative efficacy of selective serotonin reuptake inhibitors and tricyclics in the treatment of melancholia. *Am. J. Psychiatry*, **151**: 1735–1739.

165. Nair N.P., Amin M., Holm P., Katona C., Klitgaard N., Ng Ying Kin N.M., Kragh Sörensen P., Kuhn H., Leek C.A., Stage K.B. (1995) Moclobemide and

nortriptyline in elderly depressed patients. A randomized, multicentre trial against placebo. *J. Affect. Disord.*, **33**: 1–9.

166.   Lasser R., Siegel E., Dukoff R., Sunderland T. (1998) Diagnosis and treatment of geriatric depression. *CNS Drugs*, **9**: 17–30.

167.   Mitchell P. (1997) Drug interactions of clinical significance with selective serotonin reuptake inhibitors. *Drug Safety*, **17**: 390–406.

168.   Katz I.R. (1993) Drug treatment of depression in the frail elderly: discussion of the NIH Consensus Development Conference on the Diagnosis and Treatment of Depression in Late Life. *Psychopharmacol. Bull.*, **29**: 101–108.

169.   Koenig H.G., Goli V., Shelp F., Kudler H.S., Cohen H.J., Meador K.G., Blazer D.G. (1989) Antidepressant use in elderly medical inpatients: lessons from an attempted clinical trial. *J. Gen. Int. Med.*, **4**: 498–505.

170.   Schifano F., Garbin A., Renesto V., De Dominicis M.G., Trinciarelli G., Silvestri A., Magni G. (1990) A double-blind comparison of mianserin and maprotiline in depressed medically ill elderly people. *Acta Psychiatr. Scand.*, **81**: 289–294.

171.   Tan R.S.H., Barlow R.J., Abel C., Reddy S., Palmer A.J., Fletcher A.E., Nicholl C.G., Pitt B.M., Bulpitt C.J. (1994) The effect of low dose lofepramine in depressed elderly patients in general medical wards. *Br. J. Clin. Pharmacol.*, **37**: 321–324.

172.   Evans M., Hammond M., Wilson K., Lye M., Copeland J. (1997) Placebo-controlled treatment trial of depression in elderly physically ill patients. *Int. J. Geriatr. Psychiatry*, **12**: 817–824.

173.   Andersen G., Vestergaard K., Lauritzen L. (1994) Effective treatment of post-stroke depression with the selective serotonin reuptake inhibitor citalopram. *Stroke*, **25**: 1099–1104.

174.   Kernohan W.J., Chambers J.L., Wilson W.T., Daugherty J.F. (1967) Effects of nortriptyline on the mental and social adjustment of geriatric patients in a mental hospital. *J. Am. Geriatr. Soc.*, **15**: 196–202.

175.   Katz I.R., Simpson G.M., Curlik S.M., Parmelee P.A., Muhly C. (1990) Pharmacologic treatment of major depression for elderly patients in residential care settings. *J. Clin. Psychiatry*, **51** (Suppl. 7) 41–47.

176.   Lipsey J.R., Robinson R.G., Pearlson G.D., Rao K., Price T.R. (1984) Nortriptyline treatment of post-stroke depression: a double-blind study. *Lancet*, **i**: 297–300.

177.   Borson S., McDonald G.J., Gayle T., Deffenback M., Lakschminarayan S., Van Tuinen C. (1992) Improvement in mood, physical symptoms, and function with nortriptyline for depression in patients with chronic obstructive pulmonary disease. *Psychosomatics*, **33**: 190–201.

178.   Lakshmanan M., Mion L.C., Frengley J.D. (1986) Effective low dose tricyclic antidepressant treatment for depressed geriatric rehabilitation patients. A double-blind study. *J. Am. Geriatr. Soc.*, **34**: 421–426.

179.   Roose S.P., Laghrissi Thode F., Kennedy J.S., Nelson J.C., Bigger J.T. Jr, Pollock B.G., Gaffrey A., Narayan M., Flokel M.S., McCafferty J. *et al* (1998) Comparison of paroxetine and nortriptyline in depressed patients with ischemic heart disease. *JAMA*, **279**: 287–291.

180.   Small G.W., Birkett M., Meyers B.S., Koran L.M., Bystritsky A., Nemeroff C.B. (1996) Impact of physical illness on quality of life and antidepressant response in geriatric major depression. *J. Am. Geriatr. Soc.*, **44**: 1220–1225.

181.   Wallace A.E., Kofoed L.L., West A.N. (1995) Double-blind, placebo-controlled trial of methylphenidate in older, depressed, medically ill patients. *Am. J. Psychiatry*, **152**: 929–931.

182. Koenig H.G., Breitner J.C.S. (1990) Use of antidepressants in medically ill older patients. *Psychosomatics*, **31**: 22–32.
183. Reifler B.V., Teri L., Raskind M., Veith R., Barnes R., White E., McLean P. (1989) Double-blind trial of imipramine in Alzheimer's disease patients with and without depression. *Am. J. Psychiatry*, **146**: 45–49.
184. Nyth A.L., Gottfries C.G., Lyby K., Smedegaard Andersen L., Gylding Sabroe J., Kristensen M., Refsum H.E., Ofsti E., Eriksson S., Syversen S. (1992) A controlled multicenter clinical study of citalopram and placebo in elderly depressed patients with and without concomitant dementia. *Acta Psychiatr. Scand.*, **86**: 138–145.
185. Passeri M., Cucinotta D., Abate G., Senin U., Ventura A., Stramba Badiale M., Daian R., La Greca P., Le Grazie C. (1993) Oral 5'-methyltetrahydrofolic acid in senile organic mental disorders with depression: results of a double-blind multicenter study. *Aging*, **5**: 63–71.
186. Fuchs A., Hehnke U., Erhart C., Schell C., Pramshohler B., Danninger B., Schautzer F. (1993) Video rating analysis of effect of maprotiline in patients with dementia and depression. *Pharmacopsychiatry*, **26**: 37–41.
187. Roth M., Mountjoy C.Q., Amrein R. (1996) Moclobemide in elderly patients with cognitive decline and depression. An international double-blind, placebo-controlled study. *Br. J. Psychiatry*, **168**: 149–157.
188. Nyth A.L., Gottfries C.G. (1990) The clinical efficacy of citalopram in treatment of emotional disturbances in dementia disorders. A Nordic multicentre study. *Br. J. Psychiatry*, **157**: 894–901.
189. Volicer L., Rheaume Y., Cyr D. (1994) Treatment of depression in advanced Alzheimer's disease using sertraline. *J. Geriatr. Psychiatr. Neurol.*, **7**: 227–229.
190. Rovner B.W., German P.S., Brant L.J., Clark R., Burton L., Folstein M.F. (1991) Depression and mortality in nursing homes. *JAMA*, **265**: 993–996.
191. Phillips C.J., Henderson A.S. (1991) The prevalence of depression among Australian nursing home residents: results using draft ICD-10 and DSM-III-R criteria. *Psychol. Med.*, **21**: 739–748.
192. Snowdon J., Burgess E., Vaughan R., Miller R. (1996) Use of antidepressants, and the prevalence of depression and cognitive impairment in Sydney nursing homes. *Int. J. Geriatr. Psychiatry*, **11**: 599–606.
193. Trappler B., Cohen C.I. (1998) Use of SSRIs in "very old" depressed nursing home residents. *Am. J. Geriatr. Psychiatry*, **6**: 83–89.
194. Elkin I., Shea M.T., Watkins J.T., Imbec S.D., Sotsky S.M., Collins J.F., Glass D.R., Pilkonis P.A., Leber W.R., Docherty J.P. (1989) NIMH Treatment of Depression Collaboration Research Program: I. General effectiveness of treatments. *Arch. Gen. Psychiatry*, **46**: 971–982.
195. Parnetti L., Sommacal S., Morselli L.A.M., Senin U. (1993) Multicentre controlled randomized double-blind placebo study of minaprine in elderly patients suffering from prolonged depressive reaction. *Drug Invest.*, **6**: 181–188.
196. Pelicier Y., Schaeffer P. (1993) Multicenter double-blind study comparing the efficacy and tolerance of paroxetine and clomipramine in reactive depression in the elderly patient. *Encephale*, **19**: 257–261.
197. Casacchia M., Bolino F., Marola W., Pirro R., Nivoli G., Rapisarda V., Pancheri P. (1994) Controlled multicentre study of teniloxazine in mild depression of the elderly. *New Trends Exp. Clin. Psychiatry*, **10**: 187–192.
198. Scogin F., McElreath L. (1994) Efficacy of psychosocial treatments for geriatric depression: a quantitative review. *J. Consult. Clin. Psychol.*, **62**: 69–74.
199. Morris R.G., Morris L.W. (1991) Cognitive and behavioural approaches with the depressed elderly. *Int. J. Geriatr. Psychiatry*, **6**: 407–413.

200. Koder D., Brodaty H., Anstey K. (1996) Cognitive therapy for depression in the elderly. *Int. J. Geriatr. Psychiatry*, **11**: 97–107.
201. Robinson L.A., Berman J.S., Neimeyer R.A. (1990) Psychotherapy for the treatment of depression: a comprehensive review of controlled outcome research. *Psychol. Bull.*, **108**: 30–49.
202. Rybarczyk B., Gallagher-Thompson D., Rodman J., Zeiss A., Gantz F.E., Yesavage J. (1992) Applying cognitive-behavioral psychotherapy to the chronically-ill elderly: treatment issues and case illustration. *Int. Psychogeriatr.*, **4**: 127–140.
203. Mossey J.M., Knott K.A., Higgins M., Talerico K. (1996) Effectiveness of a psychosocial intervention, interpersonal counseling, for subdysthymic depression in medically ill elderly. *J. Gerontol. Biol. Sci. Med. Sci.*, **51**: M172–M178.
204. Steuer J.L., Mintz J., Hammen C.L., Hill M.A., Jarvik L.F., McCarley T., Motoike P., Rosen R. (1984) Cognitive-behavioural and psychodynamic group psychotherapy in the treatment of geriatric depression. *J. Consult. Clin. Psychol.*, **52**: 180–189.
205. Teri L., Logsdon R.G., Uomoto J., McCurry S.M. (1997) Behavioral treatment of depression in dementia patients: a controlled clinical trial. *J. Gerontol.*, **52B**: P159–P166.
206. Abraham I.L., Neundorfer M.M., Currie L.J. (1992) Effects of group interventions on cognition and depression in nursing home residents. *Nursing Res.*, **41**: 196–202.
207. Hussian R.A., Lawrence P.S. (1981) Social reinforcement of activity and problem-solving training in the treatment of depressed institutionalized elderly patients. *Cogn. Ther. Res.*, **5**: 57–69.
208. Youssef F.A. (1990) The impact of group reminiscence counseling on a depressed elderly population. *Nurse Pract.*, **15**: 35–38.
209. Zerhusen J.D., Boyle K., Wilson W. (1991) Out of the darkness: group cognitive therapy for the depressed elderly. *J. Psychosoc. Nurs. Ment. Health Serv.*, **29**: 16–21.
210. Rosen J., Rogers J.C., Marin R.S., Mulsant B.H., Shahar A., Reynolds C.F. III (1997) Control-relevant intervention in the treatment of minor and major depression in a long-term care facility. *Am. J. Geriatr. Psychiatry*, **5**: 247–257.
211. Singh N.A., Clements K.M., Fiatarone M.A. (1997) A randomized controlled trial of progressive resistance training in depressed elders. *J. Gerontol.*, **51**: M27–M35.
212. McNeil K., LeBlanc E., Joyce M. (1991) The effect of exercise on depressive symptoms in the moderately depressed elderly. *Psychol. Aging*, **3**: 487–488.
213. Hanser S.B., Thompson L.W. (1994) Effects of a music therapy strategy on depressed older adults. *J. Gerontol.*, **49**: P265–P269.
214. Kramer B.A. (1985) Use of ECT in California, 1977–1983. *Am. J. Psychiatry*, **142**: 1190–1192.
215. Brodaty H., Harris L., Wilhelm K., Hickie I., Boyce P., Mitchell P., Parker G., Eyers K. (1993) Lessons from a mood disorders unit. *Aust. N. Zeal. J. Psychiatry*, **27**: 254–263.
216. Devanand D.P., Krueger R.B. (1994) Electroconvulsive therapy in the elderly. *Curr. Opin. Psychiatry*, **7**: 359–364.
217. Clinical Research Centre Division of Psychiatry (1984) The Northwick Park ECT trial: predictors of response to real and simulated ECT. *Br. J. Psychiatry*, **144**: 227–237.
218. Hickie I., Mason C., Parker G., Brodaty H. (1996) Prediction of ECT response: validation of a refined sign-based (CORE) system for defining melancholia. *Br. J. Psychiatry*, **169**: 68–74.

219. Flint A.J., Rifat S.L. (1998) The treatment of psychotic depression in later life: a comparison of pharmacotherapy and ECT. *Int. J. Geriatr. Psychiatry*, **13**: 23–28.

220. Morris P.D. (1991) Which elderly depressives will respond to ECT? *Int. J. Geriatr. Psychiatry*, **6**: 159–163.

221. O'Leary D., Gill D., Gregory S., Shawcross C. (1995) Which depressed patients respond to ECT? The Nottingham results. *J. Affect. Disord.*, **33**: 245–250.

222. Sobin C., Prudic J., Devanand D.P., Nobler M.S., Sackheim H.A. (1996) Who responds to electroconvulsive therapy? *Br. J. Psychiatry*, **169**: 322–328.

223. Wilkinson A.M., Anderson D.N., Peters S. (1993) Age and the effects of ECT. *Int. J. Geriatr. Psychiatry*, **8**: 401–406.

224. Janicak P.G., Davis J.M., Gibbons RP., Ericksen S., Chang S., Gallagher P. (1985) Efficacy of ECT: a meta-analysis. *Am. J. Psychiatry*, **142**: 297–302.

225. O'Leary D., Gill D., Gregory S., Shawcross C. (1994) The effectiveness of real versus simulated electroconvulsive therapy in depressed elderly patients. *Int. J. Geriatr. Psychiatry*, **9**: 567–571.

226. Folkerts H.W., Michael N., Tolle R., Schonauer K., Mucke S., Schulze Monking H. (1997) Electroconvulsive therapy vs. paroxetine in treatment-resistant depression — a randomized study. *Acta Psychiatr. Scand.*, **96**: 334–342.

227. Philibert R.A., Richards L., Lynch C.F., Winokur G. (1995) Effect of ECT on mortality and clinical outcome in geriatric unipolar depression. *J. Clin. Psychiatry*, **56**: 390–394.

228. Fraser R.M., Glass I.B. (1980) Unilateral and bilateral ECT in elderly patients: a comparative study. *Acta Psychiatr. Scand.*, **62**: 13–31.

229. Gaspar D., Samarasinghe L.A. (1982) ECT in psychogeriatric practice — a study of risk factors, indications and outcome. *Compr. Psychiatry*, **23**: 170–175.

230. Karlinsky H., Shulman K.I. (1984) The clinical use of electroconvulsive therapy in old age. *J. Am. Geriatr. Soc.*, **32**: 183–186.

231. Mielke D.H., Winstead D.K., Goethe J.W., Schwartz B.D. (1984) Multiple-monitored electroconvulsive therapy: safety and efficacy in elderly depressed patients. *J. Am. Geriatr. Soc.*, **32**: 180–182.

232. Benbow S.M. (1987) The use of electroconvulsive therapy in old age psychiatry. *Int. J. Geriatr. Psychiatry*, **2**: 25–30.

233. Godber C., Rosenvinge H., Wilkinson D., Smithies J. (1987) Depression in old age: prognosis after ECT. *Int. J. Geriatr. Psychiatry*, **2**: 19–24.

234. Burke W.J., Rubin E.H., Zorumski C.F., Wetzel R.D. (1987) The safety of ECT in geriatric psychiatry. *J. Am. Geriatr. Soc.*, **35**: 516–521.

235. Kramer B.A. (1987) Electroconvulsive therapy use in geriatric depression. *J. Nerv. Ment. Dis.*, **175**: 233–235.

236. Cattan R.A., Barry P.P., Mead G., Reefe W.E., Gay A., Silverman M. (1990) Electroconvulsive therapy in octogenarians. *J. Am. Geriatr. Soc.*, **38**: 753–758.

237. Murphy E. (1983) The prognosis of depression in old age. *Br. J. Psychiatry*, **142**: 111–119.

238. Prudic J., Sackheim H.A., Devanand D.P. (1990) Medication resistance and clinical response to electroconvulsive therapy. *Psychiatry Res.*, **31**: 287–296.

239. Prudic J., Haskett R.F., Mulsant B., Malone K.M., Pettinati H.M., Stephens S., Greenberg R., Rifas S.L., Sackheim H.A. (1996) Resistance to antidepressant medications and short-term clinical response to ECT. *Am. J. Psychiatry*, **153**: 985–992.

240. Heshe J., Roeder E., Theilgaard A. (1978) Unilateral and bilateral ECT. A psychiatric and psychological study of therapeutic effect and side effects. *Acta Psychiatr. Scand.* (Suppl. 275).

241. Pettinati H.M., Mathisen K.S., Rosenberg J., Lynch J.F. (1986) Meta-analytic approach to reconciling discrepancies in efficacy between bilateral and unilateral electroconvulsive therapy. *Conv. Ther.*, **2**: 7–17.
242. Benbow S.M. (1991) ECT in late life. *Int. J. Geriatr. Psychiatry*, **6**: 401–406.
243. Sackheim H.A., Prudic J., Devanand D.P., Kiersky J.E., Fitzsimons L., Moody B.J., McElhiney M.C., Coleman E.A., Settembrino J.M. (1993) Effects of stimulus intensity and electrode placement on the efficacy and cognitive effects of electroconvulsive therapy. *N. Engl. J. Med.*, **328**: 839–846.
244. Abrams R. (1997) *Electroconvulsive Therapy*, 3rd edn, Oxford University Press, New York.
245. McCall W.V., Farah B.A., Reboussin D., Colenda C.C. (1995) Comparison of the efficacy of titrated, moderate-dose and fixed, high-dose right unilateral ECT in elderly patients. *Am. J. Geriatr. Psychiatry*, **3**: 317–324.
246. Sobin C., Sackheim H.A., Prudic J., Devanand D.P., Moody B.J., McElhiney M.C. (1995) Predictors of retrograde amnesia following ECT. *Am. J. Psychiatry*, **152**: 995–1001.
247. Stoudemire A., Hill C.D., Morris R., Martino Salzman D., Markwalter H., Lewison B. (1991) Cognitive outcome following tricyclic and electroconvulsive treatment of major depression in the elderly. *Am. J. Psychiatry*, **148**: 1336–1340.
248. Zielinski R.J., Roose S.P., Devanand D.P., Woodring S., Sackheim H.A. (1993) Cardiovascular complications of ECT in depressed patients with cardiac disease. *Am. J. Psychiatry*, **150**: 904–909.
249. Draper B., Luscombe G. (1998) Quantification of factors contributing to length of stay in an acute psychogeriatrics ward. *Int. J. Geriatr. Psychiatry*, **13**: 1–7.
250. Nelson J.P., Rosenberg D.R. (1991) ECT treatment of demented elderly patients with major depression: a retrospective study of efficacy and safety. *Conv. Ther.*, **7**: 157–165.
251. Price T.R.P., McAllister T.W. (1989) Safety and efficacy of ECT in depressed patients with dementia: a review of clinical experience. *Conv. Ther.*, **5**: 61–74.
252. Bonner D., Howard R. (1995) Treatment-resistant depression in the elderly. *Int. Psychogeriatr.*, **7** (Suppl.): 83–94.
253. Goff D.C., Jenike M.A. (1986) Treatment-resistant depression in the elderly. *J. Am. Geriatr. Soc.*, **34**: 63–70.
254. Borson S., Raskind M. (1986) Antidepressant-resistant depression in the elderly. *J. Am. Geriatr. Soc.*, **34**: 245–249.
255. Roth M. (1955) The natural history of mental disorders in old age. *J. Ment. Sci.*, **101**: 281–301.
256. Cole M.G., Bellavance F. (1997) The prognosis of depression in old age. *Am. J. Geriatr. Psychiatry*, **5**: 4–14.
257. Department of Clinical Epidemiology and Biostatistics, McMaster University (1981) How to read clinical journals. III. To learn the clinical course and prognosis of disease. *Can. Med. Ass. J.*, **124**: 869–872.
258. American Psychiatric Association (1980) *Diagnostic and Statistical Manual of Mental Disorders*, 3rd edn, American Psychiatric Association, Washington, DC.
259. O'Connor D., Blessed G., Cooper B., Jonker C., Morris J.C., Presnell I.B., Ames D., Kay D.W., Bickel H., Schaufele M. *et al* (1996) Cross-national interrater reliability of dementia diagnosis in the elderly and factors associated with disagreement. *Neurology*, **47**: 1194–1199.
260. McGorry P., Copolov D.L., Singh B. (1989) The validity of the assessment of psychopathology in the psychoses. *Aust. N. Zeal. J. Psychiatry*, **23**: 469–482.
261. Kay D., Roth M., Hopkins B. (1955) Affective disorders in the senium: their association with organic cerebral degeneration. *J. Ment. Sci.*, **101**: 302–316.

262. Post F. (1962) *The Significance of Affective Symptoms in Old Age*, Maudsley Monographs 10, Oxford University Press, London.
263. Post F. (1972) The management and nature of depressive illness in late life: a follow-through study. *Br. J. Psychiatry*, **121**: 393–404.
264. Gordon W.F. (1981) Elderly depressives: treatment and follow-up. *Can. J. Psychiatry*, **26**: 110–113.
265. Cole M.G. (1983) Age, age of onset, and course of primary depressive illness in the elderly. *Can. J. Psychiatry*, **28**: 102–104.
266. Cole M.G. (1985) The course of elderly depressed outpatients. *Can. J. Psychiatry*, **30**: 217–220.
267. Magni G., Palazzolo O., Bianchin G. (1988) The course of depression in elderly outpatients. *Can. J. Psychiatry*, **33**: 21–24.
268. Agbayewa M.O. (1990) Outcome of depression in a geriatric medical day hospital following psychiatric consultation. *Int. J. Geriatr. Psychiatry*, **5**: 33–39.
269. Meats P., Timol M., Jolley D. (1991) Prognosis of depression in the elderly. *Br. J. Psychiatry*, **159**: 659–663.
270. Burvill P.W., Hall W.D., Stampfer H.G., Emmerson J.P. (1991) The prognosis of depression in old age. *Br. J. Psychiatry*, **158**: 64–71.
271. Hinrichsen G.A. (1992) Recovery and relapse from major depressive disorder in the elderly. *Am. J. Psychiatry*, **149**: 1575–1579.
272. Baldwin R.C., Benbow S.M., Marriott A., Wilhelm K., Hickie I., Boyce P., Mitchell P., Parker G., Eyers K. (1993) Depression in old age: a reconsideration of cerebral disease in relation to outcome. *Br. J. Psychiatry*, **163**: 82–90.
273. Brodaty H., Harris L., Peters K., Wilhelm K., Hickie I., Boyce P., Mitchell P., Parker G., Eyers K. (1993) Prognosis of depression in the elderly: a comparison with younger patients. *Br. J. Psychiatry*, **163**: 589–596.
274. Old Age Depression Interest Group (1993) How long should the elderly take antidepressants? A double-blind placebo-controlled study of continuation/prophylaxis therapy with dothiepin. *Br. J. Psychiatry*, **162**: 175–182.
275. Stoudemire A., Hill C.D., Morris R., Martino-Saltzman D., Lewinson B. (1993) Long-term affective and cognitive outcome in depressed older adults. *Am. J. Psychiatry*, **150**: 896–900.
276. Freyne A., Wrigley M. (1995) Prognosis of depression in the elderly. *Irish J. Psychol. Med.*, **12**: 6–11.
277. Tuma T.A. (1996) Effect of age on the outcome of hospital treated depression. *Br. J. Psychiatry*, **168**: 76–81.
278. Lee H., Lawlor B.A. (1997) The outcome of elderly patients presenting with depressive symptoms. *Irish J. Psychol. Med.*, **14**: 8–12.
279. Flint A.J., Rifat S.L. (1998) Two-year outcome of psychotic depression in late life. *Am. J. Psychiatry*, **155**: 178–183.
280. O'Brien J., Ames D., Chiu E., Schweitzer I., Desmond P., Tress B. (1998) Severe deep white matter lesions and outcome in elderly patients with major depressive disorder: follow-up study. *Br. Med. J.*, **317**: 982–984.
281. Cole M.G., Bellavance F. (1997) Depression in elderly medical inpatients: a meta-analysis of outcomes. *Can. Med. Ass. J.*, **157**: 1055–1060.
282. Schuckit M.A., Miller P.L., Berman J. (1980) The three year course of psychiatric problems in a geriatric population. *J. Clin. Psychiatry*, **41**: 27–32.
283. Rapp S.R., Parisi S.A., Wallace C.E. (1991) Comorbid psychiatric disorders in elderly medical patients: a one year prospective study. *J. Am. Geriatr. Soc.*, **39**: 124–131.

284. Incalzi R.A., Gemma A., Capparella O., Muzzolon R., Antico L., Carbonin P.U. (1991) Effects of hospitalization on affective status of elderly patients. *Int. Psychogeriatr.*, **3**: 67–74.

285. Pomerantz A.S., deNesnera A., West A.N. (1992) Resolution of depressive symptoms in medical inpatients after discharge. *Int. J. Psychiatry Med.*, **22**: 281–289.

286. Koenig H.G., Goli V., Shelp F., Kudler H.S., Cohen H.J., Blazer D.G. (1992) Major depression in hospitalised medically ill older men: documentation, management and outcome. *Int. J. Geriatr. Psychiatry*, **7**: 25–34.

287. Evans M.E. (1993) Depression in elderly physically ill inpatients: a twelve-month prospective study. *Int. J. Geriatr. Psychiatry*, **8**: 587–592.

288. Dunham N.C., Sager M.A. (1994) Functional status symptoms of depression and the outcomes of hospitalisation in community-dwelling elderly patients. *Arch. Family Med.*, **3**: 676–681.

289. Fenton F.R., Cole M.G., Engelsmann F., Mansouri I. (1997) Depression in older medical inpatients: one-year course and outcome. *Int. J. Geriatr. Psychiatry*, **12**: 389–394.

290. Ben-Arie O., Welman M., Teggin A.F. (1990) The depressed elderly living in the community: a follow-up study. *Br. J. Psychiatry*, **157**: 425–427.

291. O'Connor D.W., Politt P.A., Roth M. (1990) Coexisting depression and dementia in a community survey of the elderly. *Int. Psychogeriatr.*, **2**: 45–53.

292. Kivelä S.L., Pahkala K., Laipbala P. (1991) A one-year prognosis of dysthymic disorder and major depression in old age. *Int. J. Geriatr. Psychiatry*, **6**: 81–87.

293. Forsell E., Jorm A.F., Winblad B. (1994) Outcome of depression in demented and non-demented elderly: observations from a three-year follow-up in a community-based study. *Int. J. Geriatr. Psychiatry*, **9**: 5–10.

294. Kivelä S.L. (1995) Long-term prognosis of major depression in old age: a comparison with prognosis of dysthymic disorder. *Int. Psychogeriatr.*, **7** (Suppl.): 69–82.

295. Livingstone G., Watkin V., Milne B., Manela M.V., Katona C. (1997) The natural history of depression and the anxiety disorders in older people: the Islington community study. *J. Affect. Disord.*, **46**: 255–262.

296. Beekman A.T.F., Deeg D.J.H., Smit J.H., van Tilburg W. (1995) Prediction and course of depression in the older population: results from a community-based study in the Netherlands. *J. Affect. Disord.*, **34**: 41–49.

297. Kennedy G.J., Kelman H.R., Thomas C. (1991) Persistence and remission of depressive symptoms in late life. *Am. J. Psychiatry*, **148**: 174–178.

298. Ames D., Ashby D., Mann A.H., Graham N. (1988) Psychiatric illness in elderly residents of Part III Homes in one London borough: prognosis and review. *Age Ageing*, **17**: 249–256.

299. Ames D. (1990) Depression among elderly residents of local authority residential homes: its nature and the efficacy of intervention. *Br. J. Psychiatry*, **156**: 667–675.

300. Ashby D., Ames D., Macdonald A., Graham N., Mann A.H. (1991) Psychiatric morbidity as predictor of mortality for residents of local authority homes for the elderly. *Int. J. Geriatr. Psychiatry*, **6**: 567–575.

301. Lindesay J. (1991) Suicide in the elderly. *Int. J. Geriatr. Psychiatry*, **6**: 355–361.

302. Baldwin R., Chiu E., Katona C., Graham N. (2002) *Guidelines on Depression in Older People: Practising the Evidence.* Dunitz, London.

Commentaries

5.1
Depression in Older Age: Diagnostic Problems, New Knowledge and Neglected Areas
John R.M. Copeland[1]

Diagnostic issues recur repeatedly throughout each section of Chiu *et al*'s review. They are real. Similar problems were tackled by the US–UK Diagnostic Project for both younger [1] and older age groups in the 1960s and 70s. Then, trans-Atlantic diagnostic disagreement arose from lack of standardized criteria. Now it seems we have a problem with the standardized criteria. The DSM system is the most discussed. The "Quick Reference" to DSM-IV makes clear that "criteria enhances agreement among clinicians and investigators", but agreement is likely to be at its highest on fully formed illnesses that are relatively severe. High specificity (probably at the expense of sensitivity) seems the aim, good for biological research. But clinicians prefer high sensitivity so as not to lose depressions likely to respond to treatment. Two classifications would be more sensible. Diseases are human concepts, not "things", so we can redefine them and their classification for our purpose. Of course, we need to keep a balance between purpose and communication. The ICD seems to recognize this and offers two sets of criteria, a general classification and one for research. However, the usefulness is lost in the attempt to harmonize the general criteria with the DSM so that it emerges as almost as exclusive. It is no wonder that those who apply DSM find few cases of depression in community samples if the criteria are set to achieve high psychiatric agreement. It does not make sense that many depressions identified by clinicians now have to be described as "subsyndromal". What clinicians and their medical teams need is a "classification of cases for intervention". Chiu *et al* point out that one purpose of epidemiology is to provide data for health care. Such a database cannot be satisfactorily provided using either DSM or ICD. There are also dangers. If one were a director of managed care, which classification would be the most appealing?

[1]*Department of Psychiatry, University of Liverpool, Liverpool L69 36A, UK*

We must, however, be aware that when we use terms such as "cases for intervention" or "subsyndromal" we are still in the area of clinical impression. As Chiu *et al* point out, it is necessary to demonstrate that the treatment of these conditions is effective. We need evidence from random controlled trials of intervention on these so-called minor cases, many of which do not seem to be so minor.

Overall, the review indicates that we are making progress rapidly, especially as research only took off during the last two decades. We must not be discouraged that our techniques do not always deliver clear answers. For example, we now know that physical problems, especially concerning mobility, have a powerful effect on outcome, as Prince *et al*'s [2] careful and elegant studies and those of others demonstrate. A number of studies now show that depression accompanying even severe physical illness can respond to treatment, so we have messages to project where once there was therapeutic nihilism.

The message on the efficacy of electroconvulsive therapy is also important, especially to those countries where well-meaning groups have all but caused it to be banned.

We must not neglect prevention. There is evidence [3] that about a fifth of older people with depression symptoms, not considered at the time as cases severe enough for intervention, become such cases in 3 years time. How can we recognize them and the proportion of cases that we know recover spontaneously in a few weeks? Feelings of loneliness have twice emerged in our studies, as a risk factor for becoming an intervention case in 2 years time. Simple prevention ought to be possible.

We still worry about levels of depression in nursing homes. Henderson *et al* [4] reported that the prevalence of depression was no greater here than in the community. We have confirmed this surprising finding, but also find that the rates of new cases occurring are many times those in the community. So the nursing homes are not off the hook. What causes this phenomenon, is it serious physical illness left untreated or the regimen of the nursing home?

The prognosis of depression is not good. Even if depression resolves, many are left with neurotic and cognitive disorders.

There is another area we seem to neglect. Not so much culture itself, which has probably been overemphasized, but the methods for recognizing and treating depression in developing countries and how their health services can be advised. This is where the majority of the world's populations live. What about, for example, the problems of rural China, where, unlike Western communities, studies appear to show higher levels of depression and suicide among older people, compared to those living in cities?

Can we not learn something of interest by examining risk factors for depression in apparent low prevalence areas? Might not developed countries also be helped by finding ways of delivering less expensive but more effective care for depression, based on the new technologies? The research opportunities make this still one of the most exciting fields of psychiatry.

REFERENCES

1. Cooper J.E., Kendell R.E., Gurland B.J., Sharpe L., Copeland J.R.M., Simon R. (1972) *Psychiatric Diagnosis in New York and London*, Oxford University Press, London.
2. Prince M.J., Harwood R.H., Blizard R.A., Thomas A., Mann A.H. (1997) Impairment, disability and handicap as risk factors for depression in old age. The Gospel Oak Project V. *Psychol. Med.*, **27**: 311–321.
3. Sharma V.K., Copeland J.R.M., Dewey M.E., Lowe D., Davidson I. (1998) Outcome of the depressed elderly living in the community in Liverpool: a 5-year follow-up. *Psychol. Med.*, **28**: 1329–1337.
4. Henderson A.S., Korten A.E., Jorm A.F., Christensen H., Mackinnon A.J., Scott L.R. (1994) Are nursing homes depressing? *Lancet*, **344**: 1091.

5.2

Depression in the Elderly is Underdiagnosed; Etiology is Multifactorial

Carl Gerhard Gottfries[1]

As is evident from the review by Chiu *et al*, depression in the elderly is a great problem. In Sweden, where there is a large number of elderly people, statistics show that around 50% of all depressed people are 65 years old or more. Depression in the elderly is thus not a narrow field, and efforts must be made to offer this group of people good treatment.

There is clearly underdiagnosis and undertreatment of elderly depressed patients. The problem is to identify the patients. Elderly depressed patients report depressed mood less often than their younger counterparts. Instead they show a higher rate of anxiety. I think, however, that there is no problem for specialists in diagnosing depression in elderly patients; the problem is that this group of people does not seek medical help. Patients, carers and health care providers often regard depressive symptoms as manifestations of normal aging and do not identify the disorder as an illness. It is also true that elderly patients have difficulties in recognizing and describing depressive symptoms. The manifestations of the disorder therefore often give an atypical clinical picture. Concomitant somatic disease and/or organic brain damage make diagnosis more difficult, especially as elderly patients preferentially seek a somatic explanation of their complaints.

[1] *Institute of Clinical Neuroscience, Department of Psychiatry and Neurochemistry, Sahlgrenska University Hospital, S-431 80 Mölndal, Sweden*

Information about depression in the elderly should be given to the community, along with more focused information to district nurses and doctors concerning the identification of this type of patient.

Assessment tools can be used to identify elderly depressed patients. Epidemiological data show that there are many depressed elderly patients among those who are seen by district doctors. In a Swedish study, the Geriatric Depression Scale was used as a screening instrument for depression [1]. This simple scale was considered very useful.

In the diagnosis of depression in elderly people, interest should also be directed to 1-carbon metabolism. This metabolism is dependent on the vitamins B12 and folic acid. Disturbance of 1-carbon metabolism is marked by an increasing homocysteine in the serum. As shown by Heilmann [2], many elderly people have low serum levels of folic acid. Low or deficient serum or blood cell folate concentrations are found in 15–38% of depressed patients [3]. For a long time it has been well known that vitamin B12 deficiency is associated with depressed mood. According to Fava et al [4], 12–14% of depressed patients have low serum B12 levels, and in a total population of elderly people, 32% had low vitamin B12 levels. Serum homocysteine is therefore an important marker in studies of the etiology of depression in the elderly and should be investigated in the diagnostic process.

The concentrations of 5-hydroxytryptamine (5-HT) in discrete brain areas are reduced in individuals over 65 years old. The concentrations of 5-hydroxyindoleacetic acid (5-HIAA) do not appear to decrease with age (for a review see [5]). As 5-HT is considered to be a marker of the number of neuron terminals and 5-HIAA a marker of metabolic activity, these findings suggest that there is a reduction in the number of nerve terminals in normal aging but that increasing metabolic activity in the remaining terminals maintains the metabolite concentration. This may be a compensatory mechanism of the brain to the change of aging. This compensatory adaptation may also occur in the noradrenergic pathway, as noradrenaline levels decline with age, but the concentration of the end metabolite 3-methoxy-4-hydroxyphenylglycol (MHPG) does not. In fact, in some studies it has been shown to be increased [6].

Interestingly, monoamine oxidase (MAO)-B activity increases significantly with age. One possible explanation of the increased MAO-B activity is that this form of the enzyme is localized primarily to extraneuronal tissue, and age-related gliosis increases the relative amount of extraneuronal tissue. The biological importance of increased MAO-B activity is still a matter of speculation, and the increase is so small that it has been assumed to be of little importance for the metabolism of the monoaminergic neurotransmitters [7].

In post-mortem studies of human brains, age-related reductions in the concentrations of 5-HIAA in the hypothalamus have been recorded [8]. These findings indicate that the serotonergic system has a reduced impact on the hypothalamus in elderly people. As the hypothalamus controls non-neurohormonal systems, this may be of importance especially in the control of stress activity.

It can be assumed that the neurochemical changes in the aging brain, concerning both serotonin and noradrenaline metabolism, reduce the thresholds for depression and other emotional disturbances.

In the treatment of elderly people, especially those with degenerative neuropsychiatric disorders, not too much effort should be made to cram the symptomatology into the boxes of DSM-IV. Many of these elderly have emotional disturbances, such as restlessness, anxiety, irritability and aggressiveness, which respond well to treatment with selective serotonin reuptake inhibitors (SSRIs).

As mentioned above, elderly people may have disturbances of 1-carbon metabolism, which is of importance for the synthesis of neurotransmitters. In fact, the synthesis of serotonin is dependent on normal supply of methyl groups. Patients with high serum homocysteine or methylmalonic acid or low levels of vitamin B12 or folic acid should receive supplementation of these vitamins concomitant with the antidepressant treatment. There are already data indicating that patients with low serum folate levels are less likely to respond to SSRIs [4, 9] and that lithium plus folic acid in prophylactic treatment reduces depressive morbidity more than lithium alone [10].

REFERENCES

1. Gottfries C.G., Noltorp S., Norgaard N. (1997) Experience with a Swedish version of the Geriatric Depression Scale in primary care centers. *Int. J. Geriatr. Psychiatry*, **12**: 1029–1034.
2. Heilmann E. (1987) In *Folsäuremangel: Ergebnisse eigene Untersuchungen an gesunden Probanden in verschiedenen Altersstufen und bei unterschiedlichen Erkrankungen* (Ed. K. Pietrzik), pp. 41–55, Zuchschwerdt Verlag, Munich.
3. Herbert V. (1962) Experimental nutritional folate deficiency in man. *Trans. Assoc. Am. Physicians*, **75**: 307–327.
4. Fava M., Borus J.S., Alpert J.E., Niernberg A.A., Rosenbaum J.F., Bottiglieri T. (1997) Folate, vitamin B12, and homocysteine in major depressive disorder. *Am. J. Psychiatry*, **154**: 426–434.
5. Gottfries C.G. (1990) Neurochemical aspects of aging and disease with cognitive impairment. *J. Neurosci. Res.*, **27**: 541–547.
6. Gottfries C.G., Adolfsson R., Aquilonius S.M., Carlsson A., Eckernäs S.Å., Nordberg A., Oreland L., Svennerholm L., Wiberg Å., Winblad B. (1983) Biochemical changes in dementia disorders of Alzheimer type (AD/SDAT) *Neurobiol. Ageing*, **4**: 261–271.
7. Oreland L., Gottfries C.G. (1986) Platelet and brain monoamine oxidase in aging and in dementia of Alzheimer's type. *Prog. Neuropsychopharmacol. Biol. Psychiatry*, **10**: 533–540.
8. Arranz B., Blennow K., Ekman R., Eriksson A., Månsson J.-F., Marcusson J. (1996) Brain monoaminergic and neuropeptidergic variations in human aging. *J. Neural. Transm.*, **103**: 101–115.

9. Alpert M., Silva R., Pouget B. (1996) Folate as a predictor of response to sertraline or nortriptyline in geriatric depression. Presented at the 36th Annual Meeting of the NCDEU, Boca Raton, USA, 28–31 May.
10. Coppen A., Abou-Saleh M.T. (1982) Plasma folate and affective morbidity during long-term lithium therapy. *Br. J. Psychiatry*, **141**: 87–89.

5.3
Depression in the Elderly: Issues in Diagnosis and Management

David L. Dunner[1]

Depression in the elderly is of clinical significance because of the increasing numbers of elderly in the population, the prevalence of depression in this age group, and difficulty with relative tolerability of antidepressant agents amongst the elderly. Depression in the elderly can be a new or first episode, usually of unipolar major depressive disorder, a recurrence of prior episodes of unipolar or bipolar disorder, or an exacerbation or continuation of either chronic major depression or dysthymic disorder [1, 2]. In addition, bereavement is a more frequent experience in the elderly than in younger individuals, and bereavement itself may be experienced as a longstanding depression. According to DSM-IV, if significant symptoms of bereavement persist for 2 months or longer, the disorder is characterized as a major depressive disorder [3].

Depression in the elderly may be easy to recognize if it is a continuation of a condition that began earlier in life and persisted, such as chronic major depression or dysthymic disease, or a recurrent episode in a patient who has been previously treated for depression. However, the recognition of first onset depression in the elderly is sometimes made difficult because of altered presentations of depression in the elderly. In my clinical practice, it is more frequent for elderly than younger patients to deny traditional depressive symptoms, making both recognition and assessment of depression difficult. Furthermore, traditional rating scales, such as the Hamilton Depression Rating Scale [4], rely on core symptoms of depression, and in my clinical experience, elderly individuals are more difficult to assess than younger individuals for these symptoms with this scale and other depression rating scales. Thus, both assessment and detection of elderly individuals with depression is difficult. Furthermore, treatment outcome studies specific for this population are problematic, because of lack of precision in symptom reporting. Additionally, medical problems in this age group may be associated with

[1]*Department of Psychiatry and Behavioral Sciences, University of Washington, 4225 Roosevelt Way NE, Suite 306C, Seattle, Washington 98105-6099, USA*

depression, and medications used to treat medical problems in this age group may be associated with depression. Thus, the differential diagnosis of depression in the elderly is frequently more complicated than in younger individuals.

Antidepressant medication selection is also problematic. There are few reports of placebo-controlled antidepressant trials in the elderly. Most of the clinical trials reported in elderly individuals are comparator studies showing that drugs work as well as other drugs — with newer drugs perhaps having less of a side-effect burden. Studies of the efficacy of psychotherapy for depression in this age group are also generally lacking. Electroconvulsive therapy remains an important treatment for elderly individuals and in many ways may be better tolerated than traditional antidepressant agents. Electroconvulsive therapy may be particularly useful in depression complicated by psychotic features and in treatment-resistant depression.

One of the issues involved in the treatment of the elderly is the treatment of individuals who were detected earlier in life with either recurrent major depressive disorder or bipolar disorder and who are undergoing maintenance therapy with either antidepressants, lithium carbonate, or other mood stabilizers. The continued use of traditional antidepressant agents, such as tricyclic antidepressants, which may have been initiated years ago for maintenance therapy, becomes problematic because of increased sensitivity to the side effects of these medications as these patients age. Also, there may be a need to adjust dosage of maintenance medications because of impaired metabolism of these medications in the elderly as individuals age [5–7].

In summary, the proper detection and treatment of mood disorders in the elderly requires greater skill than for younger patients. As our population ages (and the percentage of elderly increase and individuals live longer), these problems will become magnified. Medical training should give greater emphasis to issues regarding diagnosis, differential diagnosis, and treatment of depression in the elderly.

REFERENCES

1. Dunner D.L. (1996) Classification of mood and anxiety disorders. *Curr. Rev. Mood Anxiety Disord.*, **1**: 1–11.
2. Dunner D.L. (1997) Therapeutic considerations in treating depression in the elderly. *J. Clin. Psychiatry*, **55**: 48–59.
3. American Psychiatric Association (1994) *Diagnostic and Statistical Manual of Mental Disorders*, 4th edn, American Psychiatric Association, Washington, DC.
4. Hamilton M. (1960) A rating scale for depression. *J. Neurol. Neurosurg. Psychiatry*, **23**: 56–59.
5. Roose S.P., Bone S., Haidorfer C., Dunner D.L., Fieve R.R. (1979) Lithium treatment in older patients. *Am. J. Psychiatry*, **136**: 843–844.

6. Dunner D.L. (1982) Lithium treatment for the aged. In *Treatment of Psychopathology in the Aged* (Eds C. Eisdorfer, W.E. Fann), pp. 137–145, Springer, New York.
7. Dunner D.L., Roose S.P., Bone S. (1979) Complication of lithium treatment in older patients. In *Lithium/Controversies and Unresolved Issues* (Eds T.B. Cooper, S. Gershon, N.S. Kline, M. Schou), pp. 427–431, Excerpta Medica, Amsterdam.

5.4

Depressive Disorders in the Elderly: A Fresh Perspective

Mike Nowers[1]

For many years psychiatry of old age was a Cinderella discipline largely ignored by general psychiatrists and regularly under-resourced. In the last few years the discipline has come out of the shadows and attracted individuals of high calibre who are prepared to act as advocates for our older patients whatever the illness from which they suffer. Committed old age psychiatrists now research and publish worldwide, and systematic reviews such as that by Chiu *et al* provide vital cutting edge information for the hard-working clinician.

Chiu *et al* point out that nosological systems do not take account of age-related features. The recent research suggests an excess of somatic features, such as weight loss, constipation and hypochondriasis, over psychological features. This is borne out in the general practitioner surgeries and hospital clinics, where the elderly consistently present with a "physical ticket". It may be that the present generation of old people find it difficult to express emotions directly and resort to biological quotients to communicate their distress.

The thorny issue of the depression-dementia continuum is also explored. Despite the efforts of researchers, the picture remains muddled. It is clear that some depressed patients go on to develop a dementia, but "the who and the how" as yet defy definition. Although treatments such as electroconvulsive therapy (ECT) have been known to worsen a pre-existing dementia, evidence shows that affective symptoms can improve and individuals should not automatically be deprived of a potentially life-saving therapy on the basis of abnormal neuroradiology.

Chiu *et al* consider the prevalence of late life depression and highlight the conflicting evidence. Energy has been expended around the world to identify whether depression is less common, equivalent or more

[1]*Community Mental Health Team for the Elderly, Cosham Hospital, Lodge Road, Kingswood, Bristol BS15 1LF, UK*

common in the elderly than the young. Papers exist to suit all tastes and persuasions!

Possibly of more concern to the busy clinician are the bio-psycho-social correlates of depression in old age. A strong association exists between physical ill-health and depression, but the patients' view of their own physical health may be adversely affected by their prevailing mood. More objective measures of ill-health, such as cancer, Parkinson's disease and stroke, all produce a consistent excess of depressive illness in sufferers of these conditions. The jury is still out on the association between ill-health and minor depression.

Social factors are important in the genesis of depression in old age and would appear to effect outcome too. Adverse life events, loneliness and social isolation speak for themselves. Equally good close support structures from family and friends appear to be a major factor in protection from old age depression. It must be remembered that published work on younger patients may not be generalisable to the elderly.

Chiu *et al*, exploring aetiology, confirm the exciting future that awaits this area with the increasing sophistication of techniques. Neurochemical and neuroendocrinological studies have not yet produced results of practical use to day-to-day clinical practice. The emphasis must be on not yet! Imaging techniques such as magnetic resonance have opened new vistas of research into the neurodegenerative basis of affective disorders, with evidence suggesting that a proportion of late life depression has a basis in cerebrovascular disease.

The question "which antidepressant for the elderly?" has not yet been answered. Selective serotonin reuptake inhibitors (SSRIs) have been shown to have a gentle side-effect profile and hence tolerability in published meta-analyses, but doubt remains over their efficacy in the treatment of severe depression. Psychiatrists in clinical practice now have a wider range of pharmacological preparations but will, in all likelihood, continue to rely on a combination of research evidence and individual experience to guide their therapeutic preference in uncomplicated depression.

The interface between physical health and depression complicates therapy. It appears that antidepressants do not have a significant effect on depression in acute severe physical illness, but remain useful in depression associated with stable or chronic physical illness. Again clinical judgement should guide best practice. The efficacy of drug treatment for depression in dementia remains unclear.

The results of psychosocial interventions appear open to interpretation. They do no harm and would seem to be of use, particularly the more cognitive-behavioural methods as a component in the treatment of major depression and as first line therapy in minor depression.

ECT is not a controversial treatment for most in old age psychiatry. Week in, week out, elderly severely depressed patients make gratifyingly rapid response to this treatment. The research evidence supports the clinical perspective. The observation that the outcome of treatment with ECT in severe depression with dementia appears to be similar to non-demented depression, with cognitive worsening being transient, will be welcomed by those nervous in the management of these often coexisting pathologies!

There sadly appears little new as yet on the management of treatment-resistant depression.

Chiu *et al* review the prognosis of depression in the elderly, highlighting the need for clearly defined core validity criteria in the research. All studies were felt to have some problems, but the overall finding in general of 60% of subjects free from depression at follow-up under 2 years post-episode resonates with routine practice. Interpretation with caution is the order of the day.

Suicide is the preventable mortality of old age and has recently been the subject of review [1]. The importance of a previous episode of deliberate self-harm cannot be emphasized enough [2].

Chiu *et al*'s review gives us busy clinicians a fresh perspective on depression in the elderly, highlighting progress and deficiency and enunciating an exciting way forward for us all.

REFERENCES

1. Nowers M.P. (1998) Suicide and attempted suicide in the elderly. *Curr. Pract. Med.*, **1**: 39–41.
2. Hepple J., Quinton C. (1997) One hundred cases of attempted suicide in the elderly. *Br. J. Psychiatry*, **171**: 42–46.

5.5

Depression in the Elderly: Areas Open to Research
Clive Ballard[1]

Chiu *et al*'s paper provides a comprehensive review of depression in later life, although, as highlighted by the authors, the literature is limited in certain areas. The vast majority of studies focus upon hospital-based samples, with

[1]*MRC Neurochemical Pathology Unit, Newcastle General Hospital, Newcastle NE4 6BE, UK*

far less information available regarding patients in primary care and the community. In addition, very few studies focus upon the "older" old, who are likely to have the most complex needs. Perhaps more worrying, however, are the limited data pertaining to certain aspects of treatment outcome. Although there are more than 70 double-blind placebo-controlled trials of antidepressants in the elderly, only 9 of these [1] incorporate samples with a mean age over 75. These patients are the most likely to have concurrent physical illness, are more likely to be taking additional pharmaceutical agents and have the poorest drug tolerability. Other specific areas where our knowledge regarding treatment outcome in the elderly is inadequate include treatment resistance and chronic depression, patients with physical illness and patients with depression and dementia.

Dementia affects 1 in 5 people over the age of 80, 20% of whom will be experiencing a depressive illness at any one time [2]. Five controlled studies have examined treatment response in these patients. Only one of these, with more than 800 participants, demonstrated that antidepressant agents were significantly better than placebo [3]. The difficulty seems to lie in the high placebo response rate, over 35% combining these reports. This is not surprising as naturalistic studies indicate that two thirds of dementia patients with depression experience resolution of the depression within 3 months [4]. In clinical practice it would therefore seem appropriate only to treat depression lasting less than 3 months if it is particularly severe or distressing. In addition, treatment intervention studies should focus upon patients with severe or persistent depression.

Vascular depression is an interesting and potentially important concept. It is suggested that areas of infarction, particularly those in the left frontal lobe, or deep white matter hyperintensities identified by magnetic resonance imaging (MRI) scan (probably indicative of microvascular pathology), predispose to affective disturbance. Work from our own group has also suggested the importance of deep white matter lesions on MRI as an association of depression in Alzheimer's disease [5], and work in preparation indicates that microvascular lesions and diffuse white matter disease, identified at neuropathological examination, are significantly correlated with depression in vascular and mixed dementias. A very consistent picture is hence emerging, drawing evidence from a number of different disciplines, substantiating the concept of vascular depression in the elderly. Simpson et al [6] have suggested that these patients are more likely to be treatment resistant and to progress into a chronic depressive illness. This highlights the need for further work, particularly with regard to the treatment and prophylaxis of these disorders. Hypertension is an established risk factor for the development of white matter hyperintensities. Recent trials of antihypertensive agents have indicated that appropriate treatment may reduce the long-term incidence of dementia [7]. Additional studies evaluating the impact of antihypertensive treatments on the evolution of white matter disease and depression would be highly informative.

Cognitive deficits are evident in patients with late onset depression, which often persist after treatment [8], referred to in their most extreme form as depressive pseudo-dementia. The overlap between cognition disturbances and depression is, however, complex. Depression is common in patients with dementia, particularly in the early stages of the illness, whilst during episodes of depression, attention, concentration and motivation to undertake cognitive testing are impaired. Furthermore, some patients may be taking pharmaceutical agents which impair cognition and predispose to depression, whilst systemic (e.g. oat cell carcinoma) or cerebral (e.g. cerebral infarction) pathologies may increase vulnerability to both conditions. Although some studies have followed-up specific cohorts of depressed patients with cognitive impairments, such as those with depressive pseudo-dementia, there is a paucity of longitudinal studies evaluating outcome and neuropsychological profile over time in more representative groups of patients with late onset depression. It is this kind of study, incorporating the "messy" cases, which will provide the most important information.

The rapid evolution in the literature regarding depression in later life and related topics is encouraging, offering many important topics which could be discussed. I have selected one or two areas of personal interest, and I hope general relevance, to comment upon.

REFERENCES

1. Bartlett S., Ballard C.G. (1999) Antidepressants in the elderly: a review. Expert Opinion on Investigational Drugs (in press).
2. Ballard C.G., Bannister C., Oyebode F. (1996) Review: depression in dementia sufferers. *Int. J. Geriatr. Psychiatry*, **11**: 507–515.
3. Roth M., Mountjoy C.Q., Amrein R. (1996) Moclobemide in elderly patients with cognitive decline and depression. *Br. J. Psychiatry*, **168**: 149–157.
4. Ballard C.G., Patel A., Solis M., Lowe K., Wilcock G. (1996) A 1 year follow up study of depression in dementia sufferers. *Br. J. Psychiatry*, **168**: 287–291.
5. Barber R., Scheltens P., McKeith I., Ballard C., Gholker A., English A., Grey A., O'Brien J. (1998) A comparison of white matter lesions on MRI in dementia with Lewy bodies, Alzheimer's disease, vascular dementia and normal ageing. *Neurobiol. Ageing*, **19** (Suppl. 4): 865.
6. Simpson S., Jackson A., Baldwin R.C., Burns A. (1997) Subcortical hyperintensities in late life depression: acute response to treatment and neuropsychological impairment. *Int. Psychogeriatrics*, **9**: 257–275.
7. Forette F., Seux M.L., Staessen J.A., Lutgarde T., Birkenhäger W.H., Barbarskiene M.R., Babeanu S., Bossini A., Gil-Extremera B., Girerd X. *et al* (1998) Prevention of dementia in randomised double-blind placebo-controlled systolic hypertension in Europe (Syst-Eur) trial. *Lancet*, **352**: 1347–1351.
8. Abas M.A., Sahakian B.J. (1990) Neuropsychological deficits and CT scan changes in elderly depressives. *Psychol. Med.*, **20**: 507–520.

5.6
Filling in the Gaps about Depression in the Elderly

Dan Blazer[1]

Chiu *et al* provide an overview of the English language literature relevant to late life depression. They constitute a number of specific take home messages at the end of the section, yet I believe they provide a background for more general conclusions from the extant literature. I think a number of overall conclusions can be culled from a review of this review.

First, the authors provide insight into the longstanding controversy regarding the relative frequency of depression across the life cycle. They emphasize the importance of defining depression, noting that uncomplicated depression in late life (i.e. depression free of comorbid physical illness and cognitive dysfunction) is more similar to depression in mid-life than has been supposed in the past. The controversy as to whether depression is more or less frequent among the elderly compared to persons in mid-life, highlighted by findings from epidemiologic studies over the past two decades, in large part derives from the varied definitions of "caseness" of late life depression. Therefore the debate over relative frequency by age is often meaningless. There should be no doubt, however, that depression in the elderly is a significant public health problem which must be central to psychiatrists working with the elderly.

Our understanding of etiological factors is disappointing, because we have learned little about the etiology of late life depression in recent years. The one area where we have made significant gains is in the focus upon vascular depression, a concept that goes back at least to Felix Post. Non-reversible changes in the brain with aging not only manifest themselves via the dementing disorders; they also are the basis of depressive disorders often free of comorbid cognitive decline among the elderly. Many questions remain to be answered about vascular depression, not the least of which relate to the potential for preventing these changes through control of blood pressure and even more aggressive approaches, as we currently are witnessing in studies of the treatment and prevention of cardiovascular disease.

The past decade has witnessed both successes and disappointments in the treatment of late life depression. The success is documented in the literature which substantiates the value of combined pharmacotherapy and psychotherapy (especially the cognitive-behavioural therapies). The disappointment is the continued recognition of our failure to identify therapies which are effective in treating depression in the elderly associated with both physical and cognitive decline. Inpatient and outpatient therapy among elders with uncomplicated depression is effective, at least as effective as

---

[1]*Duke University Medical Center, Durham, NC 27710, USA*

most medical interventions for physical problems in the elderly. On the other hand, therapy of comorbid depression in acute care medical units and in long-term care facilities is not effective for the most part. Attempts to treat depression in the frail elderly are as frustrating to psychiatrists today as they were 20 years ago.

Though we have learned much about the outcome of late life depression, three questions which are most important remain unanswered: (1) does late life depression of first onset vary in outcome from the recurrence in late life of a depressive disorder beginning earlier in life? (2) to what extent does the outcome of late life depression predispose elders to other adverse health outcomes, such as cognitive decline and physical illness? (3) to what extent does the outcome of late life depression vary by gender once a first onset episode occurs? These are difficult questions to answer, for fielding a longitudinal study, even under the best of circumstances, is a difficult task. Nevertheless, these questions are critical if we are to understand the natural history of late life depression as a backdrop to future treatment and prevention studies.

I believe psychiatrists will be rewarded by reading Chiu *et al*'s review for it is cogent, concise and reflects the major findings of an explosion of literature on late life depression over the past decade.

5.7
A Clinical Point of View about Depression in the Elderly
Jean Wertheimer[1]

In spite of the epidemiological controversies about the prevalence of depression in old age, there is no doubt that the practitioner is very often confronted with such a pathology. The apparent difference between this daily experience and the low prevalence reported by recent surveys is certainly due to the methodologies employed. It is a matter of fact that the national (DSM-IV) and the international (ICM-10) classifications are not adapted to a large part of the psychiatry of the elderly. If, on one hand, some clinical pictures are common to young and old adults, on the other hand particularities often lead to atypical presentations. These variations increase in number by categories of age over 65. Interactions between multiple factors certainly explain this fact: physiological modifications, physical and psychiatric comorbidities, and changes in social conditions being the most apparent. The causal relations are predominantly circular and not linear. These factors induce consequences

[1] *Service Universitaire de Psychogeriatrie, Route de Mont, CH-1008 Prilly-Lausanne, Switzerland*

that enter subsequently into the aetiological loop, particularly those in the psychological field. Depression could, in this way, be considered as either a cause or a consequence of situations defined by multifactorial parameters.

Depression in the elderly is ubiquitous, present in the community, in hospitals, both somatic and psychiatric, in long-stay settings. It can be at the foreground or less evidently present, intermingled with physical diseases or/and dementia. Symptoms can be emotional, cognitive and somatic. Emotional disorders include sadness, anxiety, reduction of interest. Sadness is not always evident. It can be minimized or hidden behind an apparently smiling facial expression. A diminished facial mobility, caused by Parkinson's or a multi-infarct cerebral disease, could falsely suggest the presence of sad feelings. Anxiety is often conveyed by somatic complaints, for instance "pressure" on the heart or the solar plexus region, an impression of tightening in the throat. Obviously, such symptoms call for investigation for possible physical comorbidities that can coexist with the depressive disorder. A diminished interest is not a symptom restricted to depression and is also a feature observed in dementia, particularly of the frontal and of the subcortical type.

Cognitive symptoms, referring to the subjective perception induced by the disease, predominantly concern feelings of low self-esteem, of worthlessness, of helplessness and hopelessness, pessimistic thoughts with sometimes the conviction of being incurable, ideas of death and suicide, a sense of guilt. These feelings are frequently reinforced by the reality of life events and of life conditions marked by concrete losses: bereavement, social isolation, institutionalisation, physical diseases, economic problems. Most important is also the problem of memory. Concentration difficulties are often reported in depression, even by young adults. Both recording and recall are consequently disturbed. In old age the subjective perception of these troubles can be influenced by the prejudice that memory disturbances are common at that age, and by the fear of dementia. Consequently, the problem of failing memory could predominate in old age depression, constituting the so-called depressive pseudo-dementia.

Sleep disorders (insomnia, and less frequently, hypersomnia), poor appetite with loss of weight, and fatigue are the more frequent somatic symptoms observed in depression. They also raise the question of possible somatic comorbidities and of the eventual causal relations between physical illnesses and depression. Pain perception can be increased and the physician should try to find a possible objective explanation. Physical complaints are commonly the prior concern raised by old depressed patients, particularly against a background of cultural factors that can be local (rural background for example) or national (as in China for example). This tendency is also characteristic of personality profiles marked by a lack of psychological insight.

The clinical approach to depression must reckon with the complexity of these situations defined by potential multiple causal and consecutive factors.

Contextual parameters play important roles and contribute to triggering off, accentuating or maintaining emotional disturbances: family conflicts, disagreement with nursing staff, and so on. In institutional settings, depression is not evident in dependent and passive patients whose behaviour has not changed. Significant cues are, in such cases, frequently limited to appetite and sleep disorders.

Management [1] is guided by the particular characteristics of the individual situation. Major objectives are the reduction and abolition of signs and symptoms, the establishment of a new equilibrium through the creation of favourable living conditions, the reduction of risk of relapse and recurrence. The physician must always take into consideration the psychological dimension of depression, which affects not only the patient, but also his or her relatives, friends and also the caring staff. He will provide support to them, notably by favouring the expression of feelings, by explaining the nature of the symptoms and thus helping to exorcise thoughts of aggression or guilt towards the patient. Depressed patients are often unable to obtain help or care in the home, or to ask for assistance in the management of their own affairs. Support implies counselling and even requests to the community services. After the acute phase, psychotherapy will have a preventive value. It should remain in the long term as an ongoing available resource. Physical approach, occupational therapy and sociotherapy help the patient to regain a positive self-image. The prescription of antidepressant medications, of thymoregulators or of electroconvulsive therapy must be integrated into a comprehensive approach to depression in the elderly.

REFERENCE

1. World Psychiatric Association/International Committee for Prevention and Treatment of Depression (1999) *Educational Programme on Depressive Disorders, Module III, Depression in the Elderly*, NCM Publishers, New York.

5.8
Geriatric Depression: A Look to the Future
Charles F. Reynolds III[1]

The comprehensive review by Chiu *et al* underscores both recent advances and limitations in our understanding of depressive illnesses in later life. The World Health Organization (WHO) [1] has specified unipolar depression and

[1] *Mental Health Clinical Research Center for the Study of Late-Life Mood Disorders, Western Psychiatric Institute and Clinic, 3811 O'Hara Street, Pittsburgh, PA 15213, USA*

suicide as major contributors to the global burden of disability both now and over the next decade as the world's population ages. Thus, improvements in prevention, recognition, and treatment deserve high priority.

The hallmark and distinguishing features of geriatric depression include medical comorbidity and the attendant amplification of disability, cognitive impairment, reduced quality of life, increased risk for suicide, and increased health care costs. In their conclusions, the authors question whether depression in old age can be studied "effectively enough to permit modification of adverse prognostic factors." From a clinical perspective, the question can be restated to ask whether treatment can affect the long-term illness course of depression in later life.

In answer to the authors' question, we have recently completed a randomized, placebo-controlled study of maintenance therapies in late-life depression, which demonstrated the value of maintenance nortriptyline (NT, steady-state blood levels of 80–120 ng/ml) and of monthly interpersonal psychotherapy (IPT) in preventing or delaying recurrence of major depressive episodes in elderly patients with histories of recurrent, non-psychotic, unipolar major depression (15% of whom also had histories of suicide attempts) [2]. The study showed that maintenance NT and monthly IPT, both singly and in combination, worked better than placebo in preventing or delaying recurrences of depression over a 3-year period, and that treatment combining NT and IPT was better than either modality alone in assuring continued depression-free survival. The major covariate of long-term response was age at study entry. Patients 70 and older were more likely to suffer recurrence than patients 60–69, regardless of treatment assignment. Long-term response in both groups was best in the combined treatment condition.

These observations point to the importance of the psychosocial, as well as the biological, substrate of geriatric depression — especially to the issues of bereavement, role transition, interpersonal conflict, and social isolation addressed specifically in IPT. Severe life events and depletion of social support are important in the onset of geriatric depression and can likewise delay its offset, prolonging response to treatment [3].

These results highlight the clinical and scientific challenges posed by short- and long-term treatment–response variability in late-life depression. For example, time to remission of the index episode, in response to combined treatment with NT and IPT, is longer in association with greater severity of anxiety and depressive symptoms, increased psychosocial stress, decreased social support, earlier age at lifetime onset, and higher levels of rapid eye movement sleep [4]. Understanding the sources of treatment–response variability in late-life depression, finding ways of controlling and reducing that variability, and more accurately identifying which patients need which treatments are important issues facing the field.

Restated from a clinical perspective, the challenges are to accelerate treatment response, to identify quickly and reliably patients likely to be resistant to first line therapy, to maintain treatment response over longer periods of time, and to intervene more effectively in elderly primary care patients with depression (thereby hopefully reducing the incidence of completed suicide).

An opportunity for accelerating the onset of antidepressant activity and thereby reducing time to remission may reside in the use of one night of total sleep deprivation (TSD) combined with starting antidepressant medication on the night of recovery sleep [5], although this approach requires further controlled assessment. The cerebral metabolic response to therapeutic sleep deprivation, assessed via positron tomission tomography, may also represent an informative probe of the biology of treatment response and treatment resistance [6]. Treatment of long-term insomnia, a known risk factor for major depression across the life cycle, may represent a useful strategy for reducing the incidence of major depression in later life [7]. Combining antidepressant medication with interpersonal psychotherapy may represent the optimal approach for assuring continued wellness in those over age 70, although further controlled study of this approach and of its cost-effectiveness is very much needed [2].

If we can take advantage now of the opportunities for improving preventive and intervention strategies in geriatric depression, then the challenges posed by the WHO report may be met successfully over the next decade. The cost of failure, however, will be high: depression will continue to be a killer of the elderly.

ACKNOWLEDGEMENT

Supported in part by National Institute of Mental Health grants P30 MH52247 and K05 MH00295.

REFERENCES

1. World Health Organization (1996) Global Health Statistics: a compendium of incidence, prevalence and mortality estimates for over 200 conditions. In *The Global Burden of Disease*, Harvard University Press, Cambridge, MA.
2. Reynolds C.F. III, Frank E., Perel J.M., Imber S.D., Cornes C., Miller M.D., Mazumdar S., Houck P.R., Dew M.A., Stack J.A. *et al* (1999) Nortriptyline and interpersonal psychotherapy as maintenance therapies for recurrent major depression: a randomized controlled trial in patients older than 59 years. *JAMA*, **281**: 39–45.
3. Karp J.F., Frank E., Anderson B., George C.J., Reynolds C.F. III, Mazumdar S., Kupfer D.J. (1993) Time to remission in late-life depression: analysis of effects of demographic, treatment, and life-events measures. *Depression*, **1**: 250–256.

4. Dew M.A., Reynolds C.F. III, Houck P.R., Hall M., Buysse D.J., Frank E., Kupfer D.J. (1997) Temporal profiles of the course of depression during treatment: predictors of pathways toward recovery in the elderly. *Arch. Gen. Psychiatry*, **54**: 1016–1024.
5. Bump G.M., Reynolds C.F. III, Smith G., Pollock B.G., Dew M.A., Mazumdar S., Geary M., Houck P.R., Kupfer D.J. (1997) Accelerating response in geriatric depression: a pilot study combining sleep deprivation and paroxetine. *Depression and Anxiety*, **6**: 113–118.
6. Smith G., Reynolds C.F. III, Pollock B., Derbyshire S., Nofzinger E.A., Dew M.A., Houck P.R., Milko D., Meltzer C., Kupfer D.J. (1999) Cerebral glucose metabolic response to combined total sleep deprivation and antidepressant treatment in geriatric depression. *Am. J. Psychiatry*, **156**: 683–689.
7. Nowell P.D., Reynolds C.F., Buysse D.J., Dew M.A., Kupfer D.J. (1999) Paroxetine in the treatment of primary insomnia: preliminary clinical and EEG sleep data. *J. Clin. Psychiatry*, **60**: 89–95.

5.9
Depression in Late Life: Directions for Intervention Research

Barry D. Lebowitz[1]

Depression in late life is widespread, serious, and contributes to disability and suffering. Unrecognized or inadequately treated depression increases risks for morbidity and mortality and is a leading cause of suicide.

Concerns about gaps in our understanding of etiology and pathophysiology notwithstanding, our treatment armamentarium is robust, with a broad range of pharmacotherapeutic, psychotherapeutic, and somatic options available to the practicing clinician.

"Treatment works," we tell our patients and their family members. A generation of research has led to this inescapable conclusion. A vast body of literature including complete textbooks, chapters, and aggressive public and professional education campaigns fully explicate this positive message [1, 2]. Yet, among ourselves, we are generally less positive about the impact of our treatments on our patients' lives. We will agree that most patients do pretty well most of the time on most treatments. But we will also agree that this is not nearly good enough and much more needs to be learned.

Why do treatments rarely work as well in practice as they do in clinical trials? Why are the approaches to treatment that are studied in research settings rarely the ones that are used in practice? Does treatment enhance functioning? Does early treatment predict a more favorable response? How can we keep people well once they have been made well? What approaches should be used for the treatment-resistant patient?

[1]*National Institute of Mental Health, 5600 Fishers Lane, Rockville, MD 20857, USA*

These are the sorts of questions that are raised within a public health model of treatment [3]. These are questions we cannot yet answer as well as we would like, however, because treatment research has been determined by a more narrowly defined regulatory model [4].

Formally speaking, regulatory or efficacy studies define optimal treatment outcomes for narrowly selected patients treated under rigidly controlled and ideal conditions. With a primary focus on symptoms, the assessment of efficacy is based upon the degree to which the level of symptomatology is reduced or eliminated. In an efficacy trial, special clinicians provide optimal treatment with substantial resources expended to assure compliance. There is no minimum effect size or minimum proportion of responders necessary, and there is no requirement that the subject population be representative of the kind of patient seen in actual practice.

The classic efficacy trial is used to define the gold standard of the best outcome under ideal circumstances. Because of the tight standard of control required in efficacy studies, the practice relevance of these trials is limited.

In general, the rigid exclusions of most regulatory-oriented clinical trials have significantly distorted the conclusions of these studies and limited their application to clinical geriatric practice. Most studies, even those claiming to be geriatric, are largely restricted to the "young-old" population of patients in their sixties. Few older patients have ever been studied [5], despite the clear impact of advanced age on pharmacokinetics, dynamics, and drug metabolism [6] and treatment response [7].

A new direction for our field is to launch studies that are informed by a public health or "effectiveness" model. These studies bring us into the world of actual practice with time-pressured clinicians taking care of large numbers of patients with uncertain clinical presentations, complex comorbidities, and varying degrees of interference with ideal levels of compliance. The exclusive focus on symptomatology is expanded to include outcomes related to issues of function, disability, morbidity, mortality, resource use, and quality of life. The classic public health trial is used to assess the expected outcome under usual circumstances of practice.

This new approach to intervention promises to improve patient care by addressing the types of practical questions and functional outcomes that are typically brought to the attention of clinicians. This new research is directed toward defining standards of appropriate and cost-effective treatment for the diverse population of patients seen in all health care settings. This should not be taken to indicate that there is no place for the highly controlled efficacy research needed to establish that a treatment has merit. Efficacy is the beginning of a process of inquiry and not the end in the development of treatments for older persons with depression.

REFERENCES

1. Geriatric Psychiatry Alliance (1997) *Depression in Late Life: Not a Natural Part of Aging*, American Association for Geriatric Psychiatry, Bethesda, MD.
2. Niederehe G., Schneider L.S. (1998) Treatments for anxiety and depression in the aged. In *A Guide to Treatments that Work* (Eds P.E. Nathan, J.M. Gorman), pp. 270–287, Oxford University Press, New York.
3. Lebowitz B.D., Harris H.W. (1998) Treatment research in geriatric psychiatry: from regulatory to public health considerations. *Am. J. Geriatr. Psychiatry*, **6**: 101–103.
4. Leber P.D., Davis C.S. (1998) Threats to the validity of clinical trials employing enrichment strategies for sample selection. *Controlled Clin. Trials*, **19**: 178–187.
5. Salzman C., Schneider L.S., Lebowitz B.D. (1993) Antidepressant treatment of very old patients. *Am. J. Geriatr. Psychiatry*, **1**: 21–29.
6. Von Moltke L.L., Abernethy D.R., Greenblatt D.J. (1998) Kinetics and dynamics of psychotropic drugs in the elderly. In *Clinical Geriatric Psychopharmacology*, 3rd edn (Ed. C. Salzman), pp. 70–93, Williams and Wilkins, Baltimore.
7. Reynolds C.F. III, Frank E., Dew M.A., Houck P.R., Miller M., Mazumdar S., Perel J.M., Kupfer D.J. (1999) Treatment of 70(+)-year-olds with recurrent major depression. Excellent short-term but brittle long-term response. *Am. J. Geriatr. Psychiatry*, **7**: 64–69.

5.10
Treatment of Depression in the "Old-Old"

Sheldon H. Preskorn[1]

As pointed out by Chiu *et al*, only 4–30% of the elderly with clinical depression in primary care receive a trial of an antidepressant. That is likely in part due to the fact that physicians have few systematic data upon which to base treatment decisions.

The clinical trials done to support the registration of antidepressants are usually conducted in physically healthy patients aged 20–55. The databases used to support registration typically include 2500–3000 individuals of whom 300 or fewer are over the age of 65. Most of these are 65–70 (i.e. the "young-old"). Virtually no data come from the "old-old" (i.e. individuals over the age of 85). In addition, the "young-old" in these studies have to meet rigorous inclusion criteria: no unstable medical illnesses, no other psychiatric medications, and limited concomitant medications. These requirements severely limit the generalizability of the results to actual clinical practice, especially with regard to the "old-old." Yet, the "old-old" are a special population who are more sensitive to the adverse effects of medications, including antidepressants, for the following reasons.

[1] *Department of Psychiatry, University of Kansas Medical School, Wichita, KS 67214-2878, USA*

First, the "old-old" are likely to develop higher levels of the drug for the dose given than will younger individuals due to age-related and disease-related impairment in drug clearance. The increased body fat content also means that there is an increased reservoir for most psychiatric medications in the "old-old" compared to the "young-old," which can increase the time needed to reach steady-state conditions and to eliminate the drug once it is discontinued.

Second, the "old-old" are more likely to be on other medications. In a survey of four different practice settings ranging from primary care to a Veterans' Administration Medical Center (VAMC), the vast majority of patients on an antidepressant were on at least one other systematically taken prescription drug [1]. The VAMC population was older (average age 58 years). Over 70% of these patients were on three or more other drugs in addition to their antidepressant, with the average number of drugs being 6. This high frequency of multiple drug therapy (i.e. "polyphar-macy") sets the stage for clinically meaningful drug–drug interactions. Thus, the "old-old" are more likely to have adverse drug–drug inter-actions, to have an amplified adverse response (because they are frail), and to have their adverse outcome misattributed to the worsening of the underlying health problems. The latter increases the likelihood that more drugs will be added to treatment and that more health care dollars will be expended.

Like any medication, antidepressants can interact pharmacodynamically and/or pharmacokinetically with co-prescribed drugs. Pharmacodynamic interactions are the ones in which the mechanism of action of one drug amplifies or diminishes the response to the mechanism of action of another drug. Pharmacokinetic interactions are those in which one drug alters the pharmacokinetics (i.e. absorption, distribution, metabolism, or elimination) of another drug. The most common and most clinically important types of pharmacokinetically mediated drug–drug interactions are the ones medi-ated by the drug metabolizing cytochrome P450 (CYP) enzymes. A number of antidepressants, including some (i.e. fluoxetine, fluvoxamine, and parox-etine) but not all (citalopram and sertraline) selective serotonin reuptake inhibitors (SSRIs) inhibit one or more drug-metabolizing CYP enzymes to a clinically meaningful degree. For example, fluoxetine causes a 400–800% increase in the levels of co-administered drugs which are dependent on CYP 2D6 for their biotransformation as a prelude to their excretion from the body [2]. Such increases have resulted in serious adverse effects in some patients, particularly the "old-old" [3]. This issue is of particular concern when using fluoxetine in the elderly, due to the fact that the half-life of both the parent drug and its active metabolite is even longer in the physically healthy elderly versus the young [4]. For that reason, the effect of fluoxetine on the metabolism of other drugs can build up for weeks to months after it is started and can persist for weeks to months after it has been discontinued, putting the patient at risk for adverse drug–drug interactions.

Ideally, the prescriber should have information that addresses how to optimally dose various types of antidepressants in the "old-old", taking these issues into account. Unfortunately, I must echo Chiu *et al*'s conclusion, "one of disappointment at the inadequacy of our research methodology and inability to make useful links between alterable prognostic factors and outcomes." A concerted effort is needed to ensure that this area receives proper funding of research initiatives if we hope to have evidence-based treatments for such patients.

REFERENCES

1. Preskorn S.H. (1998) Debate resolved: there are differential effects of serotonin selective reuptake inhibitors on cytochrome P450 enzymes. *J. Psychopharmacol.*, **12**: S89–S97.
2. Preskorn S.H. (1998) Do you feel lucky? *J. Pract. Psychiatr. Behav. Hlth.*, **4**: 37–40.
3. Baumann P.A., Bertschy G. (1993) Pharmacodynamic and pharmacokinetic interactions of selective serotonin reuptake inhibiting antidepressants (SSRIs) with other psychotropic drugs. *Nord. J. Psychiatry*, **47** (Suppl. 30): 13–19.
4. Preskorn S.H., Shad M.U., Alderman J., Lane R. (1998) Fluoxetine: age and dose dependent pharmacokinetics and CYP 2C19 inhibition. *Am. Soc. Clin. Pharmacol. Ther.*, **63**: 166.

5.11

Suggested Priorities for Research into Depressive Disorders in the Elderly

Peter W. Burvill[1]

Chiu *et al*'s paper provides a good overview of the current state of our knowledge of depression in the elderly. I empathize with the authors' anticipation of an exciting future for the study of depression in the elderly, and with their assertion that developments in the field will herald a very vigorous body of data which will make the review obsolete in the not too distant future.

In our future research endeavours, it is important to try to identify the areas which deserve particular focus, and for which the use of available and emerging techniques are likely to be most rewarding. It is clear that evolving neuroimaging and other techniques will continue rapidly to provide exciting new knowledge regarding the biology of depression in the elderly. By comparison, we will need to give much greater priority to, and rethink our approach in regard to, methodology, about a number of other

[1]*Glendower Specialist Practice, 296 Fitzgerald Street, Perth, WA 6000, Australia*

areas. The latter include comorbid physical illness, the efficacy of treatment (including medications, cognitive therapy and psychosocial intervention) and prognosis. Molecular biology techniques are becoming increasingly sophisticated, but the absence of a review of these by the authors emphasizes that their use in the study of depression in the elderly is still in its infancy.

Certain "core" similarities of clinical features of depression in younger adults and the elderly have been identified. It is my belief that future research endeavours should focus on those features which are unique to, or at least found predominantly in, the elderly. These include cognitive impairment, neurostructural changes, physical illness both acute and chronic, associated common cerebral organic illnesses such as stroke and Parkinson's disease, and late-onset depression.

One of the major basic problems which has long hindered our research efforts into the aetiology and management of depression in all age groups has been the absence of an adequate classification. There is general agreement that depressive illness is a heterogeneous condition, but our knowledge of the components of that heterogeneity remains pathetically inadequate, despite major attention to the subject throughout much of this century. This hetero-geneity includes DSM-IV major depressive disorder and dysthymic disorder. As the review has pointed out, the syndromically defined diagnoses which have occupied nosology in the last two decades, while enhancing research vigor and reliability, unfortunately also have created an environment of "international suppression of variability" by which confounding factors (medical illnesses, heterogeneous symptom clusters) have been "defined out" of studies. This has driven research in a direction which increasingly is unre-lated to the reality of depressive disorders in the elderly. This must be rectified if research is to reach its full potential, for both younger and older age groups.

Robinson and his colleagues in Baltimore pioneered research in post-stroke depression and reported increased depressive illness when the cerebrovas-cular lesions involved the left frontal cortex and certain ganglia [1]. Although their neuroradiological and localization of lesion studies have since been crit-icized [2], it is noteworthy that recent neuroimaging studies have reported increased white matter changes in the frontal area and basal ganglia. These and other subcortical and grey matter changes have led investigators to coin the term "vascular depression". Study of patients with post-stroke depres-sion may help test the hypotheses of Hickie et al [3] that cerebrovascular insufficiency in older persons leads to changes in subcortical structures, which then provide a structural basis for the development of depression.

It has now been firmly established that depressive illness in the elderly, even in the absence of physical illness, has a two- to three-fold increased 5-year mortality rate [4, 5]. This reinforces the call of Chiu et al for a well-designed study, with good follow-up criteria, of depression in the elderly being treated energetically with liberal use of prophylactic antidepressants, to see if the mortality can be decreased. Such a study would form the basis of preventive strategies in the treatment of elderly depressed patients. This links with the challenge of Chiu *et al* to investigators in their statement that depression is the commonest disorder seen by old age psychiatrists, and if it cannot be studied effectively enough to permit modification of adverse prognostic factors, then the whole point of research in our field must be called into question.

REFERENCES

1. Robinson R.G., Starkstein S.E. (1990) Current research in affective disorders following stroke. *J. Neuropsychiatry Clin. Neurosci.*, **2**: 1–14.
2. Burvill P., Johnson G., Jamrosik K., Anderson G., Stewart-Wynne E. (1997) Risk factors for post-stroke depression. *Int. J. Geriatr. Psychiatry*, **12**: 219–226.
3. Hickie J., Scott E., Mitchell P., Wilhelm K., Austin M.-P., Bennett B. (1995) Subcortical hyperintensities on magnetic resonance imaging: clinical correlates and prognostic significance in patients with severe depression. *Biol. Psychiatry*, **37**: 151–160.
4. Murphy E., Smith R., Lindesay J., Slattery J. (1988) Increased mortality in late-life depression. *Br. J. Psychiatry*, **152**: 347–353.
5. Burvill P.W., Hall W.D. (1994) Predictors of increased mortality in elderly depressed patients. *Int. J. Geriatr. Psychiatry*, **9**: 219–227.

5.12
Comorbidity of Depression in Older People

Cornelius Katona[1]

As is apparent from the review by Chiu *et al*, there have been several epidemiological studies examining the prevalence of depressive disorders in older people, as well as many descriptions of symptom pattern in both clinical and epidemiological samples of patients with these disorders. It is perhaps surprising that few of these studies have examined the frequency with which depression coexists with other psychiatric disorders in old age, particularly since comorbidity with depression has been studied extensively in younger subjects [1].

We [2] have examined the prevalence of other psychiatric morbidity in a community sample of older adults with depression as part of a larger epidemiological study of psychiatric morbidity in people aged 65 and over conducted in the inner London borough of Islington. The sample

[1]*Department of Psychiatry and Behavioural Sciences, University College London Medical School, Wolfson Building, 48 Riding House Street, London W1N 8AA, UK*

was identified by "door knocking". An interviewer visited every house in randomly chosen streets within the borough and sought an interview with every inhabitant identified as being aged at least 65. This method has previously been established as an accurate way to gather a sampling frame within an inner-city population. A total of 774 eligible subjects were approached, of whom 700 (90%) agreed to be interviewed. The main interview instrument was the shortened version of the comprehensive assessment and referral evaluation (short-CARE, [3]). This has scales to measure depression, dementia, sleep disorder, somatic symptoms, subjective memory problems and limitation in activities of daily living. In addition, the Anxiety Disorders Scale [4] was administered. This generates diagnoses (non-hierarchically) for phobic disorder, generalized anxiety and panic disorder.

Complete interview data were available on 694 subjects (64% female) with a mean age of 76 years. Of these, 104 (15%) met short-CARE criteria for depression, 39 (5.6%) for dementia, and 105 (15%) for anxiety disorders. Within the anxiety disorder group, 84 (12% of the total sample) had phobic disorder and 33 (5%) had generalized anxiety. Only one subject had panic disorder, 243 (35%) had sleep disturbance, 172 (25%) had subjective memory complaints, 189 (27.0%) complained of somatic symptoms, and 235 (34%) needed help with day-to-day living. A total of 501 subjects (72%) had no psychiatric disorder.

Within the depressed group, 22% also had phobic disorder, compared with only 10% in the non-depressed group ($p < 0.001$). Generalized anxiety was present in 23 (22%) of the depressed group and only 2% of those free of depression. There was no association between depression and dementia (7.7% caseness in the depressed and 5.2% in the non-depressed). Subjective memory loss (43% vs. 21%; $p < 0.0001$), sleep disturbance (71% vs. 28%; $p < 0.0001$), somatic symptoms (50% vs. 31%; $p < 0.0001$) and activity limitation (49% vs. 23%; $p < 0.0005$) were all much commoner in depressed than in non-depressed subjects.

In a subsequent follow-up study a mean of 2.6 years later [5], we were able to obtain information on 45 of the depressed subjects [4]. We found 17 (27%) had died; 21 (34%) had recovered and 24 (39%) remained depressed. Continuing depression was associated with the presence at baseline of sleep disturbance ($p < 0.01$), activities of daily living limitation ($p < 0.05$) and phobic anxiety ($p < 0.05$).

These data indicate that older people who are depressed very commonly also have comorbid psychopathology—particularly phobic disorder and generalized anxiety—and/or physical symptoms. Generalized anxiety indeed is almost exclusively found comorbidly with depression, suggesting that depressive symptoms should always be looked for in older people presenting with an apparent anxiety disorder. Sleep disturbance, somatic symptoms and complaints of memory impairment are also so frequently associated with depression in older subjects as to mandate a search for depressive symptoms if these are not immediately apparent. Physically disabled older people are a further group in whom depression should be suspected.

The importance of comorbidity with depression may also be seen in prognostic terms. Our follow-up data suggest that depression complicated by other morbidity such as phobic anxiety, sleep disturbance or activity limitation is less likely to remit. This has relevance not only for clinical practice but also for the design of future controlled treatment trials.

REFERENCES

1. Wittchen H. (Ed.) (1996) Comorbidity of mood disorders. *Br. J. Psychiatry*, **168** (Suppl. 30).
2. Katona C.L.E., Manela M.V., Livingston G.A. (1997) Comorbidity with depression in older people: the Islington Study. *Aging and Mental Health*, 1: 57–61.
3. Gurland B., Golden R., Teresi J.A., Challop J. (1984) The short-CARE. An efficient instrument for the assessment of depression, dementia and disability. *J. Gerontology*, **39**: 166–169.
4. Lindesay J., Briggs C., Murphy E. (1989) The Guy's/Age Concern survey. Prevalence rates of cognitive impairment, depression and anxiety in an urban elderly community. *Br. J. Psychiatry*, 155: 317–329.
5. Livingston G., Watkin V., Milne B., Manela M.V., Katona C. (1997) The natural history of depression and the anxiety disorders in older people: the Islington community study. *J. Affect. Disord.*, **46**: 255–262.

5.13

Myth or Reality of Old Age Depression: The Example of Taiwan Studies

Mian-Yoon Chong[1]

Previous work in Taiwan reported low rates of depressive illness in the elderly community population (0.5–0.8%) [1], like many studies mentioned in Chiu *et al*'s review. This low risk of depression has been explained by the positive effect of the family supporting system in Taiwanese society, which traditionally gives high respect to the elderly. However, recent epidemiological studies of community subjects in Taiwan showed that elderly people had a higher risk of minor psychiatric morbidity [2, 3]. Moreover, available statistics in Taiwan have shown that elderly people presented a consistently increased risk of suicide [4] and many of those who committed suicide were found retrospectively to have suffered from depressive disorders [5]. In view of the drastic change of social and population structure in contemporary

[1] *Department of Psychiatry, Kaohsiung Medical College, 100 Shih-Chuan First Road, Kaohsiung 80708, Taiwan, Republic of China*

Taiwan, an epidemiological study of old age depression in 1500 randomized community subjects was conducted from mid-1996 to the end of 1998 [6]. Trained senior psychiatrists using the Geriatric Mental State Schedule (GMS) conducted all the assessments and measurements. The preliminary estimate of crude prevalence of depressive illnesses (including major depression and dysthymia) according to the GMS-AGECAT criteria was 20.9%. Being female, widowhood, low educational status, "older" ages and physical disability were associated with significantly higher risk for depression, and a higher rate was found in the urban than the rural regions [6].

The great discrepancy in prevalence rates in the above studies may be due to different methods of investigation. In the earlier studies [1], lay interviewers were employed for the collection of data, while in recent studies trained research psychiatrists conducted all the interviews. Epidemiological studies using trained psychiatrists for conducting interviews are costly, but they provide more reliable information than those using lay interviewers, since psychiatrists have little difficulty in distinguishing genuinely depressed patients from normal subjects who have some depressive symptoms.

Disability and impairment caused by ill-health was found to be the most important predictor of pervasive depression in the elderly, while the support from family and community did show some protective effect [6]. The preponderance of women in studies of depression in industrialized countries was confirmed in the study of old age depression [7] and in that of minor psychiatric morbidity [8] in Taiwan. The higher rate of old age depression in the urban region, found in the contemporary study in Taiwan, is probably related to the disintegration of the traditional Taiwanese extended family support system following modernization and industrialization.

The impact of the changes of social and cultural values might contribute to the increasing rates of depression in a developing country like Taiwan. Nevertheless, the large differences in reported rates of depression in the same community may well be a classical illustration of the methodological differences in investigations that need to be resolved in any future psychiatric research.

REFERENCES

1. Yeh E.K., Hwu H.K., Chang L.Y., Yeh Y.L. (1994) Mental disorders and cognitive impairment among the elderly community population in Taiwan. In *Principle and Practice of Geriatric Psychiatry* (Eds J.R.M Copeland., M.T. Abou-Saleh, D.G. Blazer), pp. 865–871, Wiley, London.
2. Cheng T.A. (1987) A Community Study of Minor Psychiatric Morbidity in Taiwan. Unpublished PhD Thesis, University of London, London.
3. Chong M.Y. (1992) The Six-Year Follow-up Study of Minor Psychiatric Morbidity in the Community in Taiwan. Unpublished PhD Thesis, University of London, London.

4. Chong M.Y., Cheng T.A. (1995) Suicidal behaviour observed in Taiwan: trends over four decades. In *Chinese Society and Mental Health* (Eds T.Y. Lin., W.S. Tseng, E.K. Yeh), pp. 209–218, Oxford University Press, Hong Kong.
5. Cheng T.A. (1995) Mental illness and suicide. *Arch. Gen. Psychiatry*, **52**, 594–603.
6. Chong M.Y., Tsang H.Y., Chen C.C. (1998) *Old Age Depression in the Community in Taiwan*. Research Report of the National Health Research Institute, Taiwan.
7. Pearson J.L., Conwell Y. (1996) *Suicide and Aging: International Perspectives*. Springer, New York.
8. Cheng T.A. (1989) Sex difference in prevalence of minor psychiatric morbidity: a social epidemiological study in Taiwan. *Acta Psychiatr. Scand.*, **80**, 395–407.

5.14

Depression in the Elderly: Predictors and Prognostic Factors

Sirkka-Liisa Kivelä[1]

A close relationship between the occurrence of depression, physical illnesses and disabilities has also been found in the Finnish studies. In particular the occurrence of coronary heart disease was associated with depression in the elderly [1], but no relationship was found between the occurrence of chronic obstructive pulmonary disease and depression [2].

The coexistence of depression in both elderly spouses is not uncommon. Both husband and wife were depressed in 5.7% of the married Finnish couples [3]. The husband was depressed and the wife nondepressed in 10.2% of the couples; and the husband was nondepressed and the wife depressed in 10.8% of the couples [3].

The analysis with a transverse design showed poor marital and family relations to be related to depression in married elderly Finnish couples [4]. However, the longitudinal analyses showed poor marital or family relations did not predict the subsequent occurrence of depression [4]. Thus, there is evidence to suggest that the poor marital and family relations experienced by many depressed elderly persons are usually a consequence rather than a predictor of depression.

After a 5-year follow-up of the aged subjects nondepressed at the baseline, the logistic regression analyses showed that an early loss of the mother and older age were independent predictors of depression in elderly men [5–7]. In women, an early loss of the father, the occurrence of previous depression, and poor health and not living alone as measured at the baseline were independent predictors [5–7]. Furthermore, in men, lowered functional abilities and poor health as measured at the baseline tended to independently predict depression [5–7].

---

[1]Oulu University Hospital, Unit of General Practice, P.B. 5000, 90401 Oulu, Finland

The above results from a follow-up of the aged subjects nondepressed at the baseline, and clinically interviewed and examined by physicians using the DSM-III criteria after the 5-year follow-up, support the conclusion that the psychological trauma which develops upon the experience of an early parental loss contributes to the development of depression even in old age. They also support the conclusion on a relapsing and episodic course of depression during one's lifespan. Poor health in both sexes, lowered functional abilities in men and not living alone in women may indicate psychosocial stress factors having some effects on the aetiology of depression in old age.

Previous studies analysing the predictors of the outcome of depression in old age have not usually treated the relapses and chronicity of depression as separate outcomes. By reanalysing our longitudinal community data about the 1- [8] and 5-year prognosis [9] of depression, we were able to identify factors predicting a relapse of depression after recovery during treatment in primary health care as well as factors predicting and related to chronicity of depression. After the recovery from depression during the 15 months of treatment in primary health care, the persons were followed-up for 4 years. Major depression and psychomotor retardation diagnosed at the beginning of the treatment were found to predict a relapse. Relapses were not related to the occurrence of somatic illnesses or stressful life events during the follow-up. A chronic course of depression was determined as the occurrence of depression at the beginning of the treatment in primary health care, at 15 months after the beginning of the treatment and at 5 years after the beginning of the treatment. Diurnal variation of symptoms and poor self-appreciation measured at the beginning of the treatment predicted a chronic course, and the occurrence of a severe somatic disease and the deterioration of one's health status during the 5-year follow-up were associated with a chronic course of depression. These results indicate that major depressive patients have a high risk for recurrences, and depressed elderly persons suffering from somatic diseases have a high risk for chronicity.

When the outcome was assessed in terms of mortality, major depression [10] and the symptoms of dissatisfaction, weight loss, anorexia and consti-pation, predicted higher mortality, which was not explained by the poor baseline somatic health of the depressed elderly. The mortality of dysthymic patients was also higher than that of nondepressed subjects, but this was explained by the high occurrence of physical diseases among them [11].

REFERENCES

1. Ahto M., Isoaho R., Puolijoki H., Laippala P., Romo M., Kivelä S.-L. (1997) Coro-nary heart disease and depression in the elderly — a population-based study. *Fam. Pract.*, **14**: 436–445.

2. Isoaho R., Keistinen T., Laippala P., Kivelä S.-L. (1995) Chronic obstructive pulmonary disease and symptoms related to depression in elderly persons. *Psychol. Rep.*, **76**: 287–297.
3. Kivelä S.-L., Luukinen H., Viramo P., Koski K. (1998) Depression in elderly spouse pairs. *Int. Psychogeriatr.*, **10**: 329–338.
4. Kivelä S.-L., Luukinen H., Sulkava R., Viramo P., Koski K. (1999) Marital and family relations and depression in married elder Finns. *J. Affect Disord.*, **54**: 177–182.
5. Kivelä S.-L., Köngäs-Saviaro P., Pahkala K., Kesti E., Laippala P. (1996) Health, health behaviour and functional ability predicting depression in old age: a longitudinal study. *Int. J. Geriatr. Psychiatry*, **11**: 871–877.
6. Kivelä S.-L., Köngäs-Saviaro P., Laippala P., Pahkala K., Kesti E. (1996) Social and psychosocial factors predicting depression in old age: a longitudinal study. *Int. Psychogeriatr.*, **8**: 635–644.
7. Kivelä S.-L., Luukinen H., Koski K., Viramo P., Pahkala K. (1998) Early loss of mother or father predicts depression in old age. *Int. J. Geriatr. Psychiatry*, **13**: 527–530.
8. Kivelä S.-L., Pahkala K. (1989) The prognosis of depression in old age. *Int. Psychogeriatr.*, **1**: 119–133.
9. Kivelä S.-L., Köngäs-Saviaro P., Kesti E., Pahkala K., Laippala P. (1994) Five-year prognosis for depression in old age. *Int. Psychogeriatr.*, **6**: 69–78.
10. Pulska T., Pahkala K., Laippala P., Kivelä S.-L. (1998) Major depression as a predictor of premature deaths in elderly people in Finland: a community study. *Acta Psychiatr. Scand.*, **97**: 408–411.
11. Pulska T., Pahkala K., Laippala P., Kivelä S.-L. (1998) Survival of elderly Finns suffering from dysthymic disorder: a community study. *Soc. Psychiatry Psychiatr. Epidemiol.*, **33**: 319–325.

5.15
Risk and Protective Factors in Elderly Depression

Orestes V. Forlenza[1]

The elderly are exposed to many putative risk factors, which contribute to the high prevalence of depressive symptoms in this age group. Risk factors are epidemiological inferences that can help define individuals as at higher relative risk for developing certain illnesses. Understanding their role is critical for disease prevention and treatment planning.

Depression in late life may be associated with structural and functional abnormalities within the brain. To date, however, it has not been possible to identify changes that distinguish late-life from earlier-onset depression, those that define late-life depression as a unique mood disorder of one age group, or the ones that suggest a specific treatment strategy. Furthermore, none of the neurobiological correlates or markers of late-life depression are

[1]*Department of Psychiatry, University of São Paulo, R. Dr Ovidio Pires de Campos, 05403-010 São Paulo, Brazil*

yet specific or sensitive enough to be used for clinical diagnostic purposes. The depression syndrome in the elderly can be clinically indistinguishable from the one that affects younger adults, and several underlying risk factors related to both conditions overlap [1].

Psychosocial factors play an important role in the causation and maintenance of late-life depression. Although it has been argued that the impact of major life events is greater in the younger than in the aged cohort [2], in no other age group do certain life events occur as often as in old age. The final decades of life come along with a global reduction in social perspectives, declining health, and cumulative losses. Such factors, both emotional and environmental, interact with the various biological changes related to the ageing process.

The interaction between ill-health and depression is complex and bidirectional. Whilst chronic ill-health contributes to a poor prognosis of depressive disorders, depression can likewise have a negative influence on the outcome of physical illness [3]. Controversy continues over the degree to which acute or chronic medical illness causes depression because of direct physiological effects on the brain, or because of a psychological reaction to the disability and other changes evoked by these illnesses.

The distinction between biological and psychosocial factors is helpful, provided the possibilities of interaction between the different levels are borne in mind. Late-life depression will be the heterogeneous result of distinct *predisposing* and *precipitating* factors, balanced by specific *protective* or *buffering* circumstances.

Predisposing and protective factors refer to personal assets and liabilities that alter the probability of depression. The biological changes related to the ageing process probably represent a greater vulnerability than specific predisposing factors for depression in younger patients, such as genetic susceptibility or childhood deprivations. On the other hand, the existence of good coping abilities in early life is essential to deal with the additive losses and threats of late life. Later achievements such as socioeconomic and marital status further modify the risk of depression. Chronic stress due to chronic financial problems, chronic physical illness, and caregiving, are primary examples of predisposing psychosocial factors. Social support is an illustration of a hypothesized protective factor.

Among 351 elderly volunteers assessed in a primary care setting in Brazil, female sex, being illiterate and having low income were the most consistent risk factors associated with psychiatric morbidity [4], the latter being an important source of stress in our environment, particularly when the elderly lack proper social and health support.

Precipitating agents and coping efforts are more proximate than predisposing and protective factors. Life events, such as bereavement and new ill-health episodes, are viewed as sudden sources of stress that may trigger the onset of depression, particularly in the presence of other risk factors. Coping efforts refer to the specific actions taken to confront a stressor, and are ultimately related to individual personality skills. Effective coping should reduce the negative effects of stress. The capacity for intimacy, and the presence of a confident relationship, are the so-called buffers of emotional distress. Obviously the ability of achieving intimacy is related to personality traits, representing another source of interaction between factors of different categories. Likewise, the availability of good social support can be an important resource for defusing stress.

In summary, two kinds of interaction are especially relevant to understanding the role of risk factors in the onset of depression. First, the possibility of interaction between life events and social support in a "stress-buffering" fashion, that is the former increasing and the latter decreasing the risk of morbidity. The inevitable life events can therefore be much more damaging in the absence of social support. Second, the extent to which the combined risk factors interact with *age*, to affect the risk of depression. Physical ill-health can be regarded as both a predisposing and a precipitating agent, depending on related circumstances. No single factor plays a decisive role in the aetiology of the disease, but many interact and contribute to it.

REFERENCES

1. Baldwin R.C., Tomenson B. (1995) Depression in later life. A comparison of symptoms and risk factors in early and late-onset cases. *Br. J. Psychiatry*, **167**: 649–652.
2. George L.K. (1994) Social factors and depression in late life. In *Diagnosis and Treatment of Depression in Late Life* (Eds L.S. Schneider, C.F. Reynolds, B.D. Lebowitz, A.J. Friedhoff), pp. 131–154, American Psychiatric Press, Washington, DC.
3. Murphy E., Brown G.W. (1980) Life events, psychiatric disturbance and physical illness. *Br. J. Psychiatry*, **136**: 326–338.
4. Almeida O.P., Forlenza O.V., Lima N.K.C., Bigliani V., Arcuri S.M., Gentile M., Faria M.M., Oliveira D.A.M. (1997) Psychiatric morbidity among the elderly in a primary care setting — report from a survey in São Paulo, Brazil. *Int. J. Geriatr. Psychiatry*, **12**: 728–736.

5.16

Depression in Elderly Chinese

Kua Ee Heok[1]

The systematic review by Chiu *et al* predominantly covers research in the United States and Europe. Recently there have been several studies on

[1]*Department of Psychological Medicine, National University of Singapore, 5 Lower Kent Ridge Road, Singapore*

the Asian elderly, especially in the Chinese population. Variation in the prevalence and clinical presentation of depression in different cultures has been noted in the elderly population. The salient issues in comparative studies are whether the variation is a consequence of cultural factors or due to dissimilar methodology.

A study in Singapore of elderly Chinese, using the Geriatric Mental State — AGECAT [1, 2] schedule, showed a prevalence of 5.7% [3], a rate which is lower than the figures quoted in Chiu et al's review.

In Japan, a survey of 5000 randomly selected people aged over 65 years, living in the Tokyo Prefecture [4], estimated a prevalence of 2.4% for depression and other neurotic disorders.

Somatic symptoms in depression often manifest according to how cultural belief interprets the source of human emotion. In the Chinese culture, emotion emanates from the heart and a quarter of elderly depressed Chinese in the Singapore study had chest discomfort [5].

In another community study of elderly Chinese with depression [6] 75% of the 64 cases had comorbid psychiatric symptoms, commonly anxiety (53.1%) and phobia (18.6%), but there were only 29 cases of comorbid psychiatric disorders (45.3%): 17 anxiety, 7 phobia, 3 hypochondriasis and 2 obsessional disorder.

In a follow-up study of a random sample of 612 elderly Chinese in Singapore, using the GMS-AGECAT package [7], 35 cases and 28 subthreshold cases of depressive disorder were identified. Five years later, only 31 cases could be traced; in this subsample, 10 were still depressed (32.6%), 8 had recovered (25.8%), 5 were categorized as subcases of depression (16.1%), 2 were diagnosed as having anxiety disorder (6.5%), one case was diagnosed as having dementia (3.2%) and 5 had died (16.1%). Only 25 subthreshold cases from the initial study could be traced; of these, 3 had developed depression (12.0%), 15 had recovered (60.0%), 4 remained as subcases (16.0%) and 3 had died (12.0%).

The Liverpool community study [8] surveyed 1070 elderly, and follow-up of 107 cases of depressive disorder indicated that 30.8% were still depressed. The proportion of depressed elderly in the Singapore follow-up study was 32.6%, and this was quite similar to the Liverpool result. The overall outcome of the depressed elderly subjects in Liverpool was poor — 64.5% were either dead or suffering from mental illnesses (depression 30.8%, dementia 4.7% and neurotic illness 5.6%). In the Singapore study, the outcome was also gloomy — 58.1% were dead or had other mental illnesses and 16.1% were subcases of depression.

Comparing the subcases, the Liverpool study had a poorer outcome, with 18% developing depressive disorder and 16.8% dead. The Singapore results showed that 12% had died, 12% had depressive disorder and 60% recovered. In both studies, subcases did predict later development of depressive disorder.

Cultural perception of illness, societal attitude towards the elderly and family support may explain the variation of clinical presentation of depression in late life and health-seeking behaviour. Understanding the culture of a community will certainly help in early detection of depression and establishing rapport for future treatment.

REFERENCES

1. Copeland J.R.M., Kelleher M.J., Kellett J.M., Gourlay A.J., Gurland B.J., Fleiss J.L., Sharp L. (1976) A semi-structured clinical interview for the assessment of diagnosis and mental state in the elderly: the Geriatric Mental State schedule. Development and reliability. *Psychol. Med.*, **6**: 439–449.
2. Copeland J.R.M., Dewey M.E., Griffiths-Jones H.M. (1986) Computerised psychiatric diagnostic system and case nomenclature for elderly subjects: GMS and AGECAT. *Psychol. Med.*, **16**: 89–99.
3. Kua E.H. (1992) A community study of mental disorders in elderly Singaporean Chinese using the GMS-AGECAT package. *Austr. N. Zeal. J. Psychiatry*, **26**: 502–506.
4. Hasegawa K. (1974) Aspects of community mental health care of the elderly in Japan. *Int. J. Mental Health*, **8**: 36–49.
5. Kua E.H. (1990) Depressive disorder in elderly Chinese people. *Acta Psychiatr. Scand.*, **81**: 386–388.
6. Kua E.H., Ko S.M., Fones C., Tan S.L. (1996) Comorbidity of depression in the elderly—an epidemiological study in a Chinese community. *Int. J. Geriatr. Psychiatry*, **11**: 699–704.
7. Kua E.H. (1993) The depressed elderly Chinese living in the community—a 5-year follow-up study. *Int. J. Geriatr. Psychiatry*, **8**: 427–430.
8. Copeland J.R.M., Davidson I.A., Dewey M.E., Gilmore C., Lankin B.A., McWilliam C., Saunders P.A., Scott A., Sharma V., Sullivan C. (1992) Alzheimer's disease, other dementias, depression and pseudodementia: prevalence, incidence and three-year outcome in Liverpool. *Br. J. Psychiatry*, **161**: 230–239.

5.17
Suicide in Old Age
Cécile Ernst[1]

There are considerable differences between the suicide rates found among the nations of Europe, which are difficult to explain. But all nations, whatever their suicide rate, are similar in that suicides occur far more frequently in old age than in adolescence or middle age [1]. This is particularly true for men, whose suicide risk increases very steeply with age.

[1]*Lenggstrasse 31, CH-8029, Zürich 8, Switzerland*

The main reason for suicide in the elderly is depression. A large number of psychological autopsies have been carried out on representative samples of suicides, particularly in the UK, Scandinavia, the USA, Canada and Australia [2, 3, 6]. These careful inquiries into the situation of the victims at the time of their death reveal a rate of subjects with diagnosable psychiatric disorder of around 95%. Generally speaking, there are two groups of suicides: a younger group suffering mainly from personality disorders and the abuse of legal and illegal drugs, and an older group suffering mainly from depression and, less frequently, from alcohol abuse.

Henriksson et al [2] investigated a random sample of Finnish suicides. In the group over 60 years of age, the rate of those with a disorder was 91% and in the younger 93%. In the older group the most frequent diagnosis was of a depressive syndrome, which includes all disorders with depressive mood (74%). In 44% the disorder was major depression (MDD), in another 21% depression not otherwise specified (NOS), and in 12% adjustment disorder. In accordance with the contribution of Chiu et al, this study confirms the importance of subsyndromal depression even for suicide, and thus the need to explore and define syndromes that do not fulfil the criteria of major depression.

In over 75 years olds, mood disorders were found in over 79% of the cases, of which half suffered from a first episode. A survey of the literature on suicide attempts in old age [4] confirms the importance of late-onset depression, of physical illness and of disturbed relationships with next of kin. These findings should lead to particular attention for this type of depression, where an underlying neurodegenerative process may be associated with a particular inability to cope with losses. Subsyndromal late-onset depression could be the key to the contradiction between the sharp increase in suicides of elderly males and the decline of well-defined and easily recognizable major depression [5].

In a psychological autopsy of suicides in Ontario [6], sufficient information was obtained on one third of the victims, of which 89% suffered from affective disorder. Treatment of depression was almost absent and, in the few cases that were treated, selective serotonin reuptake inhibitors (SSRIs) — though obtainable — were not used. Three-quarters of the subjects had, however, seen their general practitioner during the 4 weeks before their death, probably hoping for relief.

Under the influence of Hemlock Societies and philosophers praising assisted suicide and euthanasia, there is a general and increasing tendency to understand suicide in old age as a manifestation of autonomy and as a rational decision when life is not worth living any more. The psychological autopsies contradict this attitude: suicide in old age is a manifestation not of autonomy but of affective disorders — often of subsyndromal depression — which remain unrecognized and untreated.

REFERENCES

1. Diekstra R.F.W., Gulbinat W. (1993) The epidemiology of suicidal behaviour: a review of three continents. *Rapport Trimestriel Statistique de l'Organisation Sanitaire Mondiale*, **46**: 52–68.
2. Henriksson M.M., Marttunen M.J., Isometsä E.T., Heikkinen M.E., Aro H.M., Kuoppasalmi K.I., Lönnqvist J.K. (1995) Mental disorders in elderly suicides. *Int. Psychogeriatrics*, **7**: 275–286.
3. Conwell Y., Duberstein P.R., Herrmann J.H., Caine E.D. (1996) Relationship of age and Axis I diagnoses in victims of completed suicide: a psychological autopsy study. *Am. J. Psychiatry*, **153**: 1001–1008.
4. Draper B. (1996) Attempted suicide in old age. *Int. J. Geriatr. Psychiatry*, **11**: 577–578.
5. Ernst C. (1997) Epidemiology of depression in late life. *Curr. Opin. Psychiatry*, **10**: 107–110.
6. Duckworth G., McBride H. (1996) Suicide in old age, a tragedy of neglect. *Can. J. Psychiatry*, **41**: 217–222.

6

Costs of Depressive Disorders: A Review

Jerrold F. Rosenbaum[1] and Timothy R. Hylan[2]

[1]*Massachusetts General Hospital, Boston, USA;*
[2]*Lilly Research Laboratories, Indianapolis, USA*

INTRODUCTION

Depressive disorders place a significant economic burden on patients, families, caregivers, employers, and payers worldwide [1–4]. The costs of depression are similar in magnitude to, although differently distributed, the costs of cancer, AIDS, and coronary heart disease [3]. Currently, projections indicate that the global burden of depression alone, measured in terms of disability-adjusted life years, will rank second only to ischemic heart disease in the year 2020 [5]. Depression is often characterized by repeated relapse or recurrent episodes [6–8]. The significant disease chronicity that is associated with depression magnifies its long-term societal impact and economic burden.

Of the major chronic illnesses of our time, depression remains one of the most eminently treatable. Pharmacotherapy, psychotherapy, and electroconvulsive therapy (ECT) are common treatment choices. Psychotherapy has demonstrated efficacy in mild to moderate depression, while pharmacotherapy has demonstrated efficacy in moderate to severe depression; ECT has demonstrated efficacy in severe depression [9]. Over the past 10 years, the advent of newer antidepressants such as the selective serotonin reuptake inhibitors (SSRIs) and other new drugs, with their greater tolerability relative to the older tricyclic antidepressants (TCAs), has dramatically increased the number of pharmacological options available to treat depression. Despite these advances, only a small proportion of people with major depressive disorder receive adequate treatment [10–12]. The identification and treatment of depression in primary care and other outpatient clinic settings has been improving gradually over the last decade, but it remains suboptimal in most health care delivery systems.

Depressive Disorders, Second Edition. Edited by Mario Maj and Norman Sartorius.
© 2002 John Wiley & Sons Ltd.

Now a confluence of events — the introduction of new and more expensive antidepressants, the shift in focus of health care purchase decision-making to the aggregate population level, and concerns over rising health care expenditure — has increased the need for information regarding the economic outcomes associated with the recognition, diagnosis, and treatment of depression. Providers responsible for depression treatment of their patients and health care payers responsible for financing depression treatment for large populations, can make better, more defensible recommendations by reviewing the available economic evidence regarding the treatment of depression. This evidence can be grouped into four categories: (a) the economic burden of illness; (b) economic considerations in the recognition, diagnosis and treatment of depression; (c) economic outcomes associated with alternative treatment modalities; and (d) policy issues related to financing depression treatment. This chapter provides a review and discussion of each of these four topics, and concludes by summarizing the evidence to date and identifying areas in need of further development.

BURDEN OF DEPRESSION

Patients with major depression, minor depression, and depressive symptoms have greater functional impairment and consume greater health care resources than patients who are not depressed [13–29]. For example, in a comparison of patients with DSM-III-R anxiety or depressive disorders, subthreshold disorders, or no anxiety or depressive disorders, Simon *et al* [25] found that, after controlling for physician rating and disease severity, patients with anxiety or depression had statistically significantly higher 6-month health care expenditures relative to patients with no anxiety or depression (Figure 6.1).

Epidemiological studies have shown significant functional impairment in depressed patients as measured by lost productivity and absenteeism [20, 30, 31]. Studies have found that depressed patients in primary care generally have 2–4 disability days per month [32, 33]. Health care costs are also positively correlated with symptom severity [10, 34]. Furthermore, since depression often co-occurs with other psychiatric and non-psychiatric illnesses, it is not surprising that the outcomes of those other illnesses are poorer and costs are higher when the depression is present [9, 35, 36].

Direct and Indirect Costs

Direct medical costs are those costs related to the illness or disorder itself. In the case of depression these include the money spent on general practitioner and other outpatient visits, psychiatrist or other specialty care,

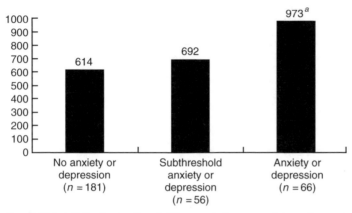

^{a}p = 0.003 statistically significant difference between anxiety or depression group and no anxiety or depression group after controlling for physician rating and chronic disease score

FIGURE 6.1   Mean 6-month health care expenditures (US$): a comparison across diagnoses
Source: from Simon *et al* [25]

pharmacotherapy, hospitalizations and other inpatient care, psychotherapy and other types of counseling, and ECT sessions. Direct non-medical costs can include costs associated with transportation to treatment centers and care provided by family and friends. Cost-of-illness studies have produced various estimates of the direct costs of depression [37–41]. Table 6.1 reports the findings of these various studies. Three out of the five studies estimated both direct and indirect costs. In general, these studies found that direct costs comprised less than 50% of the overall burden of illness with the majority of costs being indirect.

Indirect costs include the impact on productivity, days lost from work, forgone leisure time, and increased mortality. Compared with other chronic conditions, the costs associated with depression are more likely to be productivity losses caused by absenteeism and suboptimal performance in the workplace [3, 30, 37, 42]. Depressed workers can experience short- and long-term absences from work leading to reduced earnings capacity over time [43]. One study has found that the magnitude of short-term disability appears to be greater than other chronic conditions such as diabetes, back pain, and high blood pressure [44]. The costs of depression are therefore more hidden and insidious than those associated with other chronic illnesses.

Greenberg *et al* [41] estimated the costs due to lost productivity in the United States in 1990 to be $23.8bn and the costs due to depression-related suicide to be $7.5bn, for a total indirect cost impact of $31.3bn (Table 6.1). Broadhead *et al* [30] demonstrated that persons with major depression in

TABLE 6.1 Estimated direct and indirect costs of depression

	Country (year)	Direct costs[a]	Indirect costs[a]	Total[a]
Stoudemire et al, 1986 [37]	United States, 1980	$2.1bn	$14.2bn	$16.3bn
West, 1992 [38]	United Kingdom, 1986–7	£333m	n/a	n/a
Jonsson and Bebbington, 1993 [39]	United Kingdom, 1990	£222m	n/a	n/a
Kind and Sorenson, 1993 [40]	England and Wales, 1990–1	£420m	> £3bn	> £3.42bn
Greenberg et al, 1993 [41]	United States, 1990	$12.4bn	$31.3bn	$43.7bn

[a]Inflation-adjusted figures for the year shown.

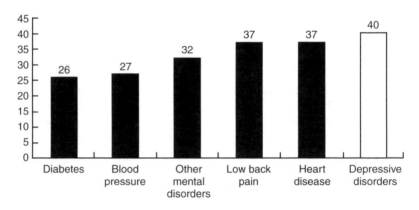

FIGURE 6.2 Days of work lost per year: average number of disability days for major diseases
Source: adapted from Conti and Burton [42]

the United States had almost five times the number of days lost from work compared with asymptomatic individuals. The same study demonstrated that persons with some depressive symptoms, but not suffering from a currently defined depressive disorder, experienced three times the number of disability days compared with asymptomatic individuals. Conti and Burton [42] estimated the average length of disability for a variety of conditions and found it to be highest for depressive disorders relative to other conditions (Figure 6.2). Other studies have found that the level of functional impairment for depressed patients exceeds that of many other general medical conditions and is higher for patients with major depression relative to those with minor depression or depressive symptoms [10, 27, 30, 45]. Other literature has found that depression is a significant risk factor for other illnesses or recovery from other illnesses such as cardiovascular disease and stroke, the economic implications of which are straightforward [46, 47]. Some authors have also argued that road traffic accidents involving depressed patients are an important source of indirect costs [48, 49]. Other research has found that the impact of learning disabilities stemming from depressive illnesses exerts a significant burden on society [50].

Quality of Life and Intangible Burdens

Depression has a substantial impact on health-related quality of life. Research has shown that depressed patients report lower physical, psychosocial, and social role functioning relative to non-depressed patients [10, 27, 51–55]. As expected, the impact of depression on quality of life is positively correlated with the severity of the depression [56–58] and is equal to or greater than the impact of other chronic medical illnesses [59]. Schonfeld *et al* [60] found that major depression was a significant determinant of reduced physical, social, and emotional functioning, as measured by the RAND Short Form-36 health scale, in primary care patients whose depressive disorder was previously unrecognized or untreated. They also found that major depression, in patients with multiple disorders, contributed more than other illnesses to compromised quality of life.

There are also other intangible burdens of depression such as the pain, suffering, and stress imposed on family, friends, relationships, and caregivers. The stigma attached to a diagnosis of depression is also an important intangible burden. At least one study has found that prescribers are likely not to record a depression diagnosis in order to reduce the associated stigma [61]. These intangibles may also manifest themselves as disruptions in daily living activities, including marital or family breakdown, and homelessness [3]. In general, intangible burdens are not measurable and therefore are omitted from burden-of-illness studies. In light of this, estimates of the direct and indirect costs of depression may represent a lower bound of the true economic impact on society.

ECONOMIC CONSIDERATIONS IN THE RECOGNITION, DIAGNOSIS AND TREATMENT OF DEPRESSION

Recognition, Diagnosis and Treatment

Studies of the treatment for depression in primary care and other outpatient clinical settings suggest a pattern that is incongruous with the magnitude of the burden of depression. It is suggested that one third of persons with depression explicitly seek treatment for their illness [12, 14]. Also, only about one half of patients with major depression who are seeking primary care for any reason are recognized by their physicians as having a psychosocial problem and less than half of these are explicitly recognized as being depressed [12, 62, 63]. Recent research has optimistically estimated that, in general medical settings, two thirds of depressed patients are actually identified by practitioners as psychologically distressed; and of these patients, slightly more than half are prescribed antidepressant medication [64]. Older results from the Medical Outcomes Study indicate that detection and treatment of depressed patients differs among practitioner types [65]. Approximately three-quarters of depressed patients who visited mental health specialists had their depression detected compared with about half of depressed patients who visited general medical clinicians even after controlling for case-mix differences.

A variety of complex interactions among patients, providers, and the health care system contribute to the under-recognition and underdiagnosis of depression [66]. At a very basic level, depressed persons may not seek help for their mood disorder symptoms. They may instead focus on somatic concerns such as gastrointestinal complaints, fatigue, or headaches. Some people may refuse to pursue treatment because of the stigma attached to a mental diagnosis or because they believe they should be able to "handle it" on their own. Other reasons for underdiagnosis of depression by providers include bias against psychiatric illnesses because of the absence of biological markers, and fear of alienating patients by suggesting that they have symptoms of depression. Finally, many general practitioners lack the time that is required to assess depression; when providers do identify the need for psychiatric evaluation, their patients may be reluctant to follow through on referrals.

At the system level, a primary reason for suboptimal treatment of depression is the lack of adequate insurance coverage for psychotherapy, ongoing psychopharmacology management, and other services by mental health professionals. The influence of health care financing arrangements has made it less attractive for providers from different specialties (e.g. a primary care physician and a psychiatrist) to collaborate with one another in treating individuals, although such an approach shows promise for treatment of depression [67, 68]. Managed care organizations which exert control over which pharmaceuticals are listed in their formularies limit the availability of a wide range of antidepressant treatment options for providers and plan members. Finally, a narrow focus on containing direct health care costs, even when the societal benefits of treatment are great, leads to the promotion of shorter term interventions that do not address the chronic and recurrent nature of depression.

Improving depression treatment can lead to improved clinical outcomes. Randomized controlled trials have shown that more intensive treatment of depression in primary care can improve outcomes [67–69]. However, some clinical trials show that less severely depressed patients can benefit from low levels of pharmacotherapy [70, 71] and at least one cohort study in clinical practice has shown that low-intensity levels of antidepressant therapy can be effective, at least in the short term [72]. Patients with short initial depression treatment duration may be at greater risk for further depressive episodes. Depression is a chronic disease for many patients and the length of antidepressant therapy is an important factor in minimizing the likelihood of relapse or recurrent episodes of depression in the longer term [8, 73]. At least one study has concluded that improving follow-up treatment and relapse prevention among those currently treated may also improve outcomes [64].

Inadequate treatment of depression can have economic consequences. Von Korff *et al* [74] reported that patients with untreated or suboptimally treated episodes of depression were more likely to use other health services, with frequent visits to primary care physicians, and excessive use of laboratory tests. In light of this finding, it is pertinent to investigate whether increasing the adequacy of depression treatment can lead to improved economic outcomes. Some studies have documented reductions in health care expenditures when depression was diagnosed and adequately treated [75–77].

Clinical trials of antidepressants indicate an efficacy rate approaching 80% response [78]. However, inadequate antidepressant treatment results in suboptimal outcomes among depressed patients. Research indicates that slightly less than half of patients receive adequate dose and duration of therapy when they are prescribed antidepressants [11, 12, 79–81]. Even for study subjects in clinical trials with moderate to severe depression, only 48–67% received prior antidepressant treatment [66]. Furthermore, the proportion of patients in clinical trials who had received adequate treatment prior to participating in the study is strikingly low — ranging from 5 to 26.8% [66]. Thus, identification and treatment of depression may be improving, but still present a significant problem. The advent of the newer antidepressants with their improved tolerability profiles may improve access to and awareness of treatment, but it is not yet clear whether the availability of these new drugs has indeed contributed to marked improvements in identification and adequate treatment of depression [82].

Economic studies of antidepressants have also compared different levels of treatment intensity to determine if a particular level of treatment is associated with lower costs. Some studies have found that an adequate dose and duration of antidepressant therapy (3–6 months) is associated with lower total direct health care expenditures relative to treatment with a shorter duration of therapy [83, 84]. However, other research [85] has found that patients who had at least 4 months of continued initial antidepressant therapy had higher health care expenditures relative to patients who had switched or augmented their initial therapy, or to those who had less than 4 months of antidepressant therapy.

Adequate treatment may have an impact on indirect costs. Mintz *et al* [86] found that improvement in depressive symptomatology and the prevention of relapse was accompanied by improved social and economic functioning, including reduced absenteeism, decreased alcoholism, increased taxable earnings, increased percentage in full-time employment, and reduced welfare receipts. Rizzo *et al* [87] found that the net benefit to employers from having workers take prescription medications for their chronic illnesses was $822 per depressed employee. Berndt *et al* [88] found that chronically and severely depressed patients had substantial improvement in workplace functioning following initiation of antidepressant treatment. The study found that this response occurred in less than 4 weeks for the majority of patients, and those with the lowest workplace function prior to treatment had the most dramatic responses.

The data are not yet conclusive that improving the adequacy of treatment leads to lower total health care expenditures overall, although the cost-effectiveness of treatment can be improved. Studies have found that initiation of depression treatment initially results in higher health care expenditures [28, 89]. In addition, other research has shown that health service utilization and expenditures do not decrease following depression recognition and initiation of treatment [25, 26, 90]. Other analysis has focused on identifying predictors of a cost-offset, finding that antidepressant therapy length and comorbid conditions are significant predictors of a reduction in health care expenditures following initiation of treatment [91]. This suggests that a reduction in health care expenditures after initiating treatment may be confined to patients with distinct characteristics. Recognition, diagnosis and treatment of depression are necessary but not sufficient for realizing a reduction in health care utilization. Improving the quality of depression treatment can, however, improve the overall cost-effectiveness or value of health care spending [92]. We return to this point below.

Antidepressant Overdose, Suicide, and Suicide Prevention

Suicidal ideation is often present in depressed patients and some depressed patients do commit suicide [93]. The indirect costs of suicide, which include the years of life forgone and the number of working years of life lost, are part of the burden of suicide [94]. In addition, the unmeasured intangible cost associated with suicide — such as the psychological impact of a suicide on surviving family and friends — is also conceivably very large. The yearly societal burden (including both direct and indirect costs) of attempted suicide as it relates to depression in the United States has been estimated at $3.6bn, while the burden of completed suicides has been estimated at $13.1bn [95]. Direct costs of suicide include health care resource utilization (hospitalization and physician costs) and autopsies after completed suicides. Runesson and Wasserman [96] estimated the direct costs of suicide attempts in Sweden at SEK42 500 ($7000) per attempt.

In light of the risk of suicidal behavior in some depressed patients, the safety of antidepressants is an important consideration. The TCAs, such as amitriptyline, desipramine, dothiepin and imipramine, generally have a higher fatality index than other antidepressants [97, 98], due to their narrow therapeutic window and greater toxicity in overdose. The TCAs represent an important risk for deaths due to overdose [99, 100]. For this reason, they are often used in low doses in clinical practice. However, there is no definitive evidence from controlled clinical trials that low doses of TCAs are efficacious [101, 102]. The use of low, possibly non-efficacious doses of antidepressants may also exacerbate, rather than improve, patient outcomes. Isacsson et al [103] studied the antidepressant prescribing patterns in Sweden of 80 individuals who later committed suicide as compared to 80 matched controls. They found that in the 3 months prior to their suicide, only 9% (vs. 13% of the controls) received antidepressants, often in low doses.

The reported frequency of overdose with SSRIs is small compared to that associated with TCAs. When SSRI overdose does occur, there is evidence that it results in lower total direct health care expenditures relative to comparable patients on a TCA [104]. A prospective, multicenter, cohort study [105] compared the hospital and physician expenditures associated with TCA and fluoxetine overdose. In a sample of 136 identified overdose patients (121 TCA and 15 fluoxetine patients), the mean hospitalization expenditures were $668 for patients with a fluoxetine overdose relative to $4691 for those with a TCA overdose. This was largely driven by differences in length of hospital stay, which were higher for TCA patients (3.59 vs. 0.73 days). Some studies have found that patients prescribed SSRIs were more likely to commit suicide than patients on TCAs [106, 107]. However, these studies did not consider the self-selection that may have been present: patients at greater perceived risk of attempting a suicide, ex ante may have been prescribed the SSRI.

Suicide and overdose in depressed patients are relatively rare events and their economic impact should be viewed in an appropriate perspective. Recent analysis has suggested that the overall suicide risk among patients treated for depression is lower than earlier estimates, which had been based on specialty and inpatient samples [108]. Undertreatment and therapeutic failure (due to the use of ineffective antidepressant doses) appear to be much larger contributors to poorer patient outcomes in clinical practice than antidepressant toxicity, overdose, or suicide [103, 109–111]. Nevertheless, given the economic burden of suicide on society, it is useful to consider the cost-effectiveness of suicide prevention. A study in the 1980s assessed the cost-effectiveness of a suicide prevention program on the island of Gotland, Sweden [112]. The intervention, initiated in 1983, was an educational program for general practitioners which focused on the diagnosis and treatment of depression. While the program was active, suicide rates on Gotland declined dramatically, although the rate increased when the program ended. For example, in 1982, there were 20 suicides per 100 000 as compared to about 8 suicides per 100 000 by 1985. The cost of the educational program was SEK369 000 ($61 000), which included SEK212 000 ($35 000) for the education program itself and SEK157 000 ($26 000) as payment to the teachers and general practitioners. Net savings totaling SEK227 000 ($37 500) resulted from a change in drug use (lower use of hypnotics and antipsychotics and increased use of antidepressants); net savings of SEK11 250 000 ($1.86m) were attributed to reduced need for inpatient care. Expenditures of general practitioner consultations remained unchanged. The remainder of the net savings were due to decreased number of inpatient days, reduction in absenteeism, and reduction in suicide rates [112]. Other studies of the effectiveness of suicide prevention programs in different settings would prove useful in assessing the generalizability of these findings.

Freemantle *et al* [113] assessed the cost-effectiveness of prescribing SSRIs as opposed to TCAs as a strategy to prevent suicide in light of tricyclic toxicity in overdose. They concluded that the cost per life year gained varied between £9000 and £173 000 and considered £50 000 as an average estimate, a much higher value than £10 000 from other life-saving and life-extending interventions [114]. From this, they concluded that a suicide prevention strategy of prescribing SSRIs instead of TCAs would not be cost-effective relative to other life-saving or life-extending interventions. Suicide is but one along with other outcome measures of antidepressant treatment such as treatment efficacy, restoration of patients' functioning and relapse or recurrence rates. Economic assessments of antidepressants should consider all the health care expenditures that can be measured that are associated with their use.

ECONOMIC OUTCOMES OF ALTERNATIVE TREATMENT MODALITIES

The most common treatment options for depression include psychotherapy, pharmacotherapy or a combination of the two, and ECT. A large body of literature has evaluated the economic outcomes of these alternative interventions within the context both of randomized controlled trials and of actual clinical practice. In light of generally higher initial total health care expenditures for depression treatment overall, it is useful to assess the economic outcomes of alternative treatments.

Randomized clinical trials (RCTs) are viewed as the "gold standard" for establishing safety and making comparisons of treatment efficacy. However, RCTs are conducted under strict, protocol-driven conditions with well-defined homogeneous patient populations, restrictions in comorbid conditions and concomitant medications, short follow-up periods, and limited sample sizes. Designed to increase internal validity, these criteria may limit RCTs' external validity (generalizability) which is important in assessing economic outcomes. The question of interest in controlled clinical trials is one of assessing therapeutic potential or clinical efficacy. "Real-world" efficacy or effectiveness in clinical practice, however, is driven by efficacy as demonstrated in clinical trials *and* how the treatments are actually used in clinical practice.

There are important limitations in generalizing from the clinical trial setting to clinical practice. A recent review [115] of controlled clinical trials for antidepressants documented certain RCT design characteristics that compromise these studies' external validity. Only 12% of the reviewed RCTs were conducted in the general practice setting, despite the fact that general practice settings are major sources of antidepressant prescribing. In addition, only 13% of the reviewed RCTs included patients with comorbid psychiatric conditions, while approximately 43% of patients in actual practice present with psychiatric comorbidity. Furthermore, only 25% of the trials had a female to male ratio of 3:1, which is the gender mix actually observed in clinical practice.

Most clinical trials are between 6 and 12 weeks in length. While this may be a sufficient length of time to detect drug therapeutic activity, it is less useful in assessing whether there will be differences in long-term real-world efficacy or effectiveness. For example, longer study time periods are necessary to detect the likelihood of achieving therapy lengths that are correlated with improved functioning [86] and prevention of relapse and recurrence [116]. Finally, patient compliance with the treatment regimen is suboptimal in actual practice [117]; even the most minor or bothersome adverse drug events can lead to important differences in patterns of actual antidepressant use between the two settings.

Economic outcomes are affected by the broader health care system in which the treatment is used and by behavioral choices that individuals make. However, RCTs often limit or eliminate individuals' behavior through the trial protocol in order to ensure a high degree of internal validity. Thus, economic outcomes observed within the clinical trial may not be replicated in clinical practice. In light of this, it is important to assess alternative treatments within the context of actual clinical practice. "Real-world" naturalistic economic clinical trials, for example, have been proposed as one way to marry the features of both clinical trials and clinical practice although these are not without their own considerations [118]. Different study designs have both their benefits and considerations. Findings which are consistent across a broad range of study designs and health care settings may be less subject to the exigencies of any one particular design or environment.

Pharmacotherapy

Tricyclic Antidepressants vs. Selective Serotonin Reuptake Inhibitors

A few randomized controlled clinical trials have made economic comparisons across specific drugs from each class. Specifically, these studies have compared the indirect costs (as measured by patients' work absenteeism) of sertraline to imipramine [119–121], but none found statistically significant difference in indirect costs between the two. Many economic comparisons of the TCAs with the SSRIs have used data from clinical trials to make assessments using meta-analyses and decision-analytic models.

Meta-analyses [113, 122–124] have generally argued that, since clinical trial efficacy and overall dropout rates are similar between the different classes, there is no difference in effectiveness either and therefore no greater cost-effectiveness of the newer agents over the TCAs. Some have extended this argument to claim that the higher drug acquisition expenditures of the newer antidepressants (e.g. the SSRIs) are not justified [122, 124]. Unfortunately, this view does not acknowledge that antidepressant use patterns, and therefore clinical outcomes and expenditures, may differ between specific antidepressants in actual clinical practice. As the authors of one recent meta-analysis [124] concluded regarding the use of data from controlled clinical trials to make inferences about cost-effectiveness, "the most obvious conclusion is that research performed to date cannot provide an answer to this problem." Thus, conclusions from RCTs or meta-analyses of clinical trial data may not be sufficient, on their own, to guide decision-making from the perspective of health care payers [125].

Most of these meta-analyses have analyzed only direct costs. Indirect costs may also be an important part of the economic impact of antidepressant selection. For example, the impact of adverse behavioral effects of TCAs on functioning may be an important source of indirect costs in so far as they increase the risk of accidents [126]. At least one researcher has argued that including the indirect costs of road traffic accidents that are attributable to poorer outcomes with TCAs would lead to the conclusion that the SSRIs are a more cost-effective treatment alternative [48]. The costs of road traffic accidents, like the costs associated with suicide, are only one component of the costs associated with antidepressant treatment.

Decision-analytic models [127–137] rely on data compiled from RCTs, meta-analyses, interviews with physicians, retrospective database studies, and other sources to assign probabilities to different treatment scenarios and their associated outcomes. By marrying results from RCTs with assumptions about usual practice pathways, decision-analytic models are intended to obviate some of the external validity problems inherent in RCT designs. These models have generally found that the SSRIs are more cost-effective relative to the TCAs. Related economic decision-analytic models of antidepressant outcomes have also focused on the use of broader, societal valuation measures. These have included the willingness-to-pay approach [138] and the cost-utility approach using quality-adjusted life years (QALYs) [139–141] or other measures of patient preferences [142].

Decision analysis provides the advantage of simultaneously modeling several different treatment pathways over a long period of time. Decision-analytic models can incorporate much longer study periods than can typically be achieved in clinical trial designs, other prospective designs, or retrospective analyses. Most decision-analytic models of antidepressant therapy, however, are sensitive to dropout rates derived from one or more clinical trials. In comparisons between TCAs and newer antidepressants, if dropout rates favor the new drug, then the analyses generally will show a favorable economic profile for the new drug because of the costs attributed to dropout and treatment failure. Although the economic effect of dropout may be relevant for severely ill and chronic patients entering clinical trial protocols, such assumptions may be less relevant for determining treatment effectiveness and associated costs of antidepressant use among the group of less severely depressed patients typically encountered in clinical practice. Because of the inherent difficulty in drawing inferences about usual practice from RCT findings, one author suggests that decision-analytic models of antidepressants uniformly overestimate the probability of treatment failure and its subsequent cost [124]. Decision-analytic models may also rely upon expert opinion and consensus groups (e.g. Delphi panels) to define parameters of the model for which data from trials and other studies do not exist. Such techniques probably are not representative of general clinical practice [118]. Moreover, the value of a model is determined by its predictive power; thus, it is important to conduct naturalistic studies of antidepressant use in clinical practice to assess how the outcomes compare with those predicted by the decision-analytic model. This is rarely done [134].

Willingness-to-pay, cost-utility, and related analyses are valuable in that they can provide an evaluation of the technology from a broader societal perspective. For example, the QALY uses a health-related quality of life measure to assess effectiveness from a societal perspective and can be used to compare across different treatments as well as across diseases. This can permit comparisons of the relative value of antidepressant treatment with that of treatments for, say, hypertension or diabetes. QALYs may be difficult to measure in the case of mental disorders such as depression, because in many cases the disease is chronic and not lethal, so that successful treatment is not likely to produce large gains in life years [143]. Moreover, depressed patients may have difficulty with the more cognitively demanding utility elicitation procedures, such as the standard gamble [143, 144]. A cost-utility approach can be useful in such situations as long as the potential short-term change in either mortality or health-related quality of life is substantial and, of course, where it is required by the government for economic assessment [145].

Clinical trials attempt to hold constant the behavioral and health system effects in order to test the efficacy of a particular treatment against a comparator. Yet it is the behavior of patients and providers interacting with the characteristics of a drug technology that ultimately leads to variability in clinical outcomes and expenditures between treatments in clinical practice [146]. Thus, study participation criteria and other design characteristics of clinical trials can limit the external validity, or generalizability, of outcomes observed in controlled clinical trials. Furthermore, because of wide variation in the underlying distribution of expenditures, the sample sizes required to detect differences in economic outcomes are typically much larger than the sample sizes needed to detect differences in clinical endpoints. Unless they are well planned, pharmacoeconomic evaluations that are incorporated in clinical trials run the risk of lacking enough statistical power to detect reliable economic differences. If there are underlying economic differences, it is also reasonable to assess whether the observed differences are sufficiently clinically or administratively relevant to prescribers and other health care decision-makers.

Two important contributions of naturalistic studies from clinical practice, including retrospective studies and prospective trials, are in identifying associations between antidepressant use and economic outcomes and in analyzing these outcomes in the context of observed patient and provider behavior. Differences in antidepressant acquisition prices are not a good predictor of broader health care expenditures. Several retrospective analyses representing a variety of health care plan settings have found that depression-related expenditures [147–150], total direct health care treatment expenditures [85, 105, 151–158], and absenteeism and work loss costs [159, 160] for patients initiating therapy with an SSRI are equal to or lower than expenditures for patients who initiate therapy with a TCA. The higher drug acquisition expenditures of SSRIs are generally offset (and in some cases more than offset) by lower expenditures for hospitalizations, additional physician visits, and other health care expenditures. Figure 6.3 depicts the expenditure differences between TCAs and SSRIs found in a representative retrospective study [85]. The figure shows that the total direct health care expenditures for patients in a privately insured sample in the United States who initiated therapy on an SSRI were statistically significantly lower than for patients who initiated therapy on a TCA. The above studies have generally

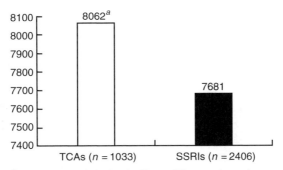

^{a}p = < 0.05; statistically significant difference in total
expenditures after controlling for both observed and
unobserved factors

FIGURE 6.3   One-year direct health care expenditures (US$) for TCAs vs. SSRIs
Source: from Crown *et al* [85]

looked at the non-elderly population. At least one study has called for further
research regarding the economic outcomes of TCAs relative to SSRIs in order
to assess the generalizability of these findings to the elderly population [161].

One consideration of retrospective studies is the non-randomization into
alternative treatments. If unobserved factors both correlated with the initial
treatment selection and subsequent outcomes are not considered, the results
may be biased. Statistical methods are available to correct for the non-
randomization inherent in retrospective data [158, 162]. Three recent retrospective studies in the United States corroborated that patients who initiated
therapy on the SSRI fluoxetine exhibited health care expenditures equal to or
lower than patients who initiated therapy on a TCA [152, 153, 158]. Unlike
other retrospective studies, these analyses used advanced econometric techniques to control for unobserved factors that might also be correlated with
both initial antidepressant selection and health care expenditures. Figure 6.4
depicts the total 1-year direct health care expenditures for a sample of patients
in a privately insured population reported by Croghan *et al* [152]. Whenever
possible, future retrospective analyses of the economic outcome associated with alternative antidepressants should employ appropriate statistical
methods to correct for non-random selection.

Another consideration of most of the above retrospective studies is the
lack of direct measures of clinical effectiveness. Many of these studies
used data from health care plan settings which did not include clinical
outcome measures. Prospective studies offer an opportunity to collect both
clinical and economic outcome data necessary to perform cost-effectiveness
analyses. To date, only one prospective, randomized, naturalistic economic
clinical trial has compared alternative antidepressant therapies [146]. This
study compared 536 patients initially randomized to either fluoxetine 20 mg

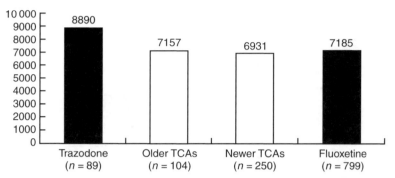

Differences were not statistically significant after controlling for observed and unobserved factors

FIGURE 6.4 One-year direct health care expenditures (US$): trazodone, TCAs and fluoxetine
Source: from Croghan *et al* [152]

($n = 173$) or a TCA (either desipramine ($n = 181$) or imipramine ($n = 182$)). After randomization, treatment was provided at the clinicians' discretion; that is, treatment was naturalistic. The study found that the 6-month clinical efficacy measures (depressive symptom scores) and total direct expenditures were not statistically different between patients who initiated therapy on fluoxetine, desipramine, or imipramine. However, those patients initiating treatment with fluoxetine reported fewer adverse events, were more likely to continue their original medication at the recommended daily dose, and were more likely to refill their prescriptions at the recommended daily dose compared with their TCA counterparts.

Of note, is that discontinuation from the original antidepressant occurred in 48% of desipramine patients and 43% of imipramine patients. The majority were switched to fluoxetine. By contrast, only 20% of fluoxetine patients switched medication. The higher than expected switch rates for TCA users, the high switch rate to fluoxetine, and the high 6-month continuation rates across all groups could have contributed to the equality of clinical efficacy rates across patient groups in the intent-to-treat design in which the subsequent outcomes are attributed to the original antidepressant.

Total direct expenditures were numerically lower for the group assigned to fluoxetine ($1967) compared with the group assigned to desipramine ($2361) or imipramine ($2105), but the difference was not statistically significant (Figure 6.5). Interestingly, the higher drug acquisition expenditures of fluoxetine were at least offset by lower outpatient visits and inpatient care. One possible interpretation of these results is that the higher switch rates among TCA users resulted in more visits to physicians relative to those who remained on their initial therapy. It is interesting to note the similarity in

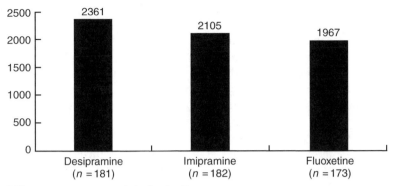

FIGURE 6.5 Six-month direct health care expenditures (US$): desipramine, imipramine and fluoxetine
Source: from Simon *et al* [146]

economic outcomes between fluoxetine and TCAs found in the Simon study [146] and the retrospective study of Croghan *et al* [152] that used statistical methods to control for potential biases due to non-randomization. The 2-year clinical and economic outcomes of the three patient cohorts in the naturalistic trial also yielded similar findings [163].

In the trial, patients were randomized to antidepressant treatment groups but not to providers, and neither the patients nor the physicians were blinded to what treatment the patient was receiving. If effectiveness and expenditures are, in part, the result of the interaction between patients and providers, then there may be remaining influences from provider characteristics that were not assessed [146]. Hybrid naturalistic trials like this one have garnered attention as a potentially optimal solution to the dilemma of maximizing both external and internal validity in pharmacoeconomic analysis. However, they also have their own set of limitations and therefore should be viewed as complementary to, rather than replacements for, the data that come from observational studies and decision models. Future randomized, naturalistic studies of clinical and economic outcomes will help to assess the contribution of this promising class of study design. To date, the most consistent finding across study designs and health care settings is that patients who initiate therapy on an SSRI have total direct health care expenditures that are equal to or lower than patients who initiate therapy on a TCA.

Comparisons Among Selective Serotonin Reuptake Inhibitors

Economic comparisons among the SSRIs have examined differences in acquisition expenditures as well as differences in utilization of a broader set of health care resources. Studies that have looked at acquisition expenditures [164–166] have generally found differences in expenditures among the antidepressants that correlate with their per unit costs. It is possible, however, that lower drug acquisition expenditures for a specific SSRI are offset by higher expenditures associated with other treatment-related health care resource utilization (e.g. coprescribing to manage adverse effects, additional physician visits). Analyses based solely on drug acquisition expenditures fail to capture the full economic impact of different treatments. Including total health care resource utilization in addition to treatment-related utilization, allows one to assess the broader economic consequences that health care decision-makers face when selecting one antidepressant vs. another.

Even depression-related expenditures may not capture the full impact of initial antidepressant selection. Patients diagnosed and treated for depression in primary care often present with non-depressive illnesses [9] and non-depression-related expenditures are generally the larger proportion of total health care expenditures [167]. Depression treatment itself is often only a small proportion of the total health care expenditures for depressed patients [25, 168]. While depression treatment itself contributes to higher expenditures, it could also reduce overall health care resource utilization in at least two ways. First, depression is often associated with comorbid illnesses [9]. If the depression treatment leads to an improvement in comorbidities common with depression, resource utilization may decrease. Second, depression leads to greater reporting of somatic symptoms [169, 170]. Improvement of the depression might also reduce the somatic complaints and their associated resource use. Thus, it is important to consider the total direct health care expenditures (both depression- and non-depression-related) when assessing the impact of alternative treatment options.

One randomized controlled clinical trial [171] compared treatment efficacy and total direct and indirect health care expenditures among patients who were randomized to treatment with either sertraline or fluoxetine, and followed those patients for 6 months. Although total health care expenditures were numerically higher for fluoxetine patients than sertraline patients, no statistical analysis was performed on the expenditure data, so it was not possible to draw firm conclusions about the expenditure differences from that study. Again, because of the exigencies of clinical trials as compared to clinical practice, it is useful to assess the economic outcomes of alternative SSRIs as they are actually used by patients and providers.

To this end, retrospective studies have explored the depression-related [172] and total health care expenditures [153, 154, 173–175] among the SSRIs. This literature has been more fully reviewed elsewhere [176–179]. As with comparisons with the TCAs, these studies find that differences in antidepressant expenditures among the SSRIs are offset [173] or more than offset [153, 154, 174, 175] by reductions in other measures of health care resource

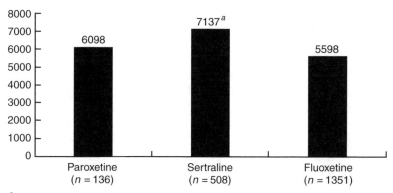

^{a}p < 0.05 (loglinear transformation) compared with fluoxetine after controlling for observed and unobserved factors

FIGURE 6.6 One-year direct health care expenditures (US$): paroxetine, sertraline and fluoxetine
Source: from Hylan *et al* [153]

utilization (i.e. concomitant therapies, physician visits, hospitalizations). For example, Hylan *et al* [153] found a statistically significant difference in the 1-year total direct health care expenditures between fluoxetine and sertraline patients after controlling for both observed and unobserved factors (Figure 6.6). Sacristan *et al* [174] estimated both the direct and indirect health care expenditures of treatment associated with the common SSRIs and venlafaxine in a primary care psychiatry setting in Spain. This study found that patients who initiated therapy on sertraline had statistically significant higher direct health care expenditures per day than patients who initiated therapy on fluoxetine. Randomized, prospective, naturalistic studies comparing the economic outcomes among the SSRIs are still needed to confirm these findings.

Other Antidepressants

Economic comparisons of other, newer antidepressants to TCAs and SSRIs have found that the use of the former results in total direct health care expenditures that are equal to or lower than those of other antidepressants. These studies include decision-analytic models comparing the cost-effectiveness of venlafaxine compared with TCAs and SSRIs [180–182] and a small hospital-based study comparing venlafaxine with TCAs and SSRIs [183]. In a retrospective database study, Sullivan *et al* [184] found that, after controlling for other observed factors through multiple regression analysis, the total direct health care expenditures for patients in a large managed care setting in the United States were similar for patients who initiated therapy on venlafaxine, a TCA, or an SSRI. Decision-analytic models have also been used to compare nefazodone with TCAs [185–187] and an extension of an earlier cost-utility model compared nefazodone with fluoxetine and imipramine [188]. Although nefazodone was found to be more cost-effective than imipramine, the cost and cost-effectiveness differences observed between nefazodone and fluoxetine were negligible. Two decision-analytic models in France and Austria compared mirtazapine with fluoxetine or amitriptyline and projected mirtazapine to be more cost-effective than the comparators [189, 190]. A cost-utility analysis of milnacipran in the prevention of recurrent depression in France [191] and a decision-analytic model comparing moclobemide and amitriptyline in Yugoslavia [192] have been performed. Finally, a recent comparative economic analysis [193] of tianeptine and fluoxetine projected cost savings by substituting fluoxetine therapy with tianeptine therapy because of lower rates of concomitant prescribing of tranquilizers with tianeptine found in a controlled clinical trial setting. Additional economic analyses of these antidepressants using data from actual clinical practice settings (like the Sullivan *et al* [184] study) are needed and may be possible as experience increases. Of particular interest are comparisons of a new antidepressant with other new antidepressants and SSRIs using data from actual clinical practice.

Despite all of these studies, it remains an open question whether these findings would be generalizable to or replicated in countries other than where the studies have currently been performed. Other countries may have different health care decision-making structures, and relative prices for different health care resources which bear on the health care expenditures realized with different antidepressants. For example, the experiences of one health maintenance organization in the United States may not be generalizable to the National Health Service in the United Kingdom. Also, in the countries where the studies above were performed, antidepressant expenditures formed a small proportion of the overall health care expenditures incurred per patient (often 10–25%). However, in some countries, a day of therapy of one of the newer, branded antidepressants may be significantly higher than even one day in the hospital or a physician's office visit. This may have a significant impact on conclusions about the relative expenditures of different antidepressant treatment options. Thus, it remains important to conduct further economic evaluations of antidepressants in other countries and health care delivery systems.

Psychotherapy

Psychotherapy (i.e. cognitive, behavioral, marital, interpersonal, brief dynamic) has demonstrated efficacy in mild to moderate depression [9]. Three approaches to economic evaluation of psychotherapy interventions have emerged: cost-consequence analysis, cost-offset analysis, and cost-effectiveness analysis. Edgell *et al* [194] examined the cost consequences of patients in a privately insured setting who had a diagnosis of depression on their medical claims form and who initiated therapy on an antidepressant, psychotherapy, a combination of antidepressant and psychotherapy, or who had a diagnosis of depression but who did not initiate treatment, the no-therapy group. Total 1-year direct health care expenditures were compared across the four cohorts. Statistical analysis was performed to correct for self-selection into the different treatment groups and for multiple comparisons. Mean total direct health care expenditures for all patients as well as the subset of patients who were seen in a mental health care setting are reported in Figure 6.7. After controlling for both observed and unobserved factors, mean total direct health care expenditures were statistically significantly lower for the no-therapy and psychotherapy cohorts relative to the combination therapy cohort. For patients who were seen in a mental health care setting, mean total direct health care expenditures were statistically significantly lower for the no-therapy and psychotherapy cohorts relative to the drug therapy cohort. No other statistical differences were found among the cohorts. This study did not contain measures of efficacy or effectiveness so it was not possible to conduct a full cost-effectiveness analysis of different treatment choices. Also, it was not possible to assess the severity of the depression diagnosis in order to determine whether appropriate therapy was given in all instances.

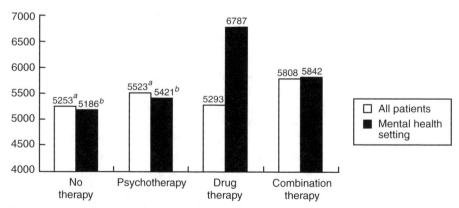

[a] Statistically significantly different from combination therapy (p < 0.008)
[b] Statistically significantly different from drug therapy (p < 0.008)

FIGURE 6.7 One-year direct health care expenditures (US$): no therapy, psychotherapy, drug therapy, combination therapy
Source: from Edgell and Hylan [194]

Some studies have assessed whether there is a "cost-offset" effect due to provision of mental heath services, particularly with regards to psychotherapy and related counseling services. The idea behind the term "cost-offset" is that, as in the case of antidepressants, savings in total medical care expenditures may outweigh the expenditures of mental health treatment. The underlying premises are that: (a) patients with untreated mental disorders frequently present with physical symptoms and somatic complaints that remit with appropriate mental health treatment; and (b) physical disorders may contribute to emotional distress which may in turn exacerbate patients' medical symptoms or delay recovery [91].

Earlier meta-analyses of this literature concluded that there was evidence of a medical cost-offset of psychotherapy treatment and that it was found mainly in inpatient expenditures [195–198]. However, there are a number of methodological problems in these studies, most notably the lack of randomization and controls for confounding variables, and the lack of an appropriate comparator. Many of the early cost-offset studies were retrospective and compared expenditures during the treatment period to a period before treatment. "Regression to the mean" is a common phenomenon upon initiation of treatment, so it is not clear whether the cost reduction was the result of the treatment or not. In addition, with retrospective data, it is important to control for not only the observed factors but also unobserved factors such as prescriber preferences and previous experience with treatment regimens, which was not done in these earlier studies [199].

To this end, a series of prospective and mostly randomized studies emerged to further investigate the cost-offset phenomenon. The results of these studies were mixed with some studies finding substantial reductions in inpatient and outpatient medical expenditures [200–204] and other studies finding no evidence of a cost-offset [25, 26, 205, 206]. A recent literature review [90] concluded that the available data identify a large potential for cost savings as the result of depression treatment, but that the studies do not clearly establish that these savings can actually be realized. They and others [207] call for more experimental studies to assess these economic outcomes.

A recent retrospective study analyzed the predictors of a medical cost-offset for patients who had an accompanying depression-related diagnosis on an insurance claim [91]. Unlike the earlier studies, this study first defined a cost-offset (a decrease in expenditures that exceeded the median cost decrease) and then assessed the predictors of the offset. The results indicated that patients with anxiety disorders, coronary artery disease, cancer, chronic fatigue syndrome, and those remaining on their initial antidepressant therapy for at least 6 months were more likely to experience significant reductions in the expenditures of medical care services. The number of psychotherapy visits was not a significant predictor of a cost-offset.

Other analyses have assessed the cost-effectiveness of various psycho-therapy interventions. Scott and Freeman [208] randomized 121 patients to antidepressant therapy prescribed by a psychiatrist, cognitive behavioral therapy provided by a psychologist, counseling and case work provided by a social worker, or routine care by a general practitioner. The researchers found that all treatment groups improved with only small differences between the groups. Specialist treatment cost at least twice as much as routine general practice. In this study, the additional expenditures associated with specialist treatment of depression in primary care were not associated with greater clinical benefits over routine general practitioner care. Likewise, a randomized clinical trial in the United Kingdom compared brief generic counseling (up to six 50-minute sessions) to usual general practitioner care, finding no clear difference in cost-effectiveness in the two interventions [209].

Kamlet *et al* [210] performed a cost-utility analysis of three maintenance treatments for recurrent depression: interpersonal therapy, imipramine drug therapy, and a combination of the two. Maintenance therapy with imipramine was found to improve expected lifetime health, to reduce direct medical expenditures, and to be cost-effective as compared with either interpersonal therapy or combination therapy. Compared with the placebo group, inter-personal therapy and combination therapy were found to improve lifetime health. However, in neither case were expected direct medical expenditures reduced.

More recently, however, Lave *et al* [211] assessed the cost-effectiveness of nortriptyline therapy or interpersonal therapy relative to usual care in a randomized controlled trial setting of primary care patients with a DSM-III-R diagnosis of major depression. The direct health care expenditures and full expenditures (which included direct health care expenditures and protocol service time and transportation expenditures) were estimated for patients completing a course of therapy on nortriptyline, interpersonal therapy, or usual care by the primary care physician. Clinical effectiveness was assessed by the Hamilton Depression Rating and the Beck Depression Inventory scales, which were used to construct a measure of depression-free days in order to obtain a measure of quality-adjusted life years.

Figure 6.8 reports the cost per quality-adjusted life year for the two treat-ment alternatives relative to usual care. Using the recommended cost per quality-adjusted life year threshold of $20 000, the authors concluded that nortriptyline was a cost-effective alternative to usual care and that inter-personal therapy was cost-effective only if its unit cost was 80% or less of the psychiatrist's government reimbursed rate (this, the authors stated, is increasingly the case in managed care fee discounting). When these cost-per-QALY results were viewed in relation to those reported for other treatments, both the nortriptyline and interpersonal therapy were cost-effective, in light of the broad range reported for other treatments. These findings were not

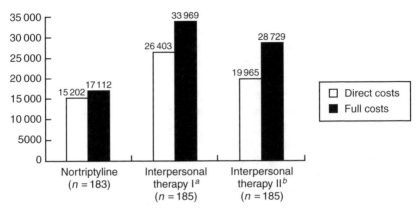

[a]Therapy I: assumes IPT sessions paid at governmentreimbursed rate for psychiatrists
[b]Therapy II: assumes IPT sessions paid at 80\% of governmentreimbursed rate for psychiatrists

FIGURE 6.8   Estimated cost per quality-adjusted life year values (US$): comparison of nortriptyline or interpersonal therapy to usual care
Source: from Lave *et al* [211]

sensitive to alternative measures of clinical outcomes or quality-adjusted life years. They corroborate those of other studies [92, 212] which find that increasing treatment consistent with guidelines costs more money but leads to improved outcomes with an increase in the overall value of care. We return to this point below.

Electroconvulsive Therapy

ECT has demonstrated efficacy for patients with severe depression [9, 213]. It has not been widely used relative to pharmacotherapy and psychotherapy; it is often reserved as treatment for patients who do not respond well to other treatments, or with concomitant psychotic symptoms or melancholia [9]. In terms of economic outcomes, while some studies [214–216] have found that ECT is associated with longer hospital stays, these studies were conducted in large, urban teaching hospitals and did not control for other baseline and pretreatment characteristics that might confound the relationship. Markowitz *et al* [217] compared patients with major depression who received ECT ($n = 19$) with those who were given tricyclic antidepressants or other medications ($n = 55$) available in the early 1980s. In terms of the outcomes, all patients who received ECT recovered from their depression; in contrast, only 49% of patients given medication recovered. The patients who had not responded to antidepressants recovered after treatment with ECT. Patients given ECT remained hospitalized a mean of

13 fewer days, which was estimated to result in a saving of more than $6400 per patient. Olfson *et al* [218] found that while ECT patients had long and costly hospital admissions, patients who received ECT within 5 days of hospital admission as compared with those who had delayed ECT or none, had significantly shorter and less costly inpatient care after controlling for other observable baseline and pretreatment factors. However, this study did not control for the possible influence of unobserved factors that might be correlated with treatment selection and outcomes, as has been done in evaluations of antidepressant therapy [85, 152, 153]. Additional studies are needed to more fully understand the economic outcomes associated with ECT compared with no treatment, psychotherapy, pharmacotherapy, or combination therapy.

POLICY ISSUES

Since 1975, health care expenditures have consumed an increasing proportion of gross domestic product (GDP) in most industrialized countries, with growth rates for health care expenditure exceeding those of GDP [219, 220]. Reasons for this include both *demand factors*, such as an aging population and a greater demand from increasing expectations for health care, and *supply factors*, such as the development and adaptation of new medical interventions and technologies. This has led to increasing health care expenditures for payers who, at the same time, face fixed or even declining budgets with which to provide health care services and treatment.

In light of increasing expenditures and resource scarcity in the 1990s, health authorities initially resorted to macroeconomic cost containment measures, such as imposing global spending limits, instituting cost controls, and tightening planning controls on major new expenditures and personnel. These reforms were unpopular because they required direct institutional or government intervention and often did not have their intended effects [219]. One reason for this is that fixed controls over one component of health care spending usually result in an increase in another component [221]. As a next wave of reforms, industrialized countries have focused on at least one or more of the following system-wide approaches: (a) redefining health objective and national health targets; (b) increasing public and private health care system partnerships; (c) requiring greater information in health care decision-making (i.e. initiatives in evidence-based medicine); and (d) implementing changes in payment system designs, such as managed care or other insurance schemes, in order to optimize the provision of health care. Even in European countries, where health care has long been provided at the national level for all citizens, there is a growing trend towards market-based approaches that seek to align incentives of various health care resource decision-makers

[219]. We focus next on the economic issues related to insurance and other payment system designs.

Financing Depression Treatment

Increasingly, national health care reforms are turning to market-oriented systems in which to finance health care in whole or in part. Health insurance is an important component of that system, and much of our understanding of the market-based economics of health insurance, and specifically, health insurance to cover depression treatment, comes from experiences and research in the United States. Historically, the financing of mental health care had been treated differently than financing of treatment for physical health problems [222]. The traditional disparity between mental health care coverage and medical care coverage can be partially explained by economic forces [223]. One force is the concept of "moral hazard." Moral hazard is the tendency for people to demand more for health services when they do not face the full price. With insurance coverage, moral hazard occurs because the price of services to the consumer does not reflect the total costs of care. Many analysts believe that the demand for mental health services is more responsive to price reductions (or insurance coverage) than is the demand for physical health services, and there is evidence of this from the RAND Health Insurance Experiment conducted in the United States during the 1970s [224]. Second, payers have only cautiously expanded coverage to include mental health care, fearing that the availability of coverage would attract "bad risks" through the process of adverse selection [222, 223]. There is some evidence that individuals' perceived mental health risk influences selection of more comprehensive insurance coverage [225].

In the recent past, when indemnity insurance plans were the norm, the insurer typically paid a fee for each service provided, and often that fee equaled what the provider charged for the service. Today, most indemnity plans have additional utilization control features. To mitigate the potential for overconsumption, indemnity plans rely upon cost-sharing mechanisms such as copayments and deductibles. The RAND Health Insurance Experiment of the mid-1970s was a large experimental study in the United States that tested the impact of alternative health insurance frameworks on the demand for medical care. The study found that full insurance coverage led to four times greater use of ambulatory mental health care [226]. In addition, the analysis found that a moderate deductible ($100–$300) with coinsurance of about 25% provided optimal insurance coverage [227]. This finding that the demand for mental health services is proportional to differences in cost-sharing has been replicated [228]. The optimal health insurance plan involves more than one pricing tool and both demand-side *and* supply-side mechanisms. In this vein, analyses of health insurance for mental health treatment have argued for a mix of both demand-side cost-sharing through a deductible, and supply-side cost-sharing, such as a prospective payment system for the provision of services [222, 229].

Throughout the 1980s and 1990s, in the United States and Europe, managed care plans have become prominent, as payers seek to better manage and predict the costs of providing health care services. In the United States, managed care plans have taken the form of health maintenance organizations (HMOs), preferred provider organizations (PPOs), independent practice associations (IPAs), and hybrid forms of these. Managed care plans attempt to promote efficient provision of health services through an internal market structure of financial incentives (e.g. capitation or discounted fee payments to providers), or restrictions on patient choice (e.g. a requirement for plan members to choose a primary care provider from the plan's provider network). Cost-sharing for managed care plan members is minimal as long as the member uses services provided by the plan's network.

One of the most dramatic trends in the US health care delivery system has been the increasing formation and use of specialty mental health plans (sometimes called "carve-outs"). In less than a decade, managed behavioral health care has changed the face of private employment-based insurance in the US. Hoping to contain costs and improve access to mental health and substance abuse services for employees, many large employers have changed their health benefit plan structures to separately manage their mental health and medical care benefits. This has allowed some employers to add mental health benefits that they previously did not provide. In addition, many state Medicaid agencies are forming public/private partnerships by contracting with private behavioral health plans to manage and provide mental health and substance abuse services.

Research on the effects of mental health carve-out plans has not kept pace with the rapidly changing market, but early evidence indicates that managed behavioral health care plans can reduce inpatient use and total expenditures without reducing access to services for plan members [230–232]. Goldman et al [232] analyzed 9 years of data for one large US employer and found that use of managed behavioral health care resulted in a 40% drop in its total cost of mental health care. This reduction in expenditures persisted from 1991 to 1996, which covered all the years of data used in the study. The authors suggest that these types of contracting arrangements should make full parity between mental health and medical/surgical benefits feasible for employers. Carve-outs, on the other hand, mitigate the effort to integrate total health care where the goal is to provide integrated medical and psychiatric treatment.

In light of these trends in financing and delivery, it is important to continually assess the impact of alternative health plan arrangements on depression treatment and outcomes. The RAND Health Insurance Experiment found no evidence of self-selection by patients into different types of health care plans (HMOs or fee-for-service). Evidence from the study also indicated that HMOs used considerably fewer resources than comparable fee-for-service plans and that the health outcomes of patients between the two types of plan were similar [233]. The Medical Outcomes Study (MOS) of the late 1980s in the United States offered an opportunity to assess the quality of care, service utilization, and economic and health outcomes of more than 20 000 adult outpatients who had a variety of chronic conditions, including depression, during a 4-year longitudinal study period in the United States. This study permitted an assessment of the impact of different payment systems and provider specialties on treatment, health outcomes, and costs of depression. The Medical Outcomes Study found that depression detection rates, intensity of mental health visits, counseling rates, and duration of antidepressant use were lower and minor tranquilizer use was higher for patients in prepaid health care plans, compared with patients in fee-for-service plans. Health outcomes were similar across the two plan types [234]. These findings, in some sense, confirm the RAND Health Insurance Experiment, but they raise questions about the detection and treatment of depression in managed care settings, and its impact on long-term outcomes for people with depression.

Capitated health care systems have been applied in other countries, although there is little evidence to date of the impact on clinical or economic outcomes. One example of this is general practitioner fundholding which was introduced in the United Kingdom in 1991 as part of a broader set of health care reforms in that country. Under this system, general practitioners and primary care teams received capitated funds that they could use to purchase secondary care directly from providers. It was thought that the introduction of a purchaser–provider split, to enable general practitioners to be more aware of the financial consequences of their clinical decisions, would lead to improved clinical and economic outcomes [235]. Evidence as to whether this approach improved both the quality and value of health care spending appears mixed at best [236].

There is a real need for current, well-designed studies that examine how treatment for depression and outcomes of care differ, not just across different types of health plans, but also according to particular delivery system characteristics. It is also important to further assess the economic consequences on both direct and indirect costs (i.e. work productivity, absenteeism, and disability) of changing the access to insurance coverage for depression treatment. One recent study [237], for example, has found that removing annual limits on mental health care coverage would increase per-worker insurance premiums by only $1.

Many countries are undergoing significant reform in methods of health care financing [238, 239]. Further assessments are needed to determine whether the findings about financing mental health care are consistent across health

care systems in other countries, particularly where health care has traditionally been provided at the national level. In these instances, individual patient
and provider decisions are inextricably related to larger government-wide
health care administrative decision-making processes. In addition, cultural
forces and social values shape a country's view towards health care and
what, how and for whom it should be provided. These factors ultimately
impact whatever financing arrangement is used.

Improving the Cost-effectiveness of Depression Treatment

Total health care costs can be thought of as the overall costs for patients
treated in a given setting. The marginal, or unit, cost refers to the cost of one
additional unit; for example, in the case of health care, the marginal cost can
be thought of as the cost of treating one additional patient. Effective health
care treatments are viewed as cost-effective if they lower the marginal cost
of treatment, thereby increasing the value of health care spending [92]. From
a health care payer's perspective, the marginal cost of treating patients is
an important consideration. Identifying and implementing those treatments
that are cost-effective (i.e. those that lower the marginal cost of treatment) can
contribute to the number of patients treated for a given health care budget
and thereby increase the value of health care spending.

In light of the large economic burden of depression and current treatment opportunities, some have argued that treatment, including preventive
treatment, can be cost-effective [240, 241]. Similarities in health outcomes
between indemnity and managed care plans, and lower resource use in
the latter, might suggest to payers that shifting people into managed care
options is a cost-effective policy. However, simply shifting groups of people
into managed care plans is not the solution to issues of mental health care
financing. Managed care plans often emphasize depression treatment by
general practitioners over treatment by specialists, and many plans may
limit access to providers for ongoing management of depression treatment.
It is more likely that opportunities for cost-effective depression treatment lie
in specific settings with specific treatment strategies rather than at a broad
macrolevel.

Sturm and Wells [92] estimated the cost and health effects of changes in
the content and quality of care for depressed patients treated in prepaid
general medical practices and mental health specialty practices. Using simulation analysis based on the Medical Outcomes Study, they estimated the
impact of three incremental treatment process strategies for depression
treatment — adequate doses of antidepressants, adequate doses and counseling therapy, and adequate doses, counseling therapy, and reduction in
the use of minor tranquilizers. Patient functioning was measured as the

number of serious limitations in daily role and physical functioning. The study found that using only the strategy of moving treatment from the specialty sector to the general medical sector resulted in lower costs, poorer functional outcomes for patients because of less appropriate treatment, and no improvement in the cost-effectiveness of care. Table 6.2 reports their findings as they relate to simulating the impact of process improvements and changing specialty mix. Their analyses found that moving patients towards treatment in general medical practices reduced costs but resulted in poorer functioning. By contrast, moving patients to the general medical sector *and* implementing process improvements resulted in lower cost-effectiveness ratios, suggesting an increase in the overall value of health care spending.

From these findings, the authors concluded that the most cost-effective strategies involved a combination of shifting care to the general medical sector *and* making quality improvements in the type of care patients received, such as improving the rates of adequate dosing and counseling. Shifting treatment from specialty care to the general medical sector reduces total costs and making quality improvements increases costs, but by a lesser amount. The study found that quality improvement such as increasing the use of counseling, use of appropriate antidepressant medications, and reducing the use of minor tranquilizers, increased the value of care. Increasing rates of detection is not a cost-effective solution in and of itself, but may be cost-effective when combined with an increase in treatment effectiveness. Other analysis has corroborated this finding [211].

The main lesson from the Medical Outcomes Study and subsequent research in the financing of mental health care is that improving the quality of depression treatment can be cost-effective even though overall total costs may increase. This could mean better care for existing patients or better access to care for a larger number of patients (or both). This is an important distinction for policy-makers who often face fixed health care budgets. Better treatment is likely to mean higher total costs in the near term, but overall efficiency can be improved if better treatment leads to a lower marginal cost of treatment in the long term. Finally, no one approach is sufficient on its own to optimize depression treatment. The right mix of payment, delivery system, and health treatment improvements can provide an opportunity to optimize the cost-effectiveness of treatment for depression [234].

Another tack to improve the value of health care spending in general has been to promote the use of information regarding the cost-effectiveness of medical technologies in decision-making. For example, some countries are increasingly considering the potential economic value of the medical technology for pricing and reimbursement or other health care purchasing decisions [145, 242–244]. Managed care organizations are also relying upon evidence of economic outcomes to inform formulary decisions. This is part of a broader movement in health care of promoting "rational prescribing"

TABLE 6.2 Effects for the system (across specialty sectors) of improved appropriateness and of a specialty shift to general medical care for severely depressed patients

Process of care	Specialty mix in medical outcomes study			New specialty mix		
	Cost per patient ($)	Reduction in functioning limitations	Cost-effectiveness ratio[a] ($)	Cost per patient ($)	Reduction in functioning limitations	Cost-effectiveness ratio[b] ($)
Care as usual	2250	0.15	5360	1825	0.09	5070
Level 1: Increase use of appropriate antidepressant medications	2490	0.27–0.35	4020–4610	2060	0.23–0.32	3490–4120
Level 2: Increase both antidepressant medication and counseling	2650	0.40–0.45	3680–3950	2240	0.38–0.43	3200–3450
Level 3a: Increase antidepressants and counseling and reduce minor tranquilizers	2580	0.40–0.56	3110–3850	2180	0.38–0.53	2730–3350
Level 3b: Increase antidepressants and counseling and reduce minor tranquilizers only in general medicine	2410	0.31–0.36	3840–4170	2050	0.31–0.37	3200–3530

*Source: From R. Sturm and K.B. Wells (1995), How can care for depression become more cost-effective? *JAMA*, **273**: 51–58. © 1995 American Medical Association, reprinted with permission.

[a] Specialty mix in Medical Outcomes Study for severely depressed (sickest quartile, according to overall psychological health): 44% general medicine, 31% psychiatry, and 25% other mental health specialties. Simulated new mix: 60% general medicine, 15% psychiatry, and 25% other mental health specialties.

[b] Average cost of removing one functioning limitation (cost-effectiveness ratio relative to no care, assuming $0 cost and −0.27 deterioration).

or "evidence-based medicine." This movement promotes the systematic use of information on the value of alternative technologies to help guide health care purchase and prescribing decisions, with the goal of improving the overall quality and value of health care spending [245, 246]. This approach does not always lead to clear answers because different studies may lead to different findings [247]. Naturally, this has spurred a great deal of debate and recommended guidelines on what kind of information, studies, and methods are appropriate to demonstrate the cost-effectiveness of health care technologies, and has led many public and private organizations and research groups to oversee, fund, conduct, review and critique these studies [145, 242, 245, 248–250].

Despite the methodological advances in the field of technology assessment in recent years, there are still challenges in implementing the findings at the health policy or purchasing level [251]. For example, identifying cost-effective treatments is a necessary but not sufficient condition for increasing the value of health care spending. Using cost-effective treatments relies critically upon the free flow of financial resources and a decision-making perspective that considers all components of health care budgets. Consider the opportunities for cost-offset demonstrated by economic outcome studies of SSRIs and TCAs. The studies described in this review, consistently using data from clinical practice, show that initiation of therapy with an SSRI results in equal or lower total direct health care expenditures compared with initiation of antidepressant therapy on a TCA. The distribution of the costs, however, may differ. With the SSRIs, drug expenditures will be higher with offsets possible in other areas of resource use (physician visits and hospitalizations). However, if payers are not able to redirect resources across different budgetary sectors, the cost-offsets may be difficult to achieve. In addition, if payment for physician visits is capitated and the supply of hospital beds is fixed, it is difficult to achieve the projected cost-offsets in the short-run. Thus, it is not sufficient to promote "evidence-based medicine" or "rational prescribing." It is also necessary for health care decision-makers to take a broader perspective when making decisions about paying for depression treatment by enabling the transfer of resources across budget components when necessary, if cost-effective solutions are to be implemented. This broader budgetary perspective is consistent with an objective of providing the greatest health care benefit for a given population and health care budget.

SUMMARY

This paper has reviewed the body of evidence regarding the costs of depressive disorders. There are several areas where the evidence is well established, but areas remain where the evidence is uncertain and open to future research.

Consistent Evidence

It is now well established that depression imposes a significant economic burden on society in terms of direct and indirect costs, quality of life, mortality and morbidity, and intangible burdens. The direct costs of depression are only a small proportion of the total economic burden; indirect costs represent the majority of burden. Depressed patients suffer from significantly lower physical, psychosocial, and social role functioning, and they consume a greater amount of health care resources than patients without depression. Overdose and suicide impose a significant economic burden on society and an intangible psychological burden on surviving families and friends. The burden as a result of ineffective treatment of depression with low dose TCAs outweighs the potential burden resulting from the possibility of suicide due to antidepressant overdose.

There appears to be little economic justification for considering TCAs as first line pharmacotherapy, given how they are actually used in clinical practice. Differences in antidepressant acquisition prices are not a good predictor of broader health care expenditures. Studies using data from clinical practice have consistently shown that patients who initiate therapy with an SSRI have total direct and indirect health care expenditures equal to or lower than patients who initiate therapy on a TCA. Differences in antidepressant acquisition expenditures are offset, and sometimes more than offset, by other health care resource utilization (e.g. physician visits, hospitalizations).

Improving the quality of antidepressant treatment most likely increases the overall total costs of depression treatment but can improve the cost-effectiveness or value of treatment. Improving the rates of usage of adequate antidepressant doses and reducing minor tranquilizer use can improve the cost-effectiveness of depression treatment. Research has also shown that shifting treatment for depression from specialty care settings to general practice settings is not cost-effective unless it is accompanied by improvements in treatment effectiveness.

That the demand for mental health services is proportional to differences in cost-sharing is a finding that has been replicated. The optimal health insurance plan involves more than one pricing tool and both demand-side and supply-side mechanisms. It is also well established that more than one policy tool is needed in order to affect the economic outcomes of depression treatment. Singular measures on their own often do not have their intended effect, because limits in one sector can have consequences in other sectors.

At least one policy tool is needed for each economic outcome measure that is targeted for change, and policy-makers need to coordinate a number of different policy tools and changes simultaneously in order to bring about the intended effect.

Incomplete Evidence

There remain areas of research where the evidence to date is uncertain. Some evidence suggests that suicide prevention may be a cost-effective intervention, but further studies are needed to assess the generalizability of these findings. In addition, most studies of the economic outcomes of antidepressants have not examined their use in elderly populations, and few have addressed their use in populations with chronic or life-threatening illnesses. Whether the findings summarized in this chapter are completely generalizable to these other populations is an open question.

Despite advances in observational study design and econometric methods addressing observed and unobserved bias, causal inferences from analyses of retrospective data are not possible. There is potential value in a research strategy that augments results from a retrospective data analysis with other research and this can be accomplished in a number of ways: (a) by replicating the same retrospective analysis in other settings; (b) by building prospective studies from samples used for retrospective data analyses; or (c) by using other creative approaches. We have yet to fully utilize the convenience and statistical power inherent in retrospective economic analysis. The debate over which study design is best to assess economic outcomes continues. Different study designs have both their benefits and their considerations. Findings which are consistent across a broad range of study designs (controlled clinical trials, meta-analyses, decision-analytic models, retrospective studies, and prospective, naturalistic economic clinical trials) and health care settings may be less subject to the exigencies of any one particular design or environment.

Some questions will remain unanswered without data from experimental studies. For example, the evidence of a cost-offset resulting from psychotherapy treatment is mixed. More experimental studies are needed to investigate this phenomenon. As with comparisons with the TCAs, studies comparing among the SSRIs and venlafaxine find that differences in antidepressant expenditures are offset or more than offset by reductions in other measures of health care resource utilization (i.e. concomitant therapies, physician visits, hospitalizations). Further corroborating research is needed, including randomized, prospective naturalistic trials comparing the economic outcomes of these drugs to confirm these findings.

Areas Still Open to Research

Finally, there are areas open to new research. Despite the many health economic studies of antidepressants, it remains an open question whether these findings would be replicated in countries whose health care decision-making structure or relative prices of health care may not be similar to countries where studies have been performed. A study of the economic outcomes of ECT compared with other treatment modalities would also be useful. Also needed are economic comparison studies among the SSRIs and other, newer antidepressants (e.g. nefazodone, milnacipran, mirtazapine, reboxetine) in actual clinical practice rather than relying upon decision analysis and data from clinical trials. Also, health economic analyses that are based on actual clinical practice have generally compared outcomes of different antidepressant treatments for only a 1-year period, with only one study to date evaluating 2-year economic outcomes.

With evidence from studies measuring outcomes over periods greater than 1 year we can answer questions about long-term cost-offset effects, and questions about how effective one antidepressant is compared with another in reducing the large indirect costs that are associated with depression. Long-term economic outcome studies of psychotherapy are also needed.

More research is needed on the economic considerations in the recognition, diagnosis, and outcomes of alternative treatments for depression in clinical practice on productivity, disability, absenteeism, and other measures of indirect costs. Much of the research to date has focused on the direct health care expenditures of treatment and alternative interventions because they have been easier to measure. As data on indirect costs become more systematically available to researchers, further research on the economic impact of depression and alternative treatment modalities on productivity may be possible. From a methodological standpoint, more refined measures of productivity losses and indirect costs are needed. Indeed, measuring more precisely the impact of depression on productivity while on the job remains a significant challenge. But as these costs remain one of the largest components of the economic burden of depression, it remains an important area to study. Studies are also needed of economic outcomes among SSRIs and newer antidepressants in measures of productivity and indirect costs in clinical practice.

Further assessments of alternative methods of financing mental health care in other countries would also help us to understand whether various schemes have similar effects. It is also important to further assess the economic consequences of changing the access to insurance coverage for depression treatment. Assessment of reforms to mental health care delivery in countries other than the United States and Europe is important in order to assess the resultant depression-economic outcomes in other countries around the world.

REFERENCES

1. Rice D.P., Kelman S., Miller L.S. (1990) *The Economic Costs of Alcohol and Drug Abuse and Mental Illnesses*, Institute for Health and Aging, University of California, San Francisco.
2. Klerman G.L., Weissman M.M. (1992) The course, morbidity, and costs of depression. *Arch. Gen. Psychiatry*, **49**: 831–834.
3. Greenberg P., Stiglin L.E., Finkelstein S., Berndt E. (1993) Depression: a neglected major illness. *J. Clin. Psychiatry*, **54**: 419–424.
4. Ansseau M. (1998) The socioeconomics of depression. *Rev. Med. Liège*, **53**: 308–310.
5. Murray C.J., Lopez A.D. (1996) *The Global Burden of Disease*, World Health Organization, Geneva.
6. Wells K.B., Burnam M., Rogers W.W., Hays R., Camp P. (1992) Course of depression for adult outpatients: results from the Medical Outcomes Study. *Arch. Gen. Psychiatry*, **49**: 788–794.
7. Keller M.B., Lavori P.W., Mueller T.I., Endicott J., Coryell W., Hirschfeld R.M.A., Shea T. (1992) Time to recovery, chronicity, and levels of psychopathology in major depression: a 5-year prospective follow-up of 431 subjects. *Arch. Gen. Psychiatry*, **49**: 809–816.
8. Kupfer D.J., Frank E., Perel J.M., Cornes C., Mallinger A.G., Thase M.E., McEachran A.B., Grochochinski V.J. (1992) Five-year outcome for maintenance therapies in recurrent depression. *Arch. Gen. Psychiatry*, **49**: 769–773.
9. Agency for Health Care Policy Research (1993) Treatment of major depression: clinical practice guidelines, no. 5, vol. 2, US Department of Health and Human Services, Rockville, MD, AHCPR Publication no. 93-0550.
10. Wells K.B., Stewart A., Hays R.D., Burnham M.A., Rogers W., Daniels M., Berry S., Greenfield S., Ware J. (1989) The functioning and well-being of depressed patients: results from the medical outcomes study. *JAMA*, **262**: 914–919.
11. Katon W., Von Korff M., Lin E., Bush T., Ormel J. (1992) Adequacy and duration of antidepressant treatment in primary care. *Med. Care*, **30**: 67–76.
12. Lepine J.P., Gastpar M., Mendlewicz J., Tylee A. (1997) Depression in the community: the first pan-European study DEPRES (Depression Research in European Society). *Int. Clin. Psychopharmacol.*, **12**: 19–29.
13. Mechanic D., Cleary P.D., Greenley J.R. (1982) Distress syndromes, illness behavior, access to care and medical utilization in a defined population. *Med. Care*, **20**: 361–372.
14. Shapiro S., Skinner E.A., Kessler L.G., Von Korff M., German P.S., Tischler G.L., Leaf P.J., Benham L., Cottler L., Regier D.A. (1984) Utilization of health and mental health services: three epidemiological catchment area sites. *Arch. Gen. Psychiatry*, **41**: 971–978.
15. McFarland B.H., Freeborn D.K., Mullooly J.P., Pope C.R. (1985) Utilization patterns among long-term enrollees in a pre-paid group practice health maintenance organization. *Med. Care*, **23**: 1221–1233.

16. Kessler L.G., Burns B.J., Shapiro S., Tischler G.I., George L.K., Hough R.L., Bodison D., Miller R.H. (1987) Psychiatric diagnoses of medical service users: evidence from the Epidemiological Catchment Area program. *Am. J. Public Health*, **77**: 18–24.
17. Koenig H.G., Shelp F., Goli V., Cohen H.J., Blazer D.G. (1989) Survival and health care utilization in elderly medical in-patients with major depression. *J. Am. Geriatr. Soc.*, **37**: 599–606.
18. Katon W., Von Korff M., Lin E., Lipscomb P., Russo J., Wagner E., Polk E. (1990) Distressed high utilizers of medical care, DSM-III-R diagnoses and treatment needs. *Gen. Hosp. Psychiatry*, **12**: 355–362.
19. Levenson J.L., Hammer R.M., Rossiter L.F. (1990) Relation of psychopathology in general medical inpatients to use and cost of services. *Am. J. Psychiatry*, **147**: 1498–1503.
20. Johnson J., Weissman M., Klerman G. (1992) Service utilization and social morbidity associated with depressive symptoms in the community. *JAMA*, **267**: 1478–1483.
21. Manning W., Wells K.B. (1992) The effects of psychosocial distress and psychological well-being on use of medical services. *Med. Care*, **30**: 541–553.
22. Callahan C.M., Wolinsky F.D. (1995) Hospitalization for major depression among older Americans. *J. Gerontol. A Biol. Sci. Med. Sci.*, **50**: M196–M202.
23. Bingefors K., Isacson D., von Knorring L., Smedby B. (1995) Prescription drug use and health care utilization among patients treated with antidepressants in a Swedish community. *Ann. Pharmacother.*, **29**: 566–570.
24. Bingefors K., Isacson D., von Knorring L., Smedby B., Ekselius L., Kupper L. (1996) Antidepressant treated patients in ambulatory care: long-term use of non-psychotropic and psychotropic drugs. *Br. J. Psychiatry*, **168**: 292–298.
25. Simon G.E., Von Korff M., Barlow W. (1995) Health care costs associated with depressive and anxiety disorders in primary care. *Am. J. Psychiatry*, **152**: 352–357.
26. Simon G.E., Von Korff M., Barlow W. (1995) Health care costs of primary care patients with recognized depression. *Arch. Gen. Psychiatry*, **52**: 850–856.
27. Judd L.L., Paulus M.P., Wells K.B., Rapaport M.H. (1996) Socioeconomic burden of subsyndromal depressive symptoms and major depression in a sample of the general population. *Am. J. Psychiatry*, **153**: 1411–1417.
28. Henk H., Katzelnick D.J., Koback K.A., Greist J.H., Jefferson J.W. (1996) Medical costs attributed to depression among patients with a history of high medical expenses in a health maintenance organization. *Arch. Gen. Psychiatry*, **53**: 899–904.
29. Unutzer J., Patrick D.L., Simon G., Grembowski D., Walker E., Rutter C., Katon W. (1997) Depressive symptoms and the cost of health services in HMO patients aged 65 years and older. A 4-year prospective study. *JAMA*, **277**: 1618–1623.
30. Broadhead W.E., Blazer D.G., George L., Tze C.K. (1990) Depression, disability days, and days lost from work in a prospective epidemiologic survey. *JAMA*, **264**: 2525–2528.
31. Kessler R., Frank R. (1997) The impact of psychiatric disorders on work loss days. *Psychol. Med.*, **27**: 861–73.
32. Ormel J., Von Korff M., Ustun T.B., Pini S., Korten A., Oldehinkel T. (1994) Common mental disorders and disability across cultures. *JAMA*, **272**: 1741–1748.
33. Spitzer R., Kroenke K., Linzer M., Hahn S.R., Williams J.B., deGruy F.V., Brody D., Davies M. (1995) Health-related quality of life in primary care patients with mental disorders. *JAMA*, **274**: 1511–1517.

34. Hu T.W., Rush A.J. (1995) Depressive disorders: treatment patterns and costs of treatment in the private sector of the United States. *Soc. Psychiatry Psychiatr. Epidemiol.*, **30**: 224–230.

35. Keitner G.I., Ryan C.E., Miller I.W., Norman W.H. (1992) Recovery and major depression: factors associated with twelve-month outcome. *Am. J. Psychiatry*, **149**: 93–99.

36. Lustman P.J., Griffith L.S., Freedland K.E., Clouse R.E. (1997) The course of major depression in diabetes. *Gen. Hosp. Psychiatry*, **19**: 138–143.

37. Stoudemire A., Frank R., Hedemark N., Kamlet M., Blazer D. (1986) The economic burden of depression. *Gen. Hosp. Psychiatry*, **8**: 387–394.

38. West R. (1992) *Depression*, Office of Health Economics, London.

39. Jonsson B., Bebbington P.E. (1993) Economic studies of the treatment of depressive illness. In *Health Economics of Depression* (Eds B. Jonsson, J. Rosenbaum), pp. 34–48, Wiley, London.

40. Kind P., Sorenson J. (1993) The cost of depression. *Int. Clin. Psychopharmacol.*, **7**: 191–195.

41. Greenberg P., Stiglin L.E., Finkelstein S., Berndt E. (1993) The economic burden of depression in 1990. *J. Clin. Psychiatry*, **54**: 405–418.

42. Conti D., Burton W. (1994) The economic impact of depression in a workplace. *J. Occup. Med.*, **36**: 983–988.

43. Ettner S.L., Frank R.G., Kessler R.C. (1997) The impact of psychiatric disorders on labor market outcomes. *Industr. Lab. Rel. Rev.*, **1**: 64–81.

44. O'Neill D.M., Bertollo D.N. (1998) Work and earnings losses due to mental illness: perspectives from three national surveys. *Admin. Policy Ment. Health*, **25**: 505–523.

45. Craig T.J., van Natta P.A. (1983) Disability and depressive symptoms in two communities. *Am. J. Psychiatry*, **140**: 598–601.

46. Musselman D.L., Evans D.L., Nemeroff C.B. (1998) The relationship of depression to cardiovascular disease: epidemiology, biology, and treatment. *Arch. Gen. Psychiatry*, **55**: 580–592.

47. Everson S.A., Roberts R.E., Goldberg D.E., Kaplan G.A. (1998) Depressive symptoms and increased risk of stroke mortality over a 29-year period. *Arch. Intern. Med.*, **158**: 1133–1138.

48. Hale A.S. (1994) The importance of accidents in evaluating the cost of SSRIs: a review. *Int. Clin. Psychopharmacol.*, **9**: 195–201.

49. Hindmarch I. (1997) Behavioral toxicity and depression: the search for optimum therapy. *Prim. Care Psychiatry*, **3** (Suppl. 1): S17–S20.

50. Smith K., Shah A., Wright K., Lewis G. (1995) The prevalence and costs of psychiatric disorders and learning disabilities. *Br. J. Psychiatry*, **166**: 9–18.

51. Weissman M.M., Paykel E.S., Siegel K., Klerman G.L. (1971) The social role performance of depressed women: comparisons with a normal group. *Am. J. Orthopsychiatry*, **41**: 390–405.

52. Parkerson G.R., Gehlbach S.H., Wagner E.H., James S.A., Clapp N.E., Muhlbaier L.H. (1981) The Duke UNC Health Profile: an adult health status instrument for primary care. *Med. Care*, **19**: 806–828.

53. Fitton F., Temple B., Acheson H.W. (1985) The cost of prescribing in general practice. *Soc. Sci. Med.*, **21**: 1097–1105.

54. Rodin G., Voshart K. (1987) Depressive symptoms and functional impairment in the medically ill. *Gen. Hosp. Psychiatry*, **9**: 251–258.

55. Gregoire J., de Leval N., Mesters P., Czarka M. (1994) Validation of the Quality of Life in Depression Scale in a population of adult depressive patients aged 60 and above. *Int. Clin. Psychopharmacol.*, **3**: 13–19.

56. Heiligenstein J.H., Ware J.E. Jr, Beusterien K.M., Roback P.J., Andrejasich C., Tollefson G.D. (1995) Acute effects of fluoxetine versus placebo on functional health and well-being in late-life depression. *Int. Psychogeriatr.*, **7** (Suppl.): 125–137.
57. Mesters P., Cosyns P., Dejaiffe G., Fanielle J., Gilles C., Godderis J., Gregoire J., de Leval N., Meire P., Mesotten F. *et al* (1993) Assessment of quality of life in the treatment of major depressive disorder with fluoxetine, 20 mg, in ambulatory patients aged over 60 years. *Int. Clin. Psychopharmacol.*, **8**: 337–340.
58. Beusterien K.M., Steinwald B., Ware J.E. (1996) Usefulness of the SF-36 Health Survey in measuring health outcomes in the depressed elderly. *J. Geriatr. Psychiatry Neurol.*, **9**: 13–21.
59. Hays R.D., Wells K.B., Sherbourne C.D., Rogers W., Spritzer K. (1995) Functioning and well-being outcomes of patients with depression compared with chronic general medical illnesses. *Arch. Gen. Psychiatry*, **52**: 11–19.
60. Schonfeld W.H., Verboncoeur C.J., Fifer S.K., Lipschutz R.C., Lubeck D.P., Buesching D.P. (1997) The functioning and well-being of patients with unrecognized anxiety disorders and major depressive disorder. *J. Affect. Disord.*, **43**: 105–119.
61. Rost K., Smith G.R., Matthews D.B., Guise B. (1994) The deliberate misdiagnosis of major depression in primary care. *Arch. Fam. Med.*, **3**: 333–337.
62. Goldberg D., Huxley P. (1980) *Mental Illness in the Community. The Pathway to Psychiatric Care*, Tavistock, London.
63. Freeling P., Rao B.M., Paykel E.S., Sireling L.I., Burton R.H. (1985) Unrecognized depression in general practice. *Br. Med. J.*, **290**: 1880–1883.
64. Simon G.E., Von Korff M. (1995) Recognition, management and outcomes of depression in primary care. *Arch. Fam. Med.*, **4**: 99–105.
65. Wells K.B., Hays R.D., Burham M.A., Rogers W., Greenfield S., Ware J.E. (1989) Detection of depressive disorder for patients receiving prepaid or fee-for-service: results from the medical outcomes study. *JAMA*, **262**: 3298–3302.
66. Hirschfeld R.M.A., Keller M.B., Panico S., Arons B.S., Barlow D., Davidoff F., Endicott J., Froom J., Goldstein M., Gorman J.M. *et al* (1997) The national depressive and manic-depressive association consensus statement on the undertreatment of depression. *JAMA*, **277**: 333–340.
67. Katon W., Von Korff M., Lin E., Bush T., Ludman E., Simon G.E., Walker E. (1995) Collaborative management to achieve treatment guidelines: impact on depression in primary care. *JAMA*, **273**: 1026–1031.
68. Katon W., Robinson P., Von Korff M., Simon G.E., Bush T., Robinson P., Russo J. (1996) A multi-faceted intervention to improve treatment of depression in primary care. *Arch. Gen. Psychiatry*, **53**: 924–932.
69. Schulberg H., Block M.R., Madonia M.J., Scott C.P., Rodriguez E., Imber S.D., Perel J., Lave J., Houck P.R., Coulehan J.L. (1996) Treating major depression in primary care practice: eight-month clinical outcomes. *Arch. Gen. Psychiatry*, **53**: 913–919.
70. Paykel E.S., Hollyman J.A., Freelin P., Sedgwick P. (1988) Predictors of therapeutic benefit from amitriptyline in mild depression: a general practice placebo controlled trial. *J. Affect. Disord.*, **14**: 83–95.
71. Elkin I., Shea T., Watkins J.T. (1989) National Institute of Mental Health Treatment of Depression Collaborative Research Program. *Arch. Gen. Psychiatry*, **46**: 971–982.
72. Simon G.E., Lin E.B., Katon W., Saunders K., von Korff M., Walker E., Bush T., Robinson P. (1995) Outcomes of "inadequate" antidepressant treatment. *J. Gen. Int. Med.*, **10**: 663–670.

73. Prien R.F., Kupfer D.J. (1986) Continuation drug therapy for major depressive disorder: how long should it be maintained? *Am. J. Psychiatry*, **143**: 18–23.
74. Von Korff M., Ormel J., Katon W., Lin E.H. (1992) Disability and depression among high utilizers of health care. A longitudinal analysis. *Arch. Gen. Psychiatry*, **49**: 91–100.
75. Verbosky L.A., Franco K., Zrull J.P. (1993) The relationship between depression and length of stay in the general hospital patient. *J. Clin. Psychiatry*, **54**: 177–181.
76. Lane R., McDonald G. (1994) Reducing the economic burden of depression. *Int. Clin. Psychopharmacol.*, **9**: 229–243.
77. Katzelnick D.J., Koback K.A., Greist J.H., Jefferson J.W., Henk J.J. (1997) Effect of primary care treatment of depression on service use by patients with high medical expenditures. *Psychiatr. Serv.*, **48**: 59–64.
78. Anderson I.M., Tomenson B.M. (1994) The efficacy of selective serotonin reuptake inhibitors in depression: a meta-analysis of studies against tricyclic antidepressants. *J. Psychopharmacol.*, **8**: 238–249.
79. Simon G.E., von Korff M., Lin E., Bush T., Ormel J. (1993) Patterns of antidepressant use in community practice. *Gen. Hosp. Psychiatry*, **15**: 399–408.
80. MacDonald T.M., McMahon A.D., Reid I.C., Fenton G.W., McDevitt D.G. (1996) Antidepressant drug use in primary care: a record linkage study in Tayside, Scotland. *Br. Med. J.*, **313**: 860–861.
81. MacDonald T.M. (1997) Treatment of depression: prescription for success? *Prim. Care Psychiatry*, **3** (Suppl. 1): S7–S10.
82. Rosholm J.U., Gram L.F., Isacsson G., Hallas J., Bergman U. (1997) Changes in the pattern of antidepressant use upon the introduction of the new antidepressants: a prescription database study. *Eur. J. Clin. Pharmacol.*, **52**: 205–209.
83. McCombs J.S., Nichol M.B., Stimmel G.L., Sclar D.A., Beasley C.M., Gross L.S. (1990) The cost of antidepressant drug therapy failure: a study of antidepressant use patterns in a Medicaid population. *J. Clin. Psychiatry*, **51**: 60–69.
84. Thompson D., Buesching D.P., Gregor K.J., Oster G. (1996) Patterns of antidepressant use and their relations to costs of care. *Am. J. Manag. Care*, **2**: 1239–1246.
85. Crown W.H., Hylan T.R., Meneades L. (1998) Antidepressant selection and use and health care expenditures: an empirical approach. *PharmacoEconomics*, **13**: 435–448.
86. Mintz J., Mintz L.I., Arruda M.J., Hwang S.S. (1992) Treatments of depression and the functional capacity to work. *Arch. Gen. Psychiatry*, **49**: 761–768.
87. Rizzo J.A., Abbott T.A., Pashko S. (1996) Labor productivity effects of prescribed medicines for chronically ill workers. *Health Econ.*, **5**: 249–265.
88. Berndt E.R., Finklestein S.N., Greenberg P.E., Howland R.H., Keith A., Rush A.J., Russell J., Keller M.B. (1998) Workplace performance effects from chronic depression and its treatment. *J. Health Econ.*, **17**: 511–535.
89. Sharfstein S. (1997) Cost-effectiveness of psychiatric care. *Am. J. Psychiatry*, **154**: 6–7.
90. Simon G.E., Katzelnick D.J. (1998) Depression, use of medical services and cost-offset effects. *J. Psychosom. Res.*, **42**: 333–344.
91. Thompson D., Hylan T.R., McMullen W., Romeis M.E., Buesching D.P., Oster G. (1998) Predictors of a medical offset effect among patients receiving antidepressant therapy. *Am. J. Psychiatry*, **155**: 824–827.
92. Sturm R., Wells K.B. (1995) How can care for depression become more cost-effective? *JAMA*, **273**: 51–58.
93. International Committee for Prevention and Treatment of Depression (1991) WPA/PTD *Educational Program on Depressive Disorders*, Geneva.

94. Wolfersdorf M., Martinez C. (1998) Suicide in depression, lost years of life and gross social consequences: what is the outcome of suicide prevention? *Psychiatr. Praxis*, **25**: 139–141.

95. Palmer C.S., Revicki D.A., Halpem M.T., Hatziandreu E.J. (1995) The cost of suicide and suicide attempts in the United States. *Clin. Neuropharmacol.*, **18**: S25–S33.

96. Runesson B., Wasserman D. (1994) Management of suicide attempters: what are the routines and the costs? *Acta Psychiatr. Scand.*, **90**: 222–228.

97. Cassidy S., Henry J.A. (1987) Fatal toxicity of antidepressant drugs in overdose. *Br. Med. J.*, **295**: 1021–1024.

98. Henry J.A., Alexander C.A., Sener E.K. (1995) Relative mortality from overdose of antidepressants. *Br. Med. J.*, **310**: 221–224.

99. Retterstol N. (1993) Deaths due to overdose of antidepressants: experiences from Norway. *Acta Psychiatr. Scand.*, **87** (Suppl. 371): 28–32.

100. Malmvik J., Lowenhielm C.G.P., Melander A. (1994) Antidepressants in suicide: differences in fatality and drug utilization. *Eur. J. Pharmacol.*, **46**: 291–294.

101. Thompson C., Thompson C.M. (1989) The prescription of antidepressants in general practice: I. A critical review. *Hum. Psychopharmacol.*, **4**: 91–107.

102. Beaumont G., Baldwin D., Lader M. (1996) A criticism of the practice of prescribing sub-therapeutic doses of antidepressants for the treatment of depression. *Hum. Psychopharmacol.*, **11**: 283–291.

103. Isacsson G., Boethius G., Bergman U. (1992) Low level of antidepressant prescription for people who later commit suicide: 15 years of experience from a population-based drug database in Sweden. *Acta Psychiatr. Scand.*, **85**: 444–448.

104. D'Mello D.A., Finkbeiner D.S., Kocher K.N. (1995) The cost of antidepressant overdose. *Gen. Hosp. Psychiatry*, **17**: 454–455.

105. Revicki D.A., Palmer C.S., Phillips S.D., Reblando J.A., Heiligenstein J.H., Brent J., Kulig K. (1997) Acute medical costs of fluoxetine versus tricyclic antidepressants: a prospective multicentre study of antidepressant drug overdoses. *PharmacoEconomics*, **11**: 48–55.

106. Edwards G. (1995) Suicide and antidepressants. *Br. Med. J.*, **310**: 205–206.

107. Jick S.S., Dean A.D., Jick H. (1995) Antidepressants and suicide. *Br. Med. J.*, **310**: 215–218.

108. Simon G.E., Von Korff M. (1998) Suicide mortality among patients treated for depression in an insured population. *Am. J. Epidemiol.*, **147**: 155–160.

109. Isacsson G., Holmgren P., Wasserman D., Bergman U. (1994) Use of antidepressants among patients committing suicide in Sweden. *Br. Med. J.*, **308**: 506–509.

110. Isacsson G., Wasserman D., Bergman U. (1995) Self-poisonings with antidepressants and other psychotropics in an urban area of Sweden. *Arch. Gen. Psychiatry*, **7**: 113–118.

111. Isacsson G., Holmgren P., Druid H., Bergman U. (1997) The utilization of antidepressants—a key issue in the prevention of suicide: an analysis of 5201 suicides in Sweden during the period 1992–1994. *Acta Psychiatr. Scand.*, **96**: 94–100.

112. Rutz W., von Knorring L., Walinder J. (1992) Long-term effects of an educational program for general practitioners by the Swedish Committee for the Prevention and Treatment of Depression. *Acta Psychiatr. Scand.*, **85**: 83–88.

113. Freemantle N., House A., Song F., Mason J., Sheldon T.A. (1994) Prescribing selective serotonin reuptake inhibitors for prevention of suicide. *Br. Med. J.*, **309**: 249–253.

114. Tubman T.R.J., Halliday H.L., Normand C. (1990) Cost of surfactant replacement treatment for severe respiratory distress syndrome: a randomized controlled trial. *Br. Med. J.*, **301**: 842–845.

115. Olufade A.O., Gregor K.J., James S. Efficacy vs. effectiveness: the generalizability of randomized controlled trials in depression. Submitted for publication.

116. Maj M., Veltro F., Pirozzi R., Lobrace S., Magliano L. (1992) Pattern of recurrence of illness after recovery from an episode of major depression: a prospective study. *Am. J. Psychiatry*, **149**: 795–800.

117. Demyttenaere K. (1997) Compliance during treatment with antidepressants. *J. Affect. Disord.*, **43**: 27–39.

118. Simon G.E., Wagner E., Von Korff M. (1995) Cost-effectiveness comparisons using real-world randomized trials — the case of new antidepressant drugs. *J. Clin. Epidemiol.*, **48**: 363–373.

119. Russell J.M., Finkelstein S.N., Berndt E.R. (1996) Economic impact of improved work performance after treatment of chronic depression. Presented at the ECNP Congress, Melbourne, 23–27 June.

120. Finkelstein S., Berndt E.R., Greenberg P. (1996) Improvement in subjective work performance after treatment of chronic depression: some preliminary results. *Psychopharmacol. Bull.*, **32**: 33–40.

121. Keith A., Berndt E.R., Finkelstein S. (1996) Improvement in subjective work performance after treatment of chronic depression, Poster, International Health Economics Association Annual Meeting, Vancouver, 19–23 May.

122. Effective Health Care Bulletin (1993) *The Treatment of Depression in Primary Care*, **5**: 1–12.

123. Song F., Freemantle N., Sheldon T.A. (1994) Selective serotonin reuptake inhibitors: meta-analysis of efficacy and acceptability. *Br. Med. J.*, **306**: 683–687.

124. Hotopf M., Lewis G., Normand C. (1996) Are SSRIs a cost-effective alternative to tricyclics? *Br. J. Psychiatry*, **168**: 404–409.

125. Hotopf M., Lewis G., Normand C. (1997) Putting trials on trial — the cost and consequences of small trials in depression: a systematic review of methodology. *J. Epidemiol. Comm. Health*, **51**: 354–358.

126. Bech P. (1995) Social aspects of treatment of depression. *Int. Clin. Psychopharmacol.*, **10** (Suppl. 1): 11–14.

127. Le Pen C., Levy E., Ravily V., Beuzen J.N., Meurgey F. (1994) The cost of treatment dropout in depression: a cost-benefit analysis of fluoxetine vs. tricyclics. *J. Affect. Disord.*, **31**: 1–18.

128. Jonsson B., Bebbington P.E. (1994) What price depression? The cost of depression and the cost-effectiveness of pharmacological treatment. *Br. J. Psychiatry*, **164**: 665–673.

129. McFarland B.H. (1994) Cost-effectiveness considerations for managed care systems: treating depression in primary care. *Am. J. Med.*, **97** (Suppl. 6A): 47S–58S.

130. Stewart A. (1994) Antidepressant pharmacotherapy: cost comparison of SSRIs and TCAs. *Br. J. Med. Econ.*, **7**: 67–79.

131. Bentkover J., Feighner J.P. (1995) Cost-analysis of paroxetine vs. imipramine in major depression. *PharmacoEconomics*, **8**: 223–232.

132. LaPierre Y., Benktover J., Schainbaum S., Manners S. (1995) Direct costs of depression: analysis of treatment costs of paroxetine vs. imipramine in Canada. *Can. J. Psychiatry*, **40**: 370–377.

133. Nuijten M., Hardens M., Soutre E. (1995) A markov process analysis comparing the cost-effectiveness of maintenance therapy with citalopram versus standard therapy in major depression. *PharmacoEconomics*, **8**: 159–168.

134. Hylan T.R., Kotsanos I.G., Anderson J.S., Brown S.H., Copley-Merriman C., Egbuonu-Davis L., Heiligenstein J.H., Overhage M., Whiteside R.E. (1996) Comparison of a decision-analytic model with results from a naturalistic economic clinical trial: an application to evaluating alternative antidepressants. *Am. J. Manag. Care*, **2**: 1211–1223.

135. John D.N., Wright T., Berti C. (1996) Is there an economic advantage in the use of SSRIs over TCAs in the treatment of depression? *J. Serotonin Res.*, **4**: 225–235.

136. Woods S., Rizzo J. (1996) Cost-effectiveness of antidepressants reassessed. *Br. J. Psychiatry*, **168**: 257–263.

137. Nuitjens M., Hadjadjeba L., Evans C., Van den Berg J. (1998) Cost-effectiveness of fluvoxamine in the treatment of recurrent depression in France. *Pharmaco-Economics*, **14**: 443–445.

138. O'Brien B.J., Novosel S., Torrance G., Streiner D. (1995) Assessing the economic value of a new antidepressant: a willingness-to-pay approach. *PharmacoEconomics*, **8**: 34–45.

139. Hatziandreu E.J., Brown R.E., Revicki D.A., Turner R., Martindale J., Levine S., Siegel J. (1994) Cost-utility of maintenance treatment of recurrent depression with sertraline versus episodic treatment with dothiepin. *PharmacoEconomics*, **5**: 249–264.

140. Kind P., Sorenson J. (1995) Modeling the cost-effectiveness of the prophylactic use of SSRIs in the treatment of depression. *Int. Clin. Psychopharmacol.*, **10** (Suppl. 1): 41–48.

141. Canadian Coordinating Office of Health Technology Assessment (1998) *A Clinical and Economic Evaluation of Selective Serotonin Reuptake Inhibitors in Major Depression*, Ontario, Canada.

142. Revicki D.A., Wood M. (1998) Patient-assigned health state utilities for depression-related outcomes: differences by depression severity and antidepressant medications. *J. Affect. Disord.*, **48**: 25–36.

143. Evers S.M.A.A., van Wijk A.S., Ament J.H.A. (1997) Economic evaluations of mental health care interventions: a review. *Health Econ.*, **6**: 161–177.

144. Patrick D.L., Mathias S.D., Elkin E.P., Fifer S.K., Buesching D.P. (1998) Health state preferences of persons with anxiety. *Int. J. Tech. Assess.*, **14**: 357–371.

145. Canadian Coordinating Office of Health Technology Assessment (1994) *Guidelines for Economic Evaluation of Pharmaceuticals*, Ontario, Canada.

146. Simon G.E., Von Korff M., Heiligenstein J.H., Revicki D.A., Grothaus L., Katon W., Wagner E.H. (1996) Initial antidepressant choice in primary care. Effectiveness and cost of fluoxetine vs. tricyclic antidepressants. *JAMA*, **275**: 1897–1902.

147. Sclar D.A., Robison L.M., Skaer T.L., Legg R.F., Nemec N.L., Galin R.S., Hughes T.E., Buesching D.P. (1994) Antidepressant pharmacotherapy: economic outcomes in a health maintenance organization. *Clin. Ther.*, **16**: 715–730.

148. Sclar D.A., Skaer T.L., Robison L.M., Galin R.S., Legg R.F., Nemec N.L. (1998) Economic outcomes with antidepressant pharmacotherapy: a retrospective intent-to-treat analysis. *J. Clin. Psychiatry*, **59** (Suppl. 2): 13–17.

149. Skaer T.L., Sclar D.A., Robison L.M., Galin R.S., Legg R.F., Nemec N.L. (1995) Economic valuation of amitriptyline, desipramine, nortriptyline, and sertraline in the management of patients with depression. *Curr. Ther. Res.*, **56**: 556–567.

150. Skaer T.L., Sclar D.A., Robison L.M., Legg R.F., Galin R.S., Nemec N.L. (1996) Antidepressant pharmacotherapy: effect on women's resource utilization within a health maintenance organization. *Appl. Therapeutics*, **1**: 45–52.

151. Forder J., Kavanagh S., Fenyo A. (1996) A comparison of the cost-effectiveness of sertraline vs. tricyclic antidepressants in primary care. *J. Affect. Disord.*, **38**: 87–111.

152. Croghan T.W., Lair T.J., Engelhart L.E., Crown W.H., Copley-Merriman C., Melfi C.A., Obenchain R.L., Buesching D.P. (1997) Effect of antidepressant therapy on health care utilization and costs in primary care. *Psychiatr. Serv.*, **48**: 1420–1426.

153. Hylan T.R., Crown W.H., Meneades L., Heiligenstein J.H., Melfi C., Croghan T.W., Buesching D.P. (1998) SSRI and TCA antidepressant selection and health care costs: a multivariate analysis. *J. Affect. Disord.*, **47**: 71–79.

154. McCombs J.S., Nichol M.B., Stimmel G.L. The role of SSRI antidepressants for treating depressed patients in the California Medicaid (Medi-Cal) program. Submitted for publication.

155. Melton S.T., Kirkwood C.K., Farrar T.W., Brink D.D., Carroll N.V. (1997) Economic evaluation of paroxetine and imipramine in depressed outpatients. *Psychopharmacol. Bull.*, **33**: 93–100.

156. Obenchain R.L., Melfi C.A., Croghan T.W., Buesching D.P. (1997) Bootstrap analyses of cost-effectiveness in antidepressant pharmacotherapy. *Pharmaco-Economics*, **11**: 464–472.

157. Simon G.E., Fishman P. (1998) Cost implications of initial antidepressant selection in primary care. *PharmacoEconomics*, **13**: 61–70.

158. Crown W.H., Obenchain R., Englehart L., Lair T., Buesching D.P., Croghan T.W. (1998) Application of sample selection models to outcomes research: the case of evaluating effects of antidepressant therapy on resource utilization. *Stat. Med.*, **17**: 1943–1958.

159. Beuzen J.N., Ravily V.F., Soutre E.F., Thomander L. (1993) Impact of fluoxetine on work loss in depression. *Int. Clin. Psychopharmacol.*, **8**: 319–321.

160. Tollefson G.D., Souetre E., Thomander L., Potvin J.H. (1993) Comorbid anxious signs and symptoms in major depression: impact on functional work capacity and comparative treatment outcomes. *Int. Clin. Psychopharmacol.*, **8**: 281–293.

161. Hughes D., Morris S., McGuire A. (1997) The cost of depression in the elderly. *Drugs Aging*, **10**: 59–68.

162. Heckman J.J., Smith J.A. (1995) Assessing the case for social experiments. *J. Econ. Perspect.*, **9**: 85–110.

163. Simon G.E., Heiligenstein J.H., Revicki D.A., Von Korff M., Katon W.J., Ludman E., Grothaus L., Wagner E. (1999) Long-term outcomes of initial antidepressant drug choice in a "real-world" randomized trial. *Arch. Fam. Med.*, **8**: 326–327.

164. Smith W., Sherrill A. (1996) A pharmacoeconomic study of the management of major depression: patients in a TennCare HMO. *Medical Interface.*, **8**: 88–92.

165. Singletary T., North D.S., Weiss M., Marman G. (1997) A cost-effective approach to the use of selective serotonin reuptake inhibitors in a Veterans' Affairs Medical Center. *Am. J. Manag. Care*, **3**: 125–129.

166. Viale G.L. (1998) An economic analysis of physicians' prescribing of selective serotonin reuptake inhibitors. *Hosp. Pharm.*, **33**: 847–850.

167. Croghan T.W., Obenchain R.L., Crown W.H. (1998) What does treatment of depression really cost? *Health Affairs*, **17**: 198–208.

168. Rost K., Zhang M., Fortney J., Smith J., Smith G.R. (1998) Expenditures for the treatment of major depression. *Am. J. Psychiatry*, **155**: 883–888.
169. Simon G.E., Von Korff M. (1991) Somatization and psychiatric disorder in the NIMH Epidemiologic Catchment Area Study. *Am. J. Psychiatry*, **148**: 1494–1500.
170. Kroenke K., Spitzer R.L., Williams J.B.W. (1994) Physical symptoms in primary care: predictors of psychiatric disorders and functional impairment. *Arch. Fam. Med.*, **3**: 774–779.
171. Boyer P., Danion J.M., Bisserbe J.C., Hotton J.M., Troy S. (1998) Clinical and economic comparison of sertraline and fluoxetine in the treatment of depression: a six-month double blind study in a primary-care setting in France. *PharmacoEconomics*, **13**: 157–169.
172. Sclar D.A., Robison L.M., Skaer T.L., Galin R.S., Legg R.F., Nemec N.L., Hughes T.E., Buesching D.P., Morgan M. (1995) Antidepressant pharmacotherapy: economic evaluation of fluoxetine, paroxetine, and sertraline in a health maintenance organization. *J. Int. Med. Res.*, **23**: 395–412.
173. Russell J.M., Berndt E.R., Miceli R., Colucci S. (1998) Course and costs of depression treatment with fluoxetine, paroxetine, and sertraline. Presented at the ECNP Congress, Paris, 31 October–4 November.
174. Sacristan J.A., Gilaberte I., Hylan T.R., Crown W.H., Bueno G., Garzon M.A., Montejo A.L. (1998) Costes del tratamiento con nuevos antidepresivos en la practica clinica habitual. *Acta Lus-Espa. Neur. Psiq. Cien. Afin.*, **26** (Suppl.): 176.
175. Ozminkowski R.J., Hylan T.R., Melfi C.A., Meneades L.M., Crown W.H., Croghan T.W., Robinson R.L. (1998) Economic consequences of selective serotonin reuptake inhibitor use with drugs also metabolized by the cyctochrome P-450 system. *Clin. Ther.*, **20**: 780–796.
176. Wilde M., Whittington R. (1995) Paroxetine: a pharmacoeconomic evaluation of its use in depression. *PharmacoEconomics*, **8**: 62–81.
177. Davis R., Wilde M. (1996) Sertraline: a pharamcoeconomic evaluation of its use in depression. *PharmacoEconomics*, **10**: 409–431.
178. Wilde M., Benfield P. (1998) Fluoxetine: a pharmacoeconomic evaluation of its use in depression. *PharmacoEconomics*, **13**: 543–561.
179. Hylan T.R., Buesching D.P., Tollefson G.D. (1998) Health economic evaluations of antidepressants: a review. *Depress. Anxiety*, **7**: 53–64.
180. Einarson T.R., Arikian S., Sweeney S., Doyle J. (1995) A model to evaluate the cost-effectiveness of oral therapies in the management of patients with major depressive disorders. *Clin. Ther.*, **17**: 136–153.
181. Einarson T.R., Addis A., Iskedjian M. (1997) Pharmacoeconomic analysis of venlafaxine in the treatment of major depression disorder. *PharmacoEconomics*, **12**: 286–296.
182. Arikian S., Einarson T.R., Casciano J.P., Doyle J.J. (1998) A health policy analysis of pharmacotherapy for major depressive disorder in Europe and the Americas. Presented at the CINP Congress, Glasgow, 12–16 July.
183. Priest R.G. (1996) Cost-effectiveness of venlafaxine for the treatment of major depression in hospitalized patients. *Clin. Ther.*, **18**: 347–358.
184. Sullivan E.M., Griffiths R.I., Frank R.G., Herbert R.J., Strauss M.J., Goldmann H.H. (1998) One-year costs of alternative second-line therapies for depression. Presented at the APA Meeting, Toronto, 30 May–4 June.
185. Anton S.F., Revicki D.A. (1995) The use of decision analysis in the pharmacoeconomic evaluation of an antidepressant: cost-effectiveness study of nefazodone. *Psychopharmacol. Bull.*, **31**: 249–258.

186. Revicki D.A., Brown R.E., Palmer W., Bakish D., Rosser W.W., Anton S.F., Feeny D. (1996) Modeling the cost effectiveness of antidepressant treatment in primary care. *PharmacoEconomics*, **8**: 524–540.

187. Montgomery S.A., Brown R.E., Clark M. (1996) Economic analysis of treating depression with nefazodone vs. imipramine. *Br. J. Psychiatry*, **168**: 768–771.

188. Revicki D.A., Brown R.E., Keller M.B., Gonzales J., Culpepper L., Hales R.E. (1997) Cost-effectiveness of newer antidepressants compared with tricyclic antidepressants in managed care settings. *J. Clin. Psychiatry*, **58**: 47–58.

189. Brown M.C.J., Guest J.F., von Loon J., Bruin R. (1998) Economic impact of using mirtazapine. *Eur. Psychiatry*, **13** (Suppl. 4): 265s.

190. Brown M.C.J., Nimmerrichter A.A., Guest J.F. (1998) Economic impact of using mirtazapine in the management of moderate and severe depression in Austria. *Eur. Psychiatry*, **13** (Suppl. 4): 266s.

191. Dardennes R., Berdeaux G., Bisserbe J.C., Lafuma A., Pribel C., Fagnani F. (1998) Cost-utility of milnacipran in the prevention of recurrent depression. *Eur. Neuropsychopharmacol.*, **8** (Suppl. 2): S136.

192. Marinkovic O., Timotijevic I. (1998) Amitripytline vs. moclobemide in depression — a pharmacoeconomic treatment analysis. *Eur. Neuropsychopharmacol.*, **8** (Suppl. 2): S136.

193. Guignard E., Allerit-Vuittenez F., Dardenne J. (1998) Economic evaluation of coprescription with antidepressants: focus on tianeptine. Presented at the CINP Congress, Glasgow, 12–16 July.

194. Edgell E.T., Hylan T.R. (1997) Economic outcomes associated with initial treatment choice in depression: a retrospective database analysis. *Am. J. Manag. Care*, **3**: S51.

195. Jones K.R., Vischi T.R. (1979) Impact of alcohol, drug abuse, and mental health treatment on medical care utilization. *Med. Care*, **17** (Dec. Suppl.): 1–82.

196. Schlesinger H.J., Mumford E., Glass G.V., Patrick G., Sharfstein S. (1983) Mental health treatment and medical care utilization in a fee-for-service system: outpatient mental health treatment following the onset of a chronic disease. *Am. J. Public Health*, **73**: 422–429.

197. Mumford E., Schlesinger H.J., Glass G.V. (1978) A critical review and indexed bibliography of the literature up to 1978 on the effects of psychotherapy on medical utilization, Report to NIMH contract NIMH-MH-77-0049, NIMH, Rockville, MD.

198. Mumford E., Schlesinger H.J., Glass G.V., Patrick C., Cuerdon T. (1984) A new look at evidence about reduced cost of medical utilization following mental health treatment. *Am. J. Psychiatry*, **141**: 1145–1158.

199. Fiedler J.L., Wight J.B. (1989) *The Medical Offset Effect and Public Health Policy: Mental Health Industry in Transition*, Praeger, New York.

200. Levitan S.J., Kornfeld D.S. (1981) Clinical and cost benefits of liaison psychiatry. *Am. J. Psychiatry*, **138**: 790–793.

201. Borus J.F., Olendzki M.C., Kessler L., Burns B.J., Brandt U.C., Broverman C.A., Henderson P.R. (1985) The "offset effect" of mental health treatment on ambulatory medical care utilization and charges. *Arch. Gen. Psychiatry*, **42**: 573–580.

202. Smith G.R., Monson R.A., Ray D.C. (1986) Psychiatric consultation in somatization disorder. *N. Engl. J. Med.*, **314**: 1407–1413.

203. Strain J.J., Lyons J.S., Hammer J.S., Fahs M., Lebovits A., Paddison P.L., Snyder S., Strauss E., Burton R., Nuber G. *et al* (1991) Cost offset from a psychiatric consultation-liaison intervention with elderly hip fracture patients. *Am. J. Psychiatry*, **148**: 1044–1049.

204. Pallack M.S., Cummings N.A., Dorken H., Henke C.J. (1993) Managed mental health, medicaid, and medical cost offset. *New Directions For Mental Health Services*, **59**: 27–40.

205. Katon W., Von Korff M., Lin E., Bush T., Russo J., Liscomb P., Wagner E. (1992) A randomized trial of psychiatric consultation with distressed high utilizers. *Gen. Hosp. Psychiatry*, **14**: 86–98.

206. Levenson J.L., Hammer R.M., Rossiter L.F. (1992) A randomized controlled study of psychiatric consultation guided by screening in general medical inpatients. *Am. J. Psychiatry*, **149**: 631–637.

207. Strain J.J., Hammer J.S., Fulop G. (1994) APM Task Force on Psychosocial Interventions in the General Hospital Setting: a review of cost-offset studies. *Psychosomatics*, **35**: 253–262.

208. Scott A.I., Freeman C.P. (1992) Edinburgh primary care depression study: treatment outcome, patient satisfaction, and cost after 16 weeks. *Br. Med. J.*, **304**: 883–887.

209. Harvey I., Nelson S.J., Lyons R.A., Unwin C., Monaghan S., Peters T.J. (1998) A randomized controlled trial and economic evaluation of counselling in primary care. *Br. J. Gen. Practice*, **48**: 1043–1048.

210. Kamlet M.S., Paul N., Greenhouse J., Kupfer K., Frank E., Wade M. (1995) Cost utility analysis of maintenance treatment for recurrent depression. *Contr. Clin. Trials*, **16**: 17–40.

211. Lave J.R., Frank R.G., Shulberg H.C., Kamlet M.S. (1998) Cost-effectiveness of treatments for major depression in primary care practice. *Arch. Gen. Psychiatry*, **55**: 645–651.

212. Von Korff M., Katon W., Bush T., Lin E.H., Simon G.E., Saunders K., Ludman E., Walker E., Unutzer J. (1998) Treatment costs, cost offset, and cost-effectiveness of collaborative management of depression. *Psychosom. Med.*, **60**: 143–149.

213. American Psychiatric Association (1990) The practice of electroconvulsive therapy: recommendations for treatment, training, and privileging: a task force report of the American Psychiatric Association, APA, Washington, DC.

214. Wilson K.G., Kraitberg N.J., Brown J.H., Bergman J.N. (1991) Electroconvulsive therapy in the treatment of depression: impact on length of stay. *Compr. Psychiatry*, **32**: 345–354.

215. Herr B.E., Abraham H.D., Anderson W. (1991) Length of stay in a general hospital psychiatric unit. *Gen. Hosp. Psychiatry*, **13**: 68–70.

216. Stotskopf C., Horn S.D. (1992) Predicting length of stay for patients with psychoses. *Health Serv. Res.*, **26**: 743–766.

217. Markowitz J., Brown R., Sweeney J., Mann J.J. (1987) Reduced length and cost of hospital stay for major depression in patients treated with ECT. *Am. J. Psychiatry*, **144**: 1025–1029.

218. Olfson M., Marcus S., Sackheim H.A., Thompson J., Pincus H.A. (1998) Use of ECT for the inpatient treatment of recurrent major depression. *Am. J. Psychiatry*, **155**: 22–29.

219. Rosleff F., Lister G. (1995) *European Healthcare Trends: Towards Managed Care in Europe*, Coopers and Lybrand Europe, United Kingdom.

220. McArthur D. (1996) *Managed Care in Europe: the Impact on the Healthcare and Pharmaceutical Sectors*, Pearson Professional, United Kingdom.

221. Horn S.D., Sharkey P.D., Tracy D.M., Horn C.E., James B., Goodwin F. (1996) Intended and unintended consequences of HMO cost-containment strategies: results from the Managed Care Outcomes Project. *Am. J. Manag. Care*, **2**: 253–264.

222. McGuire T.G. (1993) Outcomes, costs, and design of health insurance for depression. In *Health Economics of Depression* (Eds B. Jonsson, J. Rosenbaum), pp. 77–96, Wiley, London.

223. Frank R.E., Koyanagi C., McGuire T.G. (1997) The politics and economics of mental health "parity" laws. *Health Affairs*, **16**: 108–119.

224. Newhouse J.P. and the Insurance Experiment Group (1993) *Free for All? Lessons from the RAND Health Insurance Experiment*, Harvard University Press, Cambridge, MA.

225. Deb P., Wilcox-Gok V., Holmes A., Rubin J. (1996) Choice of health insurance by families of the mentally ill. *Health Econ.*, **5**: 61–76.

226. Keeler E.B. (1986) *The Demand for Episodes of Mental Health Services*, The RAND Corporation, Santa Monica, CA, Report R3432-NIMH.

227. Keeler E.B., Buchanan J.L., Rolph J.E. (1988) *The Demand for Episodes of Treatment in the Health Insurance Experiment*, The RAND Corporation, Santa Monica, CA, Report R-3454-HHS.

228. Berndt E.R., Frank R., McGuire T.G. (1997) Alternative insurance arrangements and the treatment of depression: what are the facts? *Am. J. Manag. Care*, **3**: 243–250.

229. Frank R.E., Goldman H., McGuire T.G. (1992) A model for mental health care in private insurance. *Health Affairs*, **11**: 98–117.

230. Callahan J.J., Shepard D.S., Beinecke R.H., Larson M.J., Cavanaugh D. (1995) Mental health/substance abuse treatment in managed care: the Massachusetts Medicaid experience. *Health Affairs*, **14**: 173–184.

231. Christianson J.B., Manning W., Lurie N., Stoner T.J., Gray D.Z., Popkin M., Marriott S. (1995) Utah's prepaid mental health plan: the first year. *Health Affairs*, **14**: 160–172.

232. Goldman W., McCulloch J., Sturm R. (1998) Costs and use of mental health services before and after managed care. *Health Affairs*, **17**: 40–52.

233. Phelps C. (1992) *Health Economics*, HarperCollins, New York.

234. Wells K.B., Sturm R. (1995) Care for depression in a changing environment. *Health Affairs*, **14**: 78–89.

235. Shepherd G., Muijen M., Hadley T.R., Goldman H. (1996) Effects of mental health services reform on clinical practice in the United Kingdom. *Psychiatr. Serv.*, **47**: 1351–1355.

236. Smith R.D., Wilton P. (1998) General practice fundholding: progress to date. *Br. J. Gen. Pract.*, **48**: 1253–1257.

237. Sturm R. (1997) How expensive is unlimited mental health care coverage under managed care? Working paper no. 107, Research Center on Managed Care for Psychiatric Disorders, The RAND Corporation.

238. Hutton J., Borowitz M., Oleksy I., Luce B. (1994) The pharmaceutical industry and health reform: lessons from Europe. *Health Affairs*, **13**: 98–111.

239. Shulman S.R., Lasagna L. (1996) Cost containment healthcare reform and pharmaceutical innovation: taking stock in 1995. *PharmacoEconomics*, **10** (Suppl. 2): 1–141.

240. Rupp A. (1995) The economic consequences of not treating depression. *Br. J. Psychiatry*, **166** (Suppl. 2): 29–33.

241. Weisbrod B. (1993) Economics of mental illness: costs, benefits, and incentives. In *Health Economics of Depression*, pp. 15–34, Wiley, London.

242. Langley P.C. (1996) The November 1995 revised Australian guidelines for the economic evaluation of pharmaceuticals. *PharmacoEconomics*, **9**: 341–352.

243. Spilker B. (1996) *Quality of Life and Pharmacoeconomics in Clinical Trials*. Lippincott-Raven, New York.

244. Jonsson B. (1997) Economic evaluation of medical technologies in Sweden. *Soc. Sci. Med.*, **45**: 597–604.
245. Sheldon T., Chalmers I. (1994) The UK Cochrane Centre and the NHS Centre for reviews and dissemination: respective roles within the information systems strategy of the NHS R & D programme, coordination and principles underlying collaboration. *Health Econ.*, **3**: 201–203.
246. Freemantle N., Henry D., Maynard A., Torrance G. (1995) Promoting cost-effective prescribing. *Br. Med. J.*, **310**: 955–956.
247. Kernick D.P. (1997) Which antidepressant? A commentary from general practice on evidence-based medicine and health economics. *Br. J. Gen. Pract.*, **47**: 95–98.
248. Kassirer J.P., Angell M. (1994) The "journal's" policy on cost-effectiveness analyses. *N. Engl. J. Med.*, **331**: 669–670.
249. Hillman A.L. and The Task Force on Principles for Health Care Technology (1995) Economic analysis of health care technology: a report on principles. *Ann. Int. Med.*, **122**: 60–69.
250. Gold M.R., Siegel J.E., Russell L.B., Weinstein M. (Eds) (1996) *Cost-effectiveness in Health and Medicine*, Oxford University Press, Oxford.
251. Garber A. (1994) Can technology assessment control health spending? *Health Affairs*, **13**: 115–126.

Commentaries

6.1
Economics of Depression and its Treatment: Why Are We So Interested?

Paul E. Greenberg[1]

Rosenbaum and Hylan's thorough review of the medical economics literature on depression summarizes a growing body of evidence concerning the nature and extent of resource utilization associated with this debilitating illness and its related treatment. Their summary includes attention to direct, indirect and quality of life costs of depression, economic considerations stemming from its under-recognition and undertreatment, economic outcomes resulting from alternative treatment modalities (e.g. pharmacotherapy, psychotherapy, other interventions), and health policy issues related to financing and cost-effectiveness considerations.

One of the most striking features of the large literature reviewed by Rosenbaum and Hylan is its recent growth. For example, of the 251 sources referenced in this comprehensive overview, 220 (88%) were written in the 1990s, 28 (11%) were written in the 1980s, and only 3 (1%) were written in the 1970s. This trend mirrors the recent increase in attention both to pharmacoeconomic issues generally, and to the economics of psychiatric disorders such as depression in particular.

There are a number of reasons for the increased attention to the economics of depression and its treatment, some of which are noted in the review. Several related and significant developments associated with this particular disease state, as well as health care delivery generally, have occurred during the 1990s and have resulted in greater demand for health outcomes research with respect to depression. This includes the following factors.

1. As the effects and treatability of this illness have become better understood throughout society, discussions about depression awareness, recognition, and care have become commonplace, helping to de-stigmatize it. Thus, more people are now being treated than ever before, raising the stature of depression as an important public health concern.

[1] Analysis Group/Economics, One Brattle Square, Cambridge, MA 02138, USA

2. The advent of new drugs to treat depression — for example, selective serotonin reuptake inhibitors, and selective noradrenaline reuptake inhibitors — has fundamentally changed treatment protocols. Because these new pharmaceutical agents tend to be safer than alternatives that had been developed earlier, physicians who are not mental health specialists are more comfortable in prescribing them compared with earlier generations of pharmaceutical therapy, such as tricyclics. By broadening the reach of treatment in this manner, depression is rapidly becoming a community disease alongside many highly prevalent physical disorders, as opposed to a specialty care illness.

3. Over the past decade, there have been widespread efforts throughout the industrialized world to contain health care costs. In the United States, for example, as managed care has become the dominant model for health care delivery, drug interventions prescribed by primary care physicians to a large extent have replaced other treatment modalities (e.g. cognitive-behavioural therapy provided by specialists). Changes in treatment algorithms and recommended guidelines have been seen as necessary to cost-effectively address the needs of the growing number of depressed people seeking treatment in this fundamentally changed medical environment.

4. Patient-oriented health outcomes have become much more important in recent times. Outcomes based on quality-of-life considerations (e.g. quality adjusted life years) have come to dominate the health outcomes research literature. Since the newer antidepressant medications have more favorable side-effect profiles that provide quality-of-life advantages compared with older treatments, this trend in the marketplace plays up inherent advantages of these products in a timely manner.

5. As attention to indirect costs (e.g. workplace costs) has increased in the health economics community, the enormity of the burden of depression has been reevaluated. As a result, it is now widely understood that this illness has a set of characteristics that are entirely consistent with significant adversity in the workplace. These special characteristics of depression include the following: (a) it primarily affects working-age people; (b) in many cases, it is not so debilitating that people withdraw entirely from the labor force (i.e. unlike stroke or major spinal cord injury); and (c) its symptoms, including inability to concentrate and chronic fatigue, are consistent with a sizable expected adverse impact at work. The profile of depression also results in enormous burdens on caregivers, including the family and friends of sufferers. These indirect costs may be less visible than direct cost categories, such as hospitalization or physician office visits, but are much more onerous from a societal perspective.

6. The widespread availability of inexpensive computing power has made possible the development and analysis of sophisticated datasets, based on clinical trials, administrative claims data, and other sources. This development has been pivotal in permitting serious quantitative investigation of many of the subtler aspects of the economic implications of depression. For example, it is now widely recognized that depressed patients are among the highest utilizers of the heath care system, underscoring the importance of such cost drivers as comorbidities (i.e. with other psychiatric and non-psychiatric conditions) as well as lack of early identification of this illness. In addition, the possible overuse or inappropriate use of antidepressants by some patients has been distilled from numerous large data-based studies. Furthermore, these quantitative approaches have permitted investigation of the socioeconomic implications of depression, including human capital losses due to early onset and resulting non-completion of school, early marriage and subsequent divorce, and general unhappiness with life choices given depressive symptoms over a lifetime.

Thus, numerous factors have contributed to the increased focus on the economics of depression and its treatment in recent years. This includes increasing numbers of people seeking treatment, improved quality of drugs available for treatment, cost-conscious payers needing to provide broader treatment on a cost-effective basis, characteristics of depression consistent with large indirect costs, and increasingly sophisticated data analysis capabilities. These related forces, acting in concert over the past decade, have fundamentally changed the extent to which depression has been the focus of attention by outcomes researchers, as underscored in Rosenbaum and Hylan's review. To the extent that findings from this research help us direct scarce health care resources optimally, its continued growth is vital as we strive to treat increasing numbers of depression sufferers in a cost-effective manner.

6.2
Economic Evidence and Policy Decisions
Gregory E. Simon[1]

The thorough review presented by Rosenbaum and Hylan clearly demonstrates the economic burden of depression and the potential benefits of improved treatment. Some findings deserve re-emphasis, and some probably merit a cautionary note.

[1]*Center for Health Studies, Group Health Cooperative, 1730 Minor Ave. #1600, Seattle, WA 98101, USA*

The expected costs of improved depression treatment are small compared to the economic burden of depression. Among US primary care patients, overall treatment costs (antidepressant prescriptions, outpatient visits, etc.) are typically US$50–US$75 per month [1], while the "excess" use of general medical services associated with depression is typically US$100–US$150 [1, 2]. The three to five additional days of work lost per month [3–5] account for the largest portion of overall economic burden — at least US$300 per month at prevailing wage rates.

When resource allocation decisions are made, however, the costs of depression treatment may appear large or small depending on the division of financial responsibility. For example, in US insured populations, specialty mental health expenditures typically range from US$3 to US$8 per person per month compared to general medical expenditures of approximately US$150. Increasing expenditures for depression treatment by US$1 per person per month will seem either impossible or insignificant depending on the expected source for the increase (the 3% of resources devoted to specialty mental health care or the remaining 97%). This tension regarding responsibility for financing depression treatment is magnified by "carve-out" arrangements in which responsibility for specialty mental health care is completely distinct. The controversy regarding expenditures for newer antidepressants is another illustration of this phenomenon. Rosenbaum and Hylan cite considerable evidence that higher drug acquisition costs for newer antidepressants are offset by reductions in use of other medical services [6–9]. Higher drug acquisition costs, however, are usually borne by the pharmacy budget while any resultant savings are widely distributed. I recall the response of one health plan pharmacy director to the argument that newer antidepressants would not increase overall costs: "Tell me exactly who will save the money so I can ask them to send it back to me."

While some data suggest that restricting access to specialty mental health care does not adversely affect outcomes, such findings must be interpreted carefully. Two observations cited by Rosenbaum and Hylan (one old and one recent) can be used to illustrate this point. The Health Insurance Experiment found that assignment to a health maintenance organization (HMO) [10] or to a plan with higher out-of-pocket costs [11] led to significant reductions in use of mental health services without any significant effect on clinical outcomes. More recently, evaluations of the impact of carve-out behavioral health management firms find dramatic reductions in service use without apparent reductions in indicators of access or quality of care [12, 13]. These observations should not be interpreted as evidence of excessive or unnecessary spending on mental health care. Instead, these findings support a less-than-startling conclusion: reducing access to ineffective or poorly organized care does not affect care quality or patient outcomes. Because much of current treatment provided for depression (or other mental disorders) is neither well-organized nor evidence-based, it is difficult to demonstrate negative effects of even the most draconian reductions in levels of service. While the findings cited above have been used by some to defend restrictions on mental health treatment, they should be seen instead as arguing for more organized and evidence-based services.

The data suggesting a greater "moral hazard" or price elasticity for mental health services (compared to general medical services) [14–16] should also be interpreted carefully. This finding has often been used to justify higher copayments, coinsurance, or deductibles for mental health care. The implicit assumption appears to be that mental health utilization is more price-sensitive because mental health care is more discretionary. This interpretation, however, is inconsistent with evidence that the effect of price increases on use of mental health services is just as great among those with more severe mental disorders [17, 18]. If we assume instead that mental health treatment is truly necessary, the finding of greater price sensitivity could be used to argue for lower cost-sharing for mental health care than for general medical care.

While it is important to emphasize the potential economic benefits of improved depression treatment, we must also ask whether treatment of mental disorders is being judged by a different standard than are other aspects of health care. The debate over possible "cost-offset" effects of depression treatment is one illustration of this bias. Reasonable evidence suggests that effective depression treatment may reduce use of general medical services [19, 20]. One potential danger in discussing this "cost-offset" effect, however, is the unintended implication that cost savings are the primary justification for depression treatment. It does not appear that treatments for other major health conditions (such as breast cancer, cardiovascular disease, or human immunodeficiency virus [HIV] infection) are required to pass this test. In fact, it seems almost absurd to argue that the value of expenditures in a particular medical specialty area such as gastroenterology or urology depends on cost savings in other sectors of health care. Unfortunately, resources expended on mental health treatment are often judged by this criterion alone. While it is certainly important to demonstrate the economic value of mental health treatment, we must take care not to reinforce traditional discrimination against those who suffer from mental disorders.

REFERENCES

1. Simon G.E., Von Korff M., Barlow W. (1995) Health care costs of primary care patients with recognized depression. *Arch. Gen. Psychiatry*, **52**: 850–856.
2. Henk H.J., Katzelnick D.J., Kobak K.A., Greist J.H., Jefferson J.W. (1996) Medical costs attributed to depression among patients with a history of high medical

expenses in a health maintenance organization. *Arch. Gen. Psychiatry*, **53**: 899–904.

3. Spitzer R.L., Kroenke K., Linzer M., Hahn S.R., Williams J.B.W., deGruy F.V., Brody D., Davies M. (1995) Health-related quality of life in primary care patients with mental disorders. *JAMA*, **274**: 1511–1517.

4. Ormel J., Von Korff M., Ustun T.B., Pini S., Korten A., Oldehinkel T. (1994) Common mental disorders and disability across cultures. *JAMA*, **272**: 1741–1748.

5. Von Korff M., Ormel J., Katon W.J., Lin E.H.B. (1992) Disability and depression among high utilizers of health care. *Arch. Gen. Psychiatry*, **49**: 91–100.

6. Simon G.E., Von Korff M., Heiligenstein J.H., Revicki D.A., Grothaus L., Katon W., Wagner E.H. (1996) Initial antidepressant selection in primary care: effectiveness and cost of fluoxetine vs. tricyclic antidepressants. *JAMA*, **275**: 1897–1902.

7. Simon G.E., Fishman P. (1998) Cost implications of initial antidepressant selection in primary care. *PharmacoEconomics*, **13**: 61–70.

8. Hylan T.R., Crown W.H., Meneades L., Heiligenstein J.H., Melfi C., Buesching T.W., Croghan D.P. (1998) SSRI and TCA antidepressant selection and health care costs: a multivariate analysis. *J. Affect. Disord.*, **47**: 71–79.

9. Croghan T.W., Lair T.J., Engelhart L.E., Crown W.H., Copley-Merriman C., Melfi C.A., Obenchain R.L., Buesching D.P. (1997) Effect of antidepressant therapy on health care utilization and costs in primary care. *Psychiatr. Serv.*, **48**: 1420–1426.

10. Wells K.B., Manning W.G., Valdez R.B. (1990) The effects of a prepaid group practice on mental health outcomes. *Health Serv. Res.*, **25**: 615–625.

11. Wells K.B., Manning W.G., Valdez R.B. (1989) The effects of insurance generosity on the psychological distress and psychological well-being of a general population. *Arch. Gen. Psychiatry*, **46**: 315–320.

12. Christianson J.B., Manning W., Lurie N., Stoner T.J., Gray D.Z., Popkin M., Marriott S. (1995) Utah's Prepaid Mental Health Plan: the first year. *Health Aff. (Millwood)*, **14**: 160–172.

13. Lurie N., Christianson J.B., Gray D.Z., Manning W.G., Popkin M.K. (1998) The effect of the Utah Prepaid Mental Health Plan on structure, process, and outcomes of care. *New Dir. Ment. Health. Serv.*, **78**: 99–106.

14. Wells K.B., Keeler E., Manning W.G. (1990) Patterns of outpatient mental health care over time: some implications for estimates of demand and for benefit design. *Health Serv. Res.*, **24**: 773–789.

15. Taube C.A., Kessler L.G., Burns B.J. (1986) Estimating the probability and level of ambulatory mental health services use. *Health Serv. Res.*, **21**: 321–340.

16. Horgan C.M. (1986) The demand for ambulatory mental health services from specialty providers. *Health Serv. Res.*, **21**: 291–320.

17. Landerman L.R., Burns B.J., Swartz M.S., Wagner H.R., George L.K. (1994) The relationship between insurance coverage and psychiatric disorder in predicting use of mental health services. *Am. J. Psychiatry*, **151**: 1785–1790.

18. Simon G.E., Grothaus L., Durham M.L., Von Korff M., Pabiniak C. (1996) Impact of visit copayments on outpatient mental health utilization by members of a health maintenance organization. *Am. J. Psychiatry*, **153**: 331–338.

19. Katzelnick D.J., Kobak K.A., Greist J.H., Jefferson J.W., Henk H.J. (1997) Effect of primary care treatment of depression on service use by patients with high medical expenditures. *Psychiatr. Serv.*, **48**: 59–64.

20. Mumford E., Schlesinger H.I., Glass G.V., Patrick C., Cuerdon T. (1984) A new look at evidence about reduced cost of medical utilization following mental health treatment. *Am. J. Psychiatry*, **141**: 1145–1149.

6.3
Cost-effectiveness of Treatment for Depression: Methods and Policies
Scott W. Woods[1] and C. Bruce Baker[1]

Rosenbaum and Hylan's review is impressive for its comprehensiveness and scope. We make here a few additional points about cost-effectiveness methods and about antidepressant health policy.

Cost-effectiveness analysis is subject to endless variations in how it is structured (e.g. whose perspective determines what costs and benefits are relevant, the utility weights that should be assigned to alternative outcomes), and these variations in structure heavily influence the final results of the analysis. These differences in structure explain a large part of the variations in the results of many of the studies discussed by the authors of the review. The results of such studies carry relatively little individual meaning and one can make little rational comparison across studies unless the analytic structure is made explicit [1].

Decision models are subject to analogous problems. This is illustrated in the case of decision analytic models on the cost-effectiveness of tricyclic antidepressants (TCAs) vs. selective serotonin reuptake inhibitors (SSRIs). As noted by Rosenbaum and Hylan, these models have generally concluded that newer antidepressants are most cost-effective relative to the TCAs, but some of them have found that the TCAs are more cost-effective [2–4]. Many of the decision analytic simulations which concluded that newer antidepressants were more cost-effective [5–8] used a design and assumptions very similar to those in an early SSRI vs. TCA model [9]. Our group replicated this model and revised design flaws and key assumptions that drove the results [2]. Correction of a design flaw and substitution of treatment lengths recommended by practice guidelines reversed the findings and yielded a cost-effectiveness advantage in favor of the TCAs.

This reanalysis illustrates the critical effect of varying subtle assumptions implicit in the model. Taking one simple example, it shows that varying length of treatment plays a critical role in cost-effectiveness conclusions. As Rosenbaum and Hylan note, more economic outcome studies of clinical practice among different antidepressants over periods longer than 1 year are needed. In general, the longer treatment with antidepressants is continued, the less cost-effective the newer antidepressants as first line treatment are likely to be. Longer treatment progressively increases medication acquisition costs associated with newer antidepressants as time goes on. By contrast, much of the greater cost of treatment delivery of the older drugs is expended early in the treatment, in dose titration and side-effect management visits.

[1]*Department of Psychiatry, Yale University School of Medicine, 34 Park Street, New Haven, CT 06519, USA*

Longer treatment durations progressively dilute this early cost over time. Most of the studies reviewed utilized unrealistically short time frames [10]. The two decision analytic simulations which performed analyses on treatment length [2, 3] both showed cost-effectiveness advantages for the inexpensive drug as treatment length progressed, and one simulation utilizing intermediate treatment lengths favored the TCAs [4].

Rosenbaum and Hylan report that numerous retrospective naturalistic studies indicate that costs consequent to initiating treatment with an SSRI are equal to or lower than costs following initiation of a TCA. In addition to the possibility of selection bias due to nonrandom assignment and the nonmeasurement of clinical outcomes discussed in the review, there is another potential difficulty with these methods which may be termed a "cohort effect" [10]. By cohort effect we mean that retrospective groups may not be drawn from practice in identical time frames. Apparent differences between treatments in cost may in fact be due to or confounded by changing trends in practice over time (secular trends). During the periods under study, newer antidepressants were progressively gaining market share, while at the same time health care organizations were progressively reducing other expenditures. Thus, a higher proportion of TCA starts may have occurred early in the study periods, when care was not so firmly managed, and a higher proportion of newer antidepressant starts may have occurred later in the study period, when visits and hospitalizations were more carefully scrutinized. This consideration appears to be germane to early studies of this type [10], and may be relevant to some of the later studies in the review, including the one generating the data for Figure 6.3.

Considerations of cost-offset aside, it is clear that the newer antidepressants would be more cost-effective if their prices were lower. Given the strong effect of price, it may be important from a health policy viewpoint to consider how societal mechanisms for determining price influence health outcomes. Prices charged for the newer antidepressants can vary markedly across countries, with the average price in European Union countries reported to be approximately half that in the United States [11].

Similarly, the newer antidepressants will be more cost-effective when they come off patent protection, assuming therapeutic equivalence of the generic products. In this context, it may be important from a public policy viewpoint to consider the influence of patent policy on health outcomes. Of course, the health of the public in the present must be balanced against the health of the public in the future. Shortening the duration of patent protection of new medications may increase access to these medications and thus improve the public health in the near future, but shortening the duration of patent protection for new medications could reduce incentive to develop new medications. On the other hand, it could be argued that relatively long lengths of patent protection can in some ways diminish incentive to market new medications. For example, of the companies currently marketing an SSRI in the United States, none has brought a newer antidepressant to market since their SSRI was approved.

The authors point out that identifying the most cost-effective treatment is not sufficient to make cost-effective care possible. Other necessary conditions include free redistribution of resources and basing decisions on a universal perspective of costs and benefits. However, free redistribution and a universal perspective are most likely to be possible in a unitary health care system and perhaps a political system with relatively strong central control. We would note that such systems may limit the variety of current options (e.g. in medications, in alternative structures for delivering health care) and possibly the development of future more beneficial options. These benefits can also be values one may wish to incorporate in "the greatest health care benefit for a given population and health care budget." Policy based on cost-effectiveness analysis needs to consider both the assets and the limitations of pluralistic and unitary systems.

REFERENCES

1. Gold M.E., Siegel J.E., Russell L.B., Weinstein M.C. (1996) _Cost-effectiveness in Health and Medicine_, Oxford University Press, New York.
2. Woods S.W., Rizzo J.A. (1997) Cost-effectiveness of antidepressant treatment revisited. _Br. J. Psychiatry_, **170**: 257–263.
3. McFarland B.H. (1994) Cost-effectiveness considerations for managed care systems: treating depression in primary care. _Am. J. Med._, **97** (Suppl. 6A): 47S–58S.
4. Stewart A. (1994) Anti-depressant pharmacotherapy: cost comparison of SSRIs and TCAs. _Br. J. Med. Econ._, **7**: 67–79.
5. Bentkover J.D., Feighner J.P. (1996) Cost analysis of paroxetine vs. imipramine in major depression. _PharmacoEconomics_, **8**: 223–232.
6. Lapierre Y., Bentkover J., Schainbaum S., Manners S. (1995) Direct costs of depression: analysis of treatment costs of paroxetine versus imipramine in Canada. _Can. J. Psychiatry_, **40**: 370–377.
7. Hylan T.R., Kotsanos J.G., Andersen J.S., Brown S.H., Copley-Merriman C., Egbuonu-Davis L., Heilegenstein J.H., Overhage J.M., Whiteside R.E. (1996) Comparison of a decision analytic model with results from a naturalistic economic clinical trial: an application of evaluating alternative antidepressants. _Am. J. Manag. Care_, **2**: 1211–1223.
8. Montgomery S.A., Brown R.E., Clark M. (1996) Economic analysis of treating depression with nefazodone vs. imipramine. _Br. J. Psychiatry_, **168**: 768–771.
9. Jonsson B., Bebbington P.E. (1994) What price depression? The cost of depression and the cost-effectiveness of pharmacological treatment. _Br. J. Psychiatry_, **164**: 665–673.
10. Woods S.W., Baker C.B. (1997) Cost-effectiveness of newer antidepressants. _Curr. Opin. Psychiatry_, **10**: 95–101.
11. Sasich L., Torrey E.F., Wolfe S.M. (1998) Average cost of newer medication psychotropic, antidepressant drugs twice as high in US as in Europe, study finds. _Psychiatr. Serv._, **49**: 1248.

6.4
Costs of Treating Depression: Policy Should Be Evidence-based
John Donoghue[1]

As pressures to contain the costs of health care increase worldwide, Rosenbaum and Hylan's paper is a timely review of this poorly understood aspect of depression.

Depression is characterized as a common and potentially severe illness with disproportionately high costs [1, 2]. The adverse consequences of depression on health and social functioning are well known [3], yet the "pattern of treatment is incongruous with the magnitude of the disorder and the burdens it imposes". The evidence, overwhelmingly, is of inadequate treatment [4, 5].

Rosenbaum and Hylan's review focuses inevitably on treatment with antidepressants. However, despite an extensive literature, consensus on cost-effectiveness remains elusive. There are fewer data on other treatments. Findings for psychotherapy are mixed: outcomes improve, but direct medical costs increase, with no conclusive comparative data with antidepressants. Data for electroconvulsive therapy are very limited, relating only to the length of hospital admission.

Methods of conducting health economics research, especially with antidepressants, continue to develop. Studies relying on data from controlled clinical trials — meta-analyses and decision-analytic models — are largely unreliable [6–9]. Naturalistic studies consistently find that tricyclic antidepressants (TCAs) are used suboptimally [4, 5]: such use is unlikely to be cost-effective. Other naturalistic studies have found that, in comparison, selective serotonin reuptake inhibitors (SSRIs) are associated with lower total health care costs [10–12], though these findings may be subject to selection bias. Methodologically, the most rigorous approach — the prospective "real world" trial [13, 14] — has been applied once only, with equivocal findings, probably as a result of inadequate powering coupled with crossover bias.

Generalizability of findings is a major problem. The health care system in which treatment is delivered can influence outcomes significantly. The implication is that definitive studies may be required for each different health care system in which a treatment modality is used.

Despite such problems, Rosenbaum and Hylan's review makes many convincing points. Treating depression adequately is likely to increase direct health care costs. This need not dismay us, as the purpose of health economics is not to minimize costs, but to maximize value for money [15]. However, if policy is based on cost-containment, there is little incentive to increase the effectiveness of treatment. Cost-containment ignores the complexity and

---

[1] School of Pharmacy, John Moores University, 4 Wrenfield Grove, Liverpool L17 9QD, UK

the recurrent and chronic nature of depression and the knowledge that the social costs of depression are far higher than health costs [1, 2, 16, 17].

Using cheaper antidepressants does not improve cost-effectiveness: initiating treatment with an SSRI results in direct health care costs equal to or lower than treatment with a TCA [9–12, 14]. Studies of newer antidepressants are too few to draw conclusions. The key to improving cost-effectiveness appears to lie in providing effective treatment in a less expensive setting (i.e. primary care rather than hospital). This will necessitate improving treatment with antidepressants, which seems unlikely to be achieved if cost-containment policies continue to emphasize the primacy of TCAs.

It is not enough for clinicians alone to seek to provide evidence-based treatment. Policy also needs to follow the weight of evidence that increasing the intensity of treatment is cost-effective; accepting and even promoting increased direct health care costs to achieve effective treatment, maximize health gain, and reduce global costs.

REFERENCES

1. Klerman G.L., Weissman M.M. (1992) The course, morbidity, and costs of depression. *Arch. Gen. Psychiatry*, **49**: 831–834.
2. Simon G.E., Von Korff M., Barlow W. (1995) Health care costs of primary care patients with recognized depression. *Arch. Gen. Psychiatry*, **52**: 850–856.
3. Wells K.B., Stewart A., Hays R.D., Burnham M.A., Rogers W., Daniels M., Berrey S., Greenfield S., Ware J. (1989) The functioning and well-being of depressed patients: results from the Medical Outcomes Study. *JAMA*, **262**: 914–919.
4. Beaumont G., Baldwin D., Lader M. (1996) A criticism of the practice of prescribing sub-therapeutic doses of antidepressants for the treatment of depression. *Hum. Psychopharmacol.*, **11**: 283–291.
5. Donoghue J.M. (1998) Sub-optimal use of tricyclic antidepressants in primary care. *Acta Psychiatr. Scand.*, **98**: 429–431.
6. Hotopf M., Lewis G., Normand C. (1996) Are SSRIs a cost effective alternative to tricyclics? *Br. J. Psychiatry*, **168**: 404–409.
7. Hotopf M., Lewis G., Normand C. (1997) Putting trials on trial—the costs and consequences of small trials in depression: a systematic review of methodology. *J. Epidemiol. Comm. Health*, **51**: 354–358.
8. Hotopf M. (1998) Commentary. *Evidence-based Mental Health*, **1**: 50–51.
9. Freemantle N., House A., Mason J., Song F., Sheldon T. (1995) Economics of treatment of depression. *Br. J. Psychiatry*, **166**: 397.
10. Sclar D.A., Robison L.M., Skaer T.L., Legg R.F., Nemec N.L., Galin R.S., Hughes T.E., Buesching D.P. (1994) Antidepressant pharmacotherapy: economic outcomes in a Health Maintenance Organisation. *Clin. Ther.*, **16**: 715–730.
11. Forder J., Kavanagh S., Fenyo A. (1996) A comparison of the cost-effectiveness of sertraline vs. tricyclic antidepressants in primary care. *J. Affect. Disord.*, **38**: 87–111.
12. Hylan T.R., Crown W.H., Meneades L., Heiligenstein J.H., Melfi C., Croghan T.W., Buesching D.P. (1998) SSRI and TCA antidepressant selection and health care costs: a multivariate analysis. *J. Affect. Disord.*, **47**: 71–79.

13. Simon G., Wagner E., Von Korff M. (1995) Cost-effectiveness comparisons using "real world" randomized trials: the case of new antidepressant drugs. *J. Clin. Epidemiol.*, **48**: 363–373.
14. Simon G.E., Von Korff M., Heiligenstein J.H., Revicki D.A., Grothaus S.L., Katon W., Wagner E.H. (1996) Initial antidepressant choice in primary care. *JAMA*, **275**: 1897–1902.
15. Bootman J.L. (1995) Pharmacoeconomics and outcomes research. *Am. J. Health-system Pharmacy*, **52** (Suppl. 3): S16–S19.
16. Kiloh L.G., Andrews G., Neilson M. (1988) The long-term outcome of depressive illness. *Br. J. Psychiatry*, **153**: 752–757.
17. Scott J. (1988) Chronic depression. *Br. J. Psychiatry*, **153**: 287–297.

6.5

Economic Costs and Benefits of Depression Treatment from Naturalistic Studies

Mingliang Zhang[1]

Depression is prevalent in the general population, with a 10.3% 1-year prevalence of unipolar major depression and dysthymia among community residents ages 15–54 in the United States. In addition, 11.0% of community residents who do not meet the strict criteria for either depressive disorder have substantial depressive symptoms.

Depression is costly, with estimated total economic costs of $43.7bn per year in 1990 dollars in the United States. Over 70% of these costs are indirect costs due to mortality and morbidity (disability and lost productivity) [1]. This estimate of total economic costs does not include the costs to family caregivers, the cost of lost leisure time of depressed individuals, and the cost of pain and suffering endured by depressed individuals and their families.

Effective treatment for depression improves function and it also reduces the associated costs of morbidity such as the cost of absenteeism and the cost of decreased productivity while at work. In reviewing 10 published treatment studies of depression, Mintz *et al* [2] conclude that "generally, work outcomes were good when treatment was systematically effective." Broadhead also demonstrates that depression severity is significantly related to lost work days [3].

We analyzed data collected from a community-based sample of 470 depressed patients in the state of Arkansas, United States. Consistent with the existing studies, our findings indicated that there was a greater reduction in

[1]*Outcomes Research Department, Worldwide Human Health, Merck & Co., Whitehouse Station, NJ 08889, USA*

lost earnings due to lost work days for individuals who received depression treatment during a 12-month period, compared to those who did not receive depression treatment. The reduction in dollar terms was sufficiently large to offset the costs of depression treatment. Further analysis indicated that those who received their depression treatment from mental health specialists had an even greater reduction in lost work days during the 12 months, compared to those who received their depression treatment from general medical providers [4]. In determining the economic value of depression treatment, therefore, it is necessary to include the changes in potential savings in morbidity costs, such as lost earnings.

Clinical studies of depression treatment provide information on efficacy; however, results from these studies cannot be readily used to guide policy decisions. Patients in clinical trials are selected according to stringent inclusion and exclusion criteria; therefore, they are not representative of the general population with the disorder. They are also randomized to experimental and control groups and are not allowed to choose the types of treatment as they do in reality. Policy decisions usually require information on effectiveness from naturalistic study designs that reflect the real world. In naturalistic (or observational) studies, subjects themselves decide whether and where to seek treatment for depression. These decisions lead to potential selection bias in comparing clinical and economic outcomes of treatment versus no treatment, and in comparing clinical and economic outcomes of different types of treatment. The selection bias needs to be corrected in research and in forming policy decisions.

The ever rising health care costs in most developed countries necessitate research into cost-containment measures. However, the wisdom of focusing exclusively on treatment costs in evaluating the overall economic effects of depression treatment is questionable, because only a small portion of the total economic cost of depression is treatment costs. Depression treatment is associated with savings in lost earnings. Unfortunately, community studies indicate that only 30–40% of depressed individuals receive treatment for depression during a 1-year period. To reduce the overall economic cost of depression to society, a greater proportion of depressed individuals needs to be treated for the disorder. Therefore, policies should be designed to encourage depressed individuals to seek depression treatment and to encourage providers, particularly primary care providers, to detect depression in their practices. Naturalistic studies can be used to examine the factors that influence a patient's decision to seek treatment and to seek a particular type of treatment. One such factor is the economic cost of seeking treatment, which includes out-of-pocket costs for services, travel costs, and time costs. Naturalistic studies can also be used to examine the factors that influence a provider's decision to detect and treat depression.

In today's environment of managed care, cost of treatment for mental health problems such as depression may become an easy target for cost-containment policies. However, in forming policy decisions, it is important to take into account the economic benefits of depression treatment, such as reduced lost work days and increased productivity. It is important to increase recognition of depression by the general population and by health care providers, especially primary care providers who serve as gatekeepers in managed care, so that more people who need depression treatment will get it.

REFERENCES

1. Greenberg P.E., Stiglin L.E., Finkelstein S.N., Berndt E.R. (1993) The economic burden of depression in 1990. *J. Clin. Psychiatry*, **54**: 405–418.
2. Mintz J., Mintz L.I., Arruda M.J., Hwang S.S. (1992) Treatments of depression and the functional capacity to work. *Arch. Gen. Psychiatry*, **49**: 761–768.
3. Broadhead W.E., Blazer D.G., George L.K., Tse C.K. (1990) Depression, disability days, and days lost from work in a prospective epidemiologic survey. *JAMA*, **264**: 2524–2528.
4. Zhang M., Rost K.M., Fortney J.C. (1999) Earnings changes for depressed individuals treated by mental health specialists. *Am. J. Psychiatry*, **156**: 108–114.

6.6
Compliance: Another Factor in Estimating the Cost of Depression
Russell T. Joffe[1]

Rosenbaum and Hylan have provided a scholarly, incisive and comprehensive review on all aspects of the economics of depressive disorder. The summary of their paper highlights the facts about the enormous direct and indirect economic impact that depression has on individuals and society. In particular, they provide an excellent summary of evidence that improving the rates of adequate treatment of depression, not only enhances its cost-effectiveness, but also enhances quality of life and all domains of function, as well as reducing the burden of suffering both for patients and their families.

The importance of adequate treatment in the management of depressive illness cannot be overemphasized. Several studies have shown that adherence to treatment guidelines in administering antidepressant therapy

[1]*Department of Psychiatry, Faculty of Health Sciences, McMaster University, 1200 Main Street West, Hamilton, ON, L8N 3Z5, Canada*

enhanced outcome and improved prognosis [1, 2]. For example, Melfi and collaborators [1] showed that adherence to treatment guidelines vs. early discontinuation significantly reduces the probability of relapse or recurrence in Medicaid in the United States. In their study, continued treatment, even if it involved switches to alternatives, was vastly superior to early discontinuation. Duration of treatment is an important component of adequate antidepressant therapy. In addition, the appropriate drugs, depending on the subtype of depression, at the correct dose are also important features of adequate therapy [3]. In the administration of antidepressants, selective serotonin reuptake inhibitors (SSRIs) have some advantage over drugs such as the tricyclics and also the monoamine oxidase inhibitors. Studies generally show that the SSRIs are more likely to be prescribed and, when this occurs, are more likely to be given at adequate doses, although duration of treatment still tends to be short and generally inadequate with the SSRIs as with the older classes of antidepressants [4].

There is another important component to adequate treatment which would impact on the cost-effectiveness of antidepressant therapy and the economic burden of depression. This issue, mentioned only briefly by Rosenbaum and Hylan, is compliance with antidepressant therapy. It is estimated that up to 60% of depressed patients will not comply with antidepressant therapy [5, 6]. In general, patients will discontinue treatment of their own accord or take their antidepressant medication differently from the way it was prescribed by their treating physician. However, compliance is more than just adherence to medication regimens or the absence of omission or commission errors in taking medication. It also involves complying with all treatment advice and attendance at diagnostic and therapeutic appointments [5, 6]. These latter aspects of compliance may be particularly important in psychiatric patients. Factors influencing compliance are generally complex and hard to disentangle, but can be broadly categorized as being doctor, patient and drug related [5, 6]. Many of the doctor and patient factors relate to issues of adequate communication, the nature of the doctor–patient relationship and other interactional factors. As far as other patient issues are concerned, in general, the diagnosis of depression does not increase the likelihood of non-compliance, unlike other psychiatric disorders such as schizophrenia [5, 6]. Drug factors are also important, with increased side-effect burden a definite risk factor for non-compliance [6]. In this respect, the SSRIs may have advantages over other antidepressant classes, especially the tricyclics, although the issue of sexual dysfunction related to SSRI treatment and the inevitable impact on treatment compliance requires further study.

If adequacy of treatment has an impact on the cost-effectiveness of treatment of depression, as suggested by Rosenbaum and Hylan, the importance of compliance cannot be discounted. This is an especially common occurrence with complex underpinnings which needs to be included in any models of the costs of antidepressant treatment and the economic burden of depression. Compliance issues, occurring in up to 60% of depressed patients, are a major factor which impact on the identification, diagnosis and especially treatment of depressive illness and, therefore, on its economic burden. It remains to be determined how interventions which improve compliance and therefore improve treatment adequacy may impact on the economics of depression and the cost-effectiveness of its treatment.

REFERENCES

1. Melfi C.A., Chawla A.J., Croghan T.W., Hanna M.P., Kennedy S., Svedl K. (1998) The effect of adherence to antidepressant treatment guidelines on relapse and recurrence of depression. *Arch. Gen. Psychiatry*, **55**: 1128–1132.
2. Schulberg H.C., Stock M.R., Madonia M.J., Scott C., Rodriguez E., Inber S., Perel J., Lave J., Houck P. *et al* (1996) Treating major depression in primary care practice: 8-month clinical outcomes. *Arch. Gen. Psychiatry*, **53**: 913–919.
3. Schulberg H.C., Katon W., Simon G., Rush A.J. (1998) Treating major depression in primary care practice: an update of the Agency for Health Care Policy and Research Practice Guidelines. *Arch. Gen. Psychiatry*, **55**: 1121–1127.
4. MacDonald T., McMahan A., Reid G., Fenton H., McDevitt D. (1996) Antidepressant drug use in primary care: a record linkage study in Tayside, Scotland. *Br. Med. J.*, **313**: 860–861.
5. Maddox J.C., Levi M., Thompson C. (1994) The compliance of antidepressants in general practice. *J. Psychopharmacol.*, **8**: 48–53.
6. Demyttenaere K. (1997) Compliance during treatment with antidepressants. *J. Affect. Disord.*, **43**: 27–39.

6.7

Capturing the Cost of Depressive Disorders in the Natural Laboratory of the Workplace

Daniel J. Conti[1]

Comprehensive and integrative reviews of research such as Jerrold Rosenbaum and Timothy Hylan's substantiate the overall economic impact of depressive disorders. While the subjective distress and lost opportunities that the illness brings to its sufferers cannot be adequately measured, quantification of one manifestation of depression is slowly emerging: its cost with respect to lost productivity in the workplace. These environments,

[1] First Chicago NBD Corporation, One First National Plaza, Chicago, IL 60617-0006, USA

in which behavioral output requires measurement for its compensation, provide a natural laboratory for observing the impact of depression as well as evaluating the outcomes of employer-sponsored health care plans.

The workplace is slowly awakening to the impact that mental health, and particularly depression, has on its bottom line. The few employers who track disability are discovering the impact that depression has in terms of duration and chronicity. In a study of our corporation's experience that extended the observational period of our 1994 paper [1], depressive disorders maintained their primacy over common chronic medical-surgical disorders such as heart disease, low back pain, and diabetes in terms of the average length of disability duration [2]. The likelihood of a return to disability status within 12 months of an initial disability period also remained high relative to the other disorders.

Also observed in our follow-up study was a steady, year-to-year increase in the number of psychiatric disability events, a category dominated by depressive disorders. Between 1989 and 1996, these diagnoses rose from the sixth leading cause of a disability event to the third leading cause (excluding pregnancy and childbirth). In terms of the total number of disability days, psychiatric disabilities ranked fourth in 1989, and second in 1996.

The long disability durations produced by depressive disorders are due, in part, to the nature of the disorder itself. Certainly, efficacy of treatment is also a major contributory factor. With regard to the former, the illness leaves its sufferer depleted of a key quality for successful occupational functioning: initiative. Returning depressed employees to work involves overcoming powerful forces of inertia and rekindling the drive for achievement. Add to this the depressed employee's negative self-attributions and the considerable stigma that still surrounds psychiatric illness, and the return to work situation becomes, on average, far more complex than the common medical-surgical disability situation. With regard to the amount and type of treatment given to those disabled by depression, Rosenbaum and Hylan's review documents the advancements and efficacy in pharmacotherapy and psychotherapy. But, given the complicated nature of depressive disorder in a disability situation, the need for enhanced psychosocial interventions seems undeniable. Our anecdotal research on disability management has shown that less than 15% of employees disabled by depression are receiving any treatment modality other than once-per-week outpatient sessions (including medication management visits); the same level of treatment for psychiatric disorders producing minimal impairment. Furthermore, comparisons of the lengths of psychiatric disability durations for our employees in different managed behavioral health care organizations (MBHO) revealed significant differences in disability duration which seem to correlate with differences in their treatment protocol. The MBHO that made use of a partial hospital program for psychiatrically disabled employees returned those employees back to the workplace more than 2 weeks earlier than another MBHO that made use of the common managed care approach of no more than one outpatient visit per week.

The increasing frequency of disability resulting from depressive disorders observed in our workplace is congruent with predictions made by global epidemiological studies [3]. The fact that depression is becoming a predominant occupational health issue at the beginning of the new millennium coincides with the changing nature of work. The workplace which was once dominated by a manufacturing environment has been replaced by an information management environment in which "knowledge workers" who provide efficient customer service hold the key to a company's success. Given the fact that depression can disrupt job-essential cognitive processes (e.g. slowed thinking, poor judgement, high distractibility, etc.) and negatively affect social interaction (e.g. decreased frustration tolerance, social withdrawal, increased irritability, etc.), depression's intersection with the "new" workplace authentically cripples occupational functioning. In the previous manufacturing environment, musculoskeletal problems produced a similar negative impact with workers who depended on physical strength, manual dexterity, and repetitive actions to carry out their job duties.

As the awareness of lost productivity due to depression increases, employer-sponsored insurance plans will come to be evaluated in terms of their cost-offset for not only direct costs but also indirect costs. Workplaces again provide a unique laboratory for this evaluation as tangible productivity variables can be linked to differences in plan design. Studies of this type will require workplaces to establish health data warehouses [4] where health and productivity data can be linked under the proper confidentiality and security maintenance. At this time, there seems no better situation in which to examine and quantify the relationship of direct to indirect costs of depression, and other illnesses, than the natural laboratory of the workplace.

REFERENCES

1. Conti D.J., Burton W.N. (1994) The economic impact of depression in a workplace. *J. Occup. Med.*, **36**: 983–988.
2. Conti D.J., Burton W.N. (1999) Behavioral health disability management. In *The Employee Assistance Handbook* (Ed. J. M. Oher), Wiley, New York.
3. Murray C.J., Lopez A.D. (1966) *The Global Burden of Disease*, World Health Organization, Geneva.
4. Burton W.N., Conti D.J. (1998) Use of an integrated health data warehouse to measure the employer costs of five chronic disease states. *Disease Management*, **1**: 17–26.

6.8
Depression Management: No Longer At All Costs
Gordon Parker[1]

Economics are the new religious core of public policy. [1]

For centuries, as Porter [2] recently observed, "medicine was impotent", performing its tasks with meager success. Now, argues Porter, with "mission accomplished", medicine deals with the legacy of its triumphs — inflated, unlimited and unfulfillable public expectations. Once psychiatry was also relatively impotent, offering little beyond non-specific therapeutic ingredients. It could plead "special case" status — that its compassionate approach to mental illness demonstrated the best test of a society: how it cared for those unable to articulate their own needs.

Psychiatry's remedicalization, the development of effective psychopharmacological treatments, and the demonstration of extensive psychiatric morbidity in general communities, required psychiatry to join with other medical disciplines in arguing for its place in the cost-benefit sun.

The Global Burden of Disease report [3] stirred health planners by demonstrating the extraordinary disability effected by depression, both currently and projected. It indirectly encouraged practitioners to move beyond an insular clinician argument (e.g. "My job is to do what is best for my patients, irrespective of cost") to a more integrated and population-weighted perspective. Economic parameters became more salient.

While some early economic analyses appeared "creative" in invariably "proving" the cost advantages of the particular new antidepressant under study, greater sophistication is now evident in study designs — as detailed in Jerrold Rosenbaum and Timothy Hylan's excellent review. Naturalistic studies undertaken in facilities such as Health Maintenance Organizations, where costs can be drilled down to fine detail and where efficiency is the Zeitgeist, have been particularly informative. Importantly, such studies have generally supported the newer antidepressants, while independence of many of these studies from the pharmaceutical companies has reassured us that designs have moved beyond company marketing departments.

Recent studies have produced some positive results for psychiatry — in giving some indications about those services and educational models that are likely to be effective or ineffective. Conclusions are no longer simple. For instance, improving the quality of depression treatment may be cost-effective — but total costs are likely to increase. Rosenbaum and Hylan provide many such examples of the complexities involved.

[1]*School of Psychiatry, University of New South Wales, High Street, Randwick 2031, Sydney, Australia*

Now economic issues are one integral—but not necessarily dominant—part of any strategic analysis for health care reform. For instance, Katon *et al* [4] have considered effective disease-management strategies to decrease the prevalence of major depression by mounting a population-based approach, and provide a model melding divergent innovation and convergent application.

The current review, like most individual studies, treats "depression" as an entity. We are encouraged to consider costs as emerging from depression per se. Such an Axis I preoccupation is unnecessarily and unwisely restrictive. Let me illustrate with a parallel issue. Most studies of subsyndromal depression have indicated its association with greater disability than demonstrated for major depression. Those with a subsyndromal depression may, however, be more likely to have a personality or life style both driving depressive symptoms and disability—and driving "economic costs" which may not then be most fairly costed to "depression". That is, in any costing exercise, there is wisdom in segregating the impact of "depression" from the "white noise" of an unhappy life, temperament style and other relevant factors.

Rosenbaum and Hylan make the important point that published mental health economic studies may not hold up in, or be relevant to, countries with differing health care systems. In many regions, decisions about antidepressant medications are made entirely on the basis of cost, with such decisions influencing both types of antidepressant interventions and treatment length. An antidepressant for one day may be more costly than a day in hospital. The capacity to even debate "adequate treatment" is then a luxury restricted to a minority of regions.

The "cost" of depression is not only economic—there is a personal "cost". At our Mood Disorders Unit, we are currently analyzing "costs" in patients referred with persistent and treatment-resistant depressive disorders. The percentages of patients recording costs as "severe", "extreme" or "catastrophic" were: 10% for direct financial costs; 28% for indirect financial costs such as loss of income; 27% for social costs such as loss of friends; 38% for relationship costs and 57% for "personal costs" such as loss of self-esteem and lowered confidence. That is, having a depressive episode is also "depressing", whether due to the illness itself, associated stigma or other factors, and this personal cost appears to be of greater magnitude than direct, and many indirect costs.

In a climate of economic rationalism, there would be major risks in having health managers "own" the economic analyses, with the risk being their capacity to "know the price of everything and the value of nothing". There is wisdom in health professionals designing, undertaking and interpreting such studies, as clearly demonstrated in the accompanying review.

REFERENCES

1. Saul J.R. (1995) *The Doubter's Companion*, Penguin, London.
2. Porter R. (1997) *The Greatest Benefit to Mankind. A Medical History from Antiquity to the Present*, HarperCollins, London.
3. Murray C.J., Lopez A.D. (1996) *The Global Burden of Disease*, World Health Organization, Geneva.
4. Katon W., Von Korff M., Lin E., Unutzer J., Simon G.E., Walker E., Ludman E., Bush T. (1997) Population-based care of depression: effective disease management strategies to decrease prevalence. *Gen. Hosp. Psychiatry*, **19**: 166–178.

6.9
Limitations to Cost Assessments of Depressive Disorders

Yvon D. Lapierre[1]

The extensive review of the costs of depressive disorders by Rosenbaum and Hylan provides an excellent point of reference on the economics of these illnesses. The burden of depression is becoming increasingly recognized in the industrialized world because of the high costs of health care and the negative impact that the disorder has on productivity. This is all the more important when one considers that the World Health Organization projects an increase in the incidence of depression as our societies evolve [1]. Historically, the assessment of costs has generally focused on the costs of direct intervention, be it by medication or by health care professionals, with or without additional institutional costs. Recently, a broadening of the cost base has occurred to include indirect costs which are, for all intents and purposes, astronomical.

An analysis of the indirect costs of depressive disorders is necessary to bring them into perspective. Unfortunately, these "soft" costs are susceptible to great variations in quantification. Consumer or patient assessments will inevitably differ from those of providers of care, as will these from the views of the payers of care or compensation. Though these three perspectives might possibly converge on objective reality, comprehensive studies of this type remain in the realm of utopia.

The apportionment of the costs is also subject to bias. Loss of income is often viewed as a major component of indirect costs, but is this a loss to the individual? A loss of productivity to society? Or a cost of compensation benefits? Moreover, an inability to work, resulting in job loss, has a different

───────────────
[1]*Institute of Mental Health Research, Royal Ottawa Hospital, 1145 Carling Avenue, Ottawa, Ontario K1Z 7K4, Canada*

impact in a fully employed society than in a society with a high rate of unemployment in an easily replaceable position. The loss of income is also subject to a number of variables alluded to in the chapter by Rosenbaum and Hylan. These include the incentives creating a necessity to return to work, which may vary depending on the social network available. Should there be a supportive network, the pressure to return to the former level of productivity may be less than in a society where the individual is forced into self-sufficiency.

A recently generally accepted variable in the measurement of indirect costs is the impact of a disorder on quality of life, which has been refined to quality of life years in many analyses. Quality of life is, however, extremely difficult to quantify because of its mixed subjective and objective components. The baseline assessment of quality of life may vary extensively between individuals, between conditions, and between societal groups.

Comorbidity issues are more complex than they might appear at first sight. Cost assessments must differentiate between comorbidity in the etiology and comorbidity resulting from or associated with depression. Evaluating the latter is, however, fraught with difficulties and is often highly dependent on the duration of the illness. Whether the comorbid condition antecedes depression or follows its onset, the outcome necessarily compounds the severity, duration, and cost of the depressive disorder.

Most economic systems operate on item budgets. The cost of drugs, the cost of provider services, institutional costs, other social benefits, and loss of productivity are all budgeted individually. The result is that often savings in one area lead to increased costs in the others. For example, the shifting of mental health costs to forensic or correctional costs is well documented. Unless these financing systems can be integrated, the true costs of depression will remain inadequately assessed.

Nonetheless, from the review of the studies addressing the cost of depressive disorders and their treatment, some conclusions can be drawn without hesitation. First, the costs of these disorders are progressively increasing in their impact on developed and developing societies. Second, the conclusions derived from nearly all studies on treatment costs indicate that the most expensive treatment is that which does not prevent relapse. It remains clear that the most significant cost of depression is a relapse into depression. Any manoeuvre or procedure that prevents this relapse will inevitably be the least expensive.

REFERENCE

1. Murray C.J.L., Lopez A.D. (Eds) (1996) *The Global Burden of Disease: A Comprehensive Assessment of Mortality and Disability from Diseases, Injuries, and Risk Factors in 1990 and Projected to 2020*, Harvard School of Public Health, Boston, MA.

6.10
Understanding the Economic Implications of Depression

J.A. Henry[1]

Depressive disorders produce a heavy economic burden at the personal, family and societal levels. This burden can be reduced considerably by cost-effective interventions. While suffering from depression, the individual's working capacity is considerably impaired, and depression causes more disability than any other mental disorder. One international multicentre study showed that mental disorders (depression being near the top of the list) were more strongly correlated with disability than common physical illnesses such as diabetes mellitus and hypertension in primary care settings [1]. It is thus quite clear that depressive illness is a high health management priority. However, all health care interventions have major cost implications.

Some years ago I was co-author of a publication in which we said "The relatively low cost of many of the older drugs might be considered a benefit. However, most people agree that cost should only be used as a basis for choosing between drugs once it has been decided that there is no difference between them in terms of risks and benefits" [2]. It is quite clear that although this consideration should hold in an ideal world, it is no longer acceptable. The pressures imposed by economic constraints mean that any risk-benefit analysis of drugs must take into account the cost that people are prepared to pay.

Over the last 10 years, our understanding of the financial implications of disease has advanced rapidly under the stimulus of budgetary limitations, and Jerrold Rosenbaum and Timothy Hylan have provided us with an impressive and up-to-date review of the cost implications of depressive illness. The most important factors have been the limited financial resources of health care providers, whether nationally based or private sector, and the increasing costs of drug treatment which became especially apparent of the selective serotonin reuptake inhibitors. These drugs initially had such a high price that health care providers were tempted to introduce a blacklist. Now, although they still cost considerably more than the tricyclic drugs, their price has come down steeply, but more importantly there has been a gradual change of opinion so that their additional cost has come to be regarded as justifiable by prescribers. This is in no small measure due to the influence of peer-reviewed publications in the medical literature.

[1]*Academic Department of Accident and Emergency Medicine, Imperial College School of Medicine, St Mary's Hospital, London W2 1NY, UK*

The debate about costs was initially fuelled by a landmark publication by Stoudemire *et al* in 1986 [3], which estimated the direct and indirect costs of depressive illness in the United States of America. It was this article which made the medical profession aware of the enormous burden of indirect costs which are a consequence of depressive illness. Indirect costs are borne by the individual and by society at large, but not by the health care system, and they therefore tend to be disregarded. Nevertheless the indirect costs are about seven-fold greater than the direct costs and so the overall costs of depressive illness alone could run into £2bn per year in the United Kingdom and $15bn in the United States. These figures represent a significant proportion of the gross national product for these countries, and since the treatment of depression can be highly successful, with 65–85% of cases responding to currently available medications, the cost implications of effective treatment are enormous.

The most immediate cost is the direct cost of the medication provided, and because it is so easily quantifiable this has become the biggest consideration by health care providers, who bear no responsibility for indirect costs. Rosenbaum and Hylan make it clear that short-term expenditures on treatment, if successful, would cut down the most expensive costs of depressive illness: absenteeism and low productivity in the workplace. This means that in the long run pharmacotherapy of depression is cost-effective. It is worthy of note that some national and local guidelines have now started to take indirect costs into account, and this is a major victory for commonsense. The Gotland study has shown that suicide prevention programmes, partly through prevention of suicide, but probably more importantly through reducing morbidity, could be cost-effective, even though they appear labour intensive [4].

We have moved a long way in our understanding of the costs of depressive illness. There is still much work to be done in assessing the impact of depression on quality of life and thereby influencing cost decision making even more deeply. However, the process is underway, and the next few years will deepen the rationale for cost decisions in the treatment of depressive illness.

REFERENCES

1. Ormel J., Von Korff M., Ustun T.B., Pini S., Korten A., Oldehinkel T. (1994) Common mental disorders and disability across cultures. *JAMA*, **272**: 1741–1748.
2. Henry J.A., Martin A.J. (1987) The risk-benefit assessment of antidepressants. *Med. Toxicol.*, **2**: 445–462.
3. Stoudemire A., Frank R., Hedemark N., Kamlet M., Blazer D. (1986) The economic burden of depression. *Gen. Hosp. Psychiatry*, **19**: 138–143.
4. Rutz W., von Knorring L., Walinder J. (1992) Long-term effects of an educational program for general practitioners by the Swedish Committee for the Prevention and Treatment of Depression. *Acta Psychiatr. Scand.*, **85**: 83–88.

6.11
The Burden of Depression and the Importance of Educational Programmes

Lars von Knorring[1]

The economic burden of depressive disorders ranks second only to ischaemic heart disease [1, 2]. However, self-inflicted injuries, alcohol abuse and some road traffic accidents are related to depressive disorders [3]. As these conditions are reported separately, the true burden is comparable to that of ischaemic heart disease.

Furthermore, it is often accepted that the intangible burdens are not measurable. However, some effects are possible to measure [3]. For example, 22% of the close relatives of patients involuntarily committed due to suicidal ideas had not been able to leave the patient during the month preceding the commitment and 17% had to abstain from work [3]. The losses in productivity are measurable in monetary terms, although the pain and suffering are not.

The costs are predominantly indirect, including the number of working years lost. Thus, age of onset of depressive disorders is of great importance. The age of onset seems to be decreasing, and the majority of bipolar patients have their first episode before the age of 18 [3, 4].

When all the 16 year olds in Uppsala, Sweden, were screened [4], 4.9% of the girls and 1.3% of the boys had a major depression; 14.2% of the girls and 4.8% of the boys had moderate depressive disorders. Furthermore, 7.4% of the girls and 2.4% of the boys had made an attempted suicide bid before the age of 16. Such a high prevalence of depressive disorders in adolescents will greatly influence the economic calculations concerning expected years of productive life.

Furthermore, the adolescents also had a high comorbidity with other psychic and somatic disorders, for example, panic disorder (6.5%), obsessive-compulsive disorder (27.4%), simple phobias (33.8%), eating disorder (4.3%) and conduct disorder (24.2%) [4]. Such a high comorbidity rate might result in considerable direct and indirect costs for society.

As demonstrated by DEPRES (Depression Patient Research in European Society) [5], a minority of the depressed patients will receive adequate diagnosis and treatment. Out of 100 depressed, 31 are lost without coming into contact with the health care system and 51 because they are not correctly diagnosed and treated. Thus, the most obvious results should come if the awareness of depressive disorders was increased in society and the health care personnel were better educated.

---

[1]Department of Neuroscience, Psychiatry, Uppsala University, University Hospital, SE-751 85 Uppsala, Sweden

The Defeat Depression Campaign in England [6] resulted in significant positive changes in the attitudes to depression. For example, the number of subjects who believe that depression is a medical condition like other illnesses increased from 73% to 81%.

The Gotland project is often referred to as a suicide prevention programme. However, the main emphasis was on the recognition, diagnosis and treatment of depression [7, 8]. Apart from the decrease in suicides, an increased knowledge about diagnosis and treatment of depressive disorders, a decreased number of referrals to psychiatry, decreased sick-leave due to depression, decreased prescriptions of sedatives and major tranquillisers and increased prescriptions of antidepressants were reported.

In the cost-benefit analysis [7], it was demonstrated that the programme was highly cost-effective, including when the effects on the suicide rate were omitted.

The results are considerably strengthened by the Hungarian experience [9]. A correlation was found between the rates of working physicians and diagnosed depression, and both showed a negative correlation with the suicide rate. Furthermore, when the reported and treated depressions increased 193%, the suicide rate decreased 19%.

In line with the DEPRES data and experiences from England, Sweden and Hungary, the World Health Organization (WHO) [2] has proposed the following strategies: (1) individuals' and communities' ability to recognize problems can be developed by means of information; (2) health personnel and other caregivers need to be better educated.

It is emphasized that a systematic training programme such as the Gotland study can have a major impact on the suicide rate.

REFERENCES

1. Murray C.J., Lopez A.D. (1996) *The Global Burden of Disease*, World Health Organization, Geneva.
2. World Health Organization (1998) *Health 21 — the Health for All Policy for the WHO European Region — 21 Targets for the 21st Century (EUR/RC4810)*, World Health Organization, Geneva.
3. von Knorring L., Bingefors K., Ekselius L., von Knorring A.-L., Olsson G. (1999) Cost-effectiveness in the prevention of suicide. In *Manage or Perish? The Challenges of Managed Mental Health Care in Europe* (Eds J. Guimon, N. Sartorius), pp. 295–309, Plenum Press, New York.
4. Olsson G. (1998) *Adolescent Depression. Epidemiology, Nosology, Life Stress, and Social Network*, Doctoral Dissertation from the Faculty of Medicine, No. 770, University Library, Uppsala.
5. Lepine J.P., Gastpar M., Mendlewicz J., Tylee A. (1997) Depression in the community: the first pan-European study DEPRES (Depression Research in European Society). *Int. Clin. Psychopharmacol.*, **12**: 19–29.
6. Paykel E.S., Hart D., Priest G. (1998) Changes in public attitudes to depression during the Defeat Depression Campaign. *Br. J. Psychiatry*, **173**: 519–522.

7. Rutz W., Carlsson P., von Knorring L., Wålinder J. (1992) Cost-benefit analysis of an educational program for general practitioners by the Swedish Committee for the Prevention and Treatment of Depression. *Acta Psychiatr. Scand.*, **85**: 457–464.
8. Rutz W., Wålinder J., Eberhard G., Holmberg G., von Knorring A.-L., von Knorring L., Wistedt B., Åberg-Wistedt A. (1989) An educational program on depressive disorders for general practitioners on Gotland: background and evaluation. *Acta Psychiatr. Scand.*, **79**: 19–26.
9. Rihmer Z., Rutz W., Barsi J. (1993) Suicide rate, prevalence of diagnosed depression and prevalence of working physicians in Hungary. *Acta Psychiatr. Scand.*, **88**: 391–394.

6.12
Therapy of Depression Means Less Cost Than What is Otherwise Lost

Zoltan Rihmer[1]

Rosenbaum and Hylan's comprehensive review on the costs of depressive disorders clearly shows that they cause a great economic burden, and that the cost of the diagnosis and treatment of depression (direct cost) is much lower than the negative financial consequences caused by depressions which are not treated or are undertreated (indirect cost). Moreover, the expenditure on drugs in the treatment of depression represents only 10–20% of the total direct cost. The reviewed literature also suggests that patients who initiate treatment with "expensive" selective serotonin reuptake inhibitors (SSRIs) have total direct and indirect health care costs equal to or lower than those of patients who initiate therapy on the "cheap" tricyclic antidepressants (TCAs). The advantage of SSRIs in the first line treatment of depression was supported by a recent study [1], showing that in general practice TCAs were very frequently prescribed in subtherapeutical dose (71%), while the same figure for SSRIs was only 13%.

While it is quite easy to list and count the direct costs of depression, the estimation of indirect costs is more difficult, since there are numerous hidden and intangible burdens — also mentioned tangentially in Rosenbaum and Hylan's review — rendering the loss resulting from depression higher than could be demonstrated in conventional studies. Increased cardiovascular morbidity/mortality, as well as the high prevalence of family breakdown, also belong to the most frequent hidden or intangible burdens of depression [2, 3].

There is a strong association between depression and cardiovascular disorders [4], that is depression is a risk factor for cardiovascular morbidity and it makes the prognosis of cardiac illness worse, increases mortality,

[1]*National Institute for Psychiatry and Neurology, H-1281 Budapest 27, Pf. 1, Hungary*

prolongs the days of disability and reduces the success of rehabilitation [4]. We investigated the psychiatric (co)morbidity of 164 consecutive patients at the Outpatient Department of Cardiology, Teaching Hospital, Semmelweis Medical University, Budapest. We found that 160 of them (98%) had had at least one diagnosis of cardiovascular disorder and 27 of these 160 patients (17%) had met the DSM-III-R criteria for current major depression or dysthymic disorder. Only 6 out of these 27 comorbid patients were diagnosed previously as depressed, and the majority of them (19/27 = 70%) had never been seen by a psychiatrist [5]. Given the significant and very complex relationship between cigarette smoking, depression, cardiovascular disorders and premature death [4, 6], the hidden and intangible burdens of depression-related smoking may also become the subject of further research. On the other hand, more attention should be paid to the costs of depression-related alcoholism and to the economic aspects of mania/hypomania.

The fairly high rate of divorce among depressives as well as the high prevalence of depression and bipolar disorder in the population [3, 7], particularly among suicide victims [8], are reflected in our previous finding of a significant positive association between suicide rates and divorce rates across the regions of Hungary and the USA, that is, the higher the suicide rate of the region, the higher the divorce rate [9].

Rosenbaum and Hylan point out that shifting the treatment of depression from secondary care to general practice is cost-effective only if it is accompanied by improvement of the quality of the treatment. The Gotland study — also mentioned in their review — may be a good example of this. The finding that the rate of depressive suicides among all suicides decreased significantly after the depression training programme of Gotlandian general practitioners (GPs), strongly indicates that the marked decline in suicide mortality as well as other favourable (and cost-saving) changes after the education were a direct result of the considerable decrease in depressive suicides [10]. Therefore, the scepticism about the role of GPs in suicide prevention [11] is appropriate only if GPs are not supported by health care professionals in this sort of activity.

Psychiatrists should also cooperate with health care authorities, and the most important thing they can tell health care resource decision-makers today is that early detection and adequate treatment of depression results in much lower cost than what is otherwise lost.

REFERENCES

1. Isometsä E., Seppälä I., Henriksson M., Kekki P., Lönnqvist J. (1998) Inadequate dosaging in general practice of tricyclic vs. other antidepressants for depression. *Acta Psychiatr. Scand.*, **98**: 451–454.
2. Panzarino P.J. (1998) The costs of depression: direct and indirect; treatment vs. non-treatment. *J. Clin. Psychiatry*, **59** (Suppl. 20): 11–14.

3. Kessler R.C., Walters E.E., Forthofer M.S. (1998) The social consequences of psychiatric disorders. II: Probability of marital stability. *Am. J. Psychiatry*, **155**: 1092–1096.
4. Shapiro P.A., Lidagoster L., Glassman A.H. (1997) Depression and heart disease. *Psychiatr. Ann.*, **27**: 347–352.
5. Harmati L., Rihmer Z. Psychiatric morbidity in 164 consecutive cardiological outpatients (in preparation).
6. Angst J., Clayton P.J. (1998) Personality, smoking and suicide: a prospective study. *J. Affect. Disord.*, **51**: 55–62.
7. Angst J. (1998) The emerging epidemiology of hypomania and bipolar II disorder. *J. Affect. Disord.*, **50**: 143–151.
8. Rihmer Z. (1996) Strategies of suicide prevention: focus on health care. *J. Affect. Disord.*, **39**: 83–91.
9. Lester D., Rihmer Z. (1992) Sociodemographic of suicide rates in Hungary and the United States. *Psychiat. Hung.*, **7**: 435–437.
10. Rihmer Z., Rutz W., Pihlgren H. (1995) Depression and suicide on Gotland. An intensive study of all suicides before and after a depression-training programme for general practitioners. *J. Affect. Disord.*, **35**: 147–152.
11. McDonald A. (1993) The myth of suicide prevention by general practitioners. *Br. J. Psychiatry*, **163**: 260.

6.13

Economic Aspects of Depression: the Experience of Developing Countries

R. Srinivasa Murthy[1]

Depression as a priority mental health problem has been the focus of attention of mental health professionals in developing countries in the last two decades. Until the publication of the World Health Organization (WHO) Expert Committee Report on Organisation of Mental Health Services in Developing Countries in 1975 [1], most of the care was in the institutional sphere.

A major breakthrough occurred with the WHO project "Strategies for Extending Mental Health Care", which presented data on mental disorders in primary care and demonstrated the feasibility of integrating mental health with primary health care. It is significant to note that in the seven developing countries which participated in this study there was a high prevalence of depression which was the most common mental disorder in primary care [2]. Subsequently, the WHO study on prevalence of psychiatric problems in general health care (PPGHC) confirmed this finding. In addition the study provided data relating to the disability as well as the burden of depression in primary care [3].

_____

[1]*National Institute of Mental Health, Department of Psychiatry and Neuroscience, Post Bag 2900, Bangalore, 56002-9, India*

In a study conducted in the second half of 1998, which was a collaborative effort of the Institute of Psychiatry, London, the National Institute of Mental Health and Neuroscience, Bangalore, India, and the Institute of Psychiatry, Rawalpindi, Pakistan, an attempt was made to look at the economic aspects of common mental disorders of which the depressions formed the main group. This study involved 120 patients from Bangalore, India; 133 patients from Rawalpindi, Pakistan, were identified at the level of the community. It was found that the broad group of depressions, including mild, moderate and severe depressive episode and dysthymia, accounted for more than 70% of the patients seen in the community. It was also noted that females were predominant in the patient group. An important finding was that the majority of this group of people were not receiving any care at the time of initial follow-up and all those who had received any care were receiving it mainly from the local health facility. The direct and indirect costs were found to be significant in terms of cost of taking treatment as well as the burden on the caregivers and other related factors. Patients with depression reported at the baseline that in about 2 days in a month they were unable to carry out activities and in about one day they were required to spend time in bed due to illness. At the 3-month follow-up it was noted that "alerting members of the local population to their mental health care needs (and, in the case of Sakalwara, also training primary care workers in mental health care) is not only associated with clear improvements in the outcome domains of depression, disability and quality of life, but also reduces the economic burden of mental disorder". The study concluded that it is possible to carry out economic analyses of mental health care in low income countries. There is a large unmet need in the community. The common disorders form a significant burden on the individuals and community. The major approach to providing care has to be at the local level and should emphasize integrating mental health care with primary health care.

It is important for mental health professionals not only to focus on the individual clinical issues, but also to take up the larger issues of unmet needs, the burden of depression, and the economic aspects of unmet needs as well as the cost-effectiveness of interventions [4]. Reviewing the literature from India, it is seen that there are no papers on long-term treatment of depression, as all the studies have limited themselves to the 4–6 weeks of the clinical drug trial, most often undertaken for purposes of registration prior to marketing. There have also been no systematic studies relating to the role of treatment of depression in suicide prevention and the comparison of nonpharmacological methods of treatment with drug treatment. The advent of selective serotonin reuptake inhibitors (SSRIs) is recent and their effectiveness as compared to traditional antidepressants is yet to be examined. The systematic studies of Western countries offer approaches to plan similar evaluative studies.

REFERENCES

1. World Health Organisation (1975) *Organisation of Mental Health Services in Developing Countries*, World Health Organisation, Geneva.
2. Harding T.W., De Arango N., Baltazar J., Climent C.E., Ibrahim H.H.A., Ladrido-Ignacio L., Srinivasa Murthy R., Wig N.N. (1980) Mental disorders in primary health care: a study of their frequency and diagnosis in four developing countries. *Psychol. Med.*, **10**: 231–241.
3. Ustun T.B., Sartorius N. (Eds) (1995) *Mental Illness in General Health Care: An International Study*, Wiley, Chichester.
4. Srinivasa Murthy R. (1996) Economics of mental health in developing countries. In *International Review of Psychiatry*, vol. 2 (Eds F. Lieh Mak, C.C. Nadelson), pp. 43–62, American Psychiatric Press, Washington, DC.

Acknowledgements for the First Edition

The Editors would like to thank Drs Paola Bucci, Umberto Volpe, Pasquale Saviano, Andrea Dell'Acqua, Massimo Lanzaro, Vincenzo Scarallo, Enrico Tresca, Mariangela Masella and Giuseppe Piegari, of the Department of Psychiatry of the University of Naples, for their help in the processing of manuscripts.

The publication has been supported by an unrestricted educational grant from Eli-Lilly Italia, which is hereby gratefully acknowledged.

Index